# Make NAHQ Your Professional Home

The National Association for Healthcare Quality® (NAHQ) has a mission to prepare a coordinated, competent workforce to lead and advance healthcare quality across the continuum of healthcare.

As leaders in this vital effort, NAHQ created and twice-validated the industry-standard **Healthcare Quality Competency Framework**. The comprehensive framework sets specific job requirements and capabilities across eight domains, 29 competencies, and 486 competencies-based skill statements, stratified against foundational, proficient and advanced levels.

When you leverage our competency-based training solutions, such as **HQ Solutions**, as part of your professional development plan, you are armed with a common vocabulary and knowledge that enhances your capability to advance.

In addition, NAHQ membership offers enhanced access to critical support throughout your career. When you join our network of nearly 9,000 motivated, like-minded professionals, you will receive exclusive pricing on CPHQ Prep, exam, and events. NAHQ takes pride in serving as the professional home to our members.

# CPHQ®

## Certified Professional in Healthcare Quality (CPHQ)

Thank you for adding **HQ Solutions: Resource for the Healthcare Quality Professional, Fifth Edition** to your professional development plan. When you are ready to take that next step, NAHQ provides the only accredited certification in healthcare quality, aligned to the Healthcare Quality Competency Framework: the Certified Professional in Healthcare Quality® (CPHQ). The CPHQ validates your knowledge of healthcare quality practices and competencies, providing the assurance that you possess the skills and knowledge required to succeed! For more information on training materials and scheduling for the CPHQ exam, visit **NAHQ.org**.

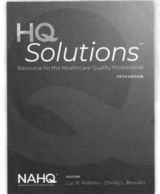

ISBN: 978-1-284-28156-9

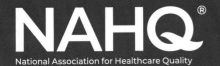

Learn more about becoming a NAHQ member by visiting **NAHQ.org**

Source Code: NAHQFlyer

# Healthcare Quality Competency Framework

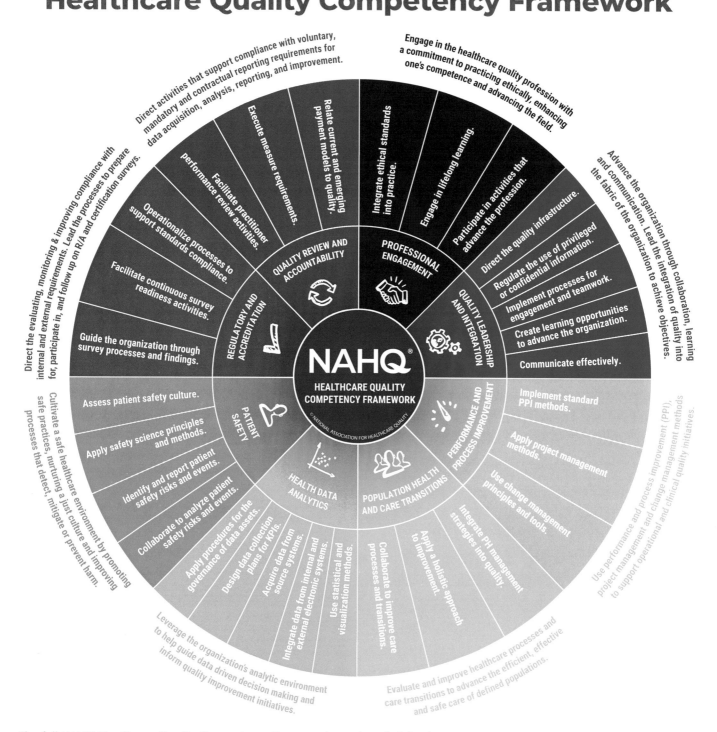

The full NAHQ Healthcare Quality Competency Framework consists of eight domains, 29 competency statements and 486 skill statements. The eight domains and 29 competency statements have been made publicly available. The skill statements, which are stratified across foundational, proficient and advanced levels, are not publicly available but are incorporated into the design of NAHQ educational program offerings, which can be purchased by individuals and healthcare organizations.

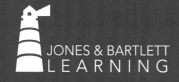

# HQ Solutions™

## Resource for the Healthcare Quality Professional

### FIFTH EDITION

**EDITORS**

Luc R. Pelletier,
MSN, APRN, PMHCNS-BC, CPHQ, FNAHQ, FAAN

Christy L. Beaudin,
PhD, LCSW, CPHQ, FNAHQ

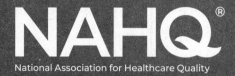

**NAHQ®**

National Association for Healthcare Quality

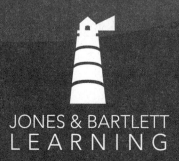

JONES & BARTLETT
LEARNING

*World Headquarters*
Jones & Bartlett Learning
25 Mall Road
Burlington, MA 01803
978-443-5000
info@jblearning.com
www.jblearning.com

Jones & Bartlett Learning books and products are available through most bookstores and online booksellers. To contact Jones & Bartlett Learning directly, call 800-832-0034, fax 978-443-8000, or visit our website, www.jblearning.com.

Substantial discounts on bulk quantities of Jones & Bartlett Learning publications are available to corporations, professional associations, and other qualified organizations. For details and specific discount information, contact the special sales department at Jones & Bartlett Learning via the above contact information or send an email to specialsales@jblearning.com.

**Production Credits**

Vice President, Product Management: Marisa R. Urbano
Vice President, Content Strategy and Implementation: Christine Emerton
Director, Product Management: Matthew Kane
Product Manager: Sophie Fleck Teague
Director, Content Management: Donna Gridley
Manager, Content Strategy: Carolyn Pershouse
Content Strategist: Tess Sackmann
Director, Project Management and Content Services: Karen Scott
Manager, Project Management: Jackie Reynen
Project Manager: Jennifer Risden
Senior Digital Project Specialist: Angela Dooley
Senior Marketing Manager: Susanne Walker
Content Services Manager: Colleen Lamy
Vice President, Manufacturing and Inventory Control: Therese Connell
Composition: Straive
Cover Design: Kristin E. Parker
Media Development Editor: Faith Brosnan
Rights & Permissions Manager: John Rusk
Rights Specialist: Maria Leon Maimone
Printing and Binding: LSC Communications

**Library of Congress Cataloging-in-Publication Data**
Names: Pelletier, Luc Reginald, editor. | Beaudin, Christy L., editor.
Title: HQ solutions : resource for the healthcare quality professional /
  Luc R. Pelletier, Christy L. Beaudin.
Description: Fifth edition. | Burlington, Massachusetts : Jones & Bartlett
  Learning, [2024] | Includes bibliographical references and index. |
Identifiers: LCCN 2022015336 | ISBN 9781284249965 (paperback)
Subjects: LCSH: Medical care–Quality control. | Total quality management.
  | BISAC: HEALTH & FITNESS / Health Care Issues
Classification: LCC RA399.A3 Q25 2024 | DDC 362.1068–dc23/eng/20220628
LC record available at https://lccn.loc.gov/2022015336

6048

Printed in the United States of America
26 25 24     10 9 8 7 6 5 4 3 2

# About the Co-Editors

**Luc R. Pelletier, MSN, APRN, PMHCNS-BC, CPHQ, FNAHQ, FAAN,** is a clinical nurse specialist at the Sharp Caster Institute for Nursing Excellence, where his research focuses on patient engagement, nursing leadership education, and the effectiveness of nurse residency programs. With over 40 years of experience, he maintains a consultancy practice and has held appointments as adjunct faculty with the University of San Diego Hahn School of Nursing and Health Science; National University; University of Phoenix; California State University, Dominguez Hills; University of California, Los Angeles; and the George Washington University. He is a graduate of Yale University (MSN) and Fairfield University (BSN). Mr. Pelletier is a technical writer and editor and publishes widely in the areas of nursing administration, quality, safety, and patient engagement, including books, book chapters, and peer-reviewed articles. He has participated in local and national initiatives focusing on safe and equitable care for persons with enduring behavioral health challenges. As a nurse expert with the U.S. Department of Justice, scientific consultant to the National Institutes of Health, and consultant to the National Quality Forum, he helped inform systems of care and national policy standards. Mr. Pelletier is a fellow of the American Academy of Nursing and the National Association for Healthcare Quality (NAHQ). For 9 years, he served as editor in chief for the *Journal for Healthcare Quality*. Mr. Pelletier received the Yale School of Nursing Distinguished Alumni Award in 2017.

**Christy L. Beaudin, PhD, LCSW, CPHQ, FNAHQ,** is senior director of quality management for Community Bridges, Inc., in Mesa, Arizona. Dr. Beaudin has worked, studied, analyzed, and practiced the art and science of healthcare quality in managed care organizations, health systems, hospitals, and community behavioral health centers for over 25 years. She is a graduate of University of California, Los Angeles; San Diego State University; and California State University, San Bernardino. She has navigated the many changes in health policy and payment in medical and behavioral health services while meeting regulatory, accreditation, and contractual requirements. Dr. Beaudin has conducted qualitative and quantitative evaluation research across the continuum of care on various topics that promote better care, smarter spending, healthier people, and joy in work. Her commitment to translational science is evidenced by authorship of over 90 peer-reviewed articles, book chapters, case studies, and reports—most tackling topics on improving human health and quality of life. Dr. Beaudin energetically serves as associate editor and panel reviewer for the *Journal for Healthcare Quality* and is an engineer for the foundational study guide for the Certified Professional in Healthcare Quality, *HQ Solutions: Resource for the Healthcare Quality Professional*, now in its fifth edition. Dr. Beaudin enjoys the benefits of being a coach and mentor to healthcare quality professionals and project teams growing from leadership experience at ValueOptions, Magellan, PacifiCare Behavioral Health, UnitedHealth, Children's Hospital Los Angeles, AIDS Healthcare Foundation, and Child & Family Center.

# About the Contributors

**Deborah J. Bulger, AAS, CPHQ,** is vice president of strategic programs at Syntellis Performance Solutions. She is responsible for the design and integration of programs that optimize the voice of the customer for a portfolio of healthcare analytics products and services. As a healthcare professional for over 35 years, her career began as a medical technologist and progressed through a series of leadership roles as laboratory manager, operational manager for ancillary services, and director of quality management in a community hospital in central Texas. Her expertise in clinical quality led to a role as a consultant for MediQual Systems, Inc., where she participated in performance improvement projects with clinicians at numerous healthcare systems, employer organizations, and business coalitions benchmarking clinical outcomes against a peer database and documenting process variation. Prior to her work at Syntellis, she was vice president of product management for McKesson Provider Technologies, leading the product management and go-to-market strategy for an integrated clinical and financial performance analytics solution for healthcare systems. Continuing her passion for quality, she has been a Certified Professional in Healthcare Quality (CPHQ) since 1986. As an active member of the National Association for Healthcare Quality, she is a frequent presenter at both local and national forums, including the past five NAHQ Next conferences. In 2017, Ms. Bulger served as a member of the NAHQ Competencies Commission and co-led HQ Essentials Quality Review and Accountability competencies development. She graduated from Navarro College and attended Dallas Baptist University.

**Cathy E. Duquette, PhD, RN, NEA-BC, CPHQ, FNAHQ,** is executive vice president for quality and safety and chief nursing executive for Lifespan. In this role, she is responsible for co-leading the system strategy for quality, patient safety, and patient experience with her physician colleague, the executive vice president and chief clinical officer, as well as leading nursing and the organization's efforts to implement Lean and Six Sigma across the health system. Her more than 30 years in healthcare includes roles as senior vice president and chief quality officer of Rhode Island Hospital, vice president of nursing and patient care services, and chief nursing officer at Newport Hospital, senior vice president at the Hospital Association of Rhode Island, and staff roles in hospital quality improvement and clinical nursing in the critical care setting. She received a BSN and an MSN from the University of Rhode Island and a PhD in nursing from the University of Massachusetts, Amherst and Worcester. Dr. Duquette is certified as a Six Sigma Black Belt and an active member of the National Association for Healthcare Quality. She serves as an associate editor for the *Journal for Healthcare Quality*. She published in professional journals and authored the leadership and management section of *HQ Solutions* for three editions. She has also served on state and national task forces involving leadership development, performance measurement, quality improvement, public reporting, and nursing workforce.

**Pradeep S.B. Podila, PhD, MHA, MS, FACHE, FHFMA, CPHQ, CPHIMS, CLSSBB,** is a health services researcher with over 15 years of combined multisectoral (federal/not-for-profit/academia) experience in health/public health informatics, and electronic health record–based clinical/operational/research data analytics. He served on the Technical Advisory Committee on the Office of National Coordinator for Health Information Technology's Project US@, a new initiative to establish a standard approach for representing patient addresses across all health IT systems to improve patient matching using accurate address information. Dr. Podila is a graduate of the Centers for Disease Control and Prevention's Public Health Informatics Fellow Program. He received master's degrees in electrical/biomedical engineering and health administration and a PhD in public health (epidemiology) from the University of Memphis. He graduated from Massachusetts Institute of Technology's applied data science program offered by the Institute for Data, Systems, and Society, and professional educational programs. He is certified in Six Sigma (Black Belt), led a team that placed third among 60+ registered teams in the seventh National SAS Data Mining Shootout Competition, and led a team that reached the finals (top three) of MIT's 2021 Policy Hackathon in the COVID-19 and healthcare track. He is a member of multiple professional organizations. He is a fellow of the American College of Healthcare Executives and the Healthcare Financial Management Association; a board member of the NAHQ Education Commission, HIMSS's professional certification board, and Exam Workstream (chair); and codeveloped a module on global health literacy within Global Health Informatics course for TIGER International task force. He serves as a reviewer for the *Journal for Healthcare Quality*.

**Jennifer Proctor, BS,** is a writer and editor, with specializations in healthcare and supply chain communications. She has written previously for the Association of American Medical Colleges and Georgetown University Medical Center. In addition, she was director of communications for the Association for Supply Chain Management, where she was editor in chief of the association's magazine. Now, Jennifer focuses on helping organizations build thought leadership and enhance member and customer value propositions. Her clients have included the Academy for Managed Care Pharmacy, the U.S. Department of Homeland Security, the Global Cold Chain Alliance, and others. Jennifer earned her journalism degree from Ohio University and resides in Falls Church, Virginia, with her husband and two children.

**Patricia Resnik, JD, MBA, FACHE,** is vice president of operations for the Center for Virtual Health, a wholly owned subsidiary of Christiana-Care, a nonprofit teaching health system located in Wilmington, Delaware, serving Delaware, Maryland, Pennsylvania, and New Jersey. Ms. Resnik has extensive experience in acute care operations; care and utilization management; population health, healthcare quality and compliance; and virtual provider practice operations. She previously served as the vice president of ChristianaCare CareVio, an award-winning, NCQA-accredited care management subsidiary supporting population health and value-based risk contracting. She is an active board member of the National Association for Healthcare

Quality. Ms. Resnik has served on several healthcare boards and committees including the Delaware Local Program Committee for the Healthcare Leadership Network of the Delaware Valley, a chapter of the American College of Healthcare Executives (ACHE); the Respiratory Care Practice Advisory Council, a committee of the Delaware Board of Medical Licensure and Discipline; and the statewide Guardianship task force for the state of Delaware. Ms. Resnik earned an MJ in health law from the Widener University Delaware Law School, and a BSN and an MBA from Widener University in Chester, Pennsylvania. She is an ACHE fellow and a past recipient of the Early Career and Senior Healthcare Executive award.

**Susan V. White, PhD, RN, CPHQ, FNAHQ, NEA-BC,** is chief of quality management at the Orlando VA Health Care System. Her areas of responsibility include quality management, performance improvement, performance measures, patient safety, risk management, continuous survey readiness, infection control, utilization management and case management, and controlled substances inspections. Prior to this role, Dr. White was associate chief nurse/quality improvement and Magnet coordinator at the James A. Haley Veterans' Hospital in Tampa, Florida. Before joining the Veterans Administration, she was vice president/quality management of the Florida Hospital Association. She was the associate executive director and director of nursing in a community hospital and developed the quality management program for a hospital within a large network. Dr. White received an MSN as well as a PhD from the University of Florida. She is a member of multiple professional organizations. She is an editorial board member for the *Journal for Healthcare Quality*. She is a NAHQ fellow. She received the Quality Award and the Author Award from the Florida Association for Healthcare Quality and the Claire Glover Quality Award from NAHQ. Dr. White served as a member of the board of directors of the Florida Center for Nursing from inception until 2009 and was an initial member of the Florida Patient Safety Corporation. Dr. White is widely published and was co-editor and author of several chapters in *Patient Safety, Principles and Practices* and has been a contributor to *HQ Solutions* for two editions.

# Advisory Panel

**Barbara Corn, RN, MA, CPHQ**
Vice President for Clinical Operations
Magellan Rx, Navigate
St. Louis, Missouri

**Tricia Elliott, DNP, MBA, CPHQ, FNAHQ**
Senior Managing Director, Measurement Science
and Application
National Quality Forum
Arlington Heights, Illinois

**Noelle Flaherty, MBA, MS, BSN, RN, CCM, CPHQ**
Director of Care Coordination & Integration
CalvertHealth Medical Center
Prince Frederick, Maryland

**Shawna Forst, MBA, CPHQ**
Performance Excellence, Quality & Risk Coordinator
MercyOne Newton Medical Center
Newton, Iowa

**Erica Natal, MHA, BSN**
Clinical Administrator
Rockford Gastroenterology
Rockford, Illinois

**Christine Nidd, MSW, CPHQ, PMP**
Manager of Quality and Compliance
Hospice of the Northwest
Mount Vernon, Washington

**Caroline Piselli, DNP, RN, MBA, FACHE**
Six Sigma Black Belt
Partner/MD, Healthcare Public Sector and
Commercial Leadership
Guidehouse, formerly PriceWaterhouseCoopers
Value Management
Vero Beach, Florida

**Jeakobe (Jake) T. Redden, DHSc, MHA, MPH, CPHQ, CPPS, FACHE**
Chief Executive Officer
Madelia Health
Madelia, Minnesota

**Michelle Scharnott, MBA, CPHQ**
National Vice President, Business Development
and Strategy
Quality, Outcomes, Research & Analytics
American Heart Association, Midwest Affiliate
Waukesha, Wisconsin

**Nidia Williams, PhD, MBB, CPHQ, FNAHQ**
Six Sigma Master Black Belt
Vice President, Quality and Safety
Lifespan
Providence, Rhode Island

# Preface

*HQ Solutions: Resource for the Healthcare Quality Professional, Fifth Edition* targets professionals and learners from across the healthcare continuum and provides critical information to develop and strengthen essential skills and knowledge. It is built on the legacy of four editions spanning nearly two decades.

Healthcare is complex, difficult to navigate, and confusing. Patients, families, and staff experience various levels of engagement in the healthcare system. Healthcare quality professionals are at the forefront to safeguard practices for patient and family-centered healthcare delivery. As leaders, healthcare quality professionals mitigate barriers to engagement and work with others to achieve the Quadruple Aim—*better care, smarter spending, healthier people, joy in work* (**Figure A**).

## Better Care

Healthcare quality professionals ensure robust infrastructures to support effective and responsive healthcare enterprises. Efforts align care, treatment, and services with evidence-based, experience-informed structures and processes yielding care that is safe, timely, effective, efficient, equitable, ethical, and person-centric. This requires developing and deploying sustainable performance and process improvement strategies. *HQ Solutions* talks to the breadth and depth of critical areas for professional development and leadership: frameworks for quality improvement, the linking of science with practice, and the translation of data into practical information to use and share with

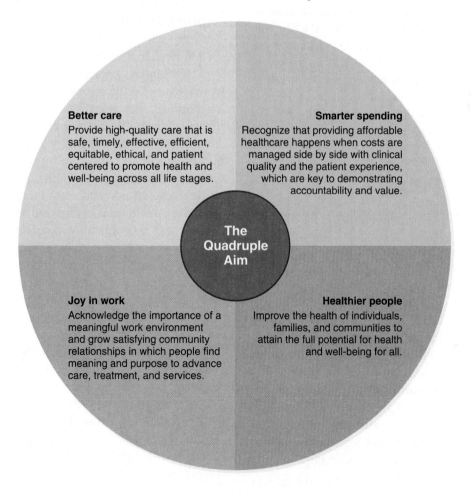

**Better care**
Provide high-quality care that is safe, timely, effective, efficient, equitable, ethical, and patient centered to promote health and well-being across all life stages.

**Smarter spending**
Recognize that providing affordable healthcare happens when costs are managed side by side with clinical quality and the patient experience, which are key to demonstrating accountability and value.

**The Quadruple Aim**

**Joy in work**
Acknowledge the importance of a meaningful work environment and grow satisfying community relationships in which people find meaning and purpose to advance care, treatment, and services.

**Healthier people**
Improve the health of individuals, families, and communities to attain the full potential for health and well-being for all.

**Figure A**

stakeholders (e.g., clinicians, third-party payers, consumers). A learning organization is sustained by fostering high reliability, creativity, and encouraging the spread of person-centric, evidence-based innovations.

## Smarter Spending

Healthcare quality professionals recognize that affordable healthcare happens when costs are managed side by side with quality and patient safety programs. Accountability and value result from high-reliability processes and standardized work. Comprehensive care ensures continuity and reduces the chance for error, unnecessary treatment, or rework. Techniques to identify and eradicate waste are an important part of the healthcare quality professional's toolkit. In this world of teeming technology, rapid innovation, and continuously expanding science, we rely on hope day in and day out—hope that political agendas will reflect the needs of patients, families, and other stakeholders, that resources will be available for the work to be done, and that fear and misinformation will not create barriers to uncovering mistakes, flaws, and failures. Armed with analytical skills and practical tools, we are a boundless force that can wildly succeed in a universe with finite resources. *HQ Solutions* talks about how data analytics are essential to understanding where things are working and where to focus efforts for improvement. Selecting the right design tool improves quality and limits costs making healthcare efficiencies possible. Prioritization conserves precious resources.

## Healthier People

Healthcare quality professionals use knowledge, experience, evidence, and tools to improve individual and population health. Effective care and positive outcomes result from care partnerships such as an empowered and engaged workforce or activated patients and families. While prevention is an important contributor to healthier populations, monitoring care, recording variance, and exploring root causes play a role in harm reduction. An enduring and just (nonpunitive) culture supports a safe workplace. *HQ Solutions* talks about how patients can be kept safe and what leaders can do to create a strong, enduring safety culture. In addition to emerging technologies and techniques, a strong, quality foundation is made possible by the collaborative relationships among stakeholders.

## Joy in Work

Healthcare is relationship based. People are our business. Mutual respect, affiliation, and accord lead to a shared mission, alignment with core values, and a sense of camaraderie. As we face complex healthcare quality challenges, there is more focus on resilience, well-being, engagement, retention, and burnout. Healthcare quality professionals can lead or partner with others on initiatives targeting new term solutions and identifying strategies to making this a priority in their organizations.

*HQ Solutions* tackles the concepts, principles, and practices associated with the delivery of care as described by the Quadruple Aim. The text anticipates what healthcare quality professionals face in their current and future work. It offers setting-agnostic quality and safety tools and techniques adaptable to organizations and daily practices. It reflects recent changes in national healthcare quality and safety imperatives and initiatives, as well as the transformation of healthcare. The *Fifth Edition* provides new content on the well-being and resilience of healthcare professionals, especially considering an unprecedented pandemic that appeared in 2019. It serves as a comprehensive and contemporary review guide to prepare for the Certified Professional in Healthcare Quality (CPHQ) exam.

*HQ Solutions* content is informed by the Healthcare Quality Certification Commission practice analysis and feedback from learners attending the CPHQ review course. The practice analysis assesses the current functions and competencies for healthcare quality professionals. Organized under the Healthcare Quality Certification Commission detailed content outline, this edition addresses these core competency domains: quality leadership and integration, quality review and accountability, regulatory and accreditation, patient safety, health data analytics, performance and process improvement, and population health and care transitions. *HQ Solutions* features critical information about the art and science of quality improvement and environmental considerations such as regulations and healthcare reform.

When we embarked on writing this edition, there was no question about the right people to make it happen. Esteemed authors and quality leaders from across the country—Deb Bulger, Cathy Duquette, Pradeep Podila, Jennifer Proctor, Patty Resnick, and Susie White—offer readers and learners core foundational knowledge and fresh, new perspectives on leadership, performance improvement, quality review and accountability, health data analytics, and population health. We also recognize past contributors—Drs. Diane Storer Brown, Jacqueline Fowler Byers, Jean A. Grube, and Robert J. Rosati.

An expert advisory panel was engaged for peer review. Their efforts are greatly appreciated. We recognize the continuous support of the NAHQ board of directors. The board allocated the necessary resources for *HQ Solutions*, which will contribute to the advancement of the healthcare quality profession in the 21st century. Our new publishing partner, Jones & Bartlett Learning, brought its infinite editorial skills to the project. Finally, Aleese Eckenrode and Carolyn Grieve from NAHQ shepherded the A–Z aspects of the book project to ensure a successful product launch.

The work and calling of healthcare quality professionals is noble. Nobility comes from our truth-seeking heritage. As stewards of truth, we strive to share quality and patient safety stories that are cogent, accurate depictions of healthcare circumstances, easily understood, and warmly received. For truth, justice, and equity in healthcare, we call on every organization and leader to

- value the contributions of healthcare quality professionals—each and every day;

- provide resources necessary to conduct investigations and to maintain reporting systems that use state-of-the-art information technologies;
- allow and support a solid infrastructure for continuous readiness, including health information technology that supports the continuous quality improvement paradigm (and is sustained after an accreditation survey, regulatory audit, or disruption);
- ensure that all organizations from the top down and bottom up are educated on the science of discovery (data, methods, analytics, and application); and
- contribute to the growing body of healthcare quality science by sharing evidence-based, outcomes-oriented quality techniques making a difference in the safety, care, and service embraced by forward-thinking, highly reliable organizations.

May you find *blessings* in every day, enduring *strength* to lead, and *health* for all.

*Luc R. Pelletier, MSN, APRN,*
*PMHCNS-BC, CPHQ, FNAHQ, FAAN*
*Indio, California*
*Christy L. Beaudin, PhD, LCSW, CPHQ, FNAHQ*
*Los Angeles, California*

# Contents

## SECTION 5 Performance and Process Improvement . . . . . . . . . 227

*Susan V. White*

## SECTION 6 Health Data Analytics . . . . . . . . . . . . . . . . . 309

**Christy L. Beaudin, Pradeep S.B. Podila, and Deborah J. Bulger**

## SECTION 7 Population Health and Care Transitions . . . . . . . . . . 375

*Patricia Resnik, Jennifer Proctor, Christy L. Beaudin, and Luc R. Pelletier*

# Quality Leadership and Integration

Cathy E. Duquette

## SECTION CONTENTS

# Introduction

Organizational leadership and management of quality and safety are critical to effective continuous quality and performance improvement programs. This section describes and discusses context for healthcare quality professionals regarding quality leadership structure and integration, frameworks and models, and healthcare organizations as complex systems. Information regarding leadership fundamentals, organizational infrastructure, strategic planning, organizational culture, and key concepts related to change and change management are provided. These structural components are presented as context to enhance the healthcare quality professional's influence on the organization's culture while linking quality, safety, and performance improvement activities to strategic goals. Specific areas covered include:

- Assessment and development of the organization's culture to support organization-wide strategic planning and linking of quality and performance improvement activities with strategic goals.
- Program and project development and evaluation, including the use of performance measures, key performance and quality indicators, and performance improvement models.
- Integration of quality and performance improvement process and results into the organization's strategic planning and explanation of the value proposition for quality and safety.
- Acknowledging the impact of burnout, wellness, resilience, and prevention on organizational leadership's ability to achieve organizational goals and objectives.

These concepts support leaders in the promotion of staff knowledge and competency so the strategic goals of healthcare organizations related to quality, safety, and continuous improvement can be achieved and sustained. See other sections for emerging practices related to patient safety, systems level performance improvement, population health and care transition considerations, approaches to data analytics to support improvement, and emerging payment models that inform the practices of the healthcare quality professional.

# Healthcare Quality Leadership and Complex Systems

Healthcare quality professionals often take on a leadership role in creating a culture of quality and safety and making the strategies to attain performance excellence operational. They are typically members of the senior leadership team and provide coaching and teaching related to principles and practices of quality, safety, and performance improvement. For the leadership team to be informed and agile in their pursuit of excellence, they must understand the concepts of organization as complex systems, leadership, culture, strategic planning, change, innovation, and creativity.

The Institute of Medicine (IOM; now the National Academy of Medicine) defines *healthcare quality* as "the degree to which health services for individuals and populations increase the likelihood of desired health outcomes and are consistent with current professional knowledge."[1(pp128-129)] Care should be based on evidence-based practice and provided in a technically and culturally competent manner with good communication and shared decision making.[2] *Quality management*, derived from *total quality management*, is "a strategic, integrated management system, which involves all managers and employees and uses quantitative methods to continuously improve an organization's processes to meet and exceed customer needs, wants, and expectations."[3(p58)]

Consumers increasingly scrutinize the U.S. healthcare delivery system and the results of their examination are not favorable. In response to the public's concern and outcry, the IOM identified six aims for healthcare improvement:

1. *Safety.* Avoid injuries to patients from care that is intended to help them.
2. *Effectiveness.* Provide services based on scientific knowledge to all who could benefit and refrain from providing services to those who are not likely to benefit (avoiding overuse and underuse).
3. *Patient-centeredness.* Provide care that is respectful of and responsive to individual patient preferences, needs, and values and ensure that patient values guide all clinical decisions.
4. *Timeliness.* Reduce waits and sometimes harmful delays for both those who receive care and those who give care.
5. *Efficiency.* Avoid waste, particularly waste of equipment, supplies, ideas, and energy.
6. *Equity.* Provide care that does not vary in quality with respect to personal characteristics, ethnicity, geographic location, or socioeconomic status.[2(p6)]

For more than 20 years, these aims have served as one framework for healthcare quality professionals when developing quality and safety strategies with senior leadership.

Leaders in healthcare organizations continuously search for ways to improve the quality and safety of the care and service provided in their organizations. The current healthcare environment, however, is complex and constantly changing, making continuous quality improvement a challenge. *Crossing the Quality Chasm: A New Health System for the 21st Century* highlighted the gap between the current and ideal state of the healthcare industry regarding the quality of patient care and framed the need to provide care to patients that focuses on the six specific aims as described earlier. This seminal work triggered a call to action for healthcare providers to develop strategies for closing the chasm in quality and safety in alignment with the IOM aims. Now, more than two decades later, while significant progress has been made, serious gaps remain, and many opportunities continue to exist to improve the healthcare delivery system.[4]

Healthcare organizations are among the most complex entities, with changing technology, new environmental pressures presenting almost daily, and complicated relationships among professionals, disciplines, departments, stakeholders, and organizations. Healthcare leaders and quality professionals must consider the science of complex systems to be effective in the management and continuous improvement of their organizations.

A *system* is a group of interacting, interpedendent, or interrelated elements that act according to a set of rules to form a unified or complex whole influenced by the environment in its functioning. The value of having a systems perspective is that systems thinking is a discipline for seeing the whole. It is a framework for seeing interrelationships rather than things; for seeing patterns of change rather than static snapshots.[5] Systems thinking is well suited for healthcare due to the increasing complexity.[5(p69)]

A list of key points for benefits of systems thinking is found in **Box 1.1**.

## Box 1.1 Key Points: Benefits of Systems Thinking

- Aiding in solving complex problems by identifying and understanding the "big picture"
- Facilitating the identification of major components in early-stage product conception and design
- Addressing recurring problems
- Identifying important relationships and providing proper stakeholder perspectives
- Avoiding excessive attention to a single part and allowing for a broad-scope solution
- Fostering integration, including who to partner with to address capability or core competency challenges
- Providing a basis for architecture, design, development, and redesign

*Complexity science*, or the study of complex adaptive systems (CASs), is a field applied to healthcare to understand complex human organizations. *Complex* implies the inclusion of a significant number of elements. *Adaptive* refers to the capacity to change and the ability to learn from experience. A *system* is a set of interdependent or connected items that are referred to in a CAS as independent agents.[6] CAS theory provides a useful alternative to the machine metaphor, which was first used by Newton to make sense of the world.[7] A Newtonian model of a machine suggests that the parts can explain the whole, whereas complexity science suggests that organizations are living systems in which the whole is not the sum of the parts. Rather than attempting to understand organizations by examination of the parts in a linear model, CAS theory is an acknowledgment that groups of people create outcomes and effects that are far greater than prediction by summing up the resources and skills available within the group. Three concepts—independent agents, distributed control, and nonlinearity—create conditions for perpetual innovation as the CAS seeks new strategies from experience. The past shapes the future.

Viewing organizations as complex systems is consistent with the principles held by quality pioneers like Deming and Juran because quality, safety, and performance improvement practices influence all processes, functions, and departments within an organization.[8,9] Making changes in one process or department naturally requires changes in other processes, functions, and departments because of their interdependencies. All the potential consequences of change need to be considered when making strategic decisions. Thus, effectiveness depends on alignment of the parts of the system. These concepts may resonate with healthcare quality professionals when reflecting on current and previous organizational experiences.

Although it is long recognized that organizations are complicated, further differentiation is necessary if one is to understand complexity and its effect on healthcare quality and safety programs. Healthcare organizations are complex adaptive systems. Because they are systems of interdependent parts or agents, such as people or departments, a significant number of connections exist between their numerous elements. Those involved can learn from the experiences of others in the system.[9]

The various agents of the system can respond in different and unpredictable ways, which can manifest as innovation, creative behavior, and errors[10]; or disruptive innovation.[11] Each person or department acts based on local knowledge and conditions, and a central body does not control the actions of the persons or departments; control is distributed throughout the CAS rather than centralized. Centralized control slows down the capacity to react and adapt. Consider that in many healthcare delivery systems, organizational executives typically work Monday through Friday predominantly during daytime business hours, although operations may be extensive as 24 hours a day, 7 days a week, 365 days a year. Complex adaptive systems may also be agents of another, larger CAS. For example, a physician is a CAS but also an agent in the department; the department is a CAS and an agent in the hospital; the hospital is a CAS and an agent in a multisystem organization; and the organization is a CAS and an agent in the healthcare system. The entire system emerges from a pattern of interactions.

Relationships between individuals are a critical component of the CAS model. Using team sports as an analogy, a team with the best individual players can lose to a team of poorer players when the second team focuses on creating outcomes that are beyond the talents or capabilities of an individual. Team members on healthcare improvement projects who use diverse thinking styles are more likely to produce innovations to solve problems or improve care.

The outcomes of a CAS emerge from a process of self-organization, which emerges from interrelationships.[9] How the system will evolve is therefore unpredictable. The coevolution of a CAS and its environment is difficult to map because it is not linear. The size of the outcome may not be correlated to the size of the input. One can relate to experiences in which a small effort resulted in huge change and, conversely, situations in which a huge effort resulted in little, if any, demonstrable or sustainable change. For example, a big push after a retreat or strategic planning session may not result in change. In contrast, one small push to the system, such as a piece of gossip or bad press, may create radical or rapid change in an organization. When social media is added to this equation, ramifications of bad press can be amplified.

Complex adaptive systems are drawn to attractors, which are patterns or areas that draw the energy of the system to it.[9] Using this concept flips change management perspectives from overcoming resistance to change or fighting against it to using the natural energy of the system. Studying CASs in nature and applying this knowledge to organizations provide insight into how change occurs in human systems.[12] A key finding is that change occurs naturally within the existing system. Reflection on how healthcare changed over the years demonstrates the natural adoption of many new procedures, medications, systems, and information and medical technologies. Change is not so much about overcoming resistance

as it is about creating attraction. What was labeled "resistance" is an attraction to factors in the current system that might not be fully understood or appreciated. Resistance is a natural, but potentially changeable, reaction of a system attracted to something else. If organizations can change the attractors or tap into existing ones that are better, the system may do the rest of the work of change on its own. The challenge for leaders is to look for and leverage the subtle attractors that may not always be obvious.

Consistent with this understanding of organizations as CASs, Zimmerman and colleagues propose practical principles of management for the real world that are ways of thinking about roles healthcare quality professionals play as quality leaders in organizations.[7] **Table 1.1** compares key characteristics of leaders in the traditional (bureaucratic) system and the CAS.

Constraints management, a management philosophy developed by Goldratt, offers another systematic approach to managing complex organizations by identifying and controlling key leverage points in a system or process to yield faster system throughput. A system constraint is anything that limits the system from attaining higher performance.[13] Put simply, the strength of any process or system is dependent upon its weakest link. Improvements to the system under constraints management aim to identify (1) what to change, (2) what to change to, and (3) how to cause the change.[13] Improvement proceeds in five general steps, namely,

1. identification of the system constraint,
2. determination of how to exploit the identified constraint,

---

**Table 1.1** Characteristics of Leaders in Traditional and Complex Adaptive Systems

| Traditional System | Complex Adaptive System |
|---|---|
| ▪ Value positions | ▪ Value persons and relationships |
| ▪ Use tight structuring | |
| ▪ Simplify | ▪ Use loose coupling |
| ▪ Socialize | ▪ Complicate or link |
| ▪ Make decisions | ▪ Diversify |
| ▪ Do planning based on forecasting | ▪ Make sense |
| | ▪ Think about the future |
| ▪ Are controlling, in charge | ▪ Are collaborative |
| ▪ Know | ▪ Listen and learn |
| ▪ Are self-preserving | ▪ Are adaptable |
| ▪ Repeat the past | ▪ Offer alternatives |

Data from Anderson RA, McDaniel RR. Managing health care organizations: where professionalism meets designing organizations. *Health Care Manage Rev.* 2000;25(1):83-92; and Center for the Study of Healthcare Management. *Applying Complexity Science to Health and Health Care.* Minneapolis, MN: Plexus Institute; 2003.

3. subordination and synchronization of the other processes in the system to maximize the capacity of the system,
4. elevation of the system constraint by investing more resources, and
5. repetition of the cycle to ensure ongoing improvement.

Key points of complex systems are summarized in **Box 1.2**.

---

**Box 1.2  Key Points: Healthcare Organizations and Complex Systems**

- Healthcare organizations are complex systems due to the ever-changing environment in which they operate.
- Healthcare organizations consider the following complex system characteristics in quality improvement:
  - Frequently changing technology
  - New and frequent external and environmental pressures
  - Multifaceted relationships between professionals, disciplines, departments, stakeholders, and other organizations
- Healthcare organizations consider the range of consequences for change—both anticipated and unanticipated—in planning as changes in one core process will likely have an impact on other processes.

---

# Leadership Frameworks and Models

Leadership and management are distinct functions. Kotter[14] notes that leadership involves coping with change by developing a vision and aligning the subsystems of the organization. In contrast, management involves coping with complexity through planning and budgeting; setting goals; organizing, staffing, and creating a structure to foster goal attainment; setting up mechanisms for monitoring; and controlling results. *Leadership* is the ability to influence an individual or group toward achievement of goals[15] and includes determining the correct direction or path. *Management* involves doing the right things to stay on that path. Both strong leadership and skilled management are necessary for high-reliability performance. Some individuals are great leaders but poor managers, whereas others are great managers but poor leaders. In some cases, an individual may thrive in both roles.

Healthcare quality professionals possess an awareness of different frameworks for driving organizational performance when working with organizational leadership. Frameworks can assist in guiding and organizing leadership activities to achieve improvement. Many

systems models exist. "The model that the manager selects is less important than how [the person] uses it to begin recognizing, understanding, and anticipating how the parts of the systems interact as a whole."[16(p73)] The healthcare quality professional assists the organizational leaders, employees, and physicians in understanding the principles and common frameworks for healthcare quality and safety strategies. Recent and classic literature point the healthcare quality professional to a wealth of evidence-based frameworks. Descriptions of some popular models and frameworks follow.

## Donabedian Model

Donabedian is credited as being the founder of the quality assurance field. As a researcher and physician at the University of Michigan, he developed a theoretical framework, with its focus on structure, process, and outcomes for patient care evaluation.[17] Donabedian's framework describes the importance of relating healthcare structures and processes to how clients fared because of their care. Structure represents the resources available for care delivery and system design, whereas *processes* involve the "set of activities that go on within and between practitioners and patients."[17(p79)] *Outcomes* include the results of that care (e.g., increased engagement, decreased morbidity, improved quality of life or well-being) or the "change in a patient's current and future health status that can be attributed to antecedent health care."[17(p83)] See **Figure 1.1** for examples.

The Donabedian model provides a framework for examining and evaluating the quality of healthcare transactions between patients and providers throughout the delivery of healthcare—structure, process, and outcomes. Seven elements of quality of medical care are considered:

1. *Efficacy.* While hard to measure, refers to care provided under optimal conditions and is the basis against which measurements should be made
2. *Effectiveness.* The outcome of interventions
3. *Efficiency.* Refers to cost reductions without compromising effects
4. *Equity.* The fairness in the distribution of healthcare in populations
5. *Optimality.* Balancing the costs and benefits of healthcare
6. *Acceptability.* Encompasses accessibility of healthcare and interpersonal patient–provider interaction
7. *Legitimacy.* The social acceptability of the healthcare institution regarding the manner in which healthcare is delivered[18]

The choice of elements and their relative prioritization should be guided by the context in which quality of care is being assessed.

| Structure | Process | Outcomes |
|---|---|---|
| Human Resources | **Technical Aspects of Care** | Clinical |
| Facilities | Diagnosis | Functional |
| Technology | Treatment | Experience |
| Financial Resources | Guidelines | Satisfaction |
| Health Coverage | **Interpersonal Aspects of Care** | Quality of Life |
| Organizational Structure | Caring Behaviors and Attitude | Financial |
| Policies and Procedures | Person-Centered Care | |
| | Patient Participation/Engagement | |
| | Communication | |
| | Situational | |

**Figure 1.1** Donabedian's Framework (Structure, Process, and Outcomes)

Donabedian was the first to describe an approach to assessing quality through a systems framework. However, the model is very basic and does not describe interrelationships. This gap led to the development of other models to illuminate the interrelationships necessary for quality performance. However, Donabedian's triad is lauded as a lasting framework for healthcare quality.[19] This evidence-based theoretical work became personal for him after he experienced the healthcare system firsthand. Donabedian shared the following in an interview published in *Health Affairs*:

> Health care is a sacred mission . . . a moral enterprise and a scientific enterprise but not fundamentally a commercial one. We are not selling a product. We don't have a consumer who understands everything and makes rational choices—and I include myself here. Doctors and nurses are stewards of something precious. . . . Ultimately the secret of quality is love. . . . If you have love, you can then work backward to monitor and improve the system.[20(p140)]

As a leader and pioneer in healthcare quality, Donabedian was always cognizant of the social, emotional, and ethical factors related to quality and safety.

## Baldrige Performance Excellence Framework

Another framework used to understand quality, safety, and performance improvement in complex systems is the 2021–2022 Baldrige Excellence Framework (Health Care) depicted in **Figure 1.2**.[21] The Malcolm Baldrige National Quality Award, named for former U.S. Secretary of Commerce Malcolm Baldrige in tribute to his managerial ability, is given to organizations demonstrating a commitment to performance excellence. In 1988, the first Baldrige National Quality Award was bestowed within manufacturing.[22] It was not until 2002 that an award was given to a healthcare organization. This framework considers core values and concepts that support principles of quality, safety, and performance improvement for the organization's

- operating environment (e.g., service offerings, vision and mission, workforce profile, assets, regulatory requirements),
- relationships (e.g., customers and stakeholders, suppliers, and partners, structure and relationship between senior leaders and the governing body), and
- specific strategic situation when developing a performance management system.

Three components of the framework—leadership, strategy, and customers—constitute the leadership triad and highlight the value of leadership focus on strategy and customers. The results triad includes workforce and operations emphasizing the impact of workforce-focused and operational process leading to results. The six elements of the leadership and results triad constitute the performance management system. The central arrows represent the important

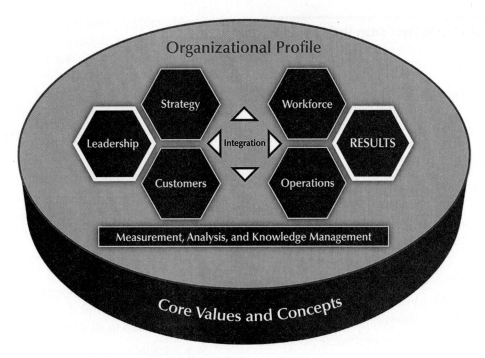

**Figure 1.2** 2021–2022 Baldrige Excellence Framework (Health Care)

Reproduced from Baldrige Performance Excellence Program 2021. *2021–2022 Baldrige Excellence Framework: Proven Leadership and Management Practices for High Performance (Health Care)*. Gaithersburg, MD: U.S. Department of Commerce, National Institute of Standards and Technology; 2021. https://www.nist.gov/baldrige/publications/baldrige-excellence-framework/health-care

integration between leadership and results where *integration* is defined as the "harmonization of plans, processes, information, resource decisions, workforce capability and capacity, actions, results, and analyses to support key organization-wide goals."[21(p49)] Integration is different from alignment. Alignment is a state of consistency among the aforementioned elements of the performance management system. Integration is attained when the elements not only are consistent but also operate as a fully interconnected unit.

Healthcare and process results reflect key healthcare and operational performance results, which demonstrate healthcare outcomes, service quality, and value that lead to patient and other customer satisfaction and engagement.

- *Healthcare outcomes.* This refers to the organization's success in delivering on its mission as a healthcare provider. It calls for the use of key data and information to demonstrate the organization's performance on healthcare outcomes and processes and in delivering healthcare. It focuses on demonstrating improving healthcare results over time.
- *Patient outcome measures.* Patient outcome measures might include decreased mortality, decreased complications, core measures, facility-associated infections, value-based payment model measures, improvement in perceived pain, resumption of activities of daily living, return to work, and long-term survival rates.

- *Service performance.* This item also emphasizes measures of healthcare service performance that serve as indicators of patients' and other customers' views and decisions relative to future interactions and relationships. These measures of service performance are derived from patient and other customer-related information gathered in patient outcome measures.
- *Healthcare process measures.* Healthcare process measures appropriate for inclusion might be based on the following: adherence to patient safety practices, treatment protocols, care plans, critical pathways, care bundles, medication administration, patient involvement in decisions, timeliness of care, information transfers and communication of treatment plans and orders, and coordination of care across practitioners and settings.

These elements are critical to the foundation of the performance management system—measurement, analysis, and knowledge management, which also serve as the foundation for effective organizational management.[22]

## The Quality Chasm

In 2001, *Crossing the Quality Chasm: A New Health System for the 21st Century*[2] offered new rules for the healthcare system. Contrasted with the then-current healthcare system approach (**Table 1.2**), the new rules were characterized as simple. Today's healthcare system, more than 20 years later, continues to struggle with adopting these

**Table 1.2** **Rules for the 21st-Century Healthcare System**

| Current Approach | New Rule |
|---|---|
| Care is based primarily on visits. | Preference is given to professional roles over the system. |
| Professional autonomy drives variability. | Care is customized based on patient needs and values. |
| Professionals control care. | The patient is the source of control. |
| Information is a record. | Knowledge is shared, and information flows freely. |
| Decision making is based on training and experience. | Decision making is evidence based. |
| "Do no harm" is an individual responsibility. | Safety is a system priority. |
| Confidentiality is necessary. | Transparency is necessary. |
| The system reacts to needs. | The system anticipates needs. |
| Cost reduction is sought. | Waste is continuously decreased. |
| Preference is given to professional roles over the system. | Cooperation among clinicians is a priority. |

Modified from Institute of Medicine, Committee on Quality of Health Care in America. *Crossing the Quality Chasm: A New Health System for the 21st Century.* Washington, DC: National Academies Press; 2001:71.

rules, with multiple sectors of the healthcare system experiencing varying degrees of success on each rule. Leaders and healthcare quality professionals consider these rules in the development and implementation of improved care delivery systems and other improvement strategies across their organizations.

## Framework for Leadership Improvement

The Institute for Healthcare Improvement's Framework for Leadership Improvement outlines five specific core leadership activities to drive improvement.[23] The activities are described in the following list (**Figure 1.3**):

*Step 1.* Establish the mission, vision, and strategy to set the direction of the organization. Organizational incentives are aligned with the purpose, and the purpose should be communicated to all stakeholders.

*Step 2.* Establish the foundation for an effective leadership system by choosing a leadership team with the right balance of skills to build relationships and improvement capability.

*Step 3.* Build will through a plan for improvement that sets aims, allocates resources, measures performance, provides encouragement,

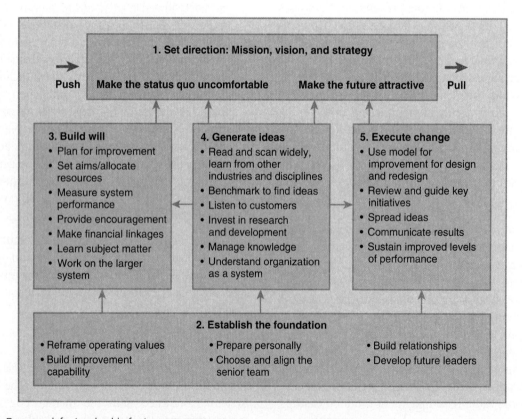

**Figure 1.3** Framework for Leadership for Improvement

Reprinted from Reinertsen JL, Bisognano M, Pugh MD. *Seven Leadership Leverage Points for Organization-Level Improvement in Health Care.* 2nd ed. IHI Innovation Series white paper. Cambridge, MA: Institute for Healthcare Improvement; 2008. www.IHI.org

and makes financial linkages to the impact of quality on cost when customer expectations are not met.

*Step 4.* Generate ideas about clinical and organizational best practices through benchmarking and listening to patients. Invest in research and development, manage knowledge, and understand the organization as a system.

*Step 5.* Execute change through a standardized approach that is used for improvement daily. Assess the effectiveness of execution efforts, spread ideas, and communicate results to sustain higher levels of performance.

# Leadership and Organizational Culture

*Culture* is defined as the set of shared attitudes, values, goals, and practices that characterize an institution or organization[24] and the social glue that holds people together.[25] At the heart of culture is the notion of shared values—what is important, and behavioral norms—how things are done.[26] Perrin defines organizational culture as "the sum of values and rituals which serve as 'glue' to integrate the members of the organization."[27(¶10)] Cultures are described as strong when the core values are intensely held and widely shared. Strong culture will promote

- a sense of identity for employees and a commitment to something larger than themselves;
- cooperation and collaboration;
- a system of informal rules spelling out how people are expected to behave; and
- distinctions between organizations, allowing a definitive competitive advantage to develop.

## Elements of Culture

Culture possesses invisible and visible elements. Invisible elements include values and norms, whereas visible elements include symbols; language, slogans, and brands; rituals and ceremonies; stories, legends, and myths; and heroes.

- *Values and norms.* The core values described in the Baldrige Excellence Framework (Health Care) criteria are one example. The role of leaders is to inspire commitment to these underlying quality values. Norms, such as how customers are greeted, are usually locally established.
- *Symbols.* Symbols are things that represent an idea. The purpose of symbols is to reflect the culture, trigger values and norms, and help people make sense of their organization. For example,

one hospital wanted to strengthen the value for reporting adverse events. To do this, staff wore buttons that said, "We care, We report, We learn." Another uses a "Stop the Line" approach to indicate staff are empowered to ensure the correct actions are taken (see Red Rules in the *Patient Safety* section).

- *Language, slogans, and brands.* Language and slogans are intended to convey cultural meaning to employees and stakeholders. They should be easy to learn, remember, and repeat (e.g., "Quality is Job 1," "Delivering health with care."). Brands help build loyalty to a product or service.
- *Rituals and ceremonies.* Rituals and ceremonies reinforce an organization's core values and goals, thereby strengthening culture. For example, healthcare quality week with annual quality and innovation forums and celebration of improvement projects conveys the importance of these activities.
- *Stories, legends, and myths.* Stories, legends, and myths are narrative examples repeated by employees to inform (often new) employees about culture. Stories are based on fact; legends are based on facts but embellished; myths are consistent with the culture but are not based on fact. For example, stories about an extraordinary event and the organization's response may illustrate a new patient safety program.
- *Heroes.* Heroes are company role models whose ideals, character, and support of the organizational culture highlight the values and norms a company wants to reinforce. Heroes provide a role model for success. For example, an employee or leader who is remembered for a transformative event may be considered an organizational hero.

By design or default, an organization develops a culture. It is better to actively direct the evolution of that culture than to try to change a strong culture that is not aligned with the organization's quality and safety goals.

## Assessing Organizational Culture

Organizations must measure their culture, provide feedback to the leadership and staff, and undertake interventions to change the culture in a way that will promote quality and reduce patient safety risk.[28] How can it be determined whether quality and safety are core values in the culture of an organization? Experts in the field of culture suggest posing the following questions[29,30]:

- Do leaders regularly pay attention to, measure, and control quality and safety?
- Are adequate resources allocated to quality, safety, and performance improvement?
- Are behaviors supporting quality, safety, and performance improvement rewarded?

- Do staff knowledge, skills, and behaviors important for quality, safety, and performance improvement figure into decisions regarding recruitment, selection, and promotion?
- Is active involvement in quality, safety, and performance improvement activities one measure of status in the organization?
- Are people spending time or being supported for spending time on quality, safety, and performance improvement?
- Does staff frequently discuss quality, safety, and performance improvement and its related activities?
- Is the prevailing attitude toward quality, safety, performance improvement, and organizational quality outdated or progressive?

Several tools exist to measure an organization's culture from the perspective of quality and safety. Healthcare quality professionals may be asked to coordinate survey processes related to a culture of safety with an outside vendor or to lead organizational efforts to measure the patient safety culture across the organization using one or more currently available survey instruments. For example, Agency for Healthcare Research and Quality (AHRQ) currently offers five surveys on patient safety culture appropriate for hospital, medical office, nursing home, community pharmacy, and ambulatory surgery settings.[31] The University of Texas has developed the Safety Attitudes Questionnaire to measure healthcare provider attitudes that are important to patient safety.[32] Additional information on culture of safety is discussed in the *Patient Safety* section. Healthcare quality professionals typically take the lead in coordinating the survey efforts and working with leaders across the organization to address identified improvement opportunities through specific actions to drive culture alignment and improvement.

## Leadership and Culture Change

Many actions for establishing and strengthening a quality culture flow from the questions used to assess an organization's culture. First, leaders must show visible support through such actions by embracing quality, safety, and performance improvement as an important part of the strategic planning process. Quality, safety, and performance improvement are everyone's responsibility. Adequate resources are allocated in the annual budget for quality, safety, and performance improvement activities; and behaviors that support quality and safety are rewarded. Second, leaders need to be evaluating and providing attention to the visible elements of culture. For example, they must accomplish the following:

- Replace old, negative stories about quality that are acting as barriers to cultural change with new, positive ones.
- Reinforce values by using symbols and creating rituals critical to quality.
- Celebrate achievements in quality, safety, and performance whether they are small, such as completing an evidence-based quality project, or large, such as receiving Magnet Recognition Program designation.

Finally, leaders invest persistent effort, knowing that culture takes a long time to change.

Although inspiring people with a vision is critical, leaders must also enable others to achieve goals and objectives. One way to enable others is to design the organization in a way that supports quality, safety, and performance improvement. Leaders must integrate healthcare safety practices into the plan for the organization's strategic direction, and goals must be developed to ensure adoption and measurement of safety practices. The organization's quality and patient safety programs are aligned with the mission, vision, core values, and goals of the organization. High-performing organizations embrace approaches that serve as a solid foundation for promoting quality and patient safety. Two examples are provided here with more detail in *Patient Safety*.

Many organizations incorporate the principles of a *just culture* to promote shared accountability and a learning environment as part of the organizational response to error. In a fair and just culture, everyone throughout the organization is aware that medical errors are inevitable, and all errors and unintended events are reported—even when the events may not cause patient injury. This culture can make the system safer. A just culture recognizes that even competent professionals make mistakes and can develop unhealthy norms such as shortcuts or routine rule violations, but a just culture has zero tolerance for reckless behavior or willful disregard for established policy and procedure. Key principles of a just culture can be summarized as follows:

- A just culture is not an effort to reduce personal accountability or discipline. It is a way to emphasize the importance of learning from mistakes and near misses to reduce errors in the future.
- In a just culture, an individual is accountable to the system, and the greatest error is to not report a mistake and thereby prevent the system and others from learning. Policies that encourage or require any healthcare provider to self-report errors are in alignment with a fair and just culture.
- Patient safety is encultured when all team members serve as safety advocates regardless of their positions within an organization. Providers and

consumers will feel safe and supported when they report medical errors or near misses and voice concerns about patient safety.

Healthcare organizations committed to a fair and just culture identify and correct the systems or processes of care that contributed to the medical error or near miss; they do not assign blame but ensure that individuals are held accountable when circumstances warrant individual action, such as events that occur because of willful disregard of policy or procedure. Another key element of a just culture involves the substitution test, which is done to determine if other competent team members with a similar level of training, faced with the same situation, could have done the same thing.[33] Feeling protected by a nonpunitive culture of medical error reporting, more healthcare professionals will report errors and near misses, which will further improve patient safety through opportunities for improvement and lessons learned.

Reducing and eliminating medical errors are major aims for most of the healthcare industry. Healthcare organizations are very complex, and variability in processes can lead to patient harm. In some organizations, leaders set the tone for patient safety as a priority through clearly articulated goals such as the aim for zero harm or in committing to the journey toward high reliability. Whether the focus is on procedure-scheduling processes, medications, or surgery, the goals are the same—to assure patients that they are being treated equally in a safe environment.

Through ongoing scans of the healthcare quality scientific literature and new and evolving regulations, healthcare quality professionals can keep the leadership team up to date and facilitate the adoption and integration of key leadership practices that support the quality and safety function within the organization. See *Patient Safety* for more discussion of concepts, safety culture, harm reduction, and mitigating risk.

A list of key points concerning organizational culture is found in **Box 1.3**.

# Strategic Planning and Performance Excellence

The environment surrounding healthcare organizations is both dynamic and complex because it changes frequently and has many constituents. With continued emphasis on improving the patient experience of care, improving the health of populations, reducing the per capita cost of healthcare, and ensuring joy in work, external forces in healthcare continue to be important. Strategic planning for healthcare quality is even more important as the impact of the shift

---

**Box 1.3  Key Points: Organizational Culture**

- Measurement of an organization's culture is critical for creating the environment where quality and patient safety are seen as priorities.
- Healthcare quality professionals typically take a leadership role in measuring and evaluating an organization's culture.
- Key factors to consider when determining if quality and safety are core values in the culture of an organization include:
  - The extent to which leaders focus on quality and safety
  - Resource allocation for quality, safety, and performance improvement
  - Reward systems in place related to behaviors supportive of quality, safety, and performance improvement
  - The level of organizational support for employee involvement in activities related to quality, safety, and performance improvement
  - Opportunities for employees to discuss quality, safety, or performance improvement activities

---

from volume-based to value-based reimbursement is felt. Other considerations are the expanded focus on the accountable care organization and the alternative payment model. There is also a significant shift from higher cost acute care settings as a focus for delivery of care to lower cost subacute, ambulatory, and primary care settings.

*Strategy* is defined as "the plans and activities developed by an organization in pursuit of its goals and objectives, particularly in regard to positioning itself to meet external demands relative to its competition."[34(p220)] Strategic planning is one way of coping with a dynamic and complex environment. The goals of strategic management are to

- provide a framework for thinking about the business;
- create a fit between the organization and its external environment;
- provide a process for coping with change and organizational renewal;
- foster anticipation, innovation, and excellence;
- facilitate consistent decision making; and
- create organizational focus.[6]

Quality, safety, and performance improvement received increased attention in recent years because organizations realize that if they are to be successful, quality and safety must be an integral part of the strategic plan. The healthcare quality professional plays a key role in strategic planning for quality and safety.

## Strategic Planning Process

The strategic planning process includes all the decisions and actions required to meet the strategic goals. Several steps are offered by various sources. **Figure 1.4** shows some of the common steps in the strategic planning process. Before a strategy is formulated, leaders consider what they want to do, what they should do, and what they can do.[35] Consideration of these three issues leads to the development of a strategic plan. Per the Baldrige Framework, strategy planning and development refer to the organization's approach to preparing for the future.[22] In developing the strategy, the level of acceptable enterprise risk is determined. Forecasts, projections, options, scenarios, knowledge, analyses, or other approaches might be used to envision the future, which aid in decision making and resource allocation.

Strategy is defined broadly and might be built around new healthcare services; differentiation of the organization's brand; new core competencies; new partnerships, alliances, or acquisitions to improve access, grow revenue, or reduce costs; and new staff or volunteer relationships.[22] The strategic planning process must include a focus on long-term organizational sustainability and consideration of the environment from competitive and collaborative perspectives.[22] Seven steps in strategic planning are described next: define and formulate goals; assess the external environment; assess the internal environment; formulate strategy; implement strategy; evaluate effectiveness of strategy and modify, if needed; and measure and monitor progress.

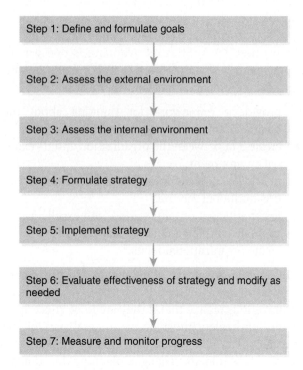

Step 1: Define and formulate goals

Step 2: Assess the external environment

Step 3: Assess the internal environment

Step 4: Formulate strategy

Step 5: Implement strategy

Step 6: Evaluate effectiveness of strategy and modify as needed

Step 7: Measure and monitor progress

**Figure 1.4** Steps in Strategic Planning Processes

### Define and Formulate Goals

In this first step of the strategic planning process, organizations determine their mission and vision, guiding principles and core values, and goals and objectives.

**Mission and Vision** Organizational executive leaders must define what they want the organization to accomplish in the future, in part, by evaluating the current state against the desired future state. Ideally, what the leaders want the organization to accomplish will be in alignment with the organization's mission and vision.

- *Mission* refers to the organization's purpose or reason for existing. It answers questions such as *Why are we here? Whom do we serve?* and *What do we do?* For example, the mission of SSM Health Care, the first healthcare Malcolm Baldrige National Quality Award recipient, awarded in 2002, is "Through our exceptional healthcare services, we reveal the healing presence of God." Its core values are compassion, respect, excellence, stewardship, and community.[36] The mission provides a long-term direction for the organization. Another example, the 2020 Baldrige recipient's (Greater Baltimore Medical Center) mission is "to provide medical care and service of the highest quality to each patient and to educate the next generation of clinicians, leading to health, healing and hope for the community" with core values of respect, excellence, accountability, teamwork, ethical behavior, and results.[37]
- *Vision* is an organization's statement of its goals for the future, described in measurable terms that clarify the direction for everyone in the organization. An organization's direction is built upon its mission and guided by its vision.

References to quality and safety are often included in organizational mission and vision statements to show that these values are priorities in what the organization wants to do. The healthcare quality professional may be expected to work with senior leaders and the governing body to evaluate and refine the mission and vision of the organization through participation in strategic planning processes. They may also be asked to assist leadership in developing the goals, objectives, and metrics for measuring the effectiveness of their mission and vision.

**Guiding Principles and Core Values** *Guiding principles* and *core values* facilitate development of leadership values and commitment to quality. They define the organization's attitudes and policies for employees and thereby help to direct the vision. The following list displays the core values and concepts identified in the Baldrige Excellence Framework (Health Care) as a set of beliefs and behaviors embraced by some organizations as a foundation for performance excellence:

- Systems perspective
- Visionary leadership
- Patient-focused excellence
- Valuing people
- Agility and resilience
- Organizational learning
- Focus on success and innovation
- Management by fact
- Societal contributions and community health
- Ethics and transparency
- Delivering value and results[22(p38)]

The organization's plans integrate the perspectives of the customer. The organization must first identify its customers. The needs of various customers, such as patients, clients, families, and other stakeholders, help the organization to refine its mission, vision, guiding principles, and core values.

**Goals and Objectives** Goals and objectives are essential components of any planning process; they guide actions and serve as a yardstick for measuring the organization's progress and performance. Confusion sometimes arises about the terms *goal* and *objective*; they differ with respect to scope and specificity. In general, goals are broad, general statements specifying a purpose or desired outcome and may be more abstract than objectives. One goal can have several objectives.

Establishing goals is the initial step in the strategic planning process and sets the direction for the activities to follow. A goal is a general statement about a desired outcome and is accompanied by one or more specific objectives that specify in precise terms exactly what is to be accomplished. Goals describe accomplishments, not tasks or activities, and need to be SMART, which stands for the following:

- Specific
- Measurable
- Achievable
- Relevant
- Time bound[38]

Objectives are specific statements that detail how the goals will be achieved through specific and measurable action; they therefore are relatively narrow and concrete. They clearly identify who is going to do what, by when, and to what extent. Objectives representing the organization's commitment to achieving specific outcomes are written as action-oriented statements. Specific activities are implemented to yield measurable and observable qualitative or quantitative performance outcomes. An example of a mission statement, a vision statement, a values statement, strategic goals, and strategic objectives can be found in **Table 1.3**.

After strategic goals and objectives are developed at the executive level, corresponding goals and objectives must be established for other levels in the organization, for example, the business level and functional level (e.g., human resources/talent management, research, and development) or the unit or departmental level (e.g., nursing, diagnostic imaging, pharmacy). Both long-term and short-term goals and corresponding objectives are established for all levels. Goal congruence is the integration of multiple goals, either within an organization or between multiple groups. Congruence is a result of the alignment of goals to achieve an overarching mission.[39]

### Assess the External Environment

Once the goals and objectives are established or revised, organizational executive leaders must look at the external environment to determine what the organization should do. On the road map, the environment is shown to influence what the organization wants to do: all organizations must adapt to the forces of the external environment to survive, stretch, and grow. In other words, the organization is one system among a variety of systems in the external environment. Adaptation includes maintaining good relationships with key constituents who can influence the organization's ability to meet the stated objectives. **Figure 1.5** depicts some of the key categories of various environmental influences on quality and safety by multiple constituents whose needs must be met and balanced with the needs of other stakeholders. The outer ring pertains to the overall environment in which the organization exists. A variety of factors—sociocultural, political, legal, economic, technologic, global, and demographic—indirectly influence the organization. For example, economic forces can influence resources available to organizations (e.g., labor, capital). For this reason, organizations must scan the general external environment looking for threats (or aspirations and results) to, or opportunities for, meeting strategic goals and objectives.

The second ring represents the immediate environment in which the organization operates. With respect to quality and safety in healthcare organizations, the key constituent is the customer as the consumer of

**Table 1.3** Example of Mission, Vision, Shared Values Statement, Strategic Goals, and Strategic Objectives

| | |
|---|---|
| **Mission** | Delivering health with care. |
| **Vision** | Lifespan will become one of the nation's leading health systems by delivering patient-centric health care that prioritizes quality, equity, access, affordability, safety and innovation through strong physician leadership, highly skilled health care teams, and dedicated employees, while achieving excellence in research and education. |
| **Shared Values Statements** | *Compassion.* Delivering care and comfort with empathy and kindness.<br>*Accountability.* Taking ownership of actions and their consequences.<br>*Respect.* Placing the highest value on every individual's well-being regardless of personal and professional differences.<br>*Excellence.* Always providing safe, high quality, innovative care, and service. |
| **Lifespan's Six Strategic Priorities and Related Strategic Goals** | *Care Transformation and Quality*<br>  1. Advance patient-centric care that prioritizes quality and innovation.<br><br>*Research and Education*<br>  2. Advance excellence and achieve distinction in research and education.<br><br>*Engagement and Culture*<br>  3. Achieve an inclusive culture of workplace excellence for physicians and staff.<br><br>*Access, Growth and Population Health*<br>  4. Improve access, advance population health, and achieve strategic growth.<br><br>*Teamwork and Patient Experience*<br>  5. Work together to consistently deliver an exceptional patient and family experience.<br><br>*Excellence in Operations and Financial Health*<br>  6. Achieve excellence in operations with resulting financial health. |
| **Selected Measures of Success for Each Strategic Objective** | *Care Transformation and Quality*<br>  1. Improve Vizient Quality & Accountability score with specific goals narrowing gap between current performance and top-decile performance—includes mortality, length of stay, readmissions, safety—hospital-acquired conditions, patient falls, patient experience.<br>  2. Improve CMS Stars and Leapfrog Safety Grade ratings.<br><br>*Research and Education*<br>  3. Monitor and increase size of Lifespan's research portfolio; activities; productivity; visibility; commercialization.<br>  4. Quantify faculty diversity and faculty development.<br><br>*Engagement and Culture*<br>  5. Improve/reduce team member turnover; improve team member retention.<br>  6. Improve overall team member vacancy rates.<br>  7. Improve Leadership Recruitment Diversity Index—race and ethnicity of candidate pool interviewing for Lifespan Leadership positions.<br><br>*Access, Growth and Population Health*<br>  8. Improve percentage of new patients seen in 14 days and reduce new patient wait times.<br>  9. Improve call center performance.<br>  10. Increase attributable lives in Rhode Island and in the Lifespan Network.<br>  11. Achieve growth targets in prioritized strategic service lines.<br>  12. Optimize Epic/LifeChart ambulatory build.<br>  13. Monitor value-based payment and population health management metrics.<br><br>*Teamwork and Patient Experience*<br>  14. Improve the patient experience with access by reducing call center abandonment rates and reducing time it takes to answer patient calls.<br>  15. Improve willingness to recommend measure across Lifespan hospitals, emergency departments, physician practices and ambulatory settings.<br>  16. Improve patient engagement in use of patient portal—MyLifespan.<br><br>*Excellence in Operations and Financial Health*<br>  17. Achieve Lifespan system operating margin (consolidated) targets.<br>  18. Develop long-range financial plan to include master facility plan.<br>  19. Adopt financial governance policies to achieve a long-term credit rating upgrade from BBB+ to A-. |

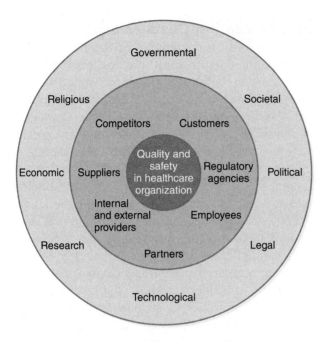

**Figure 1.5** Environmental Influences on Quality and Safety

care or service. However, other constituents also are important. For example, payers, regulatory agencies, and entities through which the patient acquires healthcare coverage are also key stakeholders.

## Assess the Internal Environment

After organizational leaders establish what they *want* the organization to do and what they believe it *should* do based on an assessment of the external environment, leaders need to know what the organization *can* realistically do to ensure effective planning for success in achieving its goals. This requires an examination of the internal environment—the resources, capabilities, and core competencies of the organization. Resources can be tangible, such as human, financial, or physical, or intangible, such as reputation. For example, if leaders want the organization to be recognized as a leader in breast cancer detection and treatment, they must ensure that the organization has qualified staff and equipment, as well as an engaged workforce and activated patients.

## Formulate Strategy

Based on the strategic goals, objectives, and evaluation of external and internal environments, strategic opportunities and threats (or aspirations and results) are identified. Generally, organizational leaders perform a gap analysis in which they evaluate the extent to which the present strategy needs change to meet the goals and objectives. Strategy formulation clearly stipulates actions to be taken to achieve goals.

Any identified gaps between the current and needed resources, capabilities, and competencies identified in the assessment of the internal environment are appropriately planned in the strategy formulation.

## Implement Strategy

Although various organizational department and service line leaders may develop their own strategies and plans, they need to align with the overall goals and objectives of the organization. Members of senior leadership can take many approaches to integrate quality, safety, and performance improvement with strategic planning and to ensure that plans and strategies are being carried out.

## Evaluate Effectiveness of Strategy and Modify as Needed

Organizational leaders establish specific measures of success to determine if the identified strategy and implementation plans are achieving desired results. Leaders may need to modify specific tactics if results are not achieved.

**Deploying Goals** *Hoshin planning*, a Japanese term that means policy deployment, is one approach for integration in a quality, safety, and performance improvement system used to ensure that the vision set forth by top management is being translated into planning objectives and actions that both management and employees will take to accomplish long-term organizational strategic goals (**Figure 1.6**). "The primary reason to undertake Hoshin planning is to focus effort and

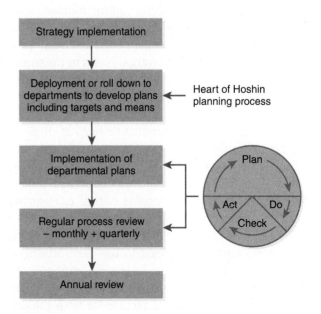

**Figure 1.6** Core Hoshin Planning Process

resources on those few strategies and processes that will best achieve the organization's survival and vision and to develop an effective process to align the goals and efforts of the organization."[40(p492)] The planning typically is performed at three levels: general (senior management), intermediate (middle management), and detailed (implementation teams). By using integrated and aligned cascading goals and objectives, individuals and groups across the organization can be guided to lead or contribute to the attainment of one of more specific goals identified as critical to success of the overall strategy. Furthermore, the *Hoshin* concept is based on the principle that high-performance organizations are those that harness the creative thinking power of all its employees. In this model, each employee is regarded as the expert at their own job, and their contributions are consistently acknowledged.[41]

### Measure and Monitor Progress

In this last step of strategic planning, management seeks to evaluate the extent to which the strategy is accomplishing the goals set forth in the first step of strategic planning and ensure that improvement opportunities are identified and corrective action is implemented. Actual performance is evaluated and compared with the performance goals and objectives established as part of the strategic plan. Gaps between desired performance and actual performance require action. Many factors influence the effectiveness of strategy. Among the most important is the need for effective leadership.

As an expert facilitator, the healthcare quality professional may be expected to facilitate one or more of the planning steps outlined earlier. The healthcare quality professional can ensure a more informed strategic planning process by ensuring that the results of quality, safety, and performance improvement processes are incorporated into various steps in the strategic planning process when they are relevant. Lessons learned from improvement efforts can inform several steps in the process. In addition, the healthcare quality professional may be expected to support or assist in strategy implementation and in measurement and control. As efforts to support the strategy are deployed throughout the organization, the expertise of the healthcare quality professional is critical to ensuring the development of appropriate metrics to monitor and evaluate success. Senior-level healthcare quality professionals are expected to use their advanced sense of organizational and situational awareness to support the strategic planning process through seeing and communicating the big picture for both present and future.[42]

**Communicating Goals** An organization's strategic goals must be communicated to all levels of the organization. Because most strategic planning processes yield a set of strategic goals that are established for a period of more than 1 year, organizational leaders and healthcare quality professionals need to conduct an annual review of key services, customer expectations, regulatory requirements, and other aspects of organizational performance to establish annual priorities and project plans for quality and safety. Leaders in high-performing/high-reliability organizations consistently demonstrate—in both words and actions— a commitment to quality.[43] Leaders can emphasize quality and safety in forums with new employees and make connections between specific daily activities and quality priorities for the organization. Healthcare quality professionals support leadership efforts by communicating organizational values and commitment to staff in daily improvement activities and huddles, connecting the dots between activities and priorities wherever possible.

## Engaging Stakeholders

Identifying key stakeholders and ensuring their engagement is an important part of leadership's role in maintaining quality, safety, and performance improvement strategies. The healthcare quality professional can also assist leadership in engaging board members, senior leaders, physicians, staff, patients, and families.

### Board of Directors

At the highest level, the organization's governing body is ultimately responsible for the quality of care provided in an organization. In most organizations, the governing body either assumes full responsibility for oversight of the organization's quality activities or delegates a large portion of the oversight responsibility to an oversight group (e.g., the quality council; the steering council; the quality, safety, and performance improvement committee; or the clinical governance committee) that consists of members of the governing body, medical staff leaders, and organizational senior leaders. Stakeholder representatives on these quality oversight committees might also sit on these committees (e.g., patients, families, and community agency representatives). The *Patient Safety* section includes additional information about board accountability.

### Executive Leaders

The organization's senior leaders perform an important role in moving the organization to achieve strategic goals tied to safety and effectiveness. All senior leaders need to be fully engaged in the safety and quality journey. The healthcare quality professional can increase the engagement of the organization's senior leaders in several ways, including the following:

- Provide periodic education on senior leaders' roles and responsibilities related to responsibility for the quality of care and service provided in the organization and on targeted quality and safety topics.
- Ensure that senior management meeting agendas are structured so that quality and safety issues receive as much attention as financial and other issues.
- Communicate the status of organizational progress on key patient safety, quality, and service measures through the dissemination of quality dashboards.

### Medical Staff

Although all members of the clinical staff are critical for patient safety and quality efforts, physicians often need focused attention to become fully engaged in quality, safety, and performance improvement efforts. Physicians are more likely to connect with quality and safety efforts that are important to them.[44] Organizations achieve success in engaging physicians in quality, safety, and performance improvement by embarking on projects that are led or co-led by physicians. A framework for engaging physicians in quality and safety can include engaged leadership, a physician compact, appropriate compensation, realignment of financial incentives, data plus enablers, and promotion.[45]

### Workforce

Leaders need to communicate that improving quality and safety is everyone's job and take steps to ensure that teamwork and collaboration are supported and rewarded. As this message spreads to the organization's frontline staffs, the healthcare quality professionals can further ensure staff engagement by ensuring appropriate frontline staff and physician representation on quality, safety, and performance improvement teams when teams are chartered. Healthcare quality professionals can provide support to frontline managers by offering suggestions for quality- and safety-related staff meeting agenda items along with data, information, stories, and other evidence to support the discussion.

### Patients and Support Systems

In patient-centered environments, patients and their families/support systems play a central role in advancing safety and quality. Many organizations add patient and family representatives to relevant committees to keep the patient's perspective visible in all discussions about quality and safety. Patients and families may need more information about their medical situation to be effective, engaged partners in their own care. With an ever-present focus on quality and safety, clinicians actively engage so patients and families understand their role and responsibilities for quality and safety. Leaders must heed the imperative to engage and activate patients.[46]

## Quality Resources for Improvement

Healthcare quality professionals may be expected to work with senior leaders across the organization to identify the resources needed to implement and evaluate the quality and safety plan. As the gap between what the organization should do and what the organization is currently doing is identified and specific goals and objectives are established, the healthcare quality professional will need to determine the staff and other resources needed to appropriately address the priority goals and objectives identified in the plan. For example, if reducing hospital-acquired conditions becomes a strategic priority as part of the quality, safety, and performance improvement plan for the organization, the healthcare quality professional will need to evaluate current performance, identify opportunities, and determine a strategy to meet the objective. The strategy will involve resources such as people, equipment, training, technology, external consultants, and other resources that need to be quantified so that appropriate resources may be allocated in the appropriate departmental budgets.

## Evaluation and Results

The organization's strategic plan takes into consideration results of the quality, safety, and performance improvement process. These results serve as the basis for objectively evaluating the gaps between what the organization is doing and could be doing. Program evaluation considers progress on these results as well as other key metrics to determine the overall effectiveness of the program. Healthcare quality professionals are involved in collecting and analyzing specific outcome metrics tied to the quality program as part of the evaluation process. The results and analyses of findings are shared internally, and action plans are developed to address opportunities using one or more of the performance improvement models accepted by the organization. Various performance improvement models are discussed in detail in the *Performance and Process Improvement* section. Results and analyses are also shared with senior leadership and the governing body so that findings may be incorporated into key steps in the next strategic planning cycle (**Box 1.4**).

---

**Box 1.4  Key Points: Strategic Planning and the Healthcare Quality Professional**

- ▪ Healthcare quality professionals have a key role in strategic planning and implementation of improvement activities within healthcare organizations. They
  - • advise organizational leadership on organizational improvement opportunities;
  - • assist organizational leaders in the development of action plans;
  - • assist in the establishment of organizational priorities;
  - • participate in activities that support the quality governance structure;
  - • work with organizational leaders to align quality and safety activities with strategic goals; and
  - • provide consultative support to the governing body and key stakeholders regarding their roles and responsibilities related to quality improvement.

---

# Organizational Infrastructure for Quality and Safety

Organizational leadership is responsible for establishing the organizational infrastructure for quality and safety. For practical purposes, day-to-day leadership is delegated to the CEO and senior leaders, elected or appointed members of the medical staff (e.g., chairs, chiefs), and administrative and clinical staff (e.g., nurses, healthcare quality professionals). Organizational senior leadership is expected to work closely with the governing body and the organized medical staff. These groups are expected to regularly communicate with each other on issues of safety and quality. Senior leaders are expected to create and maintain a culture of safety and quality throughout the organization and use organization-wide planning processes to establish structures and processes that focus on safety and quality. Organizational senior leadership is also expected to work with other leaders to effectively manage the organization's programs, services, sites, or departments. Healthcare quality professionals can be instrumental in working with organizational leadership to ensure that the quality and safety structures are organized in the most efficient and effective manner. The quality structure of an organization is defined and organized with clear linkages and reporting structures. Donabedian believed "that good structure, that is, a sufficiency of resources and proper system design,

is probably the most important means of protecting and promoting the quality of care."[17(p82)]

## Governance and Leadership

The organization's governing body (e.g., board of directors, board of trustees) bears ultimate responsibility for the setting of policy, for financial and strategic direction, and for the quality of care and service provided by all its practitioners and nonclinical staff. The role and focus of the governing body evolved from a primary focus on financial health and reputation to a focus that includes direct responsibility for the hospital's mission to provide reliable, evidence-based care.[47] Together with the organization's management and medical staff leaders, the board sets priorities for quality, safety, and performance improvement activities.

The development of meaningful board involvement in quality and safety requires assessment of the board's knowledge regarding healthcare quality. This is a key role of healthcare quality professionals, who are responsible for organizing and coordinating quality, safety, and performance improvement activities for the organization and its medical and professional staff. Healthcare quality professionals can promote the board's commitment to quality by providing useful information in a format easily understood by members who may lack familiarity with healthcare terminology and procedures.

Healthcare quality professionals work with the organization's leaders to maximize the effectiveness of the governing body's quality and safety committee. The Governance Institute offers several insights, strategies, and practices to achieve this aim.[48] Agendas and topics are organized to facilitate the governing body's quality and safety committee to focus on governance and not operations. Quality outcomes receive the same amount of focus and expectation of accountability in the governing body's quality committee as financial outcomes do in the governing body's finance committee. Clear messages about the expectation for transparency related to quality and safety come from the governing body through board adoption of policies to support fair and just culture and strong error disclosure and apology plans.

## Organized Medical Providers

In many healthcare organizations and health systems, the physicians and other licensed independent practitioners or advanced practice professionals are organized into a "medical and professional staff," and the leaders of the medical staff contribute to the leadership of the organization. In hospitals and other organizations, the medical staff functions according to a set of bylaws that are adopted by the medical staff and approved by the governing body. Bylaws establish standards for appointment, reappointment, and privileges whereby there is assurance that all members of the medical staff meet certain requirements to provide patient care. In hospitals, the organized medical staff is responsible for the quality and safety of medical care provided to patients. Medical staff departments have formal committee structures for evaluating quality of care and service provided to patients. These are critical and strengthen the organization's ability to meet its goals (e.g., clinical quality, financial). See more in the *Quality Review and Accountability* section.

In managed care networks, providers are organized as part of a healthcare delivery system to manage cost, utilization, and quality. The health plan manages the health benefits and additional services offered by a public or private third-party payer (e.g., Medicare, employer-sponsored plans). Healthcare is provided through contracted arrangements with individual and group providers. Providers go through an initial credentialing process prior to seeing health plan members and are recredentialed at set intervals (e.g., every three years). The rules for participating providers are typically informed by local, state, and national regulations and accreditation standards.

## Organizational Structure

The healthcare quality professional's role is to evaluate the effectiveness of the various structures, paying close attention to alignment, coordination, and communication. Effective quality structures with clear lines of reporting ensure ongoing effective communication between and among structures and the alignment of activities with organizational priorities.

### Operational Infrastructure

Most organizations define one or more operational-level groups of senior leaders, physicians, midlevel managers, and staff members to manage the coordination of quality, safety, and other performance improvement efforts across the organization. The number, type, and focus of these operational quality structures will vary by the size, scope, and culture of an organization. Focus areas may include, but are not limited to, clinical quality, patient safety, and patient experience through clinical quality or collaborative councils, patient safety committees, and patient experience/engagement councils.

### Quality and Performance Improvement Functions

Many operational departments within healthcare organizations advance the quality and safety agenda, and some have healthcare quality professional staff focused on one or more department-specific quality functions. However, most healthcare organizations establish an organized and staffed quality department responsible for most of the quality functions across the organization. How quality departments are staffed and structured impact how well the organization's quality, safety, and performance improvement processes are aligned, integrated, and effective.

Although limited evidence exists regarding best practices for quality functions and structures, the National Association for Healthcare Quality (NAHQ) and the Institute for Healthcare Improvement (IHI) cosponsored a research and development project that found the focus of quality departments changing from simple identification and reduction of defects to adding value to the organization. The quality department includes facilitators to educate and mentor staff to reduce variation, standardize workflow, and decrease defects in their everyday work. The department is viewed by the organization as experts in quality, safety, and performance improvement with adding value to efficiency in processes and decreasing operating costs.[49,50] How an organization's quality department is organized, structured, and staffed, as well as how it is regarded by key organizational stakeholders from a value perspective for quality, safety, and performance improvement, will influence an organization's overall ability to improve.

When designing the infrastructure to influence quality, safety, and performance improvement, leaders need to consider approaches with the greatest positive impact. Evans and Dean identified basic elements with great influence on quality.

1. focus on processes,
2. reduction in hierarchy,
3. creation of a team-based organization, and
4. use of steering committees.[51]

### Focus on Processes

A focus on processes concerns the structural elements referred to as *departmentation*, that is, how jobs are grouped together. Jobs can be grouped by function, product or service, geography, and process or customer. Quality, safety, and performance improvement tend to focus on process structure rather than functional structure, supporting both Deming and Juran, who noted that quality issues more often arise from processes than from individual worker issues. Some organizations have reorganized their organizational quality structures to assign staff resources to focus on and standardize core processes (standard work).

### Reduction in Hierarchy

One direct approach to enable others to act is modifying the structure of the organization by reducing the hierarchy. Hierarchy relates to the number of managerial levels in the organization. The trend in recent years is toward a significant flattening (reduction in the number of levels), with more focus on employee participation through cross-functional collaboration (usually in the form of teams). Flatter organizations also tend to abolish silos—replacing a department-specific focus with interdepartmental, interprofessional, and cross-functional work.

Deming maintains that improvements are more likely to be realized when frontline workers are empowered to solve problems, including changing processes and systems (most likely developed by management).[8] To work effectively, teams must be empowered. Empowerment enables people to take ownership of their jobs and make decisions concerning their department or area. People can take responsibility for their decisions and add value to their jobs. Empowerment does not mean that people can be free to do whatever they want or reassign work that they do not want to do themselves. Empowerment means regarding existing policies and practices, accepting accountability for results, and giving advice.

### Team-Based Organization

Another important structural element for quality, safety, and process improvement is creating a team-based organization. Because patient care involves multiple disciplines, the linchpin for improvement is frontline employees with regular communication and contact that allows them to coordinate and problem solve to continuously improve quality of care. The organization must develop an infrastructure within which the cycle of improvement can operate. One feature of this infrastructure is teams. Leading change through teamwork is discussed in the *Performance and Process Improvement* section.

### Steering Committees

A steering committee is usually an advisory committee consisting of key stakeholders and experts who come together to provide guidance on a specific issue or strategic objective. Steering committees are usually formed to advise and guide the development and

implementation of a major program, project, or initiative. They typically include executive sponsors, who can allocate needed resources.

A list of key points for organizational quality structures is found in **Box 1.5**.

---

**Box 1.5  Key Points: Organizational Quality Structures**

---

- Healthcare quality professionals develop, evaluate, and modify quality structures to ensure success in achieving quality and strategic priority objectives.
- Key factors in evaluating the effectiveness of organizational quality structures include the following:
  - Clear lines of reporting
  - Mechanisms for coordination, communication, and alignment of activities within the organizational structure
  - Connecting operational structure through the board of directors, executive leadership, and committees
  - Clear lines of reporting in the organization's structure (e.g., governance, executives and managers, and medical staff leadership)

---

# Change Management

Within the healthcare environment, change is not only inevitable, but it is an essential ingredient for growth. Without change, systems would stagnate, and new knowledge and technology would not be adopted. Change is constant and occurs at all levels of healthcare organizations. Each level of change requires different strategies, depending on the type of change, the people involved, and the magnitude of the behavior that must be modified to make the required change. An overview of the key concepts associated with change, models describing how change occurs, strategies to manage change, and tools to help accelerate successful change is provided. Healthcare quality professionals can use this information to help leadership facilitate successful change in their organizations.

## Change Models

Six change models will be presented to suggest different ways to think about change and the way various strategies, techniques, or tools can be used to effect change.

1. Lewin's change model
2. Palmer's change model
3. DeWeaver and Gillespie's change model
4. Galpin's human side of change model
5. Kotter's 8-step change model
6. Prochaska's transtheoretical change model

These provide foundational knowledge about change and common strategies. No single model will fit every type of change or organization. For this reason, healthcare quality professionals need a repertoire of principles and skills or a toolkit from which to draw for each situation.

Models explain a phenomenon and provide an approach for applying techniques at strategic points. The models have many common elements or similarities, such as description of movement from a current state to a future state. The impetus for this transition is dissatisfaction with the current state. Some common elements among models are readiness for change, communication of the change, and leadership for implementing the change. Using an approach in which change is planned provides the best results for a successful change.

Similarities in models also include the characteristics of the change itself and views of how these characteristics make it likely to be readily accepted by users (healthcare professionals, etc.). Common factors increasing the speed of change within an organizational setting are also identified in each model. The primary differences in the models are the scope and level of change. Most of the models address complex changes within complex organizations that often involve systems and processes, whereas other models focus on individual behavior changes.

Healthcare quality professionals are frequently asked to support or serve as change agents. A change agent is a person who helps members of an organization adapt to organizational change or creates organizational change.[52] Healthcare quality professionals can use various change models to guide them in their roles as change agents.

## Lewin

Lewin had a strong impact on the theory and practice of social and organizational psychology. Of interest in the change model is the first premise, which is motivation and readiness for change that must occur before the change takes place. The impetus to change is based on a force field of driving and restraining forces. For change to occur, the force field must be altered so that driving forces are stronger than restraining forces. A key concept of Lewin's model is that the force field—and therefore the impetus to change—could be affected more by removing restraining forces than by adding more driving force. To create the motivation to change, some level of frustration or dissatisfaction with the current situation must exist. This dissatisfaction creates a level of anxiety or creative tension that will spur the desire to change. Effective change managers will use the dissatisfaction with the status quo to begin the movement to change.

This first step in Lewin's change process, known as "unfreezing," assumes that beliefs, expectations, and norms can be remolded into new beliefs and behaviors. Through a process of learning new information, attitudes, and processes, people can redefine their current beliefs and "refreeze" these new concepts into their behaviors. This model is useful in approaching change in behaviors and identifying strategies to accelerate change and sustain new desired behaviors.

Models of change typically show movement from a current state or an old system to a new or future state. This involves first unfreezing or changing the old system and moving it out of a comfort zone so that change can occur. This progresses to a transition state or middle ground, through which the now unfrozen process is altered. Finally, a new system or future state of equilibrium emerges. This new state must be refrozen so the new change sticks. This model is used to integrate human system change with technology and work systems changes. It also can be used to create new systems to foster new activities needed by redesigned or reengineered work processes. The focus of the change effort is to invent a new status quo by directing all the activities and people involved in the change process.[53,54]

**Figure 1.7** depicts the change model of moving from a current state by unfreezing behavior, through the transition state, and finally to a future state by refreezing a new behavior.

The tool that can be used to analyze a situation or process to be changed, based on Lewin's work, is force field analysis (**Figure 1.8**). A diagram of two columns—driving forces and restraining forces—is developed to analyze opposing forces related to a specific change. Brainstorming (a verbal format) and brain writing (a written format) are tools that can be used to identify the driving and restraining forces if they are not clear. Driving forces, such as incentives and competition, tend to push change in a direction and keep it going. Restraining forces, which might include apathy or hostility, tend to

| Current State | Transition State | Future State |
|---|---|---|
| Unfreeze old behavior | Intervening change | Refreeze new behavior |

**Figure 1.7** Model for Unfreezing and Refreezing Behavior

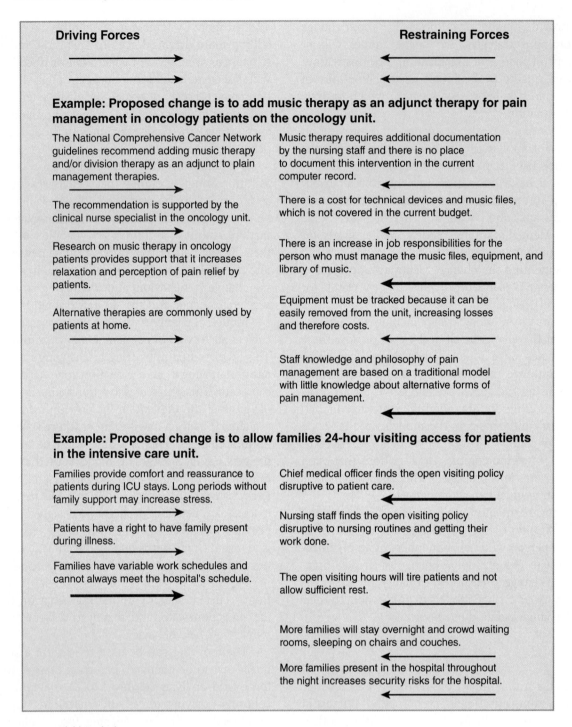

**Figure 1.8** Force Field Analysis

restrain or decrease the driving forces. For change to be possible, the driving forces must be greater than the restraining forces. However, the force field analysis shows not only the number of opposing forces but also the significance of each force. It is useful, for clarity, to indicate the relative "weights" of the opposing forces with the size of arrows. For example, if a new law requires that a change be made, this mandate, together with the threat of a large fine for noncompliance, would be a more powerful driving force than would a manager's lack of interest in the change (the lack of money could also be a strongly weighted restraining force).

A key change management strategy using force field analysis is to reduce the number of restraining forces; this approach increases the chances of success. Note, however, that adding powerful drivers does not necessarily make change happen faster.

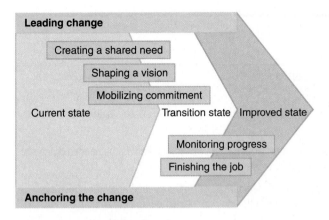

**Figure 1.9** Palmer's Change Model

## Palmer

Palmer, like Lewin, sees change involving movement from a current state through a transition state to an improved future state (**Figure 1.9**). Palmer's change model lists seven key elements of implementing change, namely,

1. leading change,
2. creating a shared need,
3. shaping a vision,
4. mobilizing commitment,
5. monitoring progress,
6. finishing the job, and
7. anchoring the change in systems and structure.[55]

**Table 1.4** assists with the assessment of failure points and indicates the needed change element for success using Palmer's model.

A key strategy to manage change using Palmer's model is to first assess readiness. By using the guidelines for change readiness listed in **Table 1.5**, one can assess an organization's readiness for change.[55,56] If a check of the elements in the guidelines does not indicate organizational readiness, then strategies are developed to achieve readiness.

## DeWeaver and Gillespie

Most change models used in healthcare follow a reductionist approach and are based on the assumptions that the change process can be broken into component parts and that healthcare quality professionals can then objectively measure the system inputs and outputs for each part. This model, described by DeWeaver and Gillespie,[57] is most useful when objective measures that can predict accurate results are in place. It depends on an orderly system in which objects behave predictably and new information can

**Table 1.4** Change Elements Necessary for Success

| Change Elements | Consequence of a Missing Model Element |
|---|---|
| Leading change | Change is slow and lacks attention and resources. |
| Creating a shared need | Change has a low priority; receives no attention; and starts, then stops. |
| Shaping a vision | Change gets off to a fast start that fizzles; there is no clear direction. |
| Mobilizing commitment | Nobody owns the change; the project is not sustainable. |
| Monitoring progress | There is no chance for feedback and improvement. |
| Finishing the job | Cynicism, naysaying, and a fad-of-the-month attitude abound. |
| Anchoring the change | Mixed signals, anxiety, and frustration increase. |

fit into existing structures. The following is a breakdown of the stages within this change model:

- *Awareness stage.* The person knows something about the change or is aware of the change and may have heard it mentioned and explained. However, the individual generally does not have a strong opinion about it and may deny that the change will affect them.
- *Curiosity stage.* The person expresses concern or curiosity about the change or asks questions about the effect of the change on them and may be defensive, resistant, or in denial about the change.
- *Visualization stage.* The person seeks to understand one's relationship to the change and the effect of the change on the person or the organization, by asking questions and seeking information.
- *Learning stage.* The person takes part in learning how to implement or use the change and may offer opinions and concerns about specifics of the change.
- *Use stage.* The person actively uses the change and integrates the change into their daily work habits and can describe or explain the change to others.[57]

Individuals progress through these stages at different rates and can revert to previous stages at any time. The model is not linear; some may never make it through all the stages. The change agent cannot force people into later stages if they have not dealt with earlier stages. Whatever actions the facilitator takes to

**Table 1.5**  **Guidelines for Assessing Change Readiness**

| Category | 10% Readiness | 50% Readiness | 90% Readiness |
|---|---|---|---|
| 1. Leading change | No one is in charge. | The leader is clear; management's commitment is clear in some areas. | The change has a clear sponsor and clear commitment from management. |
| 2. Creating shared need | Most people are happy with the status quo. | Many people think a change is needed. | Everybody knows a change is needed. |
| 3. Shaping a vision | People ask, "What vision?" | Some consensus exists on what is needed, but some apathy exists as well. | Everyone knows the needed outcome. |
| 4. Mobilizing commitment | A staffer might help someone. | Some resources have been dedicated, but more are needed to finish the job. | All the needed resources have been dedicated and are available. |
| 5. Monitoring progress | Everyone has their own opinion. | Some things are measured, but staff members also go by gut feeling sometimes. | Clear metrics exist for every activity being performed. |
| 6. Finishing the job | The situation looks like a dump and run. | Some plans have been made, but more remains to be done. | A pilot run, training, and recognition have occurred; everyone is ready. |
| 7. Anchoring the change | People ask, "Why does anything have to be done?" | Discussion about this problem has begun but hasn't been finished. | Everyone knows exactly what needs to be adjusted to embed this change. |

**Instructions for Use:**
1. Use to assess readiness in each of the categories listed and identify the corresponding percentage (e.g., if no one is in charge, then a rating of 10% is assigned).
2. After each category is assessed, total the percentages for the first three categories. If the sum of categories 1 + 2 + 3 < 50%, then the likelihood of success for the change is low, and even starting a project is risky. Consider delaying the change project until support is garnered.
3. If any category is rated < 50%, then the likelihood of success is also low (e.g., if no one is in charge, then chances of success are slim).
4. If the sum of categories 6 + 7 < 50%, then proceeding to implementation of a successful change is unlikely.
5. The greater the percentage of readiness for change, the greater the likelihood of success. This approach also demonstrates the interrelatedness of each factor for change; all elements are important.
6. Plotting the percentage of readiness by category helps planners visualize the state of readiness and consider strategies for various stages of the change project and the critical elements at different points.

assist people through the change process will need to be repeated many times for various groups of people. Some individuals may need the same process repeated several times. Others may take a "What's in it for me?" approach; they will need more time and more examples of benefits before they can commit to a change.[57]

Specific strategies can be used at each stage of the change model to increase the speed of the change process: awareness, curiosity, visualization, learning, and use.

- *Awareness stage.* Advertising in various media is used to inform people that the change is coming. Take the opportunity to highlight the positive effects of the change and link the change to meeting staff needs and eliminating problems. Increasing awareness about the change early on provides an opportunity to shape perceptions positively.
- *Curiosity stage.* Strategies for the curiosity stage include providing frequent, clear, concise

explanations and answering all questions. Taking time to elicit staff concerns and acknowledge the difficulties that the change may or will cause engenders support later in the change process. At the same time, it is important to present a viable approach to the change that acknowledges staff concerns. The curiosity stage is the time to create a level of dissatisfaction with the status quo and to generate interest in a new approach.

- *Visualization stage.* The strategy in this stage is to demonstrate the change for people and conduct user testing and reviews of the proposed changes. This gives people implementing change the opportunity to try the change before it is put into place.
- *Learning stage.* The strategy for this stage is to focus on educating staff regarding the change, conducting workshops or training sessions for as many staff members as possible, and giving them the opportunity for simulation or hands-on involvement when appropriate. An additional strategy

is to provide materials that will make the change easier to use, such as quick reference guides, frequently asked questions, troubleshooting tips, implementation teams, or help desks.

- *Use stage.* Technical assistance may be needed to make the change happen efficiently and effectively, with enough resources allocated to enable people to become experts at the new behavior.

Users will be at different stages of accepting and implementing the change. Early in the change process, facilitators meet with all stakeholder groups to communicate the change, especially discussing the reason it is needed at that time for that stakeholder group. They take time to elicit reactions to the change and be sure to correct any misunderstandings. Also, it is important to acknowledge people's reactions to the changes and ask for suggestions that will help overcome any obstacles. In summary, key strategies include multiple approaches to garner support for the change and keep people informed of the change process.

As the change is being implemented, it is important to continually assess the degree of its acceptance by the staff. This requires observing people's behavior and noting responses. Then, it is necessary to determine the stage of the change process in which people are operating. People will use many different methods to demonstrate resistance to change, and some may try to sabotage the change. It will be necessary to find ways to help people identify with the change and understand it and to anticipate and address their concerns. For change to succeed in an organization, a critical mass must support the change.

People tend to fall into three groups related to change: those who are for the change, those who are against the change, and those who are undecided. If efforts are focused on individuals who are already positively disposed to the change, they can in turn encourage those who are undecided, thereby allowing the facilitator to amass critical support. At this point, the focus turns to individuals who are not supportive, so that they can be influenced to accept the change.

Early in the change process, a communication plan must be developed to ensure that everyone becomes aware of the changes that will occur. This task may be easier to accomplish if the people's concerns are anticipated and proactively addressed. This can be achieved by providing a forum in which individuals can express their concerns openly and honestly. Forums (town halls, etc.) involve supportive stakeholders in an early demonstration of the change and include enough time for people to deal with their emotions regarding the change and to help them let go of the past and embrace the future.[57]

To summarize, key strategies that a change agent or project champion can use to accelerate change using this model include

1. assessing change readiness,
2. leading the change process proactively,
3. creating a shared need with stakeholders,
4. shaping a vision with clear goals,
5. mobilizing commitment with those who support the change,
6. monitoring progress toward completion,
7. completing the job, and
8. anchoring the change in systems and structures.

## Galpin

Traditional views of change claim that most organizations focus on the technical, financial, and operational aspects, with little regard for the human aspect.[58,59] This mindset has since shifted to a strong appreciation of the human side of change. After all, people do the work, people must make the changes, and people will support or resist the changes. Galpin's human side of change approach is based on a nine-step process in which change is a deliberate, planned process. Having a well-planned, carefully thought-out process is the best approach to change management. Except in unusual circumstances, planning for change, rather than allowing it to occur haphazardly, will ensure the greatest degree of success. Galpin's change management model involves the steps depicted in **Figure 1.10**.

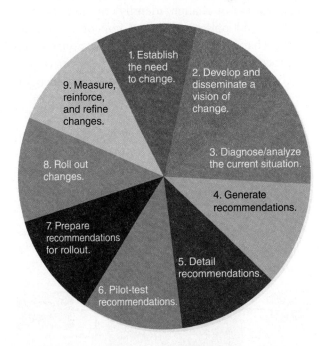

**Figure 1.10** Galpin's Change Management Process Model

Modified from Galpin TJ. *The Human Side of Change.* San Francisco, CA: Jossey-Bass; 1996: 4, with permission from John Wiley and Sons, Inc. Copyright 1996 by Jossey-Bass.

Galpin correlates these stages with suggested timeframes to guide the facilitator in planning and correlates the stages with either strategic change or grassroots change. Strategic change involves stages 1, 2, 3, 4, and 5, and grassroots change involves stages 6, 7, 8, and 9. Teams are basic infrastructure for the use of this model.[59]

Using the nine-step model, Galpin identifies four communication phases of a change effort. First is the build awareness phase (corresponding to stages 1 and 2). Next is the project status phase (corresponding to stages 3, 4, 5, 6, and 7). Then the communication plan is rolled out (corresponding to stage 8). Finally, follow-up with staff takes place at the end of the change process (corresponding to stage 9).

Galpin identified a practical change management tool, which he calls a "cultural screen." This tool focuses on the cultural aspect of change and identifies those factors associated with the culture of the organization assessed to achieve successful change. If, while using the screening tool, items that will impede the change process are found, a proactive approach to manage these specific items can be developed. If items are not identified prior to change efforts, then a risk exists that the change will be slow or arduous, or that it may even fail.

The cultural screening tool, which is used in implementing change,[58] includes the following 10 items (**Figure 1.11**):

1. *Rules and policies.* To support positive implementation of change, identify and eliminate the rules and policies that will impede or restrain the change process. Develop new policies and procedures that will reinforce or drive the change. This effort corresponds to a recognition of the restraining and driving forces in Lewin's model.
2. *Goals and measurement.* Develop clear goals and measurements that reinforce the desired change. These will help sustain change and hold gains over time.

3. *Customs and norms.* Replace the old way of doing things by making it harder to revert and reinforce the new change by making it easier to implement.
4. *Training.* Develop training and education that will reinforce the new change. Provide real-time, hands-on experience with the new process to support acceptance.
5. *Ceremonies and events.* Implement ceremonies that reinforce the new change and recognize both individual and team contributions to the success of the change effort.
6. *Management behaviors.* Publicly recognize and reward managers who support and implement the change. Link pay, merit, and promotion to desired behaviors.
7. *Rewards and recognition.* Make rewards specific to the change goals. Be sure that the performance system rewards the desired change. Rewards and recognition are key principles to successful management.
8. *Communications.* Communicate in ways that demonstrate commitment to the change. Use multiple methods to deliver a consistent message throughout the change process.
9. *Physical environment.* Ensure that the physical environment reflects and supports the change.
10. *Organizational structure.* Ensure that the organizational structure reinforces the change.[58]

In a humanistic approach to change, communication during all stages of the change process is critical for success. Communication is realistic and honest, and it must be proactive, not reactive. Change agents should link messages to the purpose of the change and repeat consistently through the entire process. Multiple avenues of communication are needed, including a feedback mechanism. This includes communication up and down as well as across the organization. Most experts on change reiterate that the most important aspect of change is communication.

Because communication is an essential aspect of Galpin's humanistic approach to change, it is important to discuss some associated pitfalls. Leaders must be clear and precise about the change. If the leaders cannot succinctly and accurately describe the change, then inaccuracies and rumors will abound throughout the organization. Leaders who believe in limiting information will quickly find that the grapevine is a powerful force and that the desired message will not be delivered as intended. Open, honest communication is important to create credibility and trust. Leaders who are promoting significant change cannot delegate communication and ownership of the change to others. A well-written communication plan with

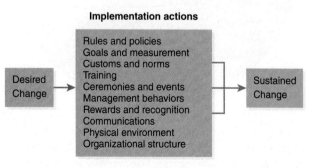

**Figure 1.11** Cultural Screening Tool

the involvement of senior leaders will be necessary throughout the entire change process. A common pitfall is to slow down communication when the process is under way. Ensuring that the change is complete and sustained is one of the more difficult tasks and is often overlooked or neglected. Providing infrastructure to maintain the change is also critical. Leaders need to communicate with staff even after the change is made to ensure that it endures.

Management strategies based on Galpin's humanistic model focus specifically on assessing the organization's culture. This approach allows for the elimination of rules and policies that hinder the change and the development of new rules that reinforce the desired approach or behavior (like restraining and driving forces). These strategies also include the development of goals and measurements that reinforce the desired changes and provide greater leverage for advancing change.

## Kotter

Kotter writes extensively on leadership and change management. Kotter and Cohen further elaborate on change management using a humanistic approach (see-feel-change). At the "heart of change" is why change happens, why organizations succeed at wide scale change, and why organizations fail.[60] Common errors of organizational change efforts include

- allowing too much complacency,
- failing to create a sufficiently powerful guiding coalition,
- underestimating the power of vision,
- undercommunicating the vision,
- permitting obstacles to block the new vision,
- failing to create short-term wins,
- declaring victory too soon, and
- neglecting to anchor changes firmly in the corporate culture.

Kotter provides an 8-step change model to proactively address errors common to organizational change efforts.[61] The first four steps in the process help "defrost" a hardened status quo, the next three steps introduce many new practices, and the last step grounds the changes in the corporate culture and helps make them stick.

1. *Increase urgency.* The first and most critical step in Kotter's model is to shake up the status quo and create a feeling of urgency. At this stage, people must be shocked into action. ("We must do something!") The major challenge at this stage is to get people ready to move. Methods that will advance this stage include dramatic presentations with compelling stories and items that people can see, touch, and feel, such as seeing a visual display of performance levels, touching a new computer, or feeling the emotional fear of job reductions. This step requires evidence that change is required.

2. *Build the guiding team.* The next step is to organize a team of influential, effective leaders. It is important to get the right people in the right place with the right change process. Team members must be fully committed to the change initiative, be well respected within the organization, and possess power and influence to drive the change effort. It is a challenge to get the right people with the best tools to be an effective, trusted team. The team makeup is diverse enough to provide multiple perspectives on the change and the stakeholders' interests.

3. *Get the vision right.* As with other models presented, a clear vision is essential. Without clear direction, the team cannot focus on the change and the implementation process. Providing this direction is leadership's responsibility. It is the vision that will steer the team into the new direction. Visioning activities about possible futures will help create strategies for the change initiative.

4. *Communicate for buy-in.* It has already been said: communicate, communicate, communicate! Once a vision and strategy are developed, they must be communicated to the organization. Sending clear, credible, and heartfelt messages about the direction of change establishes genuine, gut-level buy-in, which sets the stage for getting people to act. Keep communication simple and sincere; find out what people are feeling and address their anxiety, confusion, anger, and distrust. Rid communication channels of junk or noise so that the important message can be delivered. Constantly reassess this step throughout the change effort.

5. *Empower action.* The next step is to empower people to act by removing barriers. Removing obstacles will promote confidence in change, allowing more people to feel able to act.

6. *Create short-term wins.* Short-term wins provide visible immediate successes and inspire people to believe that the change can be implemented. The challenge is to create short-term wins and energize users about the change.

7. *Do not let up.* The process is not complete until the change is a reality. Leaders need to support the change over time, building on the momentum of short-term wins by keeping the sense of urgency alive. It is difficult to sustain excitement and energy over time and easy to become sidetracked by other tasks. Perseverance is key.

8. *Make change stick.* The end of the change process often is one of the most difficult stages. Once the change is implemented, it must be ingrained (hardwired) in the organization, so that gains can be sustained, and a return to the previous way of doing things is prevented.[60]

Successful change goes through all eight steps, usually in sequence, although it is also normal to go through multiple phases at once. Most major change initiatives are made up of several smaller projects, with each going through the multistep process. So, at any one time, people might be halfway through the overall effort, finished with a few smaller pieces, and just beginning other projects. Thus, with multiple steps and multiple projects, the result is often complex, dynamic, and messy rather than the conclusion of a simple, linear, analytical process (in other words, a CAS).

### Prochaska

Prochaska's transtheoretical approach to changing behavior is known as the transtheoretical, or stages of change, model.[62] The concepts of this model are applicable to numerous individual behavior changes including those related to maintenance of a healthy weight, smoking cessation, and substance use treatment. The stages of change explain the individual's readiness to change behavior, rather than a process change. This model is useful for working with individual staff members, patients, and providers to change behaviors.

Six stages that individuals use to change behavior (based on psychotherapy) are identified:

1. *Precontemplation.* The person has no intention to act within the next 6 months.
2. *Contemplation.* The person has an intention to act within the next 6 months.
3. *Preparation.* The person has an intention to act within the next 30 days and has taken some behavioral steps in this direction.
4. *Action.* The person's behavior changed for a period of less than 6 months.

5. *Maintenance.* The person's behavior changed for a period of more than 6 months.
6. *Termination.* The person is confident the behavior will never return and complete confidence in the ability to cope without fear of relapse.[62]

**Figure 1.12** illustrates the stages in changing behavior along a time continuum.

Prochaska led the development of measures that can be used with the transtheoretical model. Using this model requires some different strategies than those used in the other models presented. This model assumes that a person will not change their behavior until ready. Therefore, planned change is dependent on the readiness of the individual, not the organization. The person must move from a state of precontemplation to contemplation; only when this occurs can change take place. The application of this model may be useful with special populations (e.g., patients with congestive heart failure, renal failure, or diabetes) and certain health behavior changes (e.g., smoking cessation, adherence to a medication regimen, and weight loss). It also may be effective in changing the practice patterns of individual providers, for example, influencing providers to adopt a new product or technology. It is not useful for planned system change.

## Leading Change

To effect true change, one must become a compassionate leader, requiring "a paradigm shift from the present dehumanizing model of the organization as a machine to one with the organization as a living complex adaptive system."[63(p1)] Such leadership is difficult because no formula exists, and one must be willing, for starters, to change oneself. Although management involves a set of processes that can keep a complex system of people and technology running smoothly, leadership defines what the future looks like, aligns people with that vision, and inspires them to make it happen despite the obstacles.[61] This distinction is crucial, because successful transformation is 70%–90% leadership and only 10%–30% management. An emphasis on management rather than leadership is

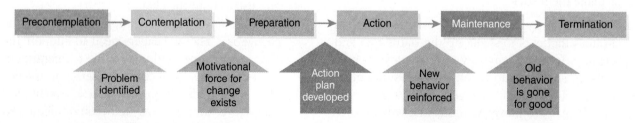

**Figure 1.12** Prochaska's Stages of Behavior Change

often institutionalized in corporate cultures that discourage employees from learning how to lead. Managing change is important because without competent management, the transformation process can go out of control. But for most organizations, the much bigger challenge is leading change. Leadership often begins with just one or two people, but that number needs to grow over time. Current organizations are far too complex to be transformed by a single individual.

The ability to manage change in a planned, productive manner is a core competency of healthcare quality professionals. It is therefore necessary to understand various aspects of change, change models, and ways to use tools to successfully manage change for improvement. One of the most important change concepts to understand is that "all changes do not lead to improvement, but all improvement requires change."[64] People may make changes that certainly disrupt routines yet have no impact on improving services or products. This reality must be clearly understood by healthcare quality professionals because of the turmoil and upheaval that constant change creates for daily workflow. When change improves services and products, healthcare quality professionals and other members of the change team can more easily and positively influence those who must make the change. Change merely for the sake of change usually causes frustration and dissatisfaction, not to mention additional work. Healthcare quality professionals play vital roles as change agents, improvement advisors, and facilitators and must be attuned to the personal side of change to manage the change process successfully.

Healthcare is a complex system in which demands change quickly. The intense competition among various healthcare organizations is intensified when resources are scarce. The question facing most organizations is not whether changes are needed, but rather how much and how often. Two factors are critical to assessing change in organizations: first, the limits of human performance in being able to respond to change, and second, the actual capacity of the systems to handle change. An organization's ability to handle frequent change depends largely upon the individuals within the organization, including its leaders.

In a Pew Research Center Survey, the top seven leadership qualities that matter most to the public included honest, intelligent, decisive, organized, compassionate, innovative, and ambitious. Women leaders were more compassionate and men more decisive.[65] Having evaluated over 30,000 leaders over 12 years, Olivo found that effective healthcare leaders exhibited these six characteristics:

1. *Directing.* Assertive yet collaborative with reasoned diplomacy and bluntness
2. *Engaging.* Verbal and social
3. *Challenging.* Very logical, but still supportive and tolerant
4. *Methodical.* Achieving and structured
5. *Adventurous.* Very ambitious, competitive, and willing to take risks
6. *Concrete.* Practical and experience based[66]

The resiliency of individuals is another critical element in an organization's ability to make changes quickly and rebound from one change to the next.

> Resilience is the process of adapting well in the face of adversity, trauma, tragedy, threats, or significant sources of stress—such as family and relationship problems, serious health problems, or workplace and financial stressors. It means 'bouncing back' from difficult experiences.[67(¶1)]

The American Psychological Association recommends that individuals follow these guidelines to build and sustain resilience, such as make connections (good relationships), avoid seeing crises as insurmountable problems, accept that change is a part of living, move toward goals, and look for opportunities for self-discovery. Although the American Psychological Association principles were developed for individuals, they are also applicable to organizational behavior. Additional information on burnout, wellness, resilience, and prevention is provided later in this section.

Although individual resiliency affects an organization's response to change, the leaders establish the culture of change, role model flexibility, and the behaviors needed to adapt to change. If participants view the change as positive, they are more likely to value the results. However, if they are not part of the change process, they probably will not accept the changes that result; this rejection will be evident in several ways. Commonly, unengaged or disgruntled staff will return to the old way of practice. They may devise workaround solutions or outright sabotage to avoid the change. Healthcare is in constant flux, and the success of healthcare organizations in the future will depend on their reliability, flexibility, resilience, and implementation of change in a purposeful, collaborative manner.

Although change generally is focused on moving people from an existing state through a transition state to a future state, no single model or tool will fit every situation in which change is desired. A repertoire of skills, knowledge, and abilities will help healthcare quality professionals understand different views of how change occurs and to use a variety of tools and techniques to effectively manage change. Reviewing a few change models that describe how change occurs, as well as some change management strategies based on their theoretical frameworks, will be useful.

## Change Concepts

The point of change is to make an improvement such as performance improvement using one or more of many tools for change, such as plan-do-study-act and plan-do-check-act.[68] Langley and colleagues[69] introduced the idea of the *change concept* as a general approach to developing specific ideas for improvement. Nine change concepts fitting the plan-do-study-act improvement cycle are identified as ways to introduce creative or innovative approaches to change and improvement. These nine change concepts, which can be further subdivided into 70 major ideas, also align with core tenets of Lean and Six Sigma:

1. Eliminate waste.
2. Improve workflow.
3. Optimize inventory.
4. Change the work environment.
5. Enhance producer–customer interface.
6. Manage time.
7. Manage variation.
8. Design error-proof systems.
9. Focus on the product or service.

This is described in more detail in the *Performance and Process Improvement* section.

## Planning and Managing Change

Planning and managing change will be described in the following three major areas:

1. Assessment of readiness for change
2. Cycles of change
3. Change concepts

Tools can assist with assessing an organization or unit for readiness to change. **Figure 1.13** simply illustrates how to assess readiness for change.

If the organization is ready and a plan is followed, chances for success are good. If the organization is not ready, the change agent must determine whether they can help make the organization ready or whether the change instead be considered later. If a change effort proceeds in an organization that is not ready, the costs of failure will be high.

It is important to reiterate that "all changes do not necessarily lead to improvement, but all improvement requires change."[68] This concept is strongly voiced by the IHI, which also provides several tools for performance improvement that will now be addressed.

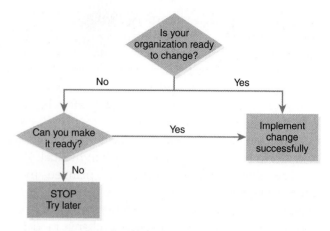

**Figure 1.13** Assessing Readiness for Change

Reprinted from Palmer B. *Making Change Work: Practical Tools for Overcoming Human Resistance to Change.* Milwaukee, WI: ASQ Quality Press; 2004, with permission from Quality Press © 2004 ASQ, www.asq.org. All rights reserved. No further distribution allowed without permission.

## Supporting and Accelerating Change

Several factors are identified as accelerators for success and can be thought about in several ways. In healthcare, there is a divide and struggle with change—spearheading fiscal progress for the organization and understanding the burden that change causes on the frontline of care. Change is accelerated when the organization's culture exhibits and encourages a capacity for continuous learning and closing the divide with executives, clinical leaders, and staff.

A recent report suggests that disconnects in transforming healthcare delivery can slow change. However,

> [the] more exposure executives and clinical leaders receive on the impact increased patient engagement and disruptors have on clinicians, the easier it will be to figure out how to alleviate system stressors. And the more clinicians see the positive impacts that patient engagement, market disruptors, and value-based care have on quality and cost outcomes, the more enthusiastic they will be about these opportunities.[70(p8)]

Having knowledge of its internal stakeholders, customers, and key business processes will allow an organization to identify driving and restraining forces quickly and move into the phases of planned change more easily. Every change requires some access to resources. The availability of resources, such as training, project materials, information systems, personnel, and financial support, will accelerate the change process. **Table 1.6** lists characteristics that accelerate change and innovation within four categories: leadership, culture, structure, and techniques.

The values of high-performing organizations outlined in the Baldrige Excellence Framework (Health

**Table 1.6** High-Performing Organizations: Factors Affecting Speed of Change

| Aspect of Organization | Accelerator of Change or Innovation |
|---|---|
| Leadership | ▪ Sets expectations for organizational performance, including a focus on creating and balancing value for patients, other customers, and other stakeholders<br>▪ Focuses on creating and balancing the value of change for patients, other customers, and other stakeholders<br>▪ Creates a focus on action that will improve the organization's performance and assesses readiness for the change<br>▪ Identifies needed actions and makes the focus or goal of the change clear<br>▪ Involves all active, visible, and supportive leaders with clear expectations for results<br>▪ Takes a direct role in motivating the workforce toward high performance and a patient, other customer, and healthcare focus, including by participating in reward and recognition programs<br>▪ Creates and promotes a culture of patient safety<br>▪ Demonstrates personal accountability for the organization's actions<br>▪ Communicates as marketplace, patient, other customer, or stakeholder requirements change<br>▪ Encourages open, two-way communication, including use of social media, when appropriate<br>▪ Communicates key decisions and needs for organizational change<br>▪ Addresses any adverse societal impacts or public concerns related to changes in healthcare services and operations |
| Culture | ▪ Fosters patient and other customer engagement<br>▪ Values relationships<br>▪ Encourages new ideas<br>▪ Supports creativity, innovation, and risk-taking<br>▪ Accepts failures (without blame), as well as successes<br>▪ Creates an environment for the achievement of mission and organizational agility<br>▪ Cultivates organizational learning, learning for people in the workforce, innovation, and intelligent risk-taking<br>▪ Supports participative structure with staff-level involvement<br>▪ Focuses on group learning<br>▪ Values continuous learning and improvement<br>▪ Supports succession planning and the development of future organizational leaders<br>▪ Encourages diversity<br>▪ Focuses on systems and processes<br>▪ Rewards individuals and teams for performance |
| Structure | ▪ Develops a strong team infrastructure and empowers team members<br>▪ Makes resources available for the change<br>▪ Enables mechanisms to obtain actionable items for desired changes, taking into consideration the voice of the customer<br>▪ Creates the means to listen to, interact with, and observe patients and other customers |
| Linkages | ▪ Makes connections between processes and the results achieved<br>▪ Measures and analyzes the strategic planning process and operations improvements<br>▪ Connects workforce planning and strategic planning<br>▪ Considers the need for patient, other customer, and market knowledge in establishing strategy and action plans<br>▪ Connects action plans with changes needed in work systems |
| Techniques | ▪ Makes tools and technology available to teams and ensures they are used<br>▪ Applies change models and concepts<br>▪ Uses constraints and forcing functions<br>▪ Replaces old ways of doing things with new customs or norms and reinforces the change<br>▪ Makes it easy to accomplish the change<br>▪ Uses training that reinforces the change<br>▪ Puts procedures in place to reinforce the change<br>▪ Evaluates sustainability of change<br>▪ Recognizes and rewards by linking promotion and pay to desired behaviors |

Data from Baldrige Performance Excellence Program 2021. *2021-2022: Baldrige Excellence Framework: A Systems Approach to Improving Your Organization's Performance.* U.S. Department of Commerce, National Institute of Standards and Technology. https://www.nist.gov/baldrige; and Fraser SW, Schall M. Accelerating the spread of better practice. Presented at the 14th Annual Institute for Healthcare Improvement Conference in Orlando, FL, December 2002.

Care; 2021) are built on the following set of interrelated core values and concepts, such as the systems perspective; visionary leadership; patient-focused excellence; valuing people; agility and resilience; organizational learning; focus on success and innovation; management by fact; societal contributions and community health, ethics and transparency; and delivering value and results.[22(p38)] Organizations exhibiting these values have a greater capacity to adapt to change and to implement innovations than organizations that do not. In the current environment, organizations must be able to adapt rapidly to changes, executing strategy more quickly than previously and with more flexibility and adaptability to survive.

In addition, healthcare organizations require increasingly robust data management systems to manage data for quality, safety, and performance improvement. As the focus of care extends beyond the walls of the individual healthcare organization, healthcare quality professionals need more complex tools for data analytics to meet the data and information needs of organizational leaders related to the overall strategy for quality and safety. A detailed discussion of data management systems to include data warehouses, business intelligence tools, and implementing health information technology is provided in the *Health Data Analytics* section.

## Resistance to Change

In managing resistance to change, three key areas need to be assessed: attitude, skill, and knowledge. Fear accompanies change, and fear cannot be eliminated, so the change strategy needs to actively address this emotion. Fear is usually associated with the unknown effects that the change will bring. This fear can be reduced by clearly identifying the effect of the change effort and communicating openly with those involved.

- Strategies to reduce resistance in people who are not willing to make the change include setting goals, measuring performance, providing coaching and feedback, and rewarding and recognizing positive efforts.
- Strategies to reduce resistance in people who are not able to perform the new change include educating and training staff in the new skills and the use of various management techniques.
- Strategies to reduce resistance in people without the necessary knowledge to make the change include
  - communicating the what, why, how, when, and who of the change process,
  - presenting a positive outlook on the proposed change,
  - having a clear focus and goal for the change and expectations of those involved,

- being flexible and adaptable during the change process,
- using a structured approach to manage ambiguity and confusion,
- planning and coordinating the change process in a systematic way with clear expectations, and
- using a proactive rather than a reactive approach.

An area that also must be considered in relation to change management is special populations. Both individuals and patient populations often require behavioral changes in healthcare practices to facilitate care transitions and thus improve the likelihood of positive outcomes. Change management approaches commonly are needed for patients with chronic conditions such as congestive heart failure, renal failure, or diabetes. Patients with complex medication or treatment schedules also may require change management. Change management can be appropriate for individuals or patient groups who need treatment or interventions for

- substance use (e.g., use of tobacco, alcohol, or illegal substances),
- conditions involving dietary and weight management (e.g., bowel disorders, obesity, eating disorders, diabetes), and
- mental health disorders (e.g., medication adherence, therapeutic behaviors).

Change management techniques also are used with specific providers, such as physicians, to engage them as champions of a change initiative or to enlist them in making a major change. Change strategies require special attention to these restraining forces and to the development of culture and methods to communicate the rationale for the change. Driving forces for this group often include a demonstration of the value of the change (the return on the investment), such as its relevance to practice or to pay-for-performance programs. The last change factor to consider with this group is accountability and how it can be applied in implementing and evaluating the change.

Key points concerning the role of stakeholders in navigating change are listed in **Box 1.6**.

## Practices for Creativity and Innovation

A *best practice* is "treatment that is accepted by medical experts as proper for a certain type of disease that is widely used by healthcare professionals. Also called standard medical care, standard of care, and standard therapy."[71] Organizational leaders need to create the environment where review, consideration, and

## Box 1.6  Key Points: Role of Stakeholders in Navigating Change

- Stakeholders exist in all healthcare settings and are the individuals and groups who play a key role in whether or not planned change is successful.
- Stakeholders include individuals, departments and services that will be affected by a planned change.
- When planning change, it is important to do the following:
  - Identify the individuals and groups of people who will be affected by the change.
  - Consider each stakeholder's level of influence over the success of the change.
  - Identify the potential impact of the change on each stakeholder as well as potential concerns that may be raised.
  - Anticipate concerns and barriers and identify key messages that will be important to communicate.
  - Engage with stakeholders to listen to their perspectives and concerns and validate your anticipated barriers.
  - Plan and implement a communication strategy that considers the key messages (i.e., what and why); the timing (i.e., when); as well as the means of communication (i.e., how) and the person who will communicate (i.e., who).
- Successful transformation is 70%–90% leadership and only 10%–30% management.

adoption or adaptation of best practices are promoted as part of quality, safety, and performance improvement. Additional details will be provided about best practices in *Performance and Process Improvement*.

If an organization desires a reliable, creative, resilient, and regenerative culture that promotes learning, then it must look at human relationships. In this context, people are more willing to change and are more adaptable when they believe that they are not alone and that together they can manage almost anything. Maher and colleagues identified seven dimensions that impact an organization's culture for innovation: (1) risk-taking, (2) resources, (3) knowledge, (4) goals, (5) rewards, (6) tools, and (7) relationships.[72] The concept of creativity corresponds to individual resiliency and capacity to change, and moving forward may be impacted by the culture.

To encourage creativity in an organization, leaders must be accessible and must acknowledge the value of people's contributions. They must create opportunities in which people can take risks and be allowed to fail. Creativity allows organizations to generate new ideas, remain competitive, and face the constant barrage of new challenges. Hundreds of ideas must be generated to find a true innovation that can be put into practice.[73] Common themes across models of creativity include the creative process (purposeful, imaginative idea generation and critical evaluation) and purposeful generation of new ideas that are directed and action oriented. Several techniques can be used to create new ideas like breaking routine ways of thinking and conducting activities to generate ideas; inspiring breakthrough performance; using brainstorming (and brain writing, its written form); using metaphors; developing prototypes and models; and using traditional tools such as fishbone (cause and effect or Ishikawa) diagrams, flowcharts, and process maps.

Creativity must be nurtured and identified as an expectation within the organizational culture. The three principles that underpin creative thinking are attention, escape, and movement. Plsek[73] described these principles in action as focusing attention, escaping the current reality, and moving mentally toward inventing or generating new ideas. The principle of attention primarily occurs in the preparation stage of creativity in which attention is focused on an idea or item in a different or uncommon way. The principle of escape allows one to see familiar objects in a new light; one must escape or abandon the tendency to oversimplify.[73]

The principle of movement involves moving away from familiar or traditional ideas toward an innovative or novel approach. Plsek identifies four general phases, or steps, in directed creativity:

1. *Preparation*. Pausing and noticing, seeking other points of view, refocusing a topic, looking closer and analyzing, searching for analogies, and creating a new world.
2. *Imagination*. Brainstorming and brain writing, using analogies, provoking imaginations, leaping, combining concepts systematically, organizing and displaying ideas, and harvesting ideas.
3. *Development*. Final harvesting.
4. *Action*. Invest the effort to implement.[73]

A structured approach within each of these four phases of directed creativity, depicted in **Figure 1.14**, guides creativity and the generation of tangible ideas and products in a cycle that starts at living with it.

Leaders and healthcare quality professionals need to foster creativity and innovation with the workforce. The Center for Creative Leadership identified important components of an innovation leadership mindset:

- *Curiosity*. Curiosity fuels the acquisition of new information.
- *Paying attention*. Paying attention is sometimes phrased as "slowing looking down" or "slowing down to power up."

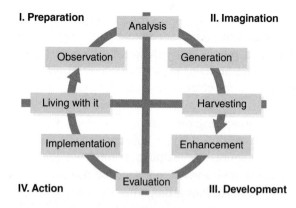

**Figure 1.14** Four Phases of Directed Creativity

Reproduced from Plsek P. Directed creativity cycle. In: Plsek P, ed. *Creativity, Innovation and Quality*. Milwaukee, WI: ASQ Quality Press; 1997. www.DirectedCreativity.com

- *Customer-centricity.* With this approach, you combine paying attention with looking through the eyes of a client—creating opportunities to adapt existing products and services or to create new ones.
- *Affirmative judgment.* Versus letting people know what you do not like, more valuable to the growth and development of the organization are leaders who take on the more difficult task of letting people know what they do like.
- *Tolerance for ambiguity.* Balance the need to move forward with the need to hold oneself open to additional possibilities.[74(pp16-17)]

When creativity and innovation are fostered and nurtured in the culture, innovations can emerge, and creative endeavors can be transformed into innovations. Baldrige's 2021–2022 Excellence Framework (Health Care) focuses on managing for *innovation*, defined as "making meaningful change to improve health care services, processes, the organization or societal well-being and create new value for stakeholders."[21(p48)] Managing for innovation leads to new dimensions of performance. Innovation builds on the knowledge of the organization and its staff. These nine rules of innovation can be adopted by the organization as strategies:

1. Innovate or imitate best performing innovative organizations.
2. Practice both research and development *and* search and development. Do not reinvent the wheel.
3. Engage in both product innovation and process innovation. (Most healthcare organizations implement process innovations.)
4. Invest in new processes and products as well as in old ones. There is a typical life span for each product and process. The usefulness of these products and processes is maximized during this period.
5. Practice both big bang (breakthrough) innovation and continuous (incremental) improvement.
6. Be both market driven and technology driven.
7. Be totally committed to innovation as a strategy.
8. Conduct both basic and applied research in a coordinated way and make basic research more application oriented.
9. Use speed strategies to bring products to market.

Creativity is necessary for innovations, and innovations depend on a creative organization with leaders who possess an innovation mindset.

## Disruptive Innovation

The theory of disruptive innovation was first introduced by Christensen's research and later popularized by the book *The Innovator's Dilemma*, published in 1997. The theory explains the phenomenon by which an innovation transforms an existing market or sector by introducing simplicity, convenience, accessibility, and affordability where complication and high cost are considered the norm. Initially, a disruptive innovation is formed in a specialized market that may appear unattractive or inconsequential to industry insiders, but eventually the new product or idea completely redefines the industry.[75] One of the most frequently cited examples of a disruptive innovation is the personal computer. Prior to its introduction, mainframes and minicomputers were the prevailing products in the computing industry. The theory of disruptive innovation helps explain how complicated, expensive products and services in healthcare are eventually converted into simpler, affordable ones.

Healthcare leaders who want to understand or even introduce disruptive innovation can explore opportunities in terms of the five Ws—who, what, when, where, and why. This involves asking the following questions about the service delivery model for a specific type of care:

**Who** is actively and substantially carrying out the process? Consider whether the patient could become a more active and substantial participant, rather than just a somewhat passive recipient, and whether clinical protocols may reduce the role of physicians in managing the process.

**What** happens in the process? Consider possible changes in the sequence of events, the content of the work, the use of different technologies, and so on.

**When** are patients able to access the service? Consider shifts in thinking regarding

24/7 access, weekends versus weekdays, and the like.

**Where** are patients able to access the service? Consider shifts that make the service accessible at home, in the community, or in a referring provider's office, rather than at a medical center.[76]

**Why** are the services offered? Why are they important in the big picture of healthcare delivery? Why does it have meaning to the patient and provider?

Nurse practitioners, general practitioners, and even patients can do things in less expensive, decentralized settings that could once be performed only by expensive specialists in centralized, inconvenient locations. Examples include remote monitoring using technology for renal transplant patients and nurse-managed healthcare clinics.

Healthcare quality professionals are in a key position to influence leadership on the importance of fostering creativity and innovation in an organization. Pradhan and Pradhan[77] identified several disruptive innovations such as Google Glass, noninvasive healthcare, automation in healthcare, 3D printing, personal health devices, gene mapping, e-patients, and digital checkups in their work describing emerging healthcare innovations.[78]

### Spread of Change and Innovation

Although generating and implementing innovative ideas take effort and can be challenging, one of the most frustrating aspects of promoting creativity and innovation is the difficulty of making sure that the innovation spreads throughout the organization.[79] Rogers and IHI offer models to facilitate the spread of innovation.[80,81,82]

# Diffusion of Innovation Model

To be widely implemented, new ideas, products, or technology must be disseminated throughout an organization. *Diffusion* is the process by which an innovation or new idea is communicated through certain channels over time among members of a social system (dissemination is synonymous with diffusion for purposes of this work). An innovation is an idea, practice, or object that is perceived as new by those who adopt it. Directed creativity activities may lead to an innovation, or the innovation may be adopted from an external source.

Rogers's diffusion model includes innovation; communication channels about the innovation; time (the time span from the point of someone first hearing of the innovation to the point of decision to accept or reject it, the number of individuals in a social system who adopt an innovation in each period, and the innovativeness of the individual or agency to determine the time needed to achieve adoption); and the social system in which an innovation is adopted.[80] The decision process on innovation consists of the following five stages for adoption:

1. *Knowledge.* Socioeconomic characteristics, personality variables, and communication behavior (the level of the person's innovativeness determines the type of adopter)
2. *Persuasion.* Attending to the perceived characteristics of the innovation: relative advantage, compatibility, complexity, trialability (suitability for trial), observability or visibility, reversibility, uncertainty
3. *Decision.* Adoption or rejection
4. *Implementation.* Direct application, reinvention, indirect application, or effect
5. *Confirmation.* Evaluation of the innovation's effectiveness to determine whether it will be continued or discontinued

Before the five stages occur, however, other factors must be considered, such as the history and culture of change in the organization, support of change given by leaders; the needs of the organization within a competitive market; the innovativeness of the organization; and the norms of the system (including the organization's culture of change, readiness for change, boundaries and relationships, channels of communication, and priorities).

The dissemination or diffusion of innovations is affected by influences in three major areas as outlined in Rogers's model:

1. Perceptions of the innovation, including the following:
   - The perceived benefit of the change or innovation (people are more likely to adopt a change or innovation if they think it can help them)
   - The compatibility of the change or innovation with the values, beliefs, history, and current needs of individuals (people are more likely to adopt a change or innovation that is consistent with their own values)
   - The complexity of the change or innovation (generally, simple changes and innovations are adopted more quickly than complicated ones)

- The trialability of the change or innovation by users (people are more likely to adopt a change or innovation that they can try before being required to use it)
- The observability of the change or innovation by people who can watch others try the change first (people are more likely to adopt a change or innovation that they can see in use before having to use it)

2. Characteristics of individuals who may (or may not) adopt the change, depending on their degree of innovativeness, including the following:
   - Innovators (2.5%)
   - Early adopters (13.5%)
   - Early majority (34%)
   - Late majority (34%)
   - Laggards (16%)

3. Managerial and contextual factors (e.g., communication, incentives, leadership, and management) within organizations involved (the rate of adoption of innovations is greater with increased communication, positive incentives, and supportive leaders).[80]

By using Rogers's model (which Berwick adapted to healthcare in 2003),[83] healthcare quality professionals can develop plans that incorporate these concepts, increasing the likelihood that desired changes and innovations will be successfully implemented. The rate of adoption of specific innovations can be affected using strategies that target specific groups of adopters. Targeting innovators and early adopters is usually sufficient to create the necessary support and momentum for adoption of a change or innovation, with the other groups following.[80] The individuals in specific adopter categories are shown in the bell curve in **Figure 1.15**.

Tools can assess the rate of adoption of innovations. The scorecard tool for new ideas (**Figure 1.16**) can be used to assess the possibility for and rate of adoption of an innovation or new change based on specific criteria defined in Rogers's model.[84] If the assessment indicates that the adoption is not likely to be successful, additional strategies can be developed to improve the odds.

Ratings are determined independently based on a five-point scale where a score of 1 signifies that the change is very weak relative to the attribute being scored and 5 signifies that the change is very strong. The higher the rating of each item on the scorecard, the greater the likelihood that a specific innovation or change will be successfully adopted. The items in the scorecard are defined as follows:

- *Relative advantage.* The degree to which an innovation is perceived as better than the idea it supersedes
- *Simplicity.* The degree to which an innovation is perceived as simple to understand and use
- *Compatibility.* The degree to which an innovation is perceived as being consistent with the existing values, experiences, beliefs, and needs of potential adopters
- *Trialability or suitability for trial.* The degree to which an innovation can be tested on a small scale
- *Observability.* The degree to which the use of an innovation and the results it produces are observable or visible to those who should consider it[85]

## Framework for Spread

This aspect of dissemination or diffusion is addressed by the IHI with a model for spreading change and innovations to promote rapid dissemination of quality, safety, and performance improvement practices across an organization. This framework (**Figure 1.17**) includes

**Figure 1.15** Categories of Adopters of Innovation

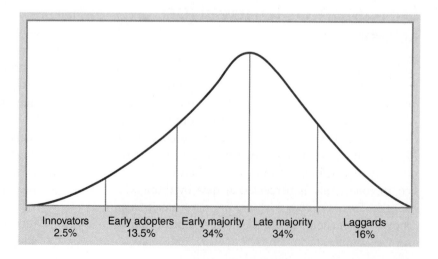

| Innovators 2.5% | Early adopters 13.5% | Early majority 34% | Late majority 34% | Laggards 16% |

| | Relative Advantage | Simplicity | Compatibility | Trialability or Suitability for Trial | Observability |
|---|---|---|---|---|---|
| | | | | | |
| Name of Innovation | Score | Score | Score | Score | Score |
| SCORING DIRECTIONS: Group exercise with individuals rating independently.<br>Score on 1–5 scale<br>1 = change is very weak relative to the attribute<br>5 = change is very strong relative to the attribute | | | | | |

**Figure 1.16** Scorecard Tool for New Ideas

Adapted from Sarah W. Fraser Associates, Aylesbury, United Kingdom. New Idea Scorecard. www.IHI.org

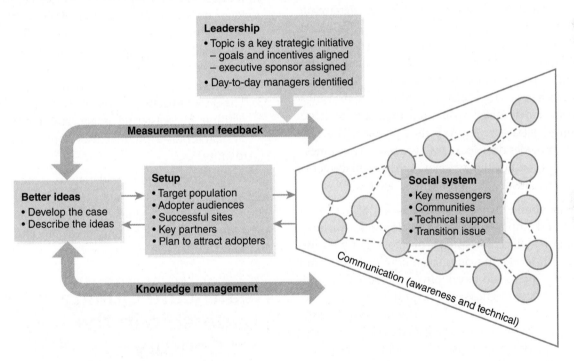

**Figure 1.17** A Framework for Spread

Massoud MR, Nielsen GA, Nola K, Schall MW, Sevin C. *A Framework for Spread: From Local Improvements to System-Wide Change.* IHI Innovation Series white paper. Cambridge, MA: Institute for Healthcare Improvement; 2006. www.IHI.org

seven major components for broad consideration and are not in a specific order.

1. *Leadership.* Leadership is required to ensure that the goal to be spread throughout the organization is aligned with strategic goals. Responsibility for day-to-day leadership must be assigned to provide guidance on the spread. Communication channels need to be established and supported by leaders as part of an ongoing process.

2. *Setup for spread (infrastructure).* The setup for spread is a structure for coordinating the activities in which the target population is identified, the sites are selected for initiating the spread, the key partners are identified, and a plan for implementation is established.

3. *Better ideas.* Better ideas are the ideas for changes or improvement with demonstrated success and are desired to be spread throughout the organization.

4. *Communication.* Communication is a key underpinning of the spread model, and communication strategies include the purpose and methods of communication for the target population.

5. *Social system.* The social system for spread includes the individuals and groups in the target population. The relationships within the social system must be understood so that problems related to communication, support, and other issues can be identified and resolved.

6. *Knowledge management.* Knowledge management is the process of collecting information about the spread with the aid of the measurement and feedback component so that the spread process can be modified as necessary. It is critical to the systems foundation that effective management be fact based and knowledge driven, permitting the system agility for improving performance and competitiveness. This enables focus on the quality and availability of data and information that result in organizational knowledge, including the sharing of best practices. Not all information is valuable, so individual organizations need to determine what information qualifies as a knowledge-based asset. The challenge of accumulating knowledge is figuring out how to recognize, generate, share, and manage it to foster innovations.

7. *Measurement and feedback.* A system for measurement and feedback is needed to ensure that the spread of the change proceeds as planned. This system provides data about the process and outcomes, and, in combination with knowledge management, allows adjustments to the spread strategy.[86]

To maximize results, a strategy is needed to spread change and improvements. These strategies include assessing readiness for spread, developing a plan for the spread, leveraging pilot sites, developing a communication plan, and developing a measurement and feedback system. These are helpful in making the business case for quality and determining investments that should be made by the organization. Employers, patients, providers, and insurers are all financial beneficiaries of quality improvement.[87] Overuse, defective, inefficient, and underuse care is not patient centered but is most often reimbursed. The business case for reducing overuse and underuse of care lies not with the healthcare organization but with self-insured employee populations and capitated plans. The business case for reducing inefficient care is derived from the benefit of reducing variation, defect, and waste and associated financial savings. However, reducing defects of care almost always improves business bottom lines, even if the defective care is reimbursed.

A business case for a healthcare improvement intervention exists if the entity that invests in the intervention realizes a financial return on its investment in a reasonable time frame, using a reasonable rate of discounting. This may be realized as bankable dollars (profit), a reduction in losses for a given program or population, or avoided costs. In addition, a business case may exist if the investing entity believes that a positive indirect effect on organizational function and sustainability will accrue within a reasonable time frame.[88(p18)] See the *Quality Review and Accountability* section for more information about making the business case for quality.

Healthcare quality professionals may be the ones in the organization who build and defend a business case for quality. The framework for establishing a business case for quality is set forth by Bailit and Dyer.[89] The framework rests on three broad categories for which a business case can be established:

1. Return on investment, the amount of financial return that an investment provides in a year, reduced expenditures or cost avoidance, and costs

2. Regulatory or contractual requirements or performance incentives (or disincentives) offered to the organization by groups such as purchasers or providers, or their alignment with explicit performance incentives (e.g., pay-for-performance initiatives)

3. The desire to gain a strategic advantage over competition by bolstering image and reputation or by marketing a product (development of brand identity)

Although strategic considerations typically focus staff members' efforts on the external world, organizations also must consider the nature of the internal environment when deciding whether to fund quality and safety initiatives.

# Healthcare Quality Leadership in the 21st Century

Leading quality and safety with an eye toward the future requires continuous learning to advise leadership on organizational opportunities. For the healthcare quality professional, there is consideration of strategy and stakeholders based on the organization type, where it sits in the continuum of care, payment streams (e.g., publicly funded, commercial product), and whether the organization stands alone or as part of a larger system.

- Strategic planning
  - Align quality and safety activities with strategic goals.
  - Establish priorities.
  - Develop action plans or projects.

- Participate in activities that support the quality governance infrastructure.
- Stakeholder engagement
  - Identify resource needs to improve quality.
  - Assess the organization's culture of quality and safety.
  - Engage stakeholders to promote quality and safety.
  - Provide consultative support to the governing body and key stakeholders regarding their roles and responsibilities related to quality improvement.
  - Promote engagement and interprofessional teamwork.

Leadership plays a critical role in shaping the culture of a healthcare organization, and approaches to guiding how to tackle the complex issues related to healthcare delivery will vary.

## Leadership Approaches

High-impact leadership provides a road map for individuals at every level of leadership in healthcare organizations to drive organization-level results from improvement efforts to achieve the Triple Aim.[90] The term Triple Aim refers to the simultaneous pursuit of improving the patient experience of care, improving the health of populations, and reducing the per capita cost of healthcare. The Triple Aim is a framework that was developed by the IHI in Cambridge, MA, and is widely referenced as a statement of purpose for healthcare system transformation to better meet the needs of people and patients. Its successful implementation will result in fundamentally new systems contributing to the overall health of populations while reducing the overall cost of care.[91] The IHI continues to promote the Triple Aim because the original emphasis was on patients, while others have added a variety of fourth dimensions and expanded the Triple Aim to the Quadruple Aim with joy in work or job satisfaction as the most common fourth aim.[92] Some organizations have identified equity or organizational readiness as the fifth aim.

Three interdependent dimensions of high-impact leadership in healthcare—new mental models, high-impact leadership behaviors, and the IHI High-Impact Leadership Framework—are depicted in **Figure 1.18** and will be described next.

High-impact leadership is critical to success for leaders shepherding the transition from volume-based to value-based care delivery systems. Success requires leaders to think differently about the world around them, to change their mental models, and to focus on value (**Figure 1.19**).

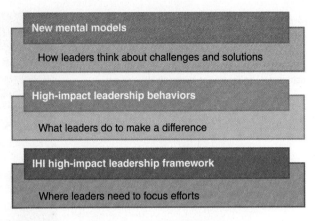

**Figure 1.18** Three Interdependent Dimensions of High-Impact Leadership in Healthcare

Swensen S, Pugh M, McMullan C, Kabcenell A. *High-Impact Leadership: Improve Care, Improve the Health of Populations, and Reduce Costs*. IHI White Paper. Cambridge, MA: Institute for Healthcare Improvement; 2013. ihi.org

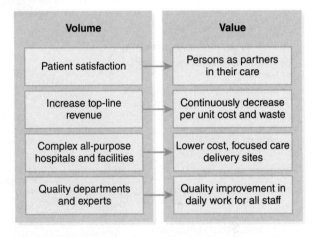

**Figure 1.19** Transitioning from Volume to Value-Based Systems

Swensen S, Pugh M, McMullan C, Kabcenell A. *High-Impact Leadership: Improve Care, Improve the Health of Populations, and Reduce Costs*. IHI White Paper. Cambridge, MA: Institute for Healthcare Improvement; 2013. ihi.org

Four new ways of thinking provide the context necessary for considering approaches to promote innovation and achieve the Triple Aim:

1. Recognize that individuals and families are partners in their care.
2. Compete on value, with continuous reduction in operating cost.
3. Reorganize services to align with new payment systems.
4. Operate from the perspective that everyone is an improver.[92(p4)]

Certain high-impact leadership behaviors are closely aligned with new ways of thinking and the High-Impact Leadership Framework. The IHI offers five behaviors to be used as a starting point for leaders who are examining their own practices as they develop efforts and strategies to achieve Triple Aim results (**Figure 1.20**): person-centeredness, frontline

**Figure 1.20** High-Impact Leadership Behaviors

Swensen S, Pugh M, McMullan C, Kabcenell A. *High-Impact Leadership: Improve Care, Improve the Health of Populations, and Reduce Costs*. IHI White Paper. Cambridge, MA: Institute for Healthcare Improvement; 2013. ihi.org

| | |
|---|---|
| 1. Person-centeredness | Be consistently person-centered in word and deed |
| 2. Frontline engagement | Be a regular authentic presence at the frontline and a visible champion of improvement |
| 3. Relentless focus | Remain focused on the vision and strategy |
| 4. Transparency | Require transparency about results, progress, aims, and defects |
| 5. Boundarilessness | Encourage and practice systems thinking and collaboration across boundaries |

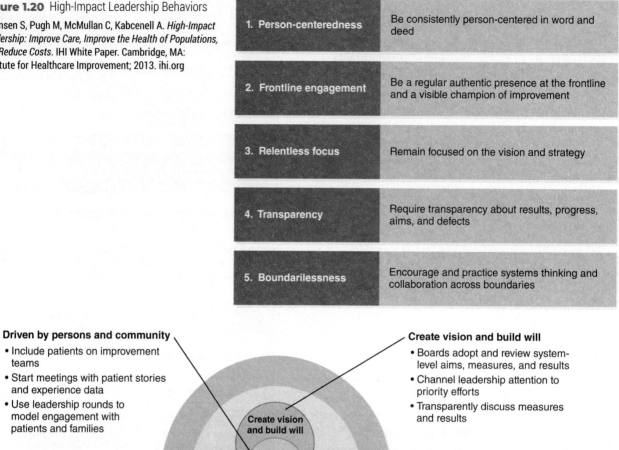

**Driven by persons and community**
- Include patients on improvement teams
- Start meetings with patient stories and experience data
- Use leadership rounds to model engagement with patients and families

**Develop capability**
- Teach basic improvement at all levels
- Invest in needed infrastructure and resources
- Integrate improvement with daily work at all levels

**Shape culture**
- Communicate and model desired behaviors
- Target leadership systems and organizational policies with desired culture
- Take swift and consistent actions against undesired behaviors

**Create vision and build will**
- Boards adopt and review system-level aims, measures, and results
- Channel leadership attention to priority efforts
- Transparently discuss measures and results

**Deliver results**
- Use proven methods and tools
- Frequently and systematically review efforts and results
- Devote resources and skilled leaders to high-priority initiatives

**Engage across boundaries**
- Model and encourage systems thinking
- Partner with other providers and community organizations in the redesign of care
- Develop cross-setting care review and coordination processes

**Figure 1.21** High-Impact Leadership Framework

Swensen S, Pugh M, McMullan C, Kabcenell A. *High-Impact Leadership: Improve Care, Improve the Health of Populations, and Reduce Costs*. IHI White Paper. Cambridge, MA: Institute for Healthcare Improvement; 2013. ihi.org

engagement, relentless focus, transparency, and boundarylessness.[90]

The IHI High-Impact Leadership Framework consists of six domains and provides a method of organizing and focusing leadership efforts for leading improvement and innovation. The following six domains are critical for leaders at all levels in healthcare to consider driving improvement and innovation to achieve the Triple Aim:

1. Driven by persons and community
2. Create vision and build will
3. Develop capability
4. Deliver results
5. Shape culture
6. Engage across boundaries

**Figure 1.21** displays the High-Impact Leadership Framework with some examples of leadership actions for each of the six domains.

Leadership styles are often presented within the context of approaches to decision making and problem solving as well as the specific tactics used to influence change. Through their own management style, leaders can influence the degree to which employees share information, knowledge, rewards, and power in the organization. Several different leadership styles are:

- *Autocratic.* The leader is directive and controlling; employees have little discretionary power in their work.
- *Participative.* The leader allows employees some degree of autonomy in completing their work while maintaining some control of the group and the decision-making process; the leader seeks input from employees and serves as facilitator.
- *Empowering.* The leader shares power and decision making with employees, enabling others by providing the necessary resources and support.
- *Transactional.* The leader views the leader–follower relationship as a process of exchange where compliance or performance is achieved through the process of giving rewards and punishment.
- *Transformational.* The leader can inspire others to change expectations and motivations to work toward common goals.[93]

Contemporary leaders tend to adapt their style to the situation, ideally resulting in a style best suited to the needs of the organization. Goleman defines six styles within situational leadership.[94]

1. *Coaching.* This style is most effective when employees understand their weaknesses and want to improve their performance and is least effective when employees are resistant to learning how to change.
2. *Pacesetting.* This style involves the leader setting high standards and then demonstrating them at times, causing many employees to feel overwhelmed.
3. *Democratic.* This style involves taking time to get employee input and works best when the leader is not certain about the solution and wants fresh ideas.
4. *Affiliative.* A key tenet of this style is a desire of the leader to keep employees satisfied and engaged. With this style, leaders place employees first.
5. *Authoritative.* In this style, the leader demonstrates self-confidence and empathy and takes charge and works to mobilize employees toward a vision.
6. *Coercive.* This style of leader just tells employees what to do and how to do it. This style works best in crisis situations.

One key to a situational leadership style is to understand and select the most effective leadership style for the situation. Healthcare quality professionals should ask themselves the following questions:

- What leadership style do I use consistently?
- In what situations might I use a different leadership style?
- How would peers and people who work for me describe my leadership style?

## Leadership Practices

An organization's leadership must be aware of the impact of both leadership styles and leadership practices on organizational performance. Several leadership practices are noted to produce a positive impact on organizational outcomes. Kouzes and Posner explored practices of exemplary leaders and identified five important general practices that apply to any type of organization.[95] An overview of the five practices follows.

1. *Model the way.* Much behavior is learned through role modeling. This practice involves setting examples by aligning actions and values. Leaders who expect employees to make changes to support quality, safety, and performance improvement must model those desired behaviors each day; actions speak louder than words. Walk the talk.
2. *Inspire a shared vision.* If a change is to be successful, leaders must be intentional in providing a vision for quality, safety, and performance improvement and influence others to share that vision. This means getting people to accept the core values underlying healthcare quality by developing a strong culture for quality and performance improvement. This effort requires more than just telling others what needs to be done; leaders need to communicate the vision in a manner that causes others to embrace it.
3. *Challenge the process.* Challenging the process means questioning the status quo and leading the way as an early adopter of innovation. It also means recognizing good ideas and demonstrating a willingness to experiment and take risks to improve the quality of care. Adoption of core values as a learning organization is key to success. Leaders ask what *should or could be* instead of accepting what *is.*
4. *Enable others to act.* This practice involves enabling others to act by sharing decision making and power in a way that enables others to move toward the direction of the vision. Along with sharing power, enabling involves having an appropriate structural design and the appropriate resources to support quality, safety, and performance improvement initiatives.

5. *Encourage the heart.* Change is difficult, even if it is done for the right reasons, and many employees need much more encouragement and feedback than many leaders realize. Encouraging the heart means recognizing the contributions that employees make and celebrating the core values and victories. The most important point of any reward system is to reward the desired behaviors.

Leaders use these five practices to keep subsystems aligned. However, leaders must first get people to support a vision of quality. One way this occurs is through the development of a strong culture of quality, safety, and performance improvement. Healthcare quality professionals typically take on a central role in defining and fostering the organization's culture of quality and safety.

The business case for quality often justifies the need for the investment in the use of external consultants and additional resources. Leaders may also use and interact with external consultants on a wide range of quality and safety-related topics. Whether one is entering an agreement with an external consultant as part of efforts toward regulatory or accreditation preparedness or working with a consultant on a focused improvement project, an external consultant is typically needed when internal resources and talent in the organization are not sufficient to address the specific need.

When the determination is made that a consultant is needed, it is helpful to check with relevant trade groups and industry partners for available options. After options are identified, the healthcare quality professional reviews available background information to help narrow the selection. The nature of the specific need may necessitate a meeting to discuss the specific expectations, scope, and deliverables of the project—what needs to be done, on what timeline, and with what resources. Relevant key organizational representatives are involved to ensure that the consultant fully understands the expectations, to work with organizational points of contact for the specific project and the consultant to establish a series of milestones and deadlines, and to address as early as possible any questions or issues that arise.

As the work progresses and the consultant offers recommendations, the healthcare quality professional should evaluate the advice offered and translate the recommendations to other leaders and colleagues. These questions are considered during the evaluation process: Has the consultant delivered what was promised? Have the core issues been addressed? Do the recommendations make sense for the organization? Finally, the healthcare quality professional needs to be clear about what the next steps are and how the consultant will be involved as recommendations are implemented.

## Wellness, Resilience, and Prevention

Organizational leaders who aim to reduce burnout and improve wellness among their team members can work to create a better work environment by aligning their commitments, leadership structures, policies, and actions with evidence-based best practices designed to reduce burnout.[96] *Burnout* is a syndrome first defined in the 1970s to describe the consequences of severe stress in helping professions and is characterized by three dimensions—emotional exhaustion, depersonalization, and decreased feelings of personal accomplishment.[97] Some researchers expanded on the IHI's Triple Aim to add a fourth aim related to focus on wellness of the workforce—joy in work.[98] The COVID-19 pandemic highlighted the need for healthcare leaders to develop and implement strategies that focus on burnout, wellness, resilience, and prevention. *Wellness* is defined as "a dynamic and ongoing process involving self-awareness and healthy choices resulting in a successful, balanced lifestyle."[99(p227)]

In 2017, the National Academy of Sciences convened an action collaborative that identified 80 factors that contribute to burnout and offered recommendations for strategies for organizational leaders to consider for implementation to address clinical burnout in their organizations.[100] The resulting 2019 report entitled *Taking Action Against Clinician Burnout: A Systems Approach to Supporting Professional Well-Being* identified clinician burnout as a threat to quality of care.[100] Others have described a model that helps organize the long list of factors to improve burnout into an easy-to-understand hierarchy based on Maslow's hierarchy.[101] The health professional wellness hierarchy consists of five levels, with strategies to address or prevent clinician burnout identified at each level:

*Level 1.* Physical and mental health

*Level 2.* Safety and security

*Level 3.* Respect

*Level 4.* Appreciation and connection

*Level 5.* Healing patients and contributing at the fullest of one's ability

Sample interventions for leadership to address burnout factors at each level are summarized in **Table 1.7**.

**Table 1.7** Interventions for Leadership to Address Burnout Factors (Level 1–Level 5)

**Level 1: Physical and Mental Health**

- Evaluate mental health of team members and the degree to which they are willing to use support systems such as employee assistance programs.
- Make support systems accessible by bringing them on-site.

**Level 2: Safety and Security**

- Train staff in de-escalation techniques.
- Increase security presence where violence is likely, such as behavioral health or emergency department areas.
- Provide for adequate staffing.

**Level 3: Respect**

- Improve the design of electronic health record systems to minimize nonvalue-added time logging in and finding information. Reduce clicks.
- Evaluate mandatory training requirements and reduce or consolidate where feasible.
- Reduce email quantity.
- Evaluate civility in the organization and take action to address incivility.
- Round with team members, listen to concerns, and act in a timely manner.

**Level 4: Appreciation and Connection**

- Evaluate compensation philosophy and maintain fair and competitive wages.
- Appreciate communication in a manner that is frequent, individualized, and specific.
- Broadly communicate major team accomplishments and responses to significant challenges.
- Facilitate community and connection through physical and virtual means.

**Level 5: Healing Patients and Contributing at the Fullest of One's Ability**

- Improve systems and processes to increase face-to-face time between team members and patients/clients.
- Support ongoing professional development to assist team members in becoming as skilled as possible.
- Resource team members to facilitate their use of new skills.

Data from Shapiro DE, Duquette C, Abbott LM, Babineau T, Pearl A, Haidet P. Beyond burnout: a physician wellness hierarchy designed to prioritize interventions at the systems level. *Am J Med*. 2019;132(5):556-563. doi:10.1016/j.amjmed.2018.11.028

**Table 1.8** Leadership Strategies for Building a Culture of Resilience

| Culture of Resilience Building Strategy | Description |
| --- | --- |
| Improve leadership effectiveness by remaining engaged. | Resilient cultures demand leaders who are engaged with and understand their team members. |
| Prioritize transparency and communication. | Open communication between leaders and team members builds the trust needed to establish a culture of resilience. |
| Build a safe and more social work environment. | Create opportunities for team members to interact as social beings to keep people engaged and connected to one another, even if it is through virtual means. |
| Be open to innovation. | Leaders should be open to adopting new strategies or technologies to respond to, recover from, or prepare for change. |
| Increase cooperation by sharing information. | Expand the use of digital tools for networking and collaboration. Team members know that knowledge is power and sharing information is empowering others. |

Data from Soundingboardinc.com. Employee resilience starts with leadership. Accessed December 15, 2021. https://www.soundingboardinc.com/blog/employee-resilience-starts-with-leadership/

*Resilience* has been defined as "the ability to use positive mental skills to remain psychologically steady and focused when faced with challenges or adversity"[102(p135)] and "the ability to withstand, recover and grow in the face of stressors and changing demands."[103(p5)] Many strategies are published in the literature to assist leaders in building a culture of resilience to mitigate or prevent burnout. Several strategies are summarized in **Table 1.8**.

Despite robust prevention strategies, during extended periods of high stress, burnout among

**Table 1.9** **Leadership Strategies to Mitigate Workforce Burnout**

| Burnout Mitigation Strategies | Examples |
|---|---|
| 1. Involve leaders from across the organization in wellness efforts. | Engage governing boards, executive leaders, and department chairs in a shared commitment to create and maintain a positive and healthy work environment. |
| 2. Build organizational will to make wellness a priority. | Identify and address the factors that contribute to burnout and allocate resources in a manner that will address them. |
| 3. Develop, communicate, and coordinate a shared focus on improving care and service across the healthcare organization. | Align organizational goals and resources and commit to a culture of teamwork and collaboration. |
| 4. Use data to continuously improve the clinical work and learning environments. | Measure and monitor team member wellness using validated instruments to measure burnout on a regular basis. Be transparent and share results. |
| 5. Create sustainable solutions to address factors driving burnout. | Cocreate solutions with team members and share successes within the organization to accelerate improvement. |

Data from National Academies of Sciences, Engineering, and Medicine. *Taking Action Against Clinician Burnout: A Systems Approach to Professional Well-Being.* Washington, DC: The National Academies Press; 2019. doi:10.17226/25521

team members may be inevitable. It is important for healthcare leaders to fully engage in wellness efforts and invest in mitigation strategies to address team member burnout. Several strategies are presented in **Table 1.9**.

Decisions about resources, constraints, incentives, and demands shape the work and the behavior of people in the organization. Healthcare quality professionals and leaders play a crucial role in developing sustainable solutions to workforce burnout.

## Summary

Organizational leadership and integration of quality and safety are the linchpins to effective continuous quality, safety, and performance improvement programs. This section described healthcare organizations as complex adaptive systems, leadership fundamentals, organizational infrastructure required to support quality and safety, strategic planning, leadership and organizational culture, and key concepts of burnout, wellness, resilience, and prevention that impact healthcare quality and safety. Change management, innovation and creativity, a business case for quality, and external consultants were reviewed. The healthcare quality professional's role is defined and described as essential to an organization's success in maintaining a quality and safe environment for patients and families. The healthcare quality professional's role in making operational the principles of leadership and management can be found in other sections of *HQ Solutions*.

Changes in the healthcare reimbursement and delivery system landscape make the role of the healthcare quality professional even more critical as value, translated in part through high-quality, reliable care and service delivery, becomes the focus for healthcare transformation. Emerging themes as they relate to the structure, process, and outcomes of healthcare delivery are shown below. This list is illustrative and by no means exhaustive.

- *Accountability.* Healthcare executives, clinical leaders, and clinicians continue to forge alliances with the organization and explore public–private partnerships. *HealthCatalyst* explored in a 2022 Insight Report "the degree to which private and public health organizations should collaborate on health services, an organization's role to produce health or health care, the responsibility of private and public health organizations for producing health or health care."[104(p4)] What is important? Shared priorities and mission; focus on coordination, collaboration, and complementary services; improved response to the needs of the community and populations served; and improved access to services regardless of ability to pay.
- *Safety.* Patient and workforce safety elevated to a primary focus given the COVID-19 pandemic under way since early 2020. Healthcare quality professionals can work to provide the framework for common risk language to support the dialogue related to managing risks; establish processes and a governance structure that promotes the early identification, assessment, and management of risks; and embed risk management principles and practices within their organization's corporate

processes to ensure that risks can be managed effectively. This requires focus that

- identifies, elevates, and manages risks so the right risks are addressed by the right people at the right time;
- fosters an organizational culture where risk identification and elevation are encouraged and rewarded; and
- creates a line of sight into risks across organizational stovepipes to create opportunities to mitigate risks with similar root causes.[105]

- *Population health.* Heightened attention to program structure, payment, and outcomes emerged in the 2010s. Important areas for the healthcare quality professionals to understand include the following:
  - Current clinical, quality, care management, analytic, legal, regulatory, policy, operational, and financial aspects of population health.
  - Knowledge about opportunities and challenges arising from population health initiatives such as maternal and child health and those programs targeting populations with significantly poorer mental health outcomes for Black people, Indigenous people, and other people of color and others with marginalized identities.
  - Navigation of the changing landscape and stakeholder implications for health systems, hospitals, provider networks, medical groups, health plans, pharmaceutical organizations, consumers, employers, regulators, and vendors.[106]

- *Care transitions.* Safety and quality are affected by care transitions and handoffs. Assuring favorable outcomes is influenced by biological, clinical, social, economic, and public policy factors. The Affordable Care Act serves as a reminder of provider accountability for care transitions through penalties and incentives for improving performance related to admissions, readmissions, and medication reconciliation.
- *Data analytics.* Successful organizations that focus on high-value data recognize that integrated data unlocks the highest value use cases, looks for reusable data that multiplies the value of data, and supports the principle that data quality evokes trust. Healthcare quality professionals are equipped to lead the application of data and translation of data to information to improve quality of care.[107]
- *Performance improvement.* Using performance improvement principles and practices, project management, and change management methods, healthcare quality professionals can support operational and clinical quality initiatives, improve performance, and achieve organizational goals. This is accomplished by implementing standardized methods for improvement and evidence-based tools.

Armed with principles, tools, and techniques, the healthcare quality professional is an invaluable resource to the healthcare enterprise as it strives to provide patient-centered, essential, safe, efficient, equitable and effective healthcare services.

# References

1. *Institute of Medicine. Medicare: A Strategy for Quality Assurance*; vol. 2. Washington, DC: National Academies Press; 2000.
2. Institute of Medicine, Committee on Quality of Health Care in America. *Crossing the Quality Chasm: A New Health System for the 21st Century*. Washington, DC: National Academies Press; 2001.
3. Stamatis DH. *Total Quality Management in Healthcare: Implementation Strategies for Optimum Results*. Chicago, IL: Irwin; 1996.
4. Dzau VJ, Shine KI. Two decades since To Err Is Human: progress, but still a "chasm." *JAMA*. 2020;324(24):2489-2490. doi:10.1001/jama.2020.23151
5. Senge PM. *Fifth Discipline: The Art and Practice of the Learning Organization*. New York, NY: Doubleday; 1990.
6. Begun J, Zimmerman B, Dooley K. Health care organizations as complex adaptive systems. In: Mick S, Wyttenbach M, eds. *Advances in Health Care Organization Theory*. San Francisco, CA: Jossey-Bass; 2003:253-258.
7. Zimmerman B, Lindberg C, Plsek P. *Edgeware: Insights From Complexity Science for Health Care Leaders*. Irving, TX: VHA; 2001.
8. Deming WE. *Out of the Crisis*. Cambridge, MA: MIT Press; 2000.
9. Juran JM. *Juran on Leadership for Quality: An Executive Handbook*. New York, NY: Free Press; 1989.
10. Plsek PE. Redesigning healthcare with insights from the science of complex adaptive systems. In: *Crossing the Quality Chasm: A New Health System for the 21st Century (Appendix B)*. Washington, DC: National Academies Press, Institute of Medicine, Committee on Quality of Healthcare in America; 2001.
11. Plsek PE. *Harnessing Disruptive Innovation in Health Care*. Rockville, MD: Agency for Healthcare Research and Quality. Accessed January 6, 2022. https://innovations.ahrq.gov/perspectives/harnessing-disruptive-innovation-health-care

12. Plsek PE, Kilo CM. From resistance to attraction: a different approach to change. *Physician Exec.* 1999;25(6):40-46.

13. Inozu B, Chauncey D, Kamataris V, Mount C. *Performance Improvement for Healthcare: Leading Change With Lean, Six Sigma, and Constraints Management.* New York, NY: McGraw-Hill; 2012.

14. Kotter JP. What leaders really do. *Harv Bus Rev.* 1990;68: 103-111.

15. Robbins S, Judge TA. *Organizational Behavior.* 16th ed. Upper Saddle River, NJ: Prentice Hall; 2015.

16. Kelly D. *Applying Quality Management in Healthcare: A Process for Improvement.* Chicago, IL: Health Administration Press; 2003.

17. Donabedian A. *The Definition of Quality and Approaches to Its Assessment.* Ann Arbor, MI: Health Administration Press; 1980.

18. Donabedian A. *An Introduction to Quality Assurance in Health Care;* vol. 1. New York, NY: Oxford University Press; 2003.

19. Ayanian JZ, Markel H. Donabedian's lasting framework for health care quality. *N Engl J Med.* 2016;375(3):205-207. doi:10.1056/NEJMp1605101

20. Mullan F. A founder of quality assessment encounters a troubled system firsthand. *Health Aff (Millwood).* 2001;20(1):137-141. doi:10.1377/hlthaff.20.1.137

21. Baldrige Performance Excellence Program. *2021-2022 Baldrige Excellence Framework (Health Care): Proven Leadership and Management Practices for High Performance.* Gaithersburg, MD: U.S. Department of Commerce, National Institute of Standards and Technology; 2021. Accessed December 2, 2021. https://www.nist.gov/baldrige-excellence-framework/health-care

22. Baldrige Performance Excellence Program. Baldrige Award recipients listing. Accessed December 1, 2021. https://www.nist.gov/baldrige/award-recipients?year=All&sector=All&title=&state=All

23. Institute for Healthcare Improvement. Seven leadership leverage points for organization-level improvement in health care (2nd ed.). Accessed January 6, 2022. http://www.ihi.org/resources/Pages/IHIWhitePapers/SevenLeadershipLeveragePointsWhitePaper.aspx

24. Merriam-Webster. Culture. Accessed December 1, 2021. https://www.merriam-webster.com/dictionary/culture

25. Siehl L, Martin J. *Learning Organizational Culture.* Palo Alto, CA: Stanford University, Graduate School of Business; 1982.

26. Rokeach M. *The Nature of Human Values.* New York, NY: Free Press; 1973.

27. Watkins MD. What is organizational culture? And why should we care? *Harv Bus Rev.* 2013. https://hbr.org/2013/05/what-is-organizational-culture

28. Agency for Healthcare Research and Quality. Culture of safety. Accessed December 1, 2021. https://psnet.ahrq.gov/primer/culture-safety

29. Schein EH. *Organizational Culture and Leadership: A Dynamic View.* 2nd ed. San Francisco, CA: Jossey-Bass; 1992.

30. Schneider B, ed. *Organizational Culture and Climate.* San Francisco, CA: Jossey-Bass; 1990.

31. Agency for Healthcare Research and Quality. Surveys on patient safety culture. SOPS Surveys. Content last reviewed November 2021. Agency for Healthcare Research and Quality, Rockville, MD. Accessed December 1, 2021. https://www.ahrq.gov/sops/surveys/index.html

32. University of Texas Health Science Center, McGovern Medical School. Center for Healthcare Quality and Safety: Generating knowledge to improve patient care: Survey; n.d. Accessed December 15, 2021. https://med.uth.edu/chqs/survey/

33. Reason, J. *Managing the Risks of Organizational Accidents.* Ashgate: Surrey, United Kingdom; 1997.

34. Shortell SM, Morrison E, Robbins S. Strategy-making in health care organizations: a framework and agenda for research. *Medical Care Rev.* 1985;2:219-266. doi:10.1177/107755878504200203

35. Luthans F, Hodgetts R, Thompson K. *Social Issues in Business: Strategic and Public Policy Perspectives.* 6th ed. Upper Saddle River, NJ: Prentice Hall.

36. SSM Health. Our mission, vision, and values. Accessed December 18, 2021. https://www.ssmhealth.com/resources/about/mission-values/

37. GBMC Healthcare. About GBMC. Accessed December 18, 2021. https://www.gbmc.org/mission

38. Minnesota Department of Health. Writing good goals and SMART objectives. Accessed November 15, 2021. https://www.health.state.mn.us/communities/practice/resources/training/docs/1601-objectives/handout_goals-objectives.pdf

39. Oxford Reference. Goal congruency. Accessed December 14, 2021. https://www.oxfordreference.com/view/10.1093/oi/authority.20110803095856963

40. Gaucher EJ, Coffey RJ. *Total Quality in Healthcare: From Theory to Practice.* San Francisco, CA: Jossey-Bass; 1993.

41. Hutchins D. *Hoshin Kanri: The Strategic Approach to Continuous Improvement.* Surrey, United Kingdom: Gower; 2016.

42. Garman A, Scribner L. Leading for quality in healthcare: development and validation of a competency model. *J Healthc Manag.* 2011;56(6):373-382.

43. Silow-Carroll S, Alteras T, Meyer JA. Hospital quality improvement: strategies and lessons learned from U.S. hospitals. Accessed December 1, 2021. http://www.commonwealthfund.org/publications/fund-reports/2007/apr/hospital-quality-improvement--strategies-and-lessons-from-u-s--hospitals

44. Botwinick L, Bisognano M, Haraden C. *Leadership Guide to Patient Safety.* IHI Innovation Series white paper. Cambridge, MA: Institute for Healthcare Improvement. Accessed November 15, 2021. http://www.ihi.org/resources/Pages/IHIWhitePapers/LeadershipGuidetoPatientSafetyWhitePaper.aspx

45. Taitz JM, Lee TH, Sequist TD. A framework for engaging physicians in quality and safety. *BMJ Qual Saf.* 2012;21:722-728. doi:10.1136/bmjqs-2011-000167

46. Pelletier LR, Stichler JE. Patient-centered care and engagement: nurse leaders' imperative for health reform. *J Nurs Adm.* 2014;44(9):473-480. doi:10.1097/NNA.0000000000000102

47. Conway J. Getting boards on board: engaging governing boards in quality and safety. *Jt Comm J Qual Patient Saf.* 2008;34(4):214-220. doi:10.1016/S1553-7250(08)34028-8

48. The Governance Institute. *Maximizing the Effectiveness of the Board's Quality Committee: Leading Practices and Lessons Learned.* San Diego, CA: The Governance Institute; 2015.

49. Institute for Healthcare Improvement. High impact leadership: improve care, improve the health of populations, and reduce costs. Accessed December 4, 2021. http://www.ihi.org/resources/pages/ihiwhitepapers/highimpactleadership.aspx

50. National Association for Healthcare Quality and Institute for Healthcare Improvement. Quality structure and functions at half the expense. Accessed December 5, 2021. https://studylib.net/doc/8181382/quality-structures-and-functions-at-half-the-expense

51. Evans JR, Dean JW. *Total Quality: Management, Organization and Strategy.* 3rd ed. Mason, OH: Thomson South-Western; 2003.

52. Oxford Reference. Change agent. Accessed August 5, 2022. https://www.oxfordreference.com/view/10.1093/oi/authority.20110803095601910

53. Schein EH. Kurt Lewin's change theory in the field and in the classroom: notes toward a model of managed learning. *Syst Pract.* 1996;9:27. doi:10.1007/BF02173417

54. Smith MK. Kurt Lewin: groups, experiential learning and action research. Accessed December 5, 2021. www.infed.org/thinkers/et-lewin.htm

55. Palmer B. *Making Change Work: Practical Tools for Overcoming Human Resistance to Change.* Milwaukee, WI: ASQ Quality Press; 2004.

56. Palmer B. Overcoming resistance to change. *Quality Progress.* 2004;37(4):35-39. doi:10.1109/EMR.2004.25109

57. DeWeaver M, Gillespie L. *Real World Project Management.* New York, NY: Quality Resources; 1997.

58. Galpin TJ. Connecting culture to organizational change. *HR Magazine.* 1996;41(30):84-89.

59. Galpin TJ. *The Human Side of Change.* San Francisco, CA: Jossey-Bass; 1996.

60. Kotter JP, Cohen DS. *The Heart of Change.* Boston, MA: Harvard Business Publishing; 2002.

61. Kotter JP. *Leading Change.* Boston, MA: Harvard Business Publishing; 1996.

62. Cancer Prevention Research Center. Transtheoretical model. Accessed December 5, 2021. http://web.uri.edu/cprc/detailed-overview/

63. De Zuelta PC. Developing compassionate leadership in healthcare: an integrative review. *J Healthcare Leadership.* 2015;8:1-10. doi:10.2147/JHL.S93724

64. Institute for Healthcare Improvement. Changes for improvement. Accessed December 5, 2021. www.ihi.org/knowledge/Pages/Changes/default.aspx

65. Pew Research Center. *Women and Leadership: Public Says Women Are Equally Qualified, But Barriers Persist.* Washington, DC: Pew Research Center; 2015. Accessed December 5, 2021. www.pewresearch.org

66. Olivo T. The profile of an effective healthcare leader. Becker's Hospital Review. Accessed December 5, 2021. http://www.beckershospitalreview.com/hospital-management-administration/the-profile-of-an-effective-healthcare-leader.html

67. American Psychological Association. Building your resilience. Accessed December 30, 2021. https://www.apa.org/topics/resilience

68. Institute for Healthcare Improvement. How to improve. Accessed December 5, 2021. www.ihi.org/knowledge/Pages/HowtoImprove/default.aspx

69. Langley GL, Nolan KM, Nolan TW, Norman CL, Provost LP. *The Improvement Guide: A Practical Approach to Enhancing Organizational Performance.* 2nd ed. San Francisco, CA: Jossey-Bass; 2009.

70. NEJM Catalyst Insights Council. Disconnects in transforming health care delivery: how executives, clinical leaders, and clinicians must bridge their divide and move forward together. Accessed December 5, 2021 https://cdn2.hubspot.net/hubfs/558940/Insights%20eBook%20Landing/Disconnects%20in%20Transforming%20Health%20Care%20Delivery%20ebook%20.pdf?t=1491409971918

71. National Cancer Institute. Dictionary of cancer terms. Accessed May 31, 2022. https://www.cancer.gov/publications/dictionaries/cancer-terms/def/best-practice

72. Maher L, Plsek P, Bevan H. *Creating the Culture for Innovation: Guide for Executives.* Coventry, UK: NHS Institute for Innovation and Improvement. Accessed December 5, 2021. https://www.england.nhs.uk/improvement-hub/wp-content/uploads/sites/44/2017/11/Creating-the-Culture-for-Innovation-Practical-Guide-for-Leaders.pdf

73. Plsek PE. Models for the creative process. Working paper. Accessed January 6, 2022. www.directedcreativity.com/pages/WPModels.html

74. Horth DM, Vhear J. *Becoming a Leader Who Fosters Innovation. White paper.* Greensboro, NC: Center for Creative Leadership; 2014.

75. Christensen CM, Bohmer RMJ, Kenagy J. Will disruptive innovations cure health care? *Harv Bus Rev.* 2000;78(5):102-112, 199.

76. Plsek P. *AHRQ innovations exchange: creating a culture of innovation.* Accessed January 6, 2022. https://innovations.ahrq.gov/article/creating-culture-innovation

77. Pradhan P, Pradhan K. Emerging health-care innovations. In: Singh VK, Lillrank P, eds. *Innovations in Healthcare Management: Cost-Effective and Sustainable Solutions.* Boca Raton, FL: CRC Press; 2015.

78. Singh VK, Lillrank P. *Innovations in Healthcare Management: Cost-Effective and Sustainable Solutions.* Boca Raton, FL: CRC Press; 2015.

79. Plsek PE. *Complexity and the adoption of innovation in health care.* Accessed December 5, 2021. https://psnet.ahrq.gov/issue/complexity-and-adoption-innovation-health-care

80. Rogers E. *The Diffusion of Innovations.* 5th ed. New York, NY: Free Press; 1995.

81. Institute for Healthcare Improvement. Linking tests of change. Accessed January 6, 2022. www.ihi.org/IHI/Topics/Improvement/ImprovementMethods/HowToImprove/rampsofchange.html

82. Institute for Healthcare Improvement. Spreading changes. Accessed January 6, 2022. www.ihi.org/knowledge/Pages/HowtoImprove/ScienceofImprovementSpreadingChanges.aspx

83. Berwick DM. Disseminating innovations in health care. *JAMA.* 2003;289(15):1969-1975. doi:10.1001/jama.289.15.1969

84. Institute for Healthcare Improvement. Tips for testing changes. Accessed January 6, 2022. www.ihi.org/knowledge/Pages/HowtoImprove/ScienceofImprovementTipsforTestingChanges.aspx

85. Institute for Healthcare Improvement. New idea scorecard. Accessed December 2, 2021. http://www.ihi.org/resources/Pages/Tools/NewIdeaScorecard.aspx

86. Massoud MR, Nielsen GA, Nola K, Schall MW, Sevin C. *A Framework for Spread: From Local Improvements to System-Wide Change.* Cambridge, MA: IHI; 2006. Accessed December 20, 2021. http://www.ihi.org/resources/Pages/IHIWhitePapers/AFrameworkforSpreadWhitePaper.aspx

87. Swensen SJ, Dilling JA, McCarty PM, Bolton JW, Harper CM. The business case for health-care quality improvement. *J Patient Saf.* 2013;9(1):44-52. doi:10.1097/PTS.0b013e3182753e33

88. Leatherman S, Berwick D, Illes D, et al. The business case for quality: case studies and an analysis. *Health Aff.* 2003;22(2):17-30. doi:10.1377/hlthaff.22.2.17

89. Bailit M, Dyer M. *Beyond Bankable Dollars: Establishing a Business Case for Improving Healthcare.* New York, NY: Commonwealth Fund; 2004.

90. Swensen S, Pugh M, McMullan C, Kabcenell A. *High-Impact Leadership: Improve Care, Improve the Health of Populations, and Reduce Costs.* IHI white paper. Cambridge, MA: Institute for Healthcare Improvement. Also available at ihi.org.

91. Institute for Healthcare Improvement. IHI triple aim initiative. Accessed November 17, 2021. http://www.ihi.org/engage/initiatives/tripleaim/pages/default.aspx

92. Institute for Healthcare Improvement. *The triple aim or the quadruple aim? Four points to help set your strategy*. Accessed November 17, 2021. http://www.ihi.org/communities/blogs/the-triple-aim-or-the-quadruple-aim-four-points-to-help-set-your-strategy

93. Burns JM. *Leadership*. New York, NY: Harper and Row; 1978.

94. Goleman D. Leadership that gets results. *Harv Bus Rev.* 2000:78-90.

95. Kouzes JM, Posner BZ. *Leadership: The Challenge*. San Francisco: Jossey-Bass; 2002.

96. Sinsky CA, Daugherty Biddison L, Mallick A, et al. *Organizational Evidence-Based and Promising Practices for Improving Clinician Well-Being*. NAM Perspectives. Discussion Paper, National Academy of Medicine, Washington, DC; 2020. doi:10.31478/202011a

97. Pines A, Maslach C. Characteristics of staff burnout in mental health settings. *Hosp Community Psychiatry*. 2006;29:233-237. doi:10.1176/ps.29.4.233

98. Bodenheimer T, Sinsky C. From triple to quadruple aim: care of the patient requires care of the provider. *Ann Fam Med.* 2014;12(6):573-576. doi:10.1370/afm.1713

99. Eckleberry-Hunt J, Van Dyke A, Lick D, Tucciarone J. Changing the conversation from burnout to wellness: physician well-being in residency training programs. *J Grad Med Educ.* 2009;1(2):225-230. doi:10.4300/JGME-D-09-00026.1

100. National Academies of Sciences, Engineering, and Medicine. *Taking Action Against Clinician Burnout: A Systems Approach to Professional Well-Being*. Washington, DC: The National Academies Press; 2019. doi:10.17226/25521

101. Shapiro DE, Duquette C, Abbott LM, Babineau T, Pearl A, Haidet P. Beyond burnout: A physician wellness hierarchy designed to prioritize interventions at the systems level. *Am J Med.* 2019;132(5):556-563. doi:10.1016/j.amjmed.2018.11.028

102. Shatte A, Perlman A, Smith B, Lynch WD. The positive effect of resilience on stress and business outcomes in difficult work environments. *J Occup Environ Med.* 2017;59(2):135-140. doi:10.1097/JOM.0000000000000914

103. American Heart Association Center for Workplace Health Research and Evaluation. Resilience in the workplace: an evidence review and implications for practice. Accessed December 23, 2021. https://www.heart.org/-/media/Data-Import/downloadables/5/2/D/RESILIENCE-IN-THE-WORKPLACE-UCM_496856.pdf

104. Bhavan KP. Public health and private health care organizations struggle to find common ground. *N Engl J Med Catalyst.* 2022;3(1). doi:10.1056/CAT.21.0432

105. Office of Inspector General. Enterprise Risk Management Framework, Version 2.0. OIG-ERM-22-02. Accessed January 23, 2022. https://www.stateoig.gov/system/files/oig-erm-22-02_state_oig_erm_framework_508.pdf

106. MCOL. Population Health News; 2022. Accessed January 23, 2022. http://www.populationhealthnews.com/resources.html

107. Brown B, Grossbart S. 2022 and beyond: navigating the road ahead in healthcare. Health Catalyst, December 2021. Accessed January 23, 2022. https://www.healthcatalyst.com/learn/webinars/2022-and-beyond-navigating-road-ahead/

## Suggested Readings

American Heart Association. Resilience in the workplace: an evidence review and implications for practice. Accessed December 22, 2021. https://www.heart.org/-/media/Data-Import/downloadables/5/2/D/RESILIENCE-IN-THE-WORKPLACE-UCM_496856.pdf

Horak BJ. *Strategic Planning in Healthcare: Building a Quality-Based Plan Step-by-Step*. Portland OR: Book News; 1999.

Jacobs LM, Brindis CD, Hughes D, Kennedy CE, Schmidt LA. Measuring consumer engagement: a review of tools and findings. *J Healthc Qual.* 2018;40(3):139-146. doi:10.1097/JHQ.0000000000000085

Kotter JP. Why transformation efforts fail. *Harv Bus Rev.* 1995(March-April):59-67.

Mackenzie SJ, Goldmann DA, Perla RJ, Parry GJ. Measuring hospital-wide mortality—pitfalls and potential. *J Healthc Qual.* 2016;38(3):187-194. doi:10.1111/jhq.12080

Mignano JL, Miner L, Cafeo C, et al. Routinization of HIV testing in an inpatient setting: a systematic process for organizational change. *J Healthc Qual.* 2016;38(3):e10-e18. doi:10.1097/01.JHQ.0000462676.94393.ee

Mitchell SE, Martin J, Holmes S, et al. How hospitals reengineer their discharge processes to reduce readmissions. *J Healthc Qual.* 2016;38(2):116-126. doi:10.1097/JHQ.0000000000000005

Montgomery AP, Azuero A, Baernholdt M, et al. Nurse burnout predicts self-reported medication administration errors in acute care hospitals. *J Healthc Qual.* 2021;43(1):13-23. doi:10.1097/JHQ.0000000000000274

National Academy of Medicine: Taking action against clinician burnout: systems approaches to professional well-being; 2019. Accessed January 6, 2022. https://www.nap.edu/catalog/25521/taking-action-against-clinician-burnout-a-systems-approach-to-professional

Neville B, Miltner RS, Shirey MR. Clinical team training and a structured handoff tool to improve teamwork, communication, and patient safety. *J Healthc Qual.* 2021;43(6):365-373. doi:10.1097/JHQ.0000000000000291

Perla RJ, Bradbury E, Gunther-Murphy C. Large-scale improvement initiatives in healthcare: a scan of the literature. *J Healthc Qual.* 2013;35(1):30-40. doi:10.1111/j.1945-1474.2011.00164.x

Perlin JB, Horner SJ, Englebright JD, Bracken RM. Rapid core measure improvement through a "Business Case for Quality." *J Healthc Qual.* 2014;36(2):50-61. doi:10.1111/j.1945-1474.2012.00218.x

Plsek PE, Greenhalgh T. The challenge of complexity in healthcare. *BMJ.* 2001;323:625-628. doi:10.1136/bmj.323.7313.625

Polancich S. Developing an organizational model for improvement: from translation to practice. *J Healthc Qual.* 2017;39(1):28-33. doi:10.1097/JHQ.0000000000000076

Ridling DA, Magyary D. Implementation science: describing implementation methods used by pediatric intensive care units in a national collaborative. *J Healthc Qual.* 2015;37(2):102-116.

Schein EH. *Organization Culture and Leadership*. San Francisco, CA: Jossey-Bass; 2004.

Zallman L, Finnegan KE, Todaro M, et al. Association between provider engagement, staff engagement, and culture of safety. *J Healthc Qual.* 2020;42(4):236-247.

# Online Resources

## *Agency for Healthcare Research and Quality (AHRQ)*

- **Quality and Patient Safety Resources**
  www.ahrq.gov/qual/patientsafetyculture
- **Education and Training for Health Professionals**
  https://www.ahrq.gov/professionals/education/index.html
- **AHRQ-Sponsored Continuing Education Activities**
  https://www.ahrq.gov/professionals/education/continuing-ed/index.html
- **Surveys on Patient Safety Culture**
  https://www.ahrq.gov/sops/index.html

## *Centers for Disease Control and Prevention—The National Institute for Occupational Safety and Health*

- **Healthcare Workers: Work Stress and Mental Health**
  https://www.cdc.gov/niosh/topics/healthcare/workstress.html
- **NIOSHTIC-2 Search Results on Burnout Based on Keywords Related to Burnout and Healthcare**
  https://www2a.cdc.gov/nioshtic-2/BuildQyr.asp?s1=(Healthcare+or+Health+care)+and+burnout&f1=*&t1=&Adv=0&terms=1&Startyear=&EndYear=&Limit=10000&D1=10&sort=&PageNo=1&View=b&n=new

## *Institute for Healthcare Improvement*

- **Education Resources**
  http://www.ihi.org/education/Pages/default.aspx
- **General Resources**
  http://www.ihi.org/resources/Pages/default.aspx

- **Transforming Moral Distress into Moral Resilience**
  http://www.ihi.org/resources/Pages/AudioandVideo/transforming-moral-distress-into-moral-resilience.aspx

## *National Academy of Medicine*

- **Clinician Well-Being COVID-19 Resource Page**
  https://nam.edu/initiatives/clinician-resilience-and-well-being/clinician-well-being-resources-during-covid-19/
- **Resources Compendium for Health Care Worker Well-Being**
  https://nam.edu/compendium-of-key-resources-for-improving-clinician-well-being/

## *National Alliance for the Mentally Ill*

- **Frontline Wellness: Healthcare Professionals**
  https://www.nami.org/Your-Journey/Frontline-Professionals/Health-Care-Professionals

## *National Association for Healthcare Quality (NAHQ) Quality Competency Framework*

  https://nahq.org/nahq-intelligence/competency-framework/

## *The Joint Commission*

- **Quick Safety: Developing Resilience to Combat Nurse Burnout**
  https://www.jointcommission.org/-/media/tjc/newsletters/quick_safety_nurse_resilience_final_7_19_19pdf.pdf

# Quality Review and Accountability

**Deborah J. Bulger**

## SECTION CONTENTS

# Introduction

With an increased focus on transparency of and accountability for healthcare quality, outcomes, cost, and value, it is essential that the healthcare quality professional understands how current and emerging payment models impact quality improvement processes, outcomes measurement, cost, and reimbursement. The healthcare quality professional must guide their leadership team toward improved clinical and financial outcomes by implementing best practices to support compliance with regulations, standards, and policies for measure reporting that advance quality improvement.

This section describes strategies and tactics to ensure data reliability, effective utilization of reporting and analytics tools, compliance with external reporting requirements, and the evaluation of technology required to support the quality, safety, and performance improvement program. Information is provided on performance review activities according to internal and external applicable regulations, standards, and policies, assembling informational resources, protecting confidentiality, and providing timely unbiased feedback to practitioners. A discussion of methods to drive multidisciplinary stakeholder collaboration across the continuum equips the healthcare quality professional with knowledge needed to become a key influencer in the quality improvement strategy.

# The Accountability Imperative

System complexity is inherent in healthcare. It is a dynamic network of interactions across diverse stakeholders who have a keen and perhaps self-centered interest in the outcome of those interactions. Patients seek illness prevention, maintenance of health, or recovery from illness; providers desire to use the best possible science to deliver evidence-based care; and payers and regulators strive to balance economic responsibility, all while adapting to social, scientific, and environmental changes beyond their control. The principles of value-based care (i.e., shared risk, improved public health, lowered cost), have prompted the industry to take greater accountability for those multistakeholder costs and outcomes with a demand for increased transparency and compliance with local, state, and national initiatives.

In 2019, healthcare spending in the United States reached $3.8 trillion, up 4.6% in 2018,[1] accounting for 17% of its gross domestic product.[2] Healthcare spending per person was $10,966, 42% higher than Switzerland, the next highest country. Payment by private insurance, by Medicare and Medicaid, and out of pocket account for roughly 80% of the healthcare spending in the United States with Medicare spending growing at a rate of nearly 7% representing over $799 billion in 2019. Of concern to consumers, out-of-pocket spending grew 4.6% in 2019, which was faster than the 3.8% growth in 2018.[1]

**Figure 2.1** shows a distribution of healthcare expenditures.

Quality review and accountability combines the science of data acquisition, data integrity, analysis, modeling, and benchmarking with the art of communication, collaboration, partnership, and behavior change to increase transparency and drive improvement. (See **Box 2.1**.) The healthcare quality professional plays an increasingly central role in the transformation of health systems to business models designed to reward cost-efficient, quality care that improves patient outcomes.

# Making the Business Case for Quality

Healthcare has roots in a cottage industry where the craft of medicine was practiced at a local level. The cost of healthcare measured in human lives lost or harmed, and the waste that will exacerbate our country's challenges to balance macroeconomic priorities, is too much to manage.[3] Today, healthcare is big business, accounting for 17% of the nation's

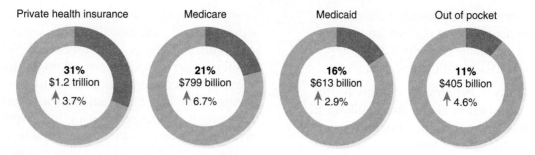

**Figure 2.1** Distribution of Healthcare Expenditures (2019)

Data from Centers for Medicare & Medicaid Services. CMS Office of the Actuary releases 2019 national health expenditures; 2020. Accessed January 10, 2022. https://www.cms.gov/newsroom/press-releases/cms-office-actuary-releases-2019-national-health-expenditures

---

### Box 2.1 Key Points: The Accountability Imperative

- The exponential growth of healthcare expenditures creates an unsustainable economic future unless significant changes are made in how healthcare value is delivered.
- The principles of value-based care place shared risk for all stakeholders, prompting the industry to promote greater accountability for lowering costs, improving population health, and improving patient experience.
- Public reporting is the foundation for transparency that holds stakeholders accountable through the publication of quality measure results of physicians, hospitals and health systems, and payers.
- Both government and private payers adopted a range of pay-for-performance strategies designed to optimize performance and align clinical outcomes with financial incentives.
- The healthcare quality professional plays an increasingly central role in the transformation from volume to value.

---

gross domestic product.[4] Ensuring healthcare quality has high stakes for patients and the U.S. economy. In 2020, medical errors were the third leading cause of death in the United States.[5] Healthcare waste, defined as failure of care delivery, failure of care coordination, overtreatment, or low-value care was cited between $760 and $935 billion annually in the United States.[6] While these statistics seem staggering, there are great strides to be made when each healthcare stakeholder—patient, provider, and payer—recognizes the contribution to managing the cost and quality of care that can be made on a local and personal level.

Making the business case for quality starts with a grassroots effort to drive the adoption of value-based care initiatives within the organization's span of control, identify productivity and efficiency gains that lead to cost reduction without compromising patient care, create a culture of safety and quality that transcends external influences like coronavirus disease 2019 (COVID-19), and reintroduce joy in the workplace. The growth of value-based reimbursement necessitates a more collaborative relationship between providers and payers of healthcare. More than ever, as accountability shifts and the potential for financial risk increases, payers and providers need to create a partnership with a common goal of identifying gaps in care, reducing cost, and promoting reliability and effectiveness while managing their respective operations, margins, and revenue. Payers and providers may renegotiate contracts on an annual basis or add or modify contract terms when market dynamics demand it. The outcome of those negotiations—specifically those related to quality—have an impact on all stakeholders. As a provider, when entering a new value-based payment contract, some key practices should be considered.

*Healthcare quality professionals at the negotiation table.* The healthcare quality professional is uniquely positioned to participate in contract negotiations to ensure that data for the quality metrics are attainable, relatable to providers, and appropriate to the organization. If providers do not understand how they are being measured or data collection and acquisition is unsustainable, they will not succeed.[7]

*Data-driven negotiations.* Healthcare quality professionals need to be prepared to demonstrate the unique value of the organization and its capacity for improvement using data to focus on centers of excellence and recent performance improvement successes. They must be realistic as impending drivers could compromise efforts to improve and set realistic and attainable goals such as the impact of COVID-19 on staffing and operations.

*Leverage payer and provider data assets.* Payers are data rich in claims from millions of bills, physician notes, appointments, procedures, and diagnostic testing. The volume of data plus the capability to apply advanced models of machine learning and artificial intelligence lends itself to the development of benchmarks, research, utilization of services, and much more. Large health plans have made significant investments in data analytics to identify gaps in care and model at a discrete population level to enable patient-centered care management outreach, particularly related to social determinants of health, according to T. Foster (personal communication, November 2021). Payer reporting can provide valuable insights that providers can use to inform, educate, and help change behaviors among physicians and patients. At the same time, providers track metrics for internal use and near real-time management of quality. Typically, the provider will have a deeper clinical data set that enables the identification of variances that may impact the outcome and can identify any data discrepancies in the payer reported metrics.

*Ongoing payer/provider communication.* An Advisory Board study estimates that 18% of rising-risk patients—those with one or more chronic diseases—escalate into the most expensive cohort of patients, the high-risk population.[8] Eliminating the gaps in care that exacerbate the patient's condition (i.e., provide preventive care and treatment) requires ongoing communication and coordination among the providers to align care across settings and among the payers to engage stakeholders in prevention and wellness, as well as to increase the patient's knowledge to manage their own health.[9]

Healthcare organizations measure financial performance using markers such as operating margin (i.e., the amount of revenue after paying for operational and overhead costs). As costs increase and revenue falls, margins decline and healthcare organizations seek additional opportunities to lower cost and sources of new revenue.[10] Value-based reimbursement models reward high quality and lower cost through financial incentives and shared savings that can boost an organization's operating margin. However, entering into a risk-sharing arrangement without first understanding the details of the cost to deliver patient care exposes an organization to unnecessary financial risk. Healthcare organizations need to have visibility to the cost of care and the impact of quality on that cost when negotiating a contract.

The debate over the relationship between cost and quality is a driving force behind healthcare reform. Conventional wisdom suggests that if quality is improved, cost reduction will automatically follow. The goal of the IHI Triple Aim is to provide high-quality, high-value healthcare at less cost; a Quadruple Aim adds joy in work. The core tenet of population health management is to guide consumers to appropriate, lower cost settings of care thus shifting away from the acute care setting (see the *Population Health and Care Transitions* section).

The correlation between cost and quality is complicated and has been difficult to quantify. However, research using a cohort of 108 New York State acute care facilities suggests there is a strong relationship in the financial performance of an organization and its ability to provide measurable quality and safety performance. This 2019 study indicates "that financially stable hospitals have better patient experience and lower readmission rates, and also show evidence of decreased risk of adverse patient quality and safety outcomes for both medical and surgical patients."[11(p13)] These findings suggest that financially stable hospitals are better able to maintain highly reliable systems and provide ongoing resources for quality and performance improvement.

These concepts build a strong case for measuring the collective outcomes of financial and clinical decisions as they impact quality. Traditionally there have been silos of information across the two disciplines, both citing concerns that the data are poorly understood and potentially misused. There is merit to this argument when the data are in fact protected, as is the case with privileged patient or physician information or sensitive financial details such as payroll. However, the correlation of cost and quality at an aggregate level can provide key indications for improvement opportunities, gains in operational efficiency, and increased margins.

Despite advancements in infection control and injury prevention, hospital-acquired conditions (HACs) continue to have a high financial burden on the healthcare system and contribute significantly to inpatient morbidity and mortality in the United States. The consequences of HACs can be serious for patients, ranging from increased length of hospital stay to worsened health outcomes or unexpected mortality.[12] Measures of HACs are included in measure programs including the Centers for Medicare & Medicaid Services (CMS) HAC Reduction Program related to payment reform.[13] In a 2017 study, the Agency for Healthcare Research and Quality (AHRQ) documented the estimated cost and mortality of 10 selected HACs as seen in **Figure 2.2**.

Current research exemplifies the impact of cost and quality. In 2021, the Centers for Disease Control and Prevention conducted research to determine the impact of the COVID-19 pandemic on healthcare-associated infection incidence in U.S. hospitals. Significant increases between 2019 and 2020 were documented in four healthcare-associated infections: central-line–associated bloodstream infections, catheter-associated urinary tract infections, ventilator-associated events, and laboratory-identified methicillin-resistant *Staphylococcus aureus*

bacteremia. Occurrences of central-line–associated bloodstream infections demonstrated the largest year-to-year magnitudes of increase (46%–47%) occurred during the third and fourth quarters, with 4460 cases reported in the third quarter of 2020.[14] At an average cost per incidence of $48,108 per the AHRQ research, this represents over $214 million in excess cost.

Historically, healthcare organizations have been reluctant to share cost information with clinicians for fear of nonclinical influences on clinical decision making.[15] However, there is some evidence that informing clinicians about the cost of medications, implants, and diagnostic procedures promotes positive decision making for both the patient and the organization. For example, for orthopedic surgeons, price awareness may reduce implant cost by 9%–11%.[16] Creating transparency to the organization's cost accounting data will also raise awareness as to the cost of care delivery and engage physicians in cost management activities. As an interdisciplinary tool, cost accounting data, when combined with the physicians' clinical expertise and administrators' insight can be an effective means of identifying variation in care practices and drive down episodic costs.[17]

| | Studies (n) | Range of Estimates | Estimate (95% CI) |
|---|---|---|---|
| **Adverse Drug Events (ADE)** | 2 | $1,277–$9,062 | $5,746 (-$3,950–$15,441) |
| **Catheter-Associated Urinary Tract Infections (CAUTI)** | 6 | $4,694–$29,743 | $13,793 ($5,019–$22,568) |
| **Central Line-Associated Bloodstream Infections (CLABSI)** | 7 | $17,896–$94,879 | $48,108 ($27,232–$68,983) |
| **Falls** | 3 | $2,680–$15,491 | $6,694 (-$1,277–$14,665) |
| **Obstetric Adverse Events (OBAE)** | 2 | $13–$1,190 | $602 (-$578–$1,782) |
| **Pressure Ulcers** | 4 | $8,573–$21,075 | $14,506 (-$14,506–$41,326) |
| **Surgical Site Infections (SSI)** | 5 | $11,778–$42,177 | $28,219 ($18,237–$38,202) |
| **Ventilator-Associated Pneumonia (VAP)** | 5 | $19,325–$80,013 | $47,238 ($21,890–$72,587) |
| **Venous Thromboembolism (VTE)** | 4 | $11,011–$31,687 | $17,367 ($11,837–$22,898) |
| ***C. difficile* Infections (CDI)** | 9 | $4,157–$32,394 | $17,260 ($9,341–$25,180) |

**Figure 2.2** Estimating the Additional Hospital Inpatient Cost and Mortality Associated With Selected Hospital-Acquired Conditions

Note: CI = confidence interval

Reproduced from Agency for Healthcare Research and Quality. *Results. Estimating the Additional Hospital Inpatient Cost and Mortality Associated with Selected Hospital-Acquired Conditions*. Rockville, MD; November 2017. https://www.ahrq.gov/hai/pfp/haccost2017-results.html

Healthcare cost accounting is a process for recording, allocating, and analyzing the detailed cost of services provided to patients (e.g., room and board, medications, lab, and radiology tests). The cost accounting functionality is part of a business decision support solution that may include components of contract modeling, productivity and budget variance analysis, and encounter analysis. While cost accounting methodologies may vary, ranging from fundamental cost to charge ratios to highly specified direct acquisition cost of supplies, measuring cost of care has become a key business requirement in today's economy. The widespread availability of business decision support technology makes this a core solution across the healthcare industry. In 2021, approximately 78% of short-term acute care hospitals in the United States reported having a cost accounting system.[18]

Leveraging cost accounting data at the patient level can produce dynamic results for measuring the impact of quality on cost. Typically managed as a division of the finance department, business decision managers are a key partner with quality, willing to share information, build integrated dashboards, and educate the team. Achieving the return on investment from quality occurs at multiple levels such as improving outcomes for patients, improving the workforce experience, improving productivity and efficiency, avoiding and reducing costs, and increasing revenue. Recognizing these multiple levels of return can also help better link the application of quality improvement to the core strategic priorities of the organization and impact on clinical, operational, and financial outcomes.[19]

For a summary of a business case for quality, see **Box 2.2**.

---

### Box 2.2  Key Points: Business Case for Quality

- Healthcare organizations need visibility to the cost of care and the impact of quality on that cost when negotiating a value-based contract.
- Cost accounting data, when combined with the physicians' clinical expertise and administrators' insight can be an effective means of identifying variation in care practices and drive down episodic costs.
- There is some evidence that informing clinicians about the cost of medications, implants, and diagnostic procedures promotes positive decision making for both the patient and the organization.
- Improvement opportunities can be identified through multidimensional analysis of contributions to cost from clinical decisions, patient severity of illness, and process variation.

---

# Quality and Payment Models

Under value-based care agreements, providers are incented to deliver an evidence-based care model that focuses on health and wellness, minimizes the effects of chronic disease, and mitigates gaps in care. Payment is based on performance derived from a combination of measures of efficiency and effectiveness. Performance-based payment models have reshaped the healthcare landscape from 2012 to 2022. In 2019, more than a third of the U.S. healthcare payments were the result of a form of value-based payment, up from 23% in 2015.[20] This relationship of cost and reimbursement to quality has redefined the role of healthcare quality measurement and management and has influenced the perception of quality in every aspect of the healthcare ecosystem.

## Quality as Policy

The COVID-19 pandemic exposed many problems in the U.S. healthcare system, including barriers to access,[21] increased incidence of hospital-acquired infections,[14] and healthcare disparity and inequity.[22] Current fee-for-service payment models pay only for specific clinical services as they are coded and billed, yet social determinants of health (SDOH), not represented in the billing process, may account for up to 80% of patient outcomes,[23] and by default, cost. An emphasis on SDOH helps to mitigate barriers to accessing preventive care in marginalized populations. For example, many screening rates, like those for cancer, are below desired levels and reflect disparities across ethnicity/race.[24] Patients benefit from outreach from providers, health plan case managers, navigators, and wellness programs provided by employers.

Policy makers are becoming increasingly aware of the need to care for the whole patient, and Medicaid programs have increased their focus by paying for health outcomes rather than volume of services. The increased focus on strategies to address social needs led 24 states to require that Medicaid managed care organizations screen beneficiaries for unmet social needs and help the patient address those needs.[25] States are prohibited from using Medicaid to directly fund nonmedical expenses, but in some cases they use case management services to enroll patients in community-based programs such as the Supplemental Nutrition Assistance Program or housing vouchers.

## Quality as a Profession

Prior to 1983, when CMS introduced the Medicare Inpatient Prospective Payment System, hospitals were paid for each unit of service.[26] Under the Inpatient Prospective Payment System, patients were grouped into diagnosis-related groups (DRGs) as a means of stratifying patients with similar diagnoses and setting payment for those DRGs, and the more accurate and specific the patient record, the greater the potential payment.[27] This first wave of payment reform elevated the medical record itself to a source of revenue and transitioned the role of medical records "librarians" as curators of the patient charts to health information management professionals whose skill can mean the difference in profit and loss.

Much like the DRG shift in the 1980s, this era of value-based reimbursement means that quality is on the critical path to profitability, and as a result, raises the visibility, responsibility, and accountability of the healthcare quality professional. The quality profession evolved from its roots in quality assurance (i.e., monitoring and reporting of measures) to a profession that is now driving quality, safety, value, and innovation in healthcare as an equal partner on the healthcare leadership.[28] Quality is no longer an afterthought but a valued advisor in the management of the organization. Chief quality officers participate in payer contract negotiations and advise on quality, safety, and performance improvement opportunities. The certification of healthcare quality professionals driven by the NAHQ Healthcare Quality Competency Framework creates awareness of the skills required to effectively lead the quality improvement and reduce the variability of quality competencies.[29]

## Quality as a Center of Excellence

Quality is not a program or a project. It is not the sole responsibility of a single individual or the quality department.[30] The principles of quality should be hardwired into every aspect of healthcare delivery with a shared desire by stakeholders at every level to achieve meaningful, sustainable improvement with the healthcare quality professional as the guide and trusted advisor. Healthcare organizations have been plagued by information silos for many years. Value-based payment models forced the dissolution of those silos across the healthcare system, empowering patients, providers, suppliers, and payers to embrace quality improvement as a center of excellence. Bringing multiple disciplines together with different skills, knowledge, attitudes, and responsibility around a common mission creates transparency and enables stakeholders to align around organizational business outcomes rather than departmental outcomes.

## Quality as an Operational Mandate

As the population ages and chronic conditions increase, so does healthcare spending. The need to provide value requires the shared clinical and financial accountability of providers and payers alike (i.e., improve health and wellness, address gaps in care, manage chronic disease, and lower spending). The introduction of alternative payment models (APMs) such as Medicare Advantage programs require provider-sponsored health plans to take responsibility for a specific subset of Medicare patients. Health plans and providers are measured on quality of care in multiple domains like care coordination, experience, and preventive health to better understand and manage disease risk.

When providers and payers share financial risk for the well-being of their constituents, patients benefit from a coordinated approach to care. Patients who have a better experience navigating the healthcare system are more prone to receive preventive services like vaccines and colonoscopies. Early detection of risk factors helps address disease progression, and chronic diseases like hypertension and diabetes are more likely to be controlled, resulting in fewer emergency department and hospital visits.[31]

## Quality as an Organizing Structure

As healthcare delivery has historically been fragmented, making it difficult to control costs and accountability, creating disruptions in the continuity of care and surprise billing for out-of-network care, the evolution of payment models may necessitate a redesign of many organizational processes to accommodate greater care coordination. A key goal of value-based healthcare models is to improve coordination of care, reimbursing the provider for overall value rather than volume and utilization.

A study using data from the AHRQ Comparative Health System Performance Initiative[32] suggests that organizational structures, composition, and other characteristics influence cost and quality performance.[33] As organizations strive to improve performance through better business alignment and assume more clinical and financial risk, it is important to understand the structure under which the organization operates. For example, multihospital systems can create economies of scale and expand their delivery network, improving access to care while potentially retaining board autonomy at the hospital level. Conversely, clinically integrated networks share a high degree of risk and rely on interdependence among network physicians to ensure cost management and quality. The clinically integrated network must share processes such as clinical protocols and information technology. **Table 2.1** provides the research findings from five integrated organizations. For more information see *Suggested Readings*.

While providers continue to be paid as a fee for service for a portion of their payment, under value-based care, they are paid a bonus for achieving cost efficiency and quality targets or incur a penalty if those performance thresholds are not met. Incentives and penalties will vary based on the level of risk accepted

by the provider. In this context, quality metrics are instrumental in developing the payment structure. However, the correlation between quality metrics and payment models is complex and evolving, and depending on the type of payment model, the contribution of the quality measures to the reimbursement model will vary. It is important for the healthcare quality professional to understand the impact of the quality measures on reimbursement and develop a plan for acquiring the data, structuring the measures, establishing a cadence of reporting, and instilling a sense of urgency around performance improvement.

Depending on the contract, the impact of quality metrics on reimbursement rules can take many forms, and it is important to dissect those rules to assess the impact. In some cases, a bonus is paid when a threshold is met, or a penalty is incurred if not. In other models, the provider must demonstrate improvement;

**Table 2.1** Key Features of the Horizontally and Vertically Integrated Structures

| Organization Type | Included Healthcare Providers and Services | Care Management Functions | Administrative Oversight of Providers |
|---|---|---|---|
| Multispecialty group practice | Physicians of various specialties<br>Varied services depending on included specialties | May facilitate patient referral, improve care coordination, and be better positioned to manage the costs of care | Multispecialty group practices share governance and infrastructure, which can result in tighter management control; however, control can vary depending on factors such as size and whether the practice is physician owned, owns a hospital, or is owned by the hospital/system. |
| Multihospital systems | Two or more hospitals<br>Primarily hospital services, which may include inpatient and ambulatory services | Varies depending on included service; if vertically integrated, may have care functions that are more analogous to integrated delivery systems | As multihospital systems are characterized by shared ownership or management, administration may have more direct control over included hospitals, including care processes, shared organizational missions, and the like. However, they may also maintain separate hospital boards and executives, despite shared asset ownership. |
| Integrated delivery system | Varies; may include hospitals, physicians, and other healthcare providers such as postacute care providers, behavioral health, community-based organizations, as well as health plans<br>Comprehensive, full continuum of care | ▪ Care coordination and information sharing along the care continuum<br>▪ Population health and care management<br>▪ Data collection, analysis, and reporting capabilities to inform quality improvement<br>▪ Health information technology capacity<br>▪ Use of evidence-based practices<br>▪ Interdisciplinary, team-based care | Providers join systems through ownership or formalized contractual agreements, which typically establish some degree of administrative control. Administrative control may vary depending on the extent to which the system centralizes management activities, engages in physician–system integration, and employs physicians. |

*(continues)*

**Table 2.1** Key Features of the Horizontally and Vertically Integrated Structures *(continued)*

| Organization Type | Included Healthcare Providers and Services | Care Management Functions | Administrative Oversight of Providers |
|---|---|---|---|
| Clinically integrated network | Primarily includes physicians but may also include hospitals and other providers such as postacute care providers<br>Varying services depending on network composition | Demonstration of integration clinically through several activities, including a program to evaluate and modify practice patterns and creation of a high degree of interdependence and cooperation among network physicians to control costs and ensure quality<br>Example features of programs include the following:<br><ul><li>Implementing systems to ensure appropriate utilization of services</li><li>Deploying evidence-based practice standards and protocols</li><li>Performance evaluation and feedback to included providers</li><li>Case management and care coordination</li></ul> | Providers are either integrated via ownership or contractual relationships; the clinical integration framework requires physicians to use consistent care protocols and to monitor quality, suggesting greater oversight and management of included providers. |
| Physician-hospital organization | Hospitals and their affiliated physicians<br>Hospitals and physician services, which vary depending on included specialties | <ul><li>Organizations facilitate managed care contracting, provide administrative services to physicians, facilitate natural referral relationships around one hospital, and manage ambulatory care facilities where physicians work.</li><li>Closed physician-hospital organizations selectively contract with physicians based on quality and cost performance and have exclusive relationships with physicians and close relationships with hospitals, which may facilitate care coordination</li><li>Organizations may provide processes and resources to support care management.</li></ul> | Physicians maintain independent ownership and management of practices, while practices contract with health plans through the organization. |

Reproduced from Heeringa J, Mutti A, Furukawa MF, Lechner A, Maurer KA, Rich E. Horizontal and vertical integration of health care providers: a framework for understanding various provider organizational structures. *Int J Integr Care*. 2020;20(1):2. doi:10.5334/ijic.4635

for example, a percentage of improvement over baseline correlates to increased reimbursement. Comparative-based measures pay bonuses for top performance in a group of eligible providers and penalties for worst performance. Regardless of the method of incentive, the rules of engagement must be understood by the healthcare quality professional to advise the organization on the best approach.

The value-based program and the quality metrics involved should be meaningful to each organization and relatable to the providers who are being measured. Assumption of risk requires all stakeholders to embrace the process. Before engaging in a risk-based contract, it is helpful to assess the organization for readiness to act on the measure results.[34]

When thinking about the impact of payment models on contracting, it is beneficial to undergo a focused assessment to determine which aspects of the business will be impacted, and particularly, what performance reporting is required that might influence the work of the healthcare quality professional.

For a summary of the impact of payment models on healthcare quality, see **Box 2.3**.

---

**Box 2.3  Key Points: Impact of Payment Models on Healthcare Quality**

- Emerging healthcare payment models redefine the role of quality measurement and management influencing the perception of quality in every aspect of the healthcare ecosystem including the impact on social policy, status of the healthcare quality profession, and operational strategies.
- Despite the promise of improvement through value-based programs, some providers are hesitant to adopt them given the need to manage multiple payment models and quality measurement approaches.
- Organizational structures, composition, and other characteristics influence how coordination of care must be understood.
- Assessing the organization's governance structure, care delivery model, technology infrastructure, and organizational performance is a prerequisite to engaging in value-based payment models.
- It is important for the healthcare quality professional to understand the impact of the quality measures on reimbursement and develop a plan for acquiring the data, structuring the measures, establishing a cadence of reporting, and instilling a sense of urgency around performance improvement.

---

# Current and Emerging Payment Models

Healthcare payment models have evolved rapidly since the introduction of the Affordable Care Act in 2010.[35] Traditionally, the fee-for-service model reimburses providers for the *quantity* of services rendered, encouraging clinicians to provide services that increase the cost of care and may not have added benefit to patient health and well-being. Lack of care coordination can result in redundancy of services, fragmented care, and lower patient satisfaction.

The transition to value-based care emphasizes *quality* of care and patient outcomes over volume, a way that accounts for the care of the patient in a financially prudent manner where all parties in the healthcare system share both the clinical and financial risk, as well as the reward. Incentives or penalties are provided to organizations and clinicians for focusing on care delivery and patient engagement. **Figure 2.3** summarizes the current landscape of payment strategies across physicians and health systems.

## Trends in Payment Reform

Many payment reform trends have been underway for quite some time. Payers and providers design, implement, and monitor program effectiveness to try to meet the objectives of the IHI Triple Aim—better health, smarter spending, healthier people. Government, state, and commercial payers have adopted a variety of alternative payment models.

### Government Payers

CMS has led the way in launching a number of new models such as the Hospital Value-Based Purchasing (VBP) Program, the Hospital Readmission Reduction Program, and the HAC Reduction Program,[36] all designed to provide financial incentives for the quality of care delivered. State Medicaid programs have increasingly included payment reforms in their waivers and Medicaid managed care contracts. Commercial payers have followed suit and have structured almost one-third of their payments as APMs.[37]

CMS has continued to test various models ranging from quality bonuses in a traditional fee-for-service model, to value-based bundles for discrete episodes of care, to full capitation in the form of patient-centered medical homes, and integrated accountable care organizations (ACOs) that take full responsibility for providing care to a specific population of patients.[38] In October 2021, the Center for Medicare and Medicaid Innovation announced its strategic direction to advance value-based care by 2030. In a white paper entitled *Innovation Center Strategy Refresh*, CMS and the Center for Medicare and Medicaid Innovation outlined the five strategic objectives upon which this vision is based, summarized in **Table 2.2**.[39] For further reading, see *Suggested Readings* at the end of the section.

| | Description | Prospective vs. retrospective | Financially discourages volume of services? | Financially encourages high quality of care? | Party that primarily bears the financial risk? | Risk adjusts for patient complexity? | Key Example |
|---|---|---|---|---|---|---|---|
| Fee-for-service (FFS) | Paid for each individual service rendered | Retrospective | No | No | Insurers / Patients (via cost-sharing; co-pays, deductibles) | No | Medicare |
| Traditional capitation (full-risk capitation, global payment) | Paid to cover all services within a specific period of time | Prospective | Yes | No, except for outcomes related to use | Primary care practices | No | Medicare Advantage HMOs |
| Pay-for-performance (P4P) exists in addition to underlying model (generally FFS or capitation) | Paid for achievement of (or improvement in) a quality measure | Both exist (most models retrospectively; however, can be paid prospectively and subsequently reconciled) | Potentially (depends on quality metrics) | Yes, for services being measured via quality metric | Depends on underlying payment model / Primary care practices, provider organizations, if targets not met | Potentially | Medicare Physician Group Practice Demonstration Project / Hospital Readmissions Reduction Program (HRRP) |
| Bundled payment (episode-of-care) | Paid for all services rendered for a given episode of care | Mixed (generally retrospectively triggered and prospectively paid) | Yes (but does not discourage volume of episodes) | No, except for outcomes related to utilization | Primary care practices, provider organizations | No | CMMI's Bundled Payments for Care Improvement |
| Shared savings | Paid based on spending below a predetermined benchmark over a period of time (contingent on meeting certain quality targets) | Mixed (prospective at level of the ACO, but providers often still paid via FFS) | Yes | Yes | ACOs | Potentially | Medicare Shared Savings Program ACOs |
| Blended FFS and capitation | Paid a predetermined amount intended to cover medical home services for a specific period of time in addition to FFS | Mixed | No (to the extent that FFS is the predominant payment mechanism) | No | Depends on underlying payment model | Potentially | Medicare Comprehensive Primary Care Initiative |
| Comprehensive (primary) care payment | Paid a risk-adjusted amount to cover all primary care services for a specific period of time; includes component of P4P | Prospective | Yes | Yes | Primary care practices | Yes | Iora Health |

**Figure 2.3** Overview of Primary Care Payment Models

Reproduced from Park B, Gold SB, Bazemore A, Liaw W. How evolving U.S. payment models influence primary care and its impact on the quadruple aim. *J Am Board Fam Med.* 2018:31(4):588-604. doi:10.3122/jabfm.2018.04.170388

**Table 2.2** Innovation Center Strategy Refresh Objectives

| Objective | Aim |
|---|---|
| Drive accountable care | Increase the number of people in a care relationship with accountability for quality and total cost of care. |
| Advance health equity | Embed health equity in every aspect of the Center for Medicare & Medicaid Innovation models and increase focus on underserved populations. |
| Support innovation | Leverage a range of supports that enable integrated, person-centered care such as actionable, practice-specific data, technology, dissemination of best practices, peer-to-peer learning collaboratives, and payment flexibilities. |
| Address affordability | Pursue strategies to address healthcare prices and affordability and reduce unnecessary or duplicative care. |
| Partner to achieve system transformation | Align priorities and policies across CMS and aggressively engage payers, purchasers, providers, states, and beneficiaries to improve quality, to achieve equitable outcomes, and to reduce healthcare costs. |

Modified from Centers for Medicare & Medicaid Services. *Innovation Center Strategy Refresh*. White paper; 2021. Accessed January 4, 2022. https://innovation.cms.gov/strategic-direction-whitepaper

| Cost of care | Access to care | Quality of care |
|---|---|---|
| Downside risk arrangements | Decrease in rural hospitals or healthcare | CMS monitoring shifts |
| Increased OOP costs | Expanding home and telehealth | Transparency promoted for patient use |
| More HSA-eligible plans and high-deductible health plans | Evolving pharmacy-based primary care services | Social determinants of health incorporated into health-system reimbursement |
| CMS indicates Centers for Medicare & Medicaid Services; HSA, health savings account; OOP, out-of-pocket. | | |

**Figure 2.4** Marketplace Change in Context of Dynamic Healthcare Issues

Reproduced from Vogenberg FR, Santilli J. Key trends in healthcare for 2020 and beyond. *Am Health Drug Benefits*. 2019;12(7):348-350.

## Commercial Markets

Programs evolve and improve as market demands change, and commercial markets tend to leverage innovation. Additionally, changes in the social and economic environment have prompted policy makers to consider the impact of cost, quality, and access to care relative to health reform and payment. **Figure 2.4** outlines marketplace changes that may drive the direction of health payment reform.

## Costs of Care

Increasing premiums and out-of-pocket costs for patients have triggered an increased interest in consumerism and transparency where patients can be more accountable for the care they choose and its financial impact. According to the Kaiser Family Foundation Benefits Survey,[40] average family premiums have increased by 55% over the past decade, at least twice as fast as wages (27%) and inflation (19%). Across all covered workers, the deductibles have increased 111%. When consumers were asked about affordability of a healthcare balance, 25% reported the inability to pay a $400+ medical bill in full, compared to $1000 in previous reports. Consumers want to make choices about how and where their healthcare dollars are spent to ensure they are getting the best value and experience for their money.[41] Visibility into both cost and quality of provider outcomes enable consumers to make more informed choices.

## Access to Care

Lack of health insurance coverage is one of the largest barriers to access to healthcare and contributes to disparities in health.[42] Approximately 1 in 10 people in the United States do not have health insurance.[43] As a result, they are less likely to have a primary care provider and more likely to neglect to seek preventive care and treatment for chronic illnesses.

The economic pressures on healthcare organizations have resulted in a number of hospital closures since 2017,[44] reducing access to inpatient and emergency care, particularly in rural areas.[45] The COVID-19 pandemic further reduced access to care, prompting the expanded use of telemedicine as an alternate tool for maintaining patient care.[46] In the first quarter of 2020, telehealth visits increased by 50% over the same period in 2019.[47] Patients have embraced digital healthcare with 76% of consumers expecting telehealth to be an ongoing option.[48] Payers continue to seek opportunities to pay for lower cost settings of care as many telehealth waivers enacted during the pandemic have become permanent. Programs have been launched, such as Hospitals Without Walls, providing hospitals the flexibility to extend acute care services at home to increase access to care.[49]

## Social Determinants of Health

The focus on social determinants of health (SDOH) for the nonmedical conditions that influence health outcomes is an emerging trend in monitoring the quality of healthcare outcomes as well as the impact on payment reform. Environments in which people are born, work, live, play, and worship can affect a wide range of health, functioning, and quality-of-life outcomes and risks.[50] Factors such as food insecurity and its impact on nutritional status, language barriers that inhibit access for ethnic and cultural populations, lack of transportation, and the inability to keep appointments or acquire prescriptions all impact patient health and the cost of care—as does recognizing and addressing these factors. Social determinants of health are inextricably linked to health equity.[51]

The COVID-19 pandemic exposed disparities in care and tested the stability of the current healthcare value chain. The increased risk of infection and death stratified along race and the prevalence of underlying conditions demonstrates the link between SDOH and disparities in care. Poverty and poor overall health combine to exacerbate those disparities and must be addressed as a component of health policy.

## Alternative Payment Models

Risk sharing is an agreement between providers and payers to share financial responsibility for the cost of patient care. The greater the risk, the greater the incentive to provide efficient, cost-effective care. Different types of risk dictate the payment structure.

- *Upside risk.* Providers share savings with the payer if the cost of care is below the benchmark. If the cost of care exceeds the benchmark, providers receive no shared savings but are also not penalized. Medicare Shared Savings Program ACOs are in an upside risk-only model.
- *Downside risk.* Providers who exceed the financial benchmark for a patient or care episode must refund the payer for all or a portion of the expense.
- *Two-sided risk.* Combined upside and downside risk. Examples include the comprehensive end-stage renal disease care model and the oncology care model (two-sided risk track).

The Health Care Payment Learning & Action Network (HCPLAN) was launched by the U.S. Department of Health & Human Services (through CMS) in March 2015 as a means to align with public and private healthcare leaders to accelerate the health system's adoption of APMs. The HCPLAN provides thought leadership and strategic direction to reduce the barriers to APM participation by providing a common nomenclature for defining and tracking U.S. healthcare payments. Based on the CMS Payment Taxonomy Framework, APMs are classified into four categories and eight subcategories forming the basis for the HCPLANs APM measurement effort (**Figure 2.5**).[52]

The HCPLAN Measurement Effort incorporates data from nearly 80% of covered Americans and provides an annual report to assess the adoption of APMs over time reporting payment data by commercial, Medicaid, Medicare Advantage, and traditional Medicare.

## Transition to New Payment Models

The transition from traditional fee-for-service payment is fueled primarily by CMS, launching many programs that shift payment toward value, including the Medicare Shared Savings Program in 2011. The passage of the Medicare Access and CHIP Reauthorization Act (MACRA) of 2015, which made significant changes to how Medicare reimburses physicians for their services, created an additional platform to drive APMs. As a result, healthcare systems across the country are

| Payment Taxonomy Framework | | | |
|---|---|---|---|
| **Category 1:**<br>*Fee for Service—No Link to Quality* | **Category 2:**<br>*Fee for Service—Link to Quality* | **Category 3:**<br>*Alternative Payment Models Built on Fee-for-Service Architecture* | **Category 4:**<br>*Population-Based Payment* |
| **Description** *Payments are based on volume of services and not linked to quality or efficiency* | *At least a portion of payments vary based on the quality or efficiency of healthcare delivery* | *Some payment is linked to the effective management of a population or an episode of care. Payment still triggered by delivery of services, but opportunities for shared savings or 2-sided risk* | *Payment is not directly triggered by service delivery so volume is not linked to payment. Clinicians and organizations are paid and responsible for the care of a beneficiary for a long period (e.g., ≥1 yr)* |
| **Medicare FFS** ▪ Limited in Medicare fee-for-service<br>▪ Majority of Medicare payments now are linked to quality | ▪ Hospital value-based purchasing<br>▪ Physician Value-Based Modifier<br>▪ Readmissions/Hospital Acquired Condition Reduction Program | ▪ Accountable care organizations<br>▪ Medical homes<br>▪ Bundled payments<br>▪ Comprehensive primary care initiative<br>▪ Comprehensive ESRD<br>▪ Medicare-Medicaid Financial Alignment Initiative Fee-For-Service Model | ▪ Eligible Pioneer accountable care organizations in years 3-5 |

**Figure 2.5** Payment Taxonomy Framework

Reproduced from Centers for Medicare & Medicaid Services. Better care. Smarter spending. Healthier people: paying providers for value, not volume. Published January 16, 2015. Accessed July 7, 2022. https://www.cms.gov/newsroom/fact-sheets/better-care-smarter-spending-healthier-people-paying-providers-value-not-volume

redesigning their delivery models to embrace value-based care and while the scope and pace of change may vary, organizations are taking steps to be more patient centered, driving health and wellness strategies into their communities.

However, the transition to value-based care continues. While CMS took the lead on performance-based payment, the healthcare industry overall is still more reliant on fee-for-service reimbursement. In a 2020 survey of 174 healthcare professionals, only 57% reported using value-based reimbursement models. This rate of adoption varies by care setting. While 70% of physician practices reported over 75% of their revenue comes from fee-for-service reimbursement, only 19% of hospitals and health systems reported the same.[53]

Understanding the impact of a payer contract before negotiation helps the organization understand the future financial impact of a new contract. During the contract term, ongoing modeling encourages compliance, prevents unexpected loss of revenue, and enables both payer and provider to identify opportunities to meet measurement thresholds, particularly those related to quality. Contract modeling is a capability within the financial decision support discipline in most hospitals that enables the organization to calculate expected payments based on the contract terms prior to receiving actual payments. Modeling what-if changes using existing or similar claims provides guidance to the amount of revenue at risk. In the example in **Figure 2.6**, the expected revenue under a standard contract for a specific patient population is calculated at $4.5 million. Modeling for penalties if the predetermined quality threshold is not met will result in an over $900,000 revenue reduction. Knowing the organization's status and its potential for improvement will minimize those losses. Contract modeling tools enable detailed analyses at the service line, department, and physician level to determine where the compliance is compromised. Working with decision support contract modeling analysts, the healthcare quality professional can develop mitigation plans for improvement. According to R. Iller, a former associate vice president of decision support, a strong collaboration between the quality, managed care, and financial leaders is a best practice that yields the most successful contract negotiation, compliance, and management for the organization (phone call with Iller, December 2021).

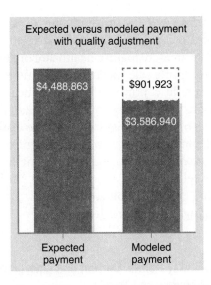

**Figure 2.6** Potential Revenue Reduction From Quality Metrics

## Forums on Healthcare Payment Reform

Healthcare policy can change rapidly, so it is necessary for the healthcare quality professional to be aware of current and pending changes to health payment reform. A change in national administration can create a sea change in which payment programs are sustained and how they are managed. Participation in external forums to learn about payment reform and its impact on quality, as well as providing input to measure development enables the healthcare quality professional to provide critical information for the strategic direction of the organization. Several external forums are available to help organizations advance healthcare quality.

For example, National Committee for Quality Assurance (NCQA) and Pharmacy Quality Alliance (PQA) develop measures used to accredit healthcare organizations and determine performance-based funding. National Quality Forum (NQF) sets scientific standards for quality measures and enforces these standards through its endorsement process. Pharmacy Quality Solutions (PQS), a healthcare quality improvement company, uses measures developed by Pharmacy Quality Alliance and others to evaluate the performance of community pharmacies.[54] These and other forums are described briefly.

- *National Committee for Quality Assurance.* NCQA accredits health plans and leads measure development for health plans and providers through the Healthcare Effectiveness Data and Information Set (HEDIS). The HEDIS measure set includes 90 measures across 6 domains of care and is used for quality improvement and reporting by entities accredited by NCQA as well as by the federal government through Medicare.

- *National Quality Forum.* NQF endorses quality measures developed by others and sets scientific standards for measure development. The federal government and other payers rely on this organization to vet measures used in performance-based payment models.[55]

- *Pharmacy Quality Alliance.* PQA is a leading developer of medication-related healthcare quality measures. It develops measures for use in Medicare Part D plans and others and is actively engaged in developing new measures for community pharmacy quality measurement.

- *National Association for Healthcare Quality.* NAHQ offers the only accredited certification in healthcare quality: the Certified Professional in Healthcare Quality. It is the professional home for more than 9000 healthcare quality professionals providing opportunities for professional growth through a variety of in-person and virtual events such as the NAHQ annual conference and ongoing learning labs. NAHQ Network enables members to share ongoing expertise and peer-to-peer learning. The *Journal for Healthcare Quality* is a peer-reviewed publication that addresses multiple facets of healthcare quality and the impact on payment strategy.[56]

- *Institute for Healthcare Improvement.* IHI is a leading innovator in healthcare improvement that collaborates with partners around the world to achieve sustainable, large-scale improvements in quality and safety, uncovering new approaches to help leaders, patients, and caregivers embrace, create, test, and implement strategies to drive change.[57] IHI offers many publications, white papers, case studies, and success stories, as well as in-person and virtual training and an annual forum featuring thought leaders in a broad array of topics from health equity to value-based care. While there are many initiatives completed or in progress, one of note is the IHI Triple Aim, a framework to improve patient experience of care, improve the health of populations, and reduce the per capita cost of healthcare.[58] The IHI Triple Aim has become a foundation for many organizations as they move toward value-based payment systems with many success stories that the healthcare quality professional can use in their daily work.

- *Healthcare Financial Management Association.* HFMA is the leading organization for managing healthcare finance. Its mission is to help financial leaders from across provider and payer organizations achieve optimal performance by providing the practical tools and solutions, education, industry analyses, and strategic guidance needed to address the many challenges that exist within the U.S. healthcare system.[59] HFMA sponsors a number of initiatives, education, and conferences and web meeting events designed to improve healthcare performance, many of which are available to the public and do not require HFMA membership. One example, the Value Project,[60] a multiyear research project in collaboration with healthcare organizations across the country designed to advance the transition from volume-based to value-based payment and care delivery, is available online. Studies are also available on a broad set of value-based care topics authored by industry thought leaders (e.g., total cost of care, outcomes-based staffing, and social determinants of care).[61]

- *National Association of Accountable Care Organizations.* NAACOS is a nonprofit organization composed of ACOs that began as a forum to ensure advocacy for ACOs in public policy deliberations. The NAACOS policy committee provides feedback to staff on rules for the Medicare Shared Savings Program and to Congress on proposed legislation. The NAACOS quality committee evaluates quality initiatives and regularly gives specific feedback on proposed regulation. The organization has evolved to include training and educational programs relevant to day-to-day ACO operations. Despite being a membership-based organization, NAACOS offers many webinars and events available to nonmembers.[62]

- *Center for Improvement in Healthcare Quality.* CIHQ is a membership-based organization composed of acute care and critical access hospitals. Its purpose is to advocate on behalf of members in shaping the accreditation and regulatory environment; educate members on standards, regulations, and the survey process; encourage professional growth through national certification; advise members on changes to standards and regulations; assist members in determining compliance to accreditation standards and certification requirements; and improve the ability of members to successfully meet the challenges of today's regulatory environment.[63]

- *American Nurses Credentialing Center.* ANCC, a subsidiary of the American Nurses Association, aims to promote excellence in nursing and healthcare globally through credentialing programs. ANCC's credentialing programs certify and recognize individual nurses in specialty practice areas; recognize healthcare organizations for promoting safe, positive work environments; and accredit continuing nursing education organizations. ANCC developed and leads the Magnet Recognition Program[64] and the Pathway to Excellence Program,[65] which recognizes healthcare organizations for quality patient care, nursing excellence, and innovations in professional nursing practice. **Box 2.4** discusses current and emerging payment models.

---

**Box 2.4 Key Points: Current and Emerging Payment Models and Trends**

- While fee-for-service delivery remains prevalent, the payment landscape is rapidly evolving to alternative payment models.
- Efforts to accelerate alternative payment models have led to the launch of the Health Care Payment Learning & Action Network (HCPLAN) to provide leadership and strategic direction for measurement.
- The Center for Medicare & Medicaid Innovation announced is strategy to advance value-based care by 2030 driving toward greater accountability, affordability, and health equity.
- Marketplace changes such as increased out-of-pocket expense, decreased access to care, and the impact of social determinants of health will impact health policy.

---

# Transparency and Quality Improvement

For many years, patient access to their own medical records was prohibited, with providers citing confidentiality, potential for misinterpretation of test results, fear of litigation, or simply inconvenience. Paper records had to be photocopied, requiring patients, insurers, and lawyers to pay a fee per page. Lack of transparency extended to patient interactions as well; a phlebotomist was not allowed to explain the tests for which a blood sample was being drawn, and nurses were not allowed to share the results of vital signs with the patient. Public reporting of provider outcomes was nonexistent as few states maintained a physician performance database, and hospital reporting was limited to state initiatives such as the Pennsylvania Health Care Cost Containment Council.[66]

Fortunately, the move to patient-centered care demands that patients are fully informed about their health status and treatment plan. Transparency enables patients to be a partner with the provider in decisions about their own care and treatment. The impact of transparency on quality is evolving as consumers have increased access to their own health records, understand the price of services, and compare hospital and physician outcomes and performance. Overall, better visibility produces better quality.

## Performance Measurement

When quality measurement reflects the care delivered, any variation from the expected measure result represents an opportunity to improve. Whether measures are sponsored by CMS, commercial payers, or the health system's internal strategic plan, improvement opportunities should be identified using appropriate analytics practices (see the *Health Data Analytics* section) and addressed through the organization's performance improvement policies and procedures. Within each value-based payer arrangement, quality improvement represents a financial incentive based on the trajectory of improvement or the achievement of a threshold. Components of performance measurement include trends and patterns, benchmarks, multidimensional analysis, physician decisions, patient contribution, and process variability.

- *Trends and patterns.* Healthcare is dynamic and subject to external influences of economic, social, and political change. As seen with the pandemic in 2020, singular events can quickly shift priorities for how, where, and when healthcare is provided. Within 4 months of the appearance of the first documented case of COVID-19, the world was engulfed by the virus with over 4 million confirmed cases and 283,271 deaths reported, overwhelming the global healthcare system.[67] To ease the disruptions to healthcare delivery, CMS instilled blanket waivers for patient screening location, verbal orders, and reporting requirements, to list a few, to ensure that hospitals could focus resources on higher patient care demands and increased patient census[68] shifting the trends of healthcare quality measurement for all providers. Comparative data within the quality measurement solutions enable each organization to account for the disruption and normalize the trends to assess improvement opportunities.
- *Benchmarks.* A key benefit of most valued-based reimbursement programs is the availability of standardized data that are aggregated, reported, and shared with the participating providers to facilitate comparative analysis. The ability to compare results to state and national benchmarks

provide insight into the magnitude of improvement needed, the urgency with which change needs to occur, and the resources needed to achieve the level of improvement required.

- *Multidimensional analysis.* Patients are not one dimensional, and neither is the analysis of their care. Variations in care found in quality measures impact financial outcomes and vice versa. For example, healthcare-associated infections such as central-line–associated bloodstream infections increase the use of intensive care unit days, impact cost, will have implications for staffing and bed availability, and may impact market perception and reimbursement. To conduct a patient-centered, multidimensional analysis, various inputs into the measure outcome must be considered.
- *Physician decisions.* Waste in healthcare is defined as failure of care delivery, failure of care coordination, overtreatment or low-value care, pricing failure, fraud and abuse, and administrative complexity.[69] In 2019, the estimated annual cost of waste in health was $935 billion with 37% of that attributed to care delivery. Unnecessary clinical variation leads to increased costs, as seen in many surgical procedures. Factors that influence and elevate costs include the use of unnecessary preoperative testing, physician preference decisions that increase implant costs or extend operating-room time, and a lack of standardized postoperative care that leads to prolonged lengths of stay and inappropriate use of postacute resources. Analyzing quality, cost, and utilization measures at the physician level can point to one source of variation, however, the analysis should not stop there.
- *Patient contribution.* Research shows that cost, length of stay, and mortality increase as severity rises and can account for between 10% and 35% variation in treatment costs.[70] As severity of illness increases, so do complexity of care and potential for unplanned outcomes. Clinicians are scientists, and any questions about how they practice must be backed by reliable, accurate, and risk-adjusted data by All Patient Refined Diagnosis Related Groups (APR-DRGs), clinical cohort, or another relevant patient-population classifier. "My patients are sicker" can be a valid input to the patient outcome and must be considered in the analysis, particularly when comparing physician peer performance. Outcome measures from both CMS and commercial payers may be severity adjusted using 3M Company APR-DRGs[71] for inpatient care or episodic groupers for outpatient and bundled care.

- *Process variability.* Patient flow and throughput not only contribute to hospital cost but can have an impact on patient quality. Delays in the emergency department can lead to total hospital length of stay, higher diversion rates, left-without-being-seen instances, and higher mortality.[72] Inefficiency in the operating room has both cost and quality implications. The average cost of an operating room minute is $62.00 according to an older study of 100 hospitals in the United States.[73] Case delays result in idle operating rooms and increase organizational cost. Furthermore, for every added minute a patient spends in the operating room (up to 10 minutes) the risk of complication increases by 1%.[74]

## Hospital Performance

In 2005, the transparency of hospital and physician quality was established with the launch of the CMS Hospital Compare initiative (now Care Compare). Since that time, public reporting of data is the norm as additional comparative data were added and consumer reporting has been improved. Additionally, data sets can be viewed in a browser, downloaded in various machine-readable formats, or accessed through an application programming interface. This enables developers to connect other applications to the data in real time using the same data that power the Medicare.gov website.[75]

The Hospital VBP Program is designed to incentivize providers for delivering high-quality care while reducing costs in the inpatient setting. Hospitals are paid for inpatient acute care services based on the quality of care. In the FY 2019–FY 2027 Hospital VBP Program, a hospital's performance is evaluated based on achievement and improvement on 24 measures across four domains.[76] Achievement points are awarded by comparing an individual hospital rate to all hospitals' rates during the performance period. Improvement points are awarded by comparing an individual hospital's rates during the performance period to its rates from the baseline period.[77] The amount earned by hospitals will depend on the actual range and distribution of all eligible/participating hospitals' total performance scores, resulting in incentives for some hospitals and penalties for others. A hospital may earn back a value-based incentive payment percentage that is less than, equal to, or more than the applicable reduction for that program year.[78] **Figure 2.7** describes measures in the clinical outcomes and clinical care domains.

The Hospital Price Transparency rule[79] states that effective January 1, 2021, each hospital operating in the United States is required to provide clear, accessible pricing information online about the items and services they provide in two ways:

1. As a comprehensive machine-readable file with all items and services to include gross charges, discounted cash prices, payer-specific negotiated charges, and deidentified minimum and maximum negotiated charges.[80]
2. A display of services in a consumer-friendly format of at least 300 shoppable services (or as many as the hospital provides if less than 300) that a healthcare consumer can schedule in advance. The display must contain plain language descriptions of the services and group them with ancillary services.[81]

This rule enables consumers to compare prices across providers and know the cost of the service prior to receiving care. For noncompliant hospitals, CMS may issue a warning notice, request a corrective action plan, and impose a civil monetary penalty and publicize the penalty on a CMS website.

The impact of pricing transparency is twofold: hospital competition and patient choice. Hospitals and payers have a line of site to the cost of services across their market, which boosts market comparisons. Patients can shop for services using a price estimator for each hospital, which enhances their ability to make choices about cost.

## Physician and Clinician Performance

Promoting interoperability (formerly meaningful use) focuses on electronic data sharing (i.e., e-prescribing, sending, and receiving orders and results to another provider through a health information exchange, queries for medication, and patient access to their charts). The 21st Century Cures Act, enacted in December 2016, included provisions to promote health information interoperability and prohibit information blocking by health information networks, health information exchanges, health information technology developers of certified health information technology, and healthcare providers.[82]

On April 5, 2021, information-blocking regulations, part of the 21st Century Cures Act, went into effect. The regulations mandate that patient electronic health information is readily available (i.e., at the same time as the physician, through the electronic health record [EHR] patient portal or an application of the patient's choice for access, exchange, or use). Penalties are established for actors[83] who engage in interference to access; all actors except providers

| Measure ID* | Measure Description | FY 2019 | FY 2020 | FY 2021 | FY 2022 | FY 2023 | FY 2024 | FY 2025 | FY 2026 | FY 2027 |
|---|---|---|---|---|---|---|---|---|---|---|
| MORT-30-AMI | Acute Myocardial Infarction (AMI) 30-Day Mortality Rate | Yes | Yes | Yes | Yes | Yes | Yes | Yes | Yes | Yes |
| MORT-30-HF | Heart Failure (HF) 30-Day Mortality Rate | Yes | Yes | Yes | Yes | Yes | Yes | Yes | Yes | Yes |
| MORT-30 PN | Pneumonia (PN) 30-Day Mortality Rate | Yes | Yes | No | No | No | No | No | No | No |
| MORT-30 PN | Pneumonia (PN) 30-Day Mortality Rate (Updated Cohort) | No | No | Yes | Yes | Yes | Yes | Yes | Yes | Yes |
| COMP-HIP-KNEE | Total Hip Arthroplasty (THA)/Total Knee Arthroplasty Complication Rate (TKA) | Yes | Yes | Yes | Yes | Yes | Yes | Yes | Yes | Yes |
| MORT-30-COPD | Chronic Obstructive Pulmonary Disease (COPD) 30-Day Mortality Rate | No | No | Yes | Yes | Yes | Yes | Yes | Yes | Yes |
| MORT-30-CABG | Coronary Artery Bypass Grafting (CABG) 30-Day Mortality Rate | No | No | No | Yes | Yes | Yes | Yes | Yes | Yes |
| **Safety Domain** | | | | | | | | | | |
| PSI-90 | Complication/Patient Safety for Selected Indicators Composite (Old Version) | No | No | No | No | No | No | No | No | No |
| PSI-90 | Patient Safety and Adverse Events Composite (New Version) | No | No | No | No | No | No | No | No | No |
| CAUTI | Catheter-Associated Urinary Tract Infection | Yes | Yes | Yes | Yes | Yes | Yes | Yes | Yes | Yes |
| CLABSI | Central Line-Associated Blood Stream Infection | Yes | Yes | Yes | Yes | Yes | Yes | Yes | Yes | Yes |
| CDI | *Clostridium difficile* Infection | Yes | Yes | Yes | Yes | Yes | Yes | Yes | Yes | Yes |
| MRSA | Methicillin-Resistant *Staphylococcus aureus* | Yes | Yes | Yes | Yes | Yes | Yes | Yes | Yes | Yes |
| SSI | SSI - Colon Surgery SSI - Abdominal Hysterectomy | Yes | Yes | Yes | Yes | Yes | Yes | Yes | Yes | Yes |
| PC-01 | Elective Delivery Prior to 39 Completed Weeks Gestation | Yes | Yes | No | No | No | No | No | No | No |

**Figure 2.7** Clinical Care Domain (FY2019) and Clinical Outcomes Domain (FY 2020 and Subsequent Fiscal Years)

Data from Centers for Medicare & Medicaid Services. *Hospital Value Based Purchasing (HVBP) Program FY 2019–2027 Measures*; 2021. Accessed January 11, 2022. https://qualitynet.cms.gov/inpatient/hvbp/measures

*(continues)*

| Efficiency and Cost Reduction Domain | | | | | | | | | | |
|---|---|---|---|---|---|---|---|---|---|---|
| MSPB | Medicare Spending Per Beneficiary | Yes | Yes | Yes | Yes | Yes | Yes | Yes | Yes | Yes |
| **Person and Community Engagement Domain HCAHPS Dimension** | | | | | | | | | | |
| Communication with Nurses | | Yes | Yes | Yes | Yes | Yes | Yes | Yes | Yes | Yes |
| Communication with Doctors | | Yes | Yes | Yes | Yes | Yes | Yes | Yes | Yes | Yes |
| Responsiveness of Hospital Staff | | Yes | Yes | Yes | Yes | Yes | Yes | Yes | Yes | Yes |
| Communication about Medicines | | Yes | Yes | Yes | Yes | Yes | Yes | Yes | Yes | Yes |
| Cleanliness and Quietness of Hospital Environment | | Yes | Yes | Yes | Yes | Yes | Yes | Yes | Yes | Yes |
| Discharge Information | | Yes | Yes | Yes | Yes | Yes | Yes | Yes | Yes | Yes |
| Overall Rating of Hospital | | Yes | Yes | Yes | Yes | Yes | Yes | Yes | Yes | Yes |
| Care Transition | | Yes | Yes | Yes | Yes | Yes | Yes | Yes | Yes | Yes |

**Figure 2.7** Clinical Care Domain (FY2019) and Clinical Outcomes Domain (FY 2020 and Subsequent Fiscal Years) *(continued)*

may be subject to civil monetary penalty fines up to $1 million per blocking violation.[84] There are exceptions such as not fulfilling access due to harm prevention, privacy, security, infeasibility, or content and manner. The impact is likely better communication between physicians and patients. As patients potentially see their information before the physician does, they can review it prior to a visit and structure questions and concerns to be addressed by the physician. This can raise the quality and outcome of the visit for both parties.

As part of the quality review process to assess clinical competence for reappraisal, reappointment, and ongoing performance improvement, practitioners must demonstrate compliance with accreditation standards, applicable bylaws, regulations, contractual obligations, and federal regulatory requirements, as well as organizational initiatives designed to improve safety, effectiveness, and efficiency. Ongoing monitoring of professional practice utilizes performance-based measures to identify improvement opportunities, communicate results to clinicians, and drive behavior change. At times, peer review is conducted to determine areas of risk and opportunities to improve. The healthcare quality professional provides oversight of these activities by partnering with the medical staff leadership, department chair, credentialing committee, and enterprise-wide committees to establish appropriate policies and procedures.

## Medical Peer Review

Peer review is an evaluation of an episode of care conducted to improve the quality of patient care or the use of healthcare resources. It is a process protected by statute in most states—although this varies—and by federal statute for federal healthcare facilities. While the protection by statute may vary, the confidentiality of the reviewer and those under review is critical to ensuring the integrity of the process. Healthcare quality professionals often coordinate and facilitate the medical review process on behalf of the medical and professional staff and are responsible for maintaining confidentiality throughout the process.

The first step is to identify an appropriate peer for the specific review. A peer is generally defined as a healthcare professional with comparable education, training, experience, licensure, or similar clinical privileges or scope of practice. The peer review process includes a criteria-based case review. The medical and professional staff establish the criteria. These reviews may include an assessment of the degree to which a standard was met or if providers in the same situation would act in the same manner. These ratings may be noted as a score or level number for tracking purposes or as a trigger for focused professional practice evaluation when continued quality concerns are identified. Results may be trended by individual provider performance or by organization system. Usually, a peer review committee manages the review and reporting function as a subcommittee of the medical executive committee. Participation in peer review is one way in which medical staff members are involved in measuring, assessing, and improving performance of licensed practitioners.

Medical staff identify criteria or circumstances that initiate a peer review, set time frames for the review to occur, identify reviewers, and provide mechanisms for participation by the person whose performance is being reviewed. Both outcomes and processes are measured. An effective peer review process includes these elements:

- Peer review is consistently conducted using defined procedures.
- Conclusions reached through the process are supported by a rationale.
- Minority opinions and views of the person being reviewed are considered and recorded.
- Peer review activities are considered in the reappointment process.
- Conclusions from peer review are tracked over time.
- Actions based on conclusions are monitored for effectiveness.
- Findings, conclusions, recommendations, and actions are communicated to appropriate entities.
- Recommendations to improve performance are implemented.

For practitioners who are granted clinical privileges, ongoing practitioner performance evaluation (OPPE) is required to monitor clinical competence and professional behavior and provides an ongoing mechanism for identifying performance issues that could impact patient care. A well-designed process supports early detection and response to performance issues that could negatively impact patient outcomes.[85]

Physician leaders have a role in improving clinical processes used for clinical privileging. As a byproduct of OPPE documentation, practitioner profiles are extremely important to maintain and are used to evaluate performance and maintain privileges. Some key aspects of these files include the following:

- Profiles are based on performance.
- Profiles are provided to each physician or provider on a regular basis.
- Organizations may use risk-adjusted software.
- Evidence-based practice determines metrics used.
- Data are timely and accurate.
- Profiles are process and outcomes focused.
- Physician data are grouped by specialty type or specific diagnoses.
- Data are reported regularly.

- Physician champions talk directly with medical staff about their data.

The physician data must be meaningful to physicians. Data represent major service lines and patient safety issues and include inpatient as well as outpatient data. When available, national targets and benchmarks are used to compare performance. For example, national rates of complications of certain procedures, when compared with a specific physician or service, can help the organization identify performance concerns about what is expected for the same procedure. Data are easily accessed and shared with the physician to improve performance; the profiles vary by the physician's specialty or area of practice. Some examples of elements that might be found in a physician profile or the OPPE might include patient volume, length of stay, conformity with system-wide initiatives (e.g., use of deep vein thrombosis or pulmonary embolism prophylaxis), legibility of records and use of unapproved abbreviations, and severity-adjusted morbidity or mortality rates. The profile or OPPE is structured along the current core competencies of the Accreditation Council for Graduate Medical Education (patient care, medical knowledge, practice-based learning and improvement, interpersonal and communication skills, professionalism, and systems-based practice; **Figure 2.8**).[86]

Finally, profiles are confidential, and there must be a mechanism to track activity when the profiles are viewed. Policies and procedures are needed to establish the system for document management and mechanisms for tracking access (e.g., date of request, reason for request, name of person reviewing, and pertinent notes). See the *Health Data Analytics* section for discussion of privacy and security of protected health information.

A discussion of practice evaluation would be incomplete without discussing advanced practice professionals (APPs) (e.g., physician assistants, nurse practitioners, certified registered nurse anesthetists, clinical nurse specialists, and certified nurse midwives) who augment the physician in both the clinical practice and the hospital. APPs are a type of midlevel practitioner trained to assess patient needs, order/interpret diagnostic tests, coordinate care, promote wellness, and formulate and implement treatment plans. In 2020, approximately 142,000 physician assistants and 325,000 nurse practitioners were licensed in the United States.[87,88] This is one of the fastest growing workforces, more than doubling in 15 years.[89] APPs are subject to the same credentialing and privileging requirements as other practitioners granted privileges by the medical staff,[90] including OPPE/focused professional practice evaluation and peer review. The APP is not assigned to a visit or discharge as an attending physician,

**Specialty:** Orthopedic surgery

**Facilities:** Hospital 1, Hospital 3, Hospital 2, Hospital 4

**Reporting Period:** July 2021 through June 2022

**Physician Roles:** Attending Physician, Admitting Physician, Discharge Physician, Operating Physician (Principal or Secondary Px)

**Patient Type:** Internal Encounter - Inpatient and Observation

**Patient Type Analysis**

| Encounter Type | # of Cases |
|---|---|
| Inpatient | 370 |
| Observation | 3 |

**Role Analysis**

| Physician Role | # of Cases |
|---|---|
| Admitting Physician | 354 |
| Attending Physician | 307 |
| Discharge Physician | 54 |
| Operating Physician (Principal or Secondary Px) | 371 |

**Professionalism and Communication**

**Doctors communicated well (Composite) (3, N)**

| # Cases | Phys. Value | Benchmark | O/E |
|---|---|---|---|
| 110 | 90.3% | 81% | 1.11 |

**Hospital rating of 9 or 10 (3, N)**

| # Cases | Phys. Value | Benchmark | O/E |
|---|---|---|---|
| 110 | 93.64% | 72% | 1.30 |

***Benchmark Profile**: Nationwide Allpayer 50th*
***Benchmark Period**: Rolling July 2021 to June 2022*

**30-Day Readmissions**

**30-Day Readmission Rate Forward (3, S)**

| # Cases | Phys. Value | Benchmark * | O/E |
|---|---|---|---|
| 370 | 4.05% | 3.51% | 1.16 |

***Benchmark Profile**: Nationwide NRD*
***Benchmark Period**: *Annual 2021*

**Mortality Rate**

**Mortality Rate (3, R)**

| # Cases | Phys. Value | Benchmark * | O/E |
|---|---|---|---|
| 373 | 0% | 0% | 0 / 0 |

***Benchmark Profile**: Nationwide Allpayer 50th*
***Benchmark Period**: *Annual 2021*

**Practice Based Learning**

**Peer Case Reviews (1, N)**

| # Cases | Phys. Value |
|---|---|
| 0 | *No Data* |

**Figure 2.8** Example of a Physician Performance Profile

Reproduced from Syntellis Performance Solutions, LLC. *Axiom clinical analytics*; 2021. https://www.syntellis.com/healthcare/clinical-analytics-software *(continues)*

| Top 5 Procedures | |
|---|---|
| **Procedure** | **Volume** |
| 0SRC0J9 - Replace of R Knee Jt with Synth Sub, Cement, Open Approach | 96 |
| 0SRD0J9 - Replace of L Knee Jt with Synth Sub, Cement, Open Approach | 74 |
| 8E0Y0CZ - Robotic Assisted Procedure of Lower Extremity, Open Approach | 35 |
| 0SR90JA - Replace of R Hip Jt with Synth Sub, Uncement, Open Approach | 27 |
| 0SRB0JA - Replace of L Hip Jt with Synth Sub, Uncement, Open Approach | 17 |
| All Other Procedures | 239 |
| Total | 488 |

| Patient Care Indicators | | | |
|---|---|---|---|
| **PSI-9 - Perioperative Hemorrhage or Hematoma Rate (3, A)** | | | |
| **# Cases** | **Phys. Value** | **Benchmark** | **O/E** |
| 363 | 0% | 0.07% | 0.00 |
| **HAC - DVT/PE after TKR - Rate (3, N)** | | | |
| **# Cases** | **Phys. Value** | **Benchmark** | **O/E** |
| 370 | 0% | 0.01% | 0.00 |
| **HAC - DVT/PE after TKR - Rate (3, N)** | | | |
| **# Cases** | **Phys. Value** | **Benchmark** | **O/E** |
| 370 | 0% | 0.01% | 0.00 |
| *Benchmark Profile: Health System* | | | |

| Length of Stay | | | |
|---|---|---|---|
| **Length of Stay (LOS) (3, S)** | | | |
| **# Cases** | **Phys. Value** | **Benchmark \*** | **O/E** |
| 373 | 1.44 | 2.70 | 0.53 |
| *Benchmark Profile: Nationwide Allpayer 50th* | | | |
| *Benchmark Period: \*Annual 2021* | | | |

| Cost | | | |
|---|---|---|---|
| **Cost - Total (3, S)** | | | |
| **# Cases** | **Phys. Value** | **Benchmark \*** | **O/E** |
| 373 | $17,119 | $15,196 | 1.13 |
| **Cost - Medical/Surgical Supplies (3, S)** | | | |
| **# Cases** | **Phys. Value** | **Benchmark †** | **O/E** |
| 373 | $10,210 | $5,294 | 1.93 |
| *Benchmark Profile: Nationwide Allpayer 50th* | | | |
| *Benchmark Period: \*Annual 2021    †Annual 2020* | | | |

**Figure 2.8** Example of a Physician Performance Profile *(continued)*

creating challenges with attribution. By working closely with medical staff leadership, organizations can identify key documents, notes, and procedures that demonstrate that the APP was functioning as the extender for the attending or consulting physician. Partnering with information technology and the clinical informatics professionals allows the transformation of that documentation into data that can be used in the traditional workflow of OPPE.

Policies and procedures ensure confidentiality during the medical peer review process. They are consistent with organizational policies and procedures (usually within the health information management/ medical records department) and may include completion of a confidentiality statement signed by staff and practitioners involved in the peer review process. The nature of the data contained in a medical record is highly confidential. Policies and procedures clearly define who may have access to a medical record and under what circumstances in accordance with medical staff bylaws, hospital policy, and applicable laws and regulations. Because of the complexity of those issues, consultation from general counsel regarding national and state statutes is critical. Practitioner profiles can be maintained as a part of the credentials file or in a separate locked file. Most states have laws governing medical peer review and its activities. When applicable, files and their contents and meeting minutes are marked as "Confidential—peer review according to statute X." A simple "CONFIDENTIAL" stamp will also suffice.

Policies and procedures define the circumstances under which copies of medical peer review information are made, such as individual physician request. In accordance with medical staff bylaws and rules and regulations, a mechanism is developed for release of information with specification of contents to be disclosed. This mechanism is in place in response to the need to evaluate a practitioner's competence for appointment and reappointment to other healthcare institutions.

Committee minutes of quality, safety, and performance improvement activities usually are protected under medical peer review statutes. Consequently, maintaining confidentiality of records extends beyond credentialing to the entire quality, safety, and performance improvement program within an organization. Therefore, maintenance of confidentiality of records extends beyond credentialing to the entire quality and performance improvement program across the organization.

A mechanism is developed to track activity on each individual practitioner profile. A log or sign-out sheet attached to each file contains the date of request, reason for request or review, name of person reviewing, and any pertinent notes such as requests for copies of the contents.

Websites such as WebMD, ZocDoc, HealthGrades, DocSpot, and CareDash (see *Online Resources* at the end of the section) provide a directory of providers with patient comments and star ratings. These sites enable provider search by specialty, location, insurance provider, language, and whether a provider is accepting new patients. Reviews by patients provide insights into patient experience and perception of the provider enabling the user to find providers that are the right fit for their needs. See **Box 2.5** for features of practitioner performance reviews.

---

**Box 2.5  Key Points: Practitioner Performance Review Features**

- OPPE is required for all credentialed practitioners including advanced practice professionals as a mechanism to monitor clinical competence and professional behavior.
- A well-designed, ongoing process supports early detection and response to performance issues that could negatively impact patient outcomes.
- Healthcare quality professionals provide oversight to both the ongoing performance evaluation and medical peer review when it becomes necessary.
- Data, measures, and reports should be meaningful to the practitioner, relevant to the organization, and shared with individual clinicians on an ongoing basis.
- Confidentiality of performance evaluations, practitioner profiles, and peer review results extends to all aspects of the organization's quality and performance improvement process and should always be respected.

---

## Public Reporting

Public reporting of quality information may be considered as one of the key external drivers for transparency and accountability.[91] Releases of public data began in the late 1980s when the Health Care Financing Administration (now Centers for Medicare & Medicaid Services) released case-mix-adjusted mortality rates for hospitals throughout the country. Eventually, these reports were no longer issued because of hospitals' criticisms of case-mix-adjusted methodology. In the early 1990s, New York State began releasing mortality data on patients who underwent open-heart surgery by hospital and ranked hospitals according to how much they deviated from case-mix-adjusted values. Hospitals were then labeled as providing either good or poor care. Hospitals with poor outcomes were encouraged to improve care processes. Eventually, New York released data on individual surgeons and other procedures such as angioplasty.

The broad implementation of mandatory public reporting was intended to guide hospitals and physicians, through incentives, toward improving the quality of care and service delivered to patients. The 2003 Hospital Inpatient Quality Reporting program aimed to provide consumers with quality information to support efforts to make informed decisions about healthcare.

The current emphasis for public reporting is on reporting structure, process, and outcome measures, and the focus of reporting is highly variable. Examples of government-sponsored reporting include CMS Care Compare efforts related to doctors and clinicians, hospitals, nursing homes, home health services, hospice care, inpatient rehabilitation facilities, long-term care hospitals, and dialysis facilities. Many private organizations emerged with varying missions around healthcare quality and safety, several of which publish different types of reports that include information about quality and safety. These reporting entities use similar, yet differing and proprietary approaches, comparing healthcare providers to national benchmarks and providing a rating as to whether care meets specific standards.

The Leapfrog Group is a not-for-profit organization founded by employers and private healthcare experts that aims to make giant leaps forward in the safety, quality, and affordability of healthcare in the United States by promoting transparency through their data collection and public reporting initiatives.[92] Healthgrades is an online resource for information about physicians and hospitals. The website reports that more than one million people a day use the site to search, compare, and connect with hospitals and physicians based on the most important factors when selecting a healthcare provider: experience, hospital quality, and patient satisfaction.[93]

Early evidence indicated that public reporting of performance data stimulates quality, safety, and performance improvement activities at the hospital level.[94] A more recent review of the available evidence indicates that public reporting programs at different levels of the healthcare sector are a challenging but rewarding public health strategy and stimulate providers to improve healthcare quality.[91]

### Incentives and Penalties

As national pressures continue to increase, new expectations emerge for leaders, including those of government agencies (e.g., CMS), public reporting groups (e.g., The Commonwealth Fund, The Leapfrog Group), accreditation agencies (e.g., The Joint Commission, DNV GL Healthcare), and third-party payers (e.g., Blue Cross Blue Shield, UnitedHealthcare, Tufts). Third-party payers implemented the practice of nonpayment for certain conditions that could have been reasonably prevented (serious reportable events), formerly known as *never events*, (e.g., pressure ulcers) and serious preventable events (e.g., leaving a sponge in the patient during surgery).

The organization's external environment relative to national and local practices that involve rewarding or penalizing organizations and providers based on specific outcomes serves as another external factor requiring consideration as part of planning for quality, safety, and performance improvement. For example, one of the key principles behind the development of The Leapfrog Group was to support value-based purchasing. The Leapfrog Group's mission is to reward healthcare providers that provide excellent care. Further, it suggests that the rewards for superior healthcare value be based on four critical ingredients: reliable use of proven methods to ensure patient safety, improved clinical information systems, routine use of modern performance improvement methods in managing and delivering care, and routine and active engagement of consumers in healthcare decision making. Purchasers are directly encouraged to shift their resources to better providers, to educate their employees about the importance of comparing the performance of healthcare providers, and to assist them in using the measures to make informed healthcare choices.

The pay-for-performance movement has expanded substantially since 2012 to include additional levels of providers. Third-party payers continue to expand their pay-for-performance initiatives through increasingly robust programs. All the major payers (including Blue Cross, Aetna, Cigna, and UnitedHealthcare) are linking reimbursement to quality in their contracts with organizations and providers.

### Customer Demands

The organization must consider what it should do from the perspective of its customers. A review of the healthcare market segments as well as an assessment of the specific needs, requirements, and expectations of various patient and stakeholder groups will help determine what the organization should do. The organization determines appropriate mechanisms for obtaining information from its customers (i.e., hard copy and online surveys, focus groups, etc.).

### Value-Based Service Delivery

As the healthcare delivery system transforms from fee-for-service to value-based service, organizations plan, evaluate, and refine their strategy in response to the ever-changing healthcare market, and understanding where an organization is in the transition is critical to determining the impact of the external demands on the organization relative to planning. To meet external demands and optimize performance and align clinical outcome priorities with current quality and revenue-cycle opportunities, healthcare quality professionals need to understand and demonstrate key competencies related to population-health management and care transitions to best guide leaders in understanding the healthcare quality implications of this external force (see the *Population Health and Care Transitions* section).

# Quality Measurement Programs

The landscape of quality measurement programs associated with value-based care is extensive and requires diligence on the part of the healthcare quality professional to maintain a current understanding of the programs and how those impact the organization. To better understand the landscape of various performance-based measure requirements, it is important to discuss who pays for healthcare. In the United States, nearly half of the almost $4 trillion spent on healthcare annually is paid by state and federal governments. This means that CMS leads the industry in quality and payment research and innovation.

The healthcare quality professional brings unique skills to advise leadership on the costs and benefits of participating in both mandatory and voluntary measure reporting programs. While the list of reporting programs that follows is not exhaustive, participation in multiple value-based programs requires an understanding of the measure collection and submission requirements, how various measures are reported and interpreted, and the value to be gained for patients, providers, and practices.

## CMS Quality Measures

CMS uses quality measures in its various quality initiatives that include quality improvement, pay for reporting, and public reporting. Quality measures are tools that measure or quantify healthcare processes, outcomes, patient perceptions, and organizational structure and/or systems that are associated with the ability to provide high-quality healthcare and/or that relate to one or more quality goals for healthcare.[95] These goals, including effective, safe, efficient, patient-centered, equitable, and timely care, are described in **Table 2.3**.

The Measures Management System (MMS) is a standardized system for developing and maintaining the quality measures used in various CMS initiatives and programs.[96] The CMS Measure Inventory Tool (see *Online Resources*) lists 2318 measures across 44 programs.[97] This interactive tool provides details on measure definitions, type, NQF status, and programs. It enables the user to search on specific measures; filter by data sources, condition, and care settings; and compare measures.

**Table 2.3** Six Domains of Healthcare Quality

| Goal | Definition | Measure Example |
|------|-----------|-----------------|
| Safe | The culture of patient safety should be systemic, identifying and mitigating risk as a matter of practice to reduce harm to patients. | Perioperative pulmonary embolism or deep vein thrombosis rate |
| Effective | Patients receive treatment to effectively manage their condition based on best available evidence and current best practices. | Readmission rates |
| Efficient | Waste in healthcare delivery such as overuse of services, patient flow bottlenecks, and poor supply management result in unnecessary costs to the organization and the consumer. | % chest X-rays for asthma patients |
| Patient centered | Care should be individualized for each patient considering social determinants of care and other factors | Doctors/nurses listened carefully |
| Equitable | Appropriate care should be delivered to all regardless of race, ethnicity, language, sexual orientation, and gender identity | Number of referrals |
| Timely | Reduce barriers that delay timely treatment, diagnosis, or preventative care | Patient wait times |

Data from Agency for Healthcare Research and Quality. *Six domains of health care quality*. Rockville, MD: Agency for Healthcare Research and Quality; 2018. Accessed January 11, 2022. https://www.ahrq.gov/talkingquality/measures/six-domains.html

# Hospital Readmissions Reduction Program

Reducing avoidable readmissions requires coordination of care across inpatient and outpatient services and patient-centered discharge planning. The Hospital Readmissions Reduction Program aims to encourage hospitals to improve patient care by reducing payment for excess readmissions in the following six 30-day, procedure specific, risk-adjusted categories:

1. Acute myocardial infarction
2. Chronic obstructive pulmonary disease
3. Heart failure
4. Pneumonia
5. Coronary artery bypass graft surgery
6. Elective primary total hip arthroplasty and/or total knee arthroplasty.[98]

Payment reduction is capped at 3%. In fiscal year 2021, Medicare reduced its payments to 2499 hospitals, or 47% of all facilities, saving the government over $521 million in the fiscal year.[99] Online resources are available to look up penalties by hospital. See *Online Resources* at the end of the section.

## Hospital-Acquired Condition Reduction Program

Hospital-acquired conditions impact patient outcomes, experience of care, and costs for the hospital encounter. CMS encourages hospitals to reduce those conditions through the Hospital-Acquired Condition Reduction Program by reducing the payment for all Medicare discharges for hospitals in the worst performing quartile for HACs.[100] Hospitals with a total HAC score greater than the 75th percentile receive a 1% payment reduction. CMS uses the total HAC score to determine the worst performing quartile of all subsection (d) hospitals based on data for six quality measures.

## Quality Payment Program

The MACRA value-based payment system incorporates quality measurement into payments with the goal of creating an equitable payment system for physicians. Collectively referred to as the Quality Payment Program that started in 2017, this federally mandated program includes two participation tracks from which eligible clinicians can choose (1) the Merit-Based Incentive Payment System (MIPS) linked to performance including following defined, evidence-based clinical quality measures or (2) advanced alternative payment models that provide financial incentives to clinicians to provide high-quality and cost-efficient care.[101] Clinicians can choose from these two tracks based on their practice size, specialty, location, or patient population.

MACRA replaced legacy programs for physicians, including the Physician Quality Reporting System, the Value-Based Payment Modifier (Value Modifier), and the Medicare EHR Incentive Program (known also as Meaningful Use or MU) (**Figure 2.9**).[102]

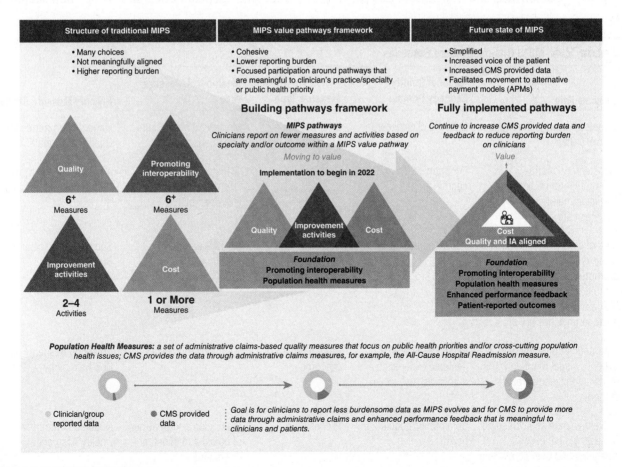

**Figure 2.9** MIPS Value Pathways

Reproduced from Centers for Medicare & Medicaid Services. MIPS Value Pathways Diagrams. Accessed June 6, 2022. https://qpp.cms.gov/resources/resource-library

MIPS performance is measured across four performance categories: quality, cost, promoting interoperability, and improvement activities, with 40% of the score attributed to quality.[103] A total of 209 MIPS quality measures were finalized for 2021, including two new administrative claims-based measures.[104]

1. Hospital-wide, 30-day, all-cause unplanned readmission rate for the MIPS-eligible clinicians groups
2. Risk-standardized complication rate following elective primary total hip arthroplasty and/or total knee arthroplasty for MIPS

**Table 2.4** shows the subset of the 2021 quality measures demonstrating examples by domain, type, meaningful measure area, and primary measure steward. A complete list of measures with definitions and other attributes may be found in the CMS 2021 MIPS Quality Measures List.

## Accountable Care Organizations

ACOs are groups of doctors, hospitals, and other healthcare providers, who come together voluntarily to give coordinated high-quality care to the Medicare patients they serve. Coordinated care helps ensure that patients, especially those with enduring and chronic illness, get the right care at the right time, with the goal of avoiding unnecessary duplication of services and preventing medical errors. When an ACO succeeds in both delivering high-quality care and spending healthcare dollars more wisely, it will share in the savings it achieves for the Medicare program.[105] ACOs use alternative payment models and ties provider reimbursements to quality metrics and reductions in the cost of care.

To participate in the Medicare Shared Savings Program, ACOs must submit quality measures across multiple domains.[106] For performance year 2020, CMS will measure quality of care using 23 nationally recognized quality measures that span four key domains:

1. Patient/caregiver experience (ten measures)
2. Care coordination/patient safety (four measures)
3. Preventive health (six measures)
4. At-risk population (three measures)

In the coming years, ACOs participating in the Medicare Shared Savings Program will see changes in the measures that are used and the way they are reported. This multiyear process is an effort to reduce the data collection and reporting burdens and drive improved patient outcomes. The new reporting

**Table 2.4** MIPS Quality Measure Examples

| Measure Title | National Quality Strategy Domain | Measure Type | Meaningful Measure Area | Primary Measure Steward |
|---|---|---|---|---|
| Diabetes: Hemoglobin A₁c poor control (>9%) | Effective clinical care | Intermediate outcome | Management of chronic conditions | National Committee for Quality Assurance |
| Diabetic retinopathy: Communication with the physician managing ongoing diabetes care | Communication and care coordination | Process | Transfer of health information and interoperability | American Academy of Ophthalmology |
| Rate of carotid endarterectomy (CEA) for asymptomatic patients, without major complications (discharged to home by postoperative day no. 2) | Patient safety | Outcome | Appropriate use of healthcare | Society for Vascular Surgeons |
| Cataracts: Improvement in patient's visual function within 90 days following cataract surgery | Person and caregiver-centered experience and outcomes | Patient reported outcome | Functional outcomes | American Academy of Ophthalmology |
| Preventive care and screening: Unhealthy alcohol use screening and brief counseling | Community/population health | Process | Prevention and treatment of opioid and substance use disorders | National Committee for Quality Assurance |

Data from Centers for Medicare & Medicaid Services. MIPS quality measures. 2021. Accessed February 1, 2022.  https://qpp-cm-prod-content.s3.amazonaws.com/uploads/1246/2021%20MIPS%20Quality%20Measures%20List.xlsx process, the APM Performance Pathway, will align with the MIPS Value Pathway and move away from siloed reporting. For MIPS eligibility, the provider needs to determine their eligibility (**Figure 2.10**).

Beginning in 2025, CMS will shift to mandatory reporting of APM Performance Pathway quality measures.[107] Performance category weights will differ from traditional MIPS and the quality measure set is illustrated in **Figure 2.11**.

## Clinical Quality Registries

Clinical quality registries are established with the purpose of monitoring quality of care, providing feedback, benchmarking performance, describing a pattern of treatment, reducing variation, and serving as a tool for conducting research as a means of improving health outcomes and reducing healthcare costs.[108] Clinical registries can serve a number of purposes from research and clinical trials to documentation of comparative therapies and benchmarking and generally fall into two categories: those collecting data on patients who are exposed to particular health services for a relatively short period of time and those tracking diseases or conditions over time or across multiple providers and/or health services. Importantly, both capture exposures and outcomes of interest to healthcare providers or healthcare systems.[109]

A cancer registry, for example, is a systematic collection of data about cancer and tumor diseases. Cancer registrars capture a complete summary of patient

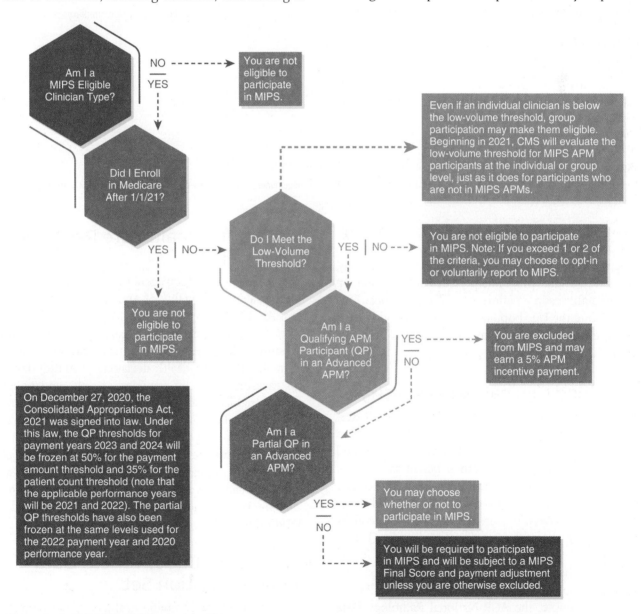

**Figure 2.10** 2021 MIPS Eligibility Decision Tree

Reproduced from Centers for Medicare & Medicaid Services. *Am I Eligible to Participate in the Merit-based Incentive Payment System (MIPS) in the 2021 Performance Year?* 2021. Accessed January 31, 2022. https://qpp-cm-prod-content.s3.amazonaws.com/uploads/1162/2021%20MIPS%20Eligibility%20 Decision%20Tree.pdf

| Measure # and Title | Collection Type | Submitter Type |
|---|---|---|
| **Quality ID#: 001** Diabetes: Hemoglobin A1c (HbA$_{1c}$) Poor Control | eCQM, MIPS CQM, Medicare Part B Claims | - MIPS Eligible Clinician<br>- Representative of a Practice<br>- APM Entities<br>- Third Party Intermediary |
| **Quality ID#: 134** Preventive Care and Screening: Screening for Depression and Follow-up Plan | eCQM, MIPS CQM, Medicare Part B Claims | - MIPS Eligible Clinician<br>- Representative of a Practice<br>- APM Entities<br>- Third Party Intermediary |
| **Quality ID#: 236** Controlling High Blood Pressure | eCQM, MIPS CQM, Medicare Part B Claims | - MIPS Eligible Clinician<br>- Representative of a Practice<br>- APM Entities<br>- Third Party Intermediary |
| **Quality ID#: 321** CAHPS for MIPS | CAHPS for MIPS Survey | - Third Party Intermediary |
| **Measure#: 479** Hospital-Wide, 30-day, All-Cause Unplanned Readmission (HWR) Rate for MIPS Eligible Clinician Groups | Administrative Claims | N/A |
| **Measure#: 484** Clinician and Clinician Group Risk-standardized Hospital Admission Rates for Patients with Multiple Chronic Conditions | Administrative Claims | N/A |

**Figure 2.11** Payment Year 2022 APP Quality Requirements Quality Measures Set

Reproduced from Centers for Medicare & Medicaid Services. Quality Measures: APP Requirements: What quality data should I submit?; 2022. https://qpp.cms.gov/mips/app-quality-requirements

history, diagnosis, treatment, and status for every cancer patient in the United States and other countries. One such program, the Surveillance, Epidemiology, and End Results program, provides information on cancer statistics in an effort to reduce the cancer burden among the U.S. population.[110] A list of additional registries may be found at the National Institutes of Health website.[111]

## Qualified Clinical Data Registry

A qualified clinical data registry (QCDR) is a CMS-approved vendor that collects clinical data from an individual clinician, group, and/or virtual group and submits the data to CMS on their behalf as a part of the MIPS. These organizations may include specialty societies, regional health collaboratives, and large health systems or software vendors working in collaboration with one of these medical entities.[112] QCDRs can develop and/or submit measures to CMS for its approval. These entities must self-nominate and successfully complete a qualification process with CMS.[113]

For example, the ACR National Radiology Data Registry was a CMS-approved QCDR for the MIPS for 2021. Fourteen QCDR measures spanning across two data registries have been approved for inclusion in the QCDR, along with 48 MIPS measures.[114]

## Agency for Healthcare Research and Quality

AHRQ is the lead federal agency charged with improving the safety and quality of America's healthcare system. AHRQ develops the knowledge, tools, and data needed to improve the healthcare system and help consumers, healthcare professionals, and policy makers make informed health decisions.[115] AHRQ develops measures used by providers, payers, and policy makers enabled by the development of the Healthcare Cost and Utilization Project,[116] a publicly available, comprehensive, all-payer database. The AHR Quality Indicators[117] website lists 62 measures under 4 quality and safety indicator sets (**Table 2.5**).[118] These measures use readily available administrative data; AHRQ software is free and may be downloaded from the AHRQ website.[119]

## Healthcare Effectiveness Data and Information Set

NCQA evaluates and accredits health plans based on the quality of care patients receive, how happy patients are with their care, and health plans' efforts to keep improving.[120] HEDIS is a comprehensive set of standardized performance measures designed to provide purchasers

**Table 2.5** AHRQ Quality and Research Measure Category Descriptions

| Indicator Set | Description | Usage | Measure Examples |
|---|---|---|---|
| Prevention quality indicators (PQIs) | Identify issues of access to outpatient care | ▪ Flag potential healthcare quality problem areas that need further investigation<br>▪ Provide a quick check on primary care access or outpatient services in a community<br>▪ Help organizations identify unmet needs in their communities | PQI 01—Diabetes, short-term complications admission rate<br>PQI 02—Perforated appendix admission rate<br>PQI 05—Chronic obstructive pulmonary disease (COPD) or asthma in older adults admission rate |
| Inpatient quality indicators (IQIs) | Assess quality of care inside the hospital | ▪ Inpatient mortality for surgical procedures and medical conditions<br>▪ Utilization of procedures for which there are questions of overuse, underuse, and misuse | IQI 12—Coronary artery bypass graft (CABG) mortality rate<br>IQI 22—Vaginal birth after cesarean (VBAC) delivery rate, uncomplicated<br>IQI 23—Laparoscopic cholecystectomy rate |
| Patient safety indicators (PSIs) | Assess incidence of adverse events and in-hospital complications | Potential in-hospital complications and adverse events following surgeries, procedures, and childbirth | PSI 21—Retained surgical item or unretrieved device fragment rate<br>PSI 22—Iatrogenic pneumothorax rate<br>PSI 23—Central venous catheter-related bloodstream infection rate |
| Pediatric quality indicators (PDIs) | Assess potentially preventable complications and iatrogenic events for pediatric patients treated in hospitals | ▪ Identify problems in pediatric hospital care that may need further study<br>▪ Evaluate preventive care for children in outpatient settings | PDI14—Asthma admissions<br>PDI15—Diabetes short-term complications<br>Pediatric heart surgery mortality<br>PDI 07—Pediatric heart surgery volume |

Data from Agency for Healthcare Research and Quality. AHRQ QI Software. Updated July 20, 2021. Accessed December 21, 2021. https://qualityindicators.ahrq.gov/Software/Default.aspx

and consumers with the information they need for reliable comparison of health plan performance used in the accreditation process.[121] Measures are designed to identify gaps in care and opportunities to improve patient engagement and represent six domains of care.

1. Effectiveness of care
2. Access/availability of care
3. Experience of care
4. Utilization and risk-adjusted utilization
5. Health plan descriptive information
6. Measures reported using electronic clinical data systems

NCQA publishes an annual report card for health plans (commercial, Medicare, Medicaid, and Exchange), healthcare clinicians and practices, and other organizations such as credentialing verification organizations using standardized measures to rate and compare performance.[122] Details about HEDIS can be found in the *HEDIS Volume 2 Technical Specifications*.

## Hospital Consumer Assessment of Healthcare Providers and Systems

The Hospital Consumer Assessment of Healthcare Providers and Systems (HCAHPS) is a survey instrument and data collection methodology adopted by CMS for measuring patients' perceptions of their hospital experience.[123,124] Overall goals of the survey are to provide objective hospital-to-hospital comparisons for what patients care about and create incentives to improve quality and accountability through public reporting. The survey asks discharged patients 29 questions about their recent hospital stay, including communication with doctors and nurses, responsiveness of hospital staff, communication about medicines, cleanliness and quietness of the hospital, discharge information, transition to posthospital care, and overall rating of the hospital. The survey also includes three items to direct patients to relevant questions, five items to adjust for the mix of patients across hospitals, and two items that support congressionally mandated reports. Surveys are administered between 2 and 42 days after discharge to a random sample of adult patients through four approved modes: mail, telephone, mail with telephone follow-up, and interactive voice response. **Table 2.6** lists the 2021 survey questions.

## CAHPS Clinician & Group Survey

The CAHPS Clinician & Group Survey (CG-CAHPS) assesses patient experiences with providers and staff in primary care and specialty care settings to determine the need for improvement activities and to equip consumers with knowledge to make choices about providers, physician practices, or medical groups.[125]

**Table 2.6** Hospital Consumer Assessment of Healthcare Providers and Systems Survey Instrument

| Domain | Questions |
|---|---|
| Your care from nurses | 1. During this hospital stay, how often did nurses treat you with <u>courtesy and respect</u>? |
| | 2. During this hospital stay, how often did nurses <u>listen carefully to you</u>? |
| | 3. During this hospital stay, how often did nurses explain things in a way you could understand? |
| | 4. During this hospital stay, after you pressed the call button, how often did you get help as soon as you wanted it? |
| Your care from doctors | 1. During this hospital stay, how often did doctors treat you with courtesy and respect? |
| | 2. During this hospital stay, how often did doctors listen carefully to you? |
| | 3. During this hospital stay, how often did doctors explain things in a way you could understand? |
| The hospital environment | 1. During this hospital stay, how often were your room and bathroom kept clean? |
| | 2. During this hospital stay, how often was the area around your room quiet at night? |
| Your experiences in this hospital | 1. During this hospital stay, did you need help from nurses or other hospital staff in getting to the bathroom or in using a bedpan? |
| | 2. How often did you get help in getting to the bathroom or in using a bedpan as soon as you wanted? |
| | 3. During this hospital stay, did you need medicine for pain? |
| | 4. During this hospital stay, how often was your pain well controlled? |
| | 5. During this hospital stay, how often did the hospital staff do everything they could to help you with your pain? |
| | 6. During this hospital stay, were you given any medicine that you had not taken before? |
| | 7. Before giving you any new medicine, how often did hospital staff tell you what the medicine was for? |
| | 8. Before giving you any new medicine, how often did hospital staff describe possible side effects in a way you could understand? |
| When you left the hospital | 1. After you left the hospital, did you go directly to your own home, to someone else's home, or to another health facility? |
| | 2. During this hospital stay, did doctors, nurses, or other hospital staff talk with you about whether you would have the help you needed when you left the hospital? |
| | 3. During this hospital stay, did you get information in writing about what symptoms or health problems to look out for after you left the hospital? |
| Overall rating of the hospital | 1. Using any number from 0 to 10, where 0 is the worst hospital possible and 10 is the best hospital possible, what number would you use to rate this hospital during your stay? |
| | 2. Would you recommend this hospital to your friends and family? |

*(continues)*

**Table 2.6** Hospital Consumer Assessment of Healthcare Providers and Systems Survey Instrument *(continued)*

| Domain | Questions |
| --- | --- |
| About you | 1. In general, how would you rate your overall health? |
| | 2. What is the highest grade or level of school that you have completed? |
| | 3. Are you of Spanish, Hispanic, or Latino origin or descent? |
| | 4. What is your race? Please choose one or more. |
| | 5. What language do you mainly speak at home? |

Modified from Centers for Medicare & Medicaid Services. HCAHPS Survey: survey instructions. 2021. Accessed January 11, 2022. https://hcahpsonline.org/globalassets/hcahps/survey-instruments/mail/effective-december-1-2021-and-forward-discharges/2021_survey-instruments_english_mail_updateda.pdf

All surveys officially designated as CAHPS surveys have been approved by the CAHPS Consortium, which is overseen by the AHRQ. **Figure 2.12** outlines the survey questions from measures from the adult survey versions 3.0 and 3.1. Organizations reporting the results can use the labels and descriptions of the composite and rating measures in reports for consumers and other audiences.

**Box 2.6** summarizes the key points of quality measurement programs.

---

### Box 2.6 Key Points: Quality Measurement Programs

- The landscape of quality measure programs associated with value-based care is extensive and requires diligence on the part of the healthcare quality professional to maintain a current understanding of the programs and how those impact the organization.
- While the Centers for Medicare & Medicaid Services (CMS) leads the way for value-based programs as the leading payer of healthcare, the landscape of various programs is broad and must be monitored.
- Sponsors of value-based programs, such as the ACO Medicare Shared Savings Program, continue to evaluate opportunities to reduce reporting burden and increase the impact on cost and quality.
- The healthcare quality professional must maintain constant awareness of changes to program reporting, data collection, and added or removed measures.

---

## Performance Measurement and Improvement

New payment models and the frequency with which measures can change impact the entire organization creating demand for interprofessional relationships across all stakeholders—providers, payers, pharmacies, and patients. Electronic clinical quality measures (eCQMs) measure many aspects of care for eligible professionals, eligible hospitals, and critical access hospitals to ensure that the system is delivering effective, safe, efficient, patient-centered, equitable, and timely care.[126] Electronic CQMs provide access to a greater set of clinical data such as laboratory results by leveraging data from the EHR to supplement claims information for quality measure calculation and reporting. This reduces the burden of time-consuming manual data collection and provides greater accuracy and specificity to quality measures. Successful implementation and adoption of eCQMs requires collaboration across many stakeholders to interpret specifications for electronic measure reporting.

## Information Technology

The use of electronic data requires that health IT systems adhere to requirements designed by CMS quality programs in which the organization participates for the acquisition and analysis of data. Healthcare quality professionals must collaborate with IT stakeholders to ensure systems data are readily available for reporting and analysis and establish standards to minimize security breaches while enabling access to patient data. In the event of mergers and acquisitions, IT must have a mechanism for adding new data sets as other providers are added or as new measures become available. As the organization grows and data volumes increase, databases will need to scale to accommodate more information.

The healthcare quality professional should communicate timeliness and frequency requirements for data acquisition and data transmission of quality measures to internal and external reporting initiatives. Information technology (IT) is responsible for ensuring system uptime and communicates a plan for system downtime that supports those initiatives. As more

| Getting Timely Appointments, Care, and Information | | |
|---|---|---|
| The survey asked patients how often they got appointments for care as soon as needed and timely answers to questions when they contacted the office. | | |
| Q6 | Patient got appointment for urgent care as soon as needed | **Response Options** |
| Q8 | Patient got appointment for non-urgent care as soon as needed | • Never<br>• Sometimes |
| Q10 | Patient got answer to medical question the same day he/she contacted provider's office | • Usually<br>• Always |
| **How Well Providers Communicate with Patients** | | |
| The survey asked patients how often their providers explained things clearly, listened carefully, showed respect, and spent enough time with the patient. | | |
| Q11 | Provider explained things in a way that was easy to understand | **Response Options** |
| Q12 | Provider listened carefully to patient | • Never<br>• Sometimes |
| Q14 | Provider showed respect for what patient had to say | • Usually |
| Q15 | Provider spent enough time with patient | • Always |
| **Providers' Use of Information to Coordinate Patient Care** | | |
| The survey asked patients how often their providers knew their medical history, followed up to give results of tests, and asked about prescription medications being taken. | | |
| Q13 | Provider knew important information about patient's medical history | **Response Options** |
| Q17 | Someone from provider's office followed up with patient to give results of blood test, x-ray, or other test | • Never<br>• Sometimes |
| Q20 | Someone from provider's office talked about all prescription medications being taken | • Usually<br>• Always |

**Figure 2.12** Selected Measures from the CAHPS Clinician & Group Adult Survey, Versions 3.0 and 3.1

Reproduced from Agency for Healthcare Research and Quality. *Guidelines for Using the CAHPS Clinician & Group Survey*. 2021. Accessed January 12, 2022. https://www.ahrq.gov/sites/default/files/wysiwyg/cahps/surveys-guidance/cg/guidance-cg-cahps.pdf

organizations support bring-your-own-device policies so that clinicians can have real-time access to key operational and quality measures, the healthcare quality professional collaborates with IT to ensure protected health information security and privacy. As the digital transformation has created access to new data, the Internet of Things opens more access to data not historically captured, such as smart watches, insulin pens, and continuous glucose monitoring devices. Collaboration with IT can bring innovative solutions to the efforts of quality.

## Business Intelligence

Tools that provide dashboards, interactive visualization, and self-serve data analysis create transparency for key stakeholders across the organization. Business intelligence (BI) tools have the capability to ingest, aggregate, and display information using data from disparate sources across the organization including eCQMs generated by the EHR or quality management system. A well-designed visualization of quality and cost outcomes can reduce the dependency on IT and reporting resources by providing decision makers with high-reliability data in a timely and effective manner. Contemporary BI tools augment the reporting of quality measures beyond the quality management reporting tool. BI solutions assign roles and privileges to specify what data can be accessed by each stakeholder. For example, the financial team should be able to view aggregated cost and quality data. However, organizations may choose to limit that view to only the highest level and disallow access to patient or physician data. The collaboration with the BI team can establish levels of access and allows for organizational transparency without compromising protected health information.

## Clinical Informatics

Domain expertise in clinical documentation is a key success factor in the secondary utilization of EHR data for quality measure reporting. The EHR was initially designed as a digital version of the patient's paper chart providing secure transactional data for authorized users, and the data were not necessarily optimized for reporting and analytics.[127] Clinical informatics focuses on how data are acquired, structured, stored, processed, retrieved, analyzed, presented, and communicated.[128] Clinical informatics specialists (or informaticists) understand how data must be structured in such a way that it can be retrieved for reporting and analytics. The healthcare quality professional in partnership with clinical informatics optimizes how data are retrieved for accuracy, annual updates to evidence-based medicine, code sets, and measure logic. Successful access to reliable data makes quality reporting a by-product of patient care.

In addition to data expertise, the clinical informaticist is instrumental in the implementation of quality measures as well. They are familiar with user-centered design and workflow methods that ensure adoption by the clinician and data accuracy and completeness for care delivery. They may work across departments to educate users and promote best practices for documentation and ultimately for data retrieval. When improvement opportunities are identified through the quality review process, they can be a method for the healthcare quality professional to adapt clinician behaviors and documentation workflows to ensure that quality measures reflect care outcomes and processes.

## EHR Vendor

The EHR vendor plays a strategic role in the ability to structure data so healthcare providers can easily retrieve and exchange patient information. Healthcare providers participating in the Promoting Interoperability Programs (formerly the Medicare and Medicaid EHR Incentive Programs) must use certified electronic health record technology to qualify for the program and demonstrate meaningful use.[129] Healthcare IT vendors who provide certified technology supporting this program have a responsibility to meet standards established by CMS and the Office of the National Coordinator for Health Information Technology.[130] For performance year 2021, organizations are required to use an EHR that meets the 2015 edition certification criteria,[131] 2015 edition Cures Act update[132] certification criteria, or a combination of both for participation in this performance category. For eligible providers, interoperability accounts for 25% of the composite score representing a significant portion of the clinician's Medicare Part B payment.[133] The healthcare quality professional must maintain current knowledge of these requirements to ensure ongoing readiness for potential rule changes by working in collaboration with the organization's IT department and the EHR vendor.

## Education

When modifications must be made to the EHR or the documentation as a result of measure changes, many stakeholders are impacted. Clinicians need coaching on how and where to input data, reporting analysts need to understand the data model and select the appropriate fields for reporting, and consumers of the reports need exposure to the purpose of the change and how it impacts measurement. Communication between the healthcare quality professional and the education department is a must to plan for the release, define the educational content, identify stakeholders, determine the method of delivering the education, and ensure modifications are made to new hire onboarding curricula.

## Marketing

Healthcare is a competitive business with organizations competing for patients, payers, staff, market share, and mind share. Large health systems typically have a chief marketing officer and a percentage of revenue allocated for the marketing budget. The average physician practice may allocate anywhere from 8% to 12% of their total revenue to promoting their brand.[134] Healthcare marketing is designed to build the organization brand, create an expectation of a high level of service and satisfaction, and support the strategic plan of the organization. Healthcare organizations build their brand by creating unique and memorable proposals to differentiate themselves. A marketing message must be true, superior to the competition, important to the target audience, easy to remember, and difficult to copy by the competition.[135] This means that collaboration with healthcare quality professionals is essential to ensuring that the message is consistent with reality. Whether the campaign is a billboard advertising Leapfrog Group rating results or a digital campaign promoting a new service line, collaboration between marketing and quality leadership is instrumental to driving organizational growth and brand.

Key points for performance measurement and improvement are listed in **Box 2.7**.

---

### Box 2.7  Key Points: Performance Measurement and Improvement

- Multiple data sources are required for measure development, including claims, clinical, and survey data, and understanding the strengths and limitations of each helps to better utilize the measures for improvement purposes.
- Best practices for staying informed of quality measure changes include participation in webinars and events sponsored by CMS, payers, EHR vendors, and thought leadership organizations.
- Reporting activities for various payment programs should be identified and managed to ensure critical timelines are met.

---

# Data Management and Reporting

Data management is a broad concept that encompasses multiple aspects of data access, storage, security, distribution, quality, and so on.[136] Given the complexity of quality reporting and the dynamic nature of quality metrics across multiple programs managing data across the vast number of data sources requires the engagement of the organization's data governance strategy. Data governance is a discipline adopted and managed by the organization's IT department in partnership with other functional areas within the organization. The U.S. Government Accountability Office (GAO) notes effective data governance helps to maintain and improve the quality and transparency of data, which can be accomplished through a framework or structure for ensuring that data assets are transparent, accessible, and of sufficient quality. Data governance activities include "authorities, roles, responsibilities, organizational structures, policies, processes, standards, and resources for the definition, stewardship, production, security and use of data."[137(p.6)] This is illustrated in **Figure 2.13**.

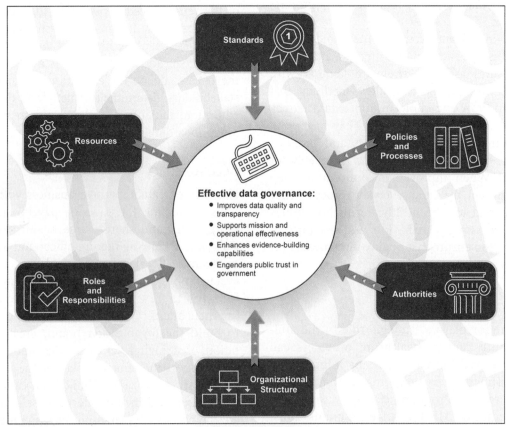

Sources: GAO analysis of GAO, OMB, and non-federal reports.  |  GAO-21-152

**Figure 2.13** Data Governance

Reproduced from United States Government Accountability Office. *Data Governance: Agencies Made Progress in Establishing Governance, but Need to Address Key Milestones.* GAO-21-152 December 2020. Accessed July 7, 2022. https://www.gao.gov/assets/gao-21-152.pdf

While data governance is a broad discipline, there are some key areas in which the quality professional should actively participate.

*Data modeling and design.* Healthcare generates massive amounts of data. It is suggested that the U.S. healthcare system generated 150 exabytes of data in 2011.[138] This exponential growth of data in healthcare spawned the development of new platforms and technologies in which to harness big data. To make data useful for quality measure reporting, it must be optimized for reporting, meaning the data model must be configured to enable queries against standard tables, mapping, dimensions, and relationships defined by the measure.

*Data quality.* Ensuring data accuracy is likely the most important aspect of measuring and reporting on the quality of patient care. It only takes one instance of inaccurate data to call into question an entire reporting initiative. Engaging the clinical informaticist helps to ensure that data are documented and extracted from the appropriate source for the required report.

*Documents and content.* Due to ongoing changes in regulations regarding measure requirements, the organization should regularly review and revise data content policies to determine what data are required and available for quality reporting. As eCQMs become more prevalent, the healthcare quality professional should be involved in those reviews.

Internal reporting activities for quality measures should be embedded in the routine reporting schedule based on the measures and are likely monthly or quarterly in nature and are a core competency of the healthcare quality professional. External reporting activities will vary depending on the value-based program. For commercial payers, in general, claims data are submitted, measures are calculated by the payer and results returned to the provider. Payment strategies are negotiated with the payer. However, value-based program reporting is largely retrospective, with significant delays in reporting that are not conducive to near real-time process improvement. For example, for the Hospital Readmission Reduction Program, CMS calculates the payment reduction for each hospital based on its performance during the Hospital Readmission Reduction Program performance period (July 1, 2017, to December 1, 2019, for FY 2022) using administrative data to measure the excess readmission ratio against weighted peer groups.[139] These reports add value to internal reporting by publishing comparative ratings, raise the visibility of the organization, and illustrate the overall relevance of the healthcare quality profession. Adhering to some best practices—outlined next—to the management of reporting activities for different payment programs will make reporting more efficient and effective.

*Maintain a program inventory.* Document all voluntary and mandatory value-based reporting programs in which the organization participates, including program name, sponsor (i.e., Medicare, Aetna), local initiative, data sources, submission process, tools, dates, and owner. Include any supporting documentation such as relevant websites, educational and thought leadership organizations, and internal executive sponsors.

*Assign a primary owner.* Measure management and reporting is a team effort; however, assigning a single point of contact will ensure accountability. This resource has responsibility for maintaining and sharing knowledge about the program changes, updates, or risks with executive and other stakeholders. Partnering the primary owner with appropriate IT and data acquisition staff ensures continuity of the process. The primary owners will be the foundation of the reporting team.

*Publish a reporting calendar.* Create transparency to the reporting process for each program by publishing a calendar of relevant activities such as data submission dates, review and correction time frames, and public release dates. For CMS programs, the hospital has 30 days to review hospital-specific reports data and respond with corrections prior to public reporting.[140] Visibility to these dates will ensure adequate staff expertise is available during that time frame. Utilizing tools such as SharePoint or Microsoft Teams promotes visibility to all stakeholders.

*Establish a cadence of communication.* No one needs more meetings but scheduling well-planned communication will add value to the reporting practices. The primary program owner should meet on a weekly basis with IT counterparts. These can be 15-minute stand-up meetings or briefings to discuss current risks or barriers to reporting. The reporting team should meet monthly to identify any cross-functional barriers, share best practices, and evaluate measure results. Communication with the executive leadership team is a standard process; include measure reporting on the agenda particularly in relation to the public release of reports.

*Prepare a consumer facing response.* As many programs make measure results publicly available, it is a best practice for quality leaders to engage the organization's marketing and legal departments to create consumer-facing messaging about the results. For example, The Leapfrog Group encourages hospitals to advertise its A ratings for quality and safety. However, if reports are less than favorable, the organization should have a policy on how it will respond to inquiries from the media and patients and who is authorized to respond.

Value-based and targeted incentive programs use quality measures in their quality improvement, public reporting, and pay-for-reporting programs for specific healthcare providers. Using CMS as an example, understanding the measure construct and life cycle enables the healthcare quality professional to better analyze the data, make improvement recommendations, and monitor progress. **Figure 2.14** outlines the CMS measure life cycle.

CMS provides a highly structured mechanism for developing measures as clarity, reliability, and repeatability are vital when producing measures on a national scale. However, the definitions are applicable when defining local measures that the organization uses to reflect quality. CMS identified five critical steps in measure development:

1. Define the data source(s).
2. Develop specification and definitions.
3. Specify codes and code systems.
4. Aggregate and calculate measures.
5. Document measures.

Payment programs will provide a compendium of measures under which an organization will be evaluated. It is important to understand the data sources and acquisition requirements for each to ensure that the organization has both the data to support the measures and the infrastructure to acquire the data. This may be through the manual collection of data, patient surveys, or secondary use of electronic data.

Data can be acquired from several sources, the strength of each lending varying levels of reliability and usability for the measure. It is helpful to understand the types of data acquisition that may be needed. **Figure 2.15** outlines the type of data sources typically available with additional discussion on more common sources.

## Administrative Data

Administrative data, also known as patient billing data, is created as a by-product of the patient care process. The National Uniform Billing Committee established standardized methodology for submitting Medicare claims[141] that includes patient demographics, type and volume of service, care location, amount billed and reimbursed, and diagnosis and procedure codes. Because this data set is available electronically across all payers and is easily accessible, it is commonly used as a foundation for public reporting. Despite the time lag and limited clinical information, quality experts view administrative data as a useful source for measuring hospital quality.[142] With the expansion of eCQMs and the use of electronic data, manual data collection has dropped to a minimum.

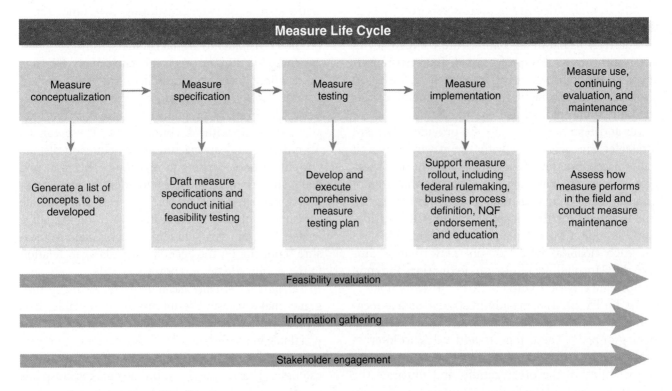

**Figure 2.14** CMS Measure Life Cycle

| Type of Data Source | Strengths | Limitations |
|---|---|---|
| **Claims** | • Readily available<br>• Uses standard coding system(s)<br>• Offers information not usually found in a clinical database<br>• Less burdensome to measured entities or data collection<br>• Drawn from large populations | • Only includes information recorded for billing purposes and not specifically for quality measurement<br>• Varying degrees of clinical detail<br>• Often limited in content, completeness, timeliness, and accuracy |
| **Electronic Clinical Data** | • Reduced cost of accessing clinical information from the patient medical record or personal health device (e.g., home blood glucose monitor) | • Identifying test sites to serve as data sources can be difficult<br>• Extracting the data requires expertise, time, and money<br>• Continued use of paper notes for point of care documentation presents an obstacle<br>• Device data may be external to the patient medical record<br>• Still only partially implemented in most settings |
| **Instruments/Standardized Patient Assessments** | • Well validated and tested | • Potential for bias because some have mixed use for determining reimbursement, meeting conditions of participation, and assessing quality<br>• May be proprietary |
| **Paper Patient Medical Records** | • Detailed clinical data with a rich description of care<br>• Includes clinically relevant information | • Labor-intensive and expensive to abstract<br>• Subjectivity and consistency concerns during abstraction<br>• Difficult to identify test sites |
| **Electronic Patient Medical Records** | • Detailed clinical data with a rich description of care<br>• Reduced cost of accessing clinical information | • Difficult to identify test sites<br>• Inconsistent adoption of EHRs<br>• Data extraction requires special expertise<br>• Structured data fields and drop-downs can reduce the richness of the clinical data |
| **Surveys** | • Established way of collecting patient perspective/experience<br>• Structured data far reporting<br>• Unique data source | • Limited scope<br>• May be labor-intensive and costly to implement<br>• Need validated and reliable instruments, which may be proprietary |
| **Registries** | • Includes detailed clinical information in structured fields<br>• Multiple data sources and care settings<br>• Can be available for electronic upload | • High cost of use<br>• Typically limited to specific clinical areas<br>• Unknown how registry requirements impact workflow<br>• Feasibility of data collection is determined by the data requirements imposed by the registry |

**Figure 2.15** Type of Data Source, Strengths, and Limitations for Measure Development

Reproduced from Centers for Medicare & Medicaid Services. *Quality Measures: How They Are Developed, Used, & Maintained.* September. 2021:11. Accessed January 11, 2022. https://www.cms.gov/files/document/quality-measures-how-they-are-developed-used-maintained.pdf

There remain some instances where medical record review is required to gather data that is either not available electronically or needs a more qualitative review. In this case, a clear definition of the data collection rules is required, including source, key terms, exclusions, timeframe, and so on.

## Claims

Claims data differ from administrative data in that it typically describes what the payer reimbursed the provider for care. The data must be acquired from the payer and can be as much as 45 days old. It is the source of data that insurers rely on for HEDIS reporting. Since the data reflect what is paid for a specific population (i.e., patients enrolled in a specific payer plan regardless of where the care was delivered), it can be used to determine if care was delivered out of network.

## Electronic Health Record

The Health Information Technology for Economic and Clinical Health Act of 2009 helped advance the adoption and meaningful use of EHRs.[143] In 2021, 72.3% of office-based physicians used a certified EHR/electronic medical record system.[144] As of 2016, 98% of all hospitals had demonstrated meaningful use and/or adopted an EHR.[145] The widespread use of the EHR has improved the ability to acquire rich clinical detail and lend credibility to quality measurement and reporting. When claims data are augmented by clinical data, the measure has a greater degree of specificity.

## Patient Surveys

Surveys provide direct access to the patient to assess experience and satisfaction with the healthcare provider and provides critical data needed to improve services, understand perceptions of care, and signal potential disparities in care. The Affordable Care Act of 2010 included HCAHPS as one of the measures to calculate results in the Hospital Value-Based Purchasing program, beginning with discharges in October 2012.[146] Organizations use a certified third party to survey clients directly or use a third party to capture the information by mail, telephone, or website.

## Patient-Reported Outcomes

Patient-reported outcomes are a mechanism for patients to self-report on health condition, functional status, symptoms, and health behaviors. The data come directly from the patient and are a rich source for measuring outcomes. The Patient-Reported Outcomes Measurement Information System tool is one example of an instrument to administer the survey and collect the data.[147]

## Meaningful Measures

With hundreds of quality metrics across dozens of government, commercial, and internal programs, data acquisition and measure curation has been burdensome and time consuming for clinicians as well as those who aggregate and report on the data. Introduced in 2017, the Meaningful Measures' objective was to reduce the number of Medicare quality measures, ease the burden on users, and prioritize patients over paperwork. As of March 2021, CMS reduced the number of Medicare

quality measures by 18%, saving more than 3 million hours of time and a projected $128 million.[148]

Meaningful Measures 2.0 moves from measure reduction to measure modernization with the following objectives:

- Focus on key quality domains and measures of highest value and impact cutting across all settings of care.
- Align measures across value-based programs and across partners, including CMS, federal agencies, private entities, and registries.
- Prioritize outcomes and patient-reported measures.
- Transform measures to fully digital by 2025 and incorporate all-payer data by accelerating to fully electronic measures.
- Develop and implement measures that reflect social and economic determinants.

An important aspect of the Meaningful Measures initiative is the move toward self-reported health and the voice of the patient in quality of care. An example of using the patient's voice is embedding measures into the workflow using the Patient-Reported Outcomes Measurement Information System tools to capture health status in real time, such as patient-reported pain, fatigue, emotional distress, functional status, and social role participation.[149] **Figure 2.16** illustrates the framework.

Meaningful measures are not intended to replace any measure initiatives but are designed to increase measure alignment across CMS programs and other public and private initiatives to focus attention on measuring what matters. Key points for data management and reporting are listed in **Box 2.8**.

---

### Box 2.8  Key Points: Considerations for Data Management and Reporting

- Data governance is a core competency of the health IT discipline, components of which should involve the quality professional to ensure data accuracy, access, and reporting capabilities.
- Collaboration with multiple stakeholders, including technical, education, business intelligence, and marketing, is required to successfully manage the transition to eCQMs.
- CMS provides a highly structured mechanism for developing measures because clarity, reliability, and repeatability are vital when producing measures on a national scale.
- The CMS Measure Inventory Tool is a key resource for identifying status of measures, measure definitions, and calculations.
- The Meaningful Measures 2.0 program is reducing the number of measures and focusing key domains, outcome priorities, and measure alignment across multiple programs with the goal to transform measures to fully digital by 2025.

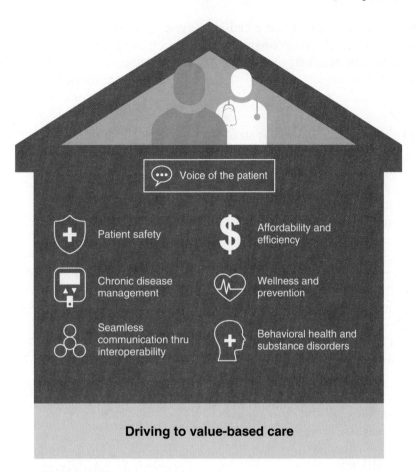

**Figure 2.16** Meaningful Measures Framework 2.0

Reproduced from Centers for Medicare & Medicaid Services. *Meaningful Measures 2.0: Moving from Measure Reduction to Modernization.* March 31, 2021. Accessed January 11, 2022. https://www.cms.gov/meaningful-measures-20-moving-measure-reduction-modernization

# Quality and Accountability

In May 2001, The Joint Commission announced four initial core measurement areas for hospitals, which included acute myocardial infarction and heart failure.[150] This initiative to create standardized quality measures was soon joined by CMS in a joint effort to align measure specifications across both entities. Commercial quality management solutions, initially designed to support the collection, aggregation, and submission of data to regulatory agencies, flooded the market. Today, through vendor consolidation, these solutions have evolved into a range of robust tools that may combine quality management, risk management, case management, and patient safety management with comparative data and advanced analytics. The healthcare quality professional is uniquely positioned to evaluate those solutions and advise leadership on quality tools that

- best fit in their organizational systems,
- enable improved performance on quality metrics, and
- support both internal and external reporting needs.

There are some key capabilities of the vendor/product that the organization should consider in the evaluation of a quality management solution.

## Organizational Structure

Size and scope of the buying organization will drive the capabilities required in a quality management solution. Quality management solutions range in functionality from regulatory reporting-only solutions to fully integrated quality, risk, safety, and case management solutions, and the type of system required depends on organizational structure, budget, and overall quality management strategy. Integrated solutions (quality, risk, care management, etc.) offer the promise of streamlined data acquisition of the core patient data (i.e., collect data once and use for multiple applications). This strategy can be especially impactful for the large integrated health networks who need to scale across many entities. However, organizations who participate in more complex value-based programs will need to look closely at the capabilities of the solution to ensure that it can support the more complex value-based programs. When organizations have budget and staffing constraints, a careful review of requirements may determine that only regulatory reporting capabilities are needed.

## Interoperability

Organizations may lean toward a single vendor strategy, centered around the EHR, to limit the number of suppliers, improve interoperability, and lower IT costs, yet there are several reasons that a quality management solution should augment the EHR. While the EHR clinical decision support capabilities are essential to quality management, the EHR may not contain a fully integrated suite of products for quality *measurement*. Furthermore, while errors are documented in the medical record, the incident report and follow-up actions are stored outside the EHR. Electronic clinical quality measures rely on electronic submissions of data to CMS and should be available to the quality management solution for additional reporting and analytics. It is therefore important that the quality management solution supports interactive data exchange to and from the EHR and other critical systems used by the organization.

## Analytics Capabilities

Any quality management system will have standard reports for viewing results. Digital distribution of reports with user-specific security is important to ensure stakeholder access to the measures. The export of calculated measures to other systems such as business decision support or other visualization tools provides the framework for an integrated view of quality, cost, and revenue outcomes. Beyond the standard reports, healthcare quality professionals should determine the level of analytics available—for example, multiple layers of segmentation—and they should drill through functionality to view different slices of data, flexible date ranges, guided analytics, and robust, flexible, embedded statistical process control graphical display. Usability is a key feature that will increase utilization and ensure adoption of the measures results. Online training enables users to refresh their knowledge on a just-in-time basis and provides an efficient method of educating new users.

## Vendor Support

In addition to product capabilities, it is important to assess the vendor from both a support and service perspective to determine the focus on continuous improvement and investment in the product life cycle. Quality management vendors must stay up to date on regulatory reporting requirements and are accountable for providing the most current measure definitions to their customers on a timely basis. Product delivery delays can impact the organization's ability to comply with regulatory standards and result in a financial impact. Vendors may also be asked by the organization to provide documentation of their security and privacy infrastructure to address technical, physical, and administrative safeguards.[151]

The service philosophy of a vendor is important to understand as it may impact the skill sets needed by the organization. The importance of tactics such as availability of support staff, customer portals for self-service support and peer-to-peer networking, and service line agreements for support turnaround and escalations should be considered. Vendors may offer additional fee-for-service consultation consisting of subject matter experts who can assist in gaining higher return on investment and greater value for the organization. Vendors may also provide optimization services at no cost, aimed at increasing product adoption and utilization.

## Decision Making

Conducting due diligence on any potential product purchase and soliciting the collaboration of strategic, financial, and technical stakeholders will empower the healthcare quality professional to advise leadership in the decision-making process. **Table 2.7** provides a sample checklist for matching the organization's strategic needs with solution capabilities. This is not an exhaustive list. Features and capabilities should be agreed upon by the decision-making team.

## Continuous Learning

With the multitude of reporting requirements across payment models and the magnitude of change that occurs in the measures, maintaining compliance with regulations, standards, and policies for measure reporting can be challenging for the healthcare organization. It is the role of the healthcare quality professional to adopt a practice of staying informed about changes that impact payment and quality measures. According to S. McClain (verbal communication, November 2021), a day in the life of the healthcare quality professional includes some form of continuing education on regulatory changes and the management of quality measures,

**Table 2.7** Evaluation Checklist for Quality Management Product Selection

| Capability Set | Y | Partial | No | Future |
|---|---|---|---|---|
| Prebuilt indicators for regulatory reporting and submission | ☐ | ☐ | ☐ | ☐ |
| Intuitive, self-serve reporting | ☐ | ☐ | ☐ | ☐ |
| Data visualization and configuration | ☐ | ☐ | ☐ | ☐ |
| Breadth and depth of benchmarking | ☐ | ☐ | ☐ | ☐ |
| Workflow for uploading and accessing data | ☐ | ☐ | ☐ | ☐ |
| Timeliness of data | ☐ | ☐ | ☐ | ☐ |
| Data integration and aggregation from multiple sources | ☐ | ☐ | ☐ | ☐ |
| Statistical analysis | ☐ | ☐ | ☐ | ☐ |
| Timely regulatory updates | ☐ | ☐ | ☐ | ☐ |
| Integration with safety, risk, and case management solutions | ☐ | ☐ | ☐ | ☐ |
| Risk adjustment | ☐ | ☐ | ☐ | ☐ |
| Scalability | ☐ | ☐ | ☐ | ☐ |
| Consultation, optimization available | ☐ | ☐ | ☐ | ☐ |
| Support availability | ☐ | ☐ | ☐ | ☐ |
| Service level agreement for support turnaround and escalations | ☐ | ☐ | ☐ | ☐ |
| Self-service support | ☐ | ☐ | ☐ | ☐ |
| Consultation and access to subject matter experts | ☐ | ☐ | ☐ | ☐ |
| Availability of optimization services | ☐ | ☐ | ☐ | ☐ |
| Online peer-to-peer networking | ☐ | ☐ | ☐ | ☐ |
| Virtual or on-site user forums | ☐ | ☐ | ☐ | ☐ |
| Other | ☐ | ☐ | ☐ | ☐ |

such as attending webinars, reading newsletters, or reviewing the *Federal Register*. The more information that can be curated, the better prepared the organization will be to adopt the necessary changes. Some best practices with sources of information are outlined next.

- *CMS email list and* MLN Connects *newsletter.* Subscribing to the CMS distribution list provides information of program requirements and milestones, policy changes, upcoming events, answers to frequently asked questions, official resources, and more. Subscribers can set or change as many preferences as desired, for example, they can subscribe to the Promoting Interoperability Program, CMS Coverage, or Measures Management System, and they can receive email notifications in real time, daily, or weekly.[152]

- *CMS webinars and events.* As part of the CMS Measure Management System, CMS sponsors the MMS Info Sessions at the official CMSHHS-gov channel on YouTube.[153] The objective of this forum is to engage stakeholders and the public in the design and development of quality measures that impact patient outcomes and value-based payment. The ongoing library of topics utilizes tutorials and videos to present topics such as digital measures, patient-centered quality measures, measures under review, technical assistance, resources for code set updates, and much more. Additional offerings from the MMS Info Sessions team include the following:
  - Annual series of webinars on high-priority CMS topics
  - Ongoing webinars
  - Stakeholder electronic mailing lists
  - Development and promotion of emerging tools and resources
  - MACRA-specific education and outreach

- *Public comment process.* Another best practice is to participate on the development of measures by providing input based on expertise for new or continuing measures. CMS depends on users of a measure to offer support, differing perspectives, or alternatives. As part of the rule making process to develop and finalize quality measures, CMS provides a mechanism for interested parties to comment on a measure. The request usually occurs as the measure is under development or undergoing maintenance. The measure developer posts requests for comment on the MMS website and the public is invited to comment on measures in development, under consideration, proposed for adoption, or under maintenance. Calls for comments are usually posted online for 2 weeks, making it essential that healthcare quality professionals enroll to receive notifications results from CMS.

- *The Joint Commission.* The Commission offers educational measurement-related webinars on topics such as performance measures, reporting requirements, and topics focused on clinical, technical, and statistical aspects of both eCQMs and chart-abstracted measures used for accreditation and certification purposes. On-demand topics include a library of eCQM expert-to-expert sessions to help hospitals improve eCQM data use, short 2- to 3-minute videos defining technical aspects of eCQMs, and general sessions that provide information by pioneers in quality on such topics as measurement requirements and changes in reporting.[154]

- *EHR vendor.* Any certified EHR vendor must provide regulatory software updates in a timely manner. As a result, each vendor has a regulatory team that is knowledgeable about upcoming regulations requiring modification to the software or the documentation. Vendors will typically provide weekly education to the healthcare organization to make stakeholders aware of changes, and, when necessary, software changes will be available. The EHR vendor will provide guidance or consultation to organizations to ensure that the required documentation is available and that reports are updated to meet reporting and data submission guidelines.

- *Regulatory and compliance team.* Because of the dynamic nature of measure regulations, establishing a team of subject matter experts across multiple disciplines reduces the risk of missing a critical update or depending on a single source of this knowledge to maintaining regulatory updates. Communication with this team is vital. Establishing a cadence of meetings with subject matter experts to provide measure updates and discuss and resolve issues is a best practice.

Key points on quality and accountability are listed in **Box 2.9**.

# Sharing Performance Results

Healthcare leaders are faced with unprecedented amounts of information and dozens of decisions

---

**Box 2.9  Key Points: Quality and Accountability**

- The growth of value-based reimbursement necessitates a more collaborative relationship between providers and payers of healthcare.
- Modeling the impact of new payment contracts for revenue gained or lost, combined with cost and quality of care provides insights into the value of the program.
- Strong collaboration between the quality, managed care, and financial leaders is a best practice that yields the most successful contract negotiation, compliance, and management for the organization.
- Healthcare policy can change rapidly, so it is necessary for the healthcare quality professional to be aware of current and pending changes to health payment reform by being aware of external forums and thought leadership organizations.
- The healthcare quality professional is uniquely positioned to evaluate quality management solutions and advise leadership on quality tools that are a best fit in their organizational systems, that can enable improved performance on quality metrics, and that support both internal and external reporting needs.

---

to make every day. The processing capacity of the conscious mind has been estimated at 120 bits per second—the information "speed limit." Listening to one person speak requires half of that bandwidth.[155] When multiplied by the number of stakeholders in a board meeting, for example, where complex decisions need to be made, the difficulty of concentration and understanding becomes exponential. While the brain can filter and process the information overload, it can have trouble sorting through that which is most important and urgent.

Communication of organizational performance is a key competency of the healthcare quality professional as a function of accountability. Achieving measurable results in healthcare performance requires putting meaningful information in the hands of accountable stakeholders to instill knowledge and inspire action. This activity transcends the scheduled distribution of weekly or monthly reports and requires the healthcare quality professional to play an active role in ensuring that quality measures are understood, relevant, and actionable by the stakeholder.

Effective communication is a skill that can and should be practiced and perfected. There are myriad publications, websites, and workshops that offer advice on skills and methods to improve communication. Healthcare organizations may offer training and education on how to improve interpersonal communications with patients, peers, and physicians. However, the healthcare quality professional faces a unique set of challenges when it comes to communicating the findings and required actions from multiple measures and numerous programs to a diverse set of stakeholders.

## Know the Audience

The two hemispheres of the human brain specialize in distinct mental functions—for example, different aspects of visual perception. In general, the left hemisphere controls a person's logical and verbal functions, while the right hemisphere is in charge of nonverbal and intuitive functions; however, most behaviors and abilities require activity in both halves of the brain.[156] The healthcare organization functions in much the same way with a "central nervous system" where multiple disciplines, each with a different mental model, need to connect to make strategic decisions. The healthcare quality professional brings a unique perspective to the decision-making table because of the multidisciplinary interactions that must occur to gain consensus on a desired action or outcome. When communicating the results of quality measures, it is important to know the audience, and appreciate its span of control and how it perceives the data.

Financial leaders may view *outcomes* through an organizational lens of cost, revenue, and margin, while the clinical leaders hold a patient perspective of human caring, mortality, or return to functional status. A conversation about readmissions may evoke failed transitions of care for any readmission for the clinician, while the finance leaders are concerned with penalties incurred for the subset of patients targeted by the CMS Readmissions Reduction Program.

For healthcare quality professionals, it is important to appreciate the nuance of healthcare finance.[157] Learning the financial vocabulary will enrich the conversations across disciplines and increase the credibility of the quality professional as a valued voice in healthcare business decisions. **Table 2.8** describes some common perspectives.

## Build a Common Vocabulary

Language barriers across countries, dialects, even regional accents, and the use of slang can lead to misinterpretation of meaning in the process of communication. Healthcare is no different in that it is laden with its own vocabulary intended to convey meaning in a concise manner. Abbreviations and acronyms are so common in healthcare that organizations prohibit the use of those that can be confusing and dangerous. An example is The Joint Commission's Do Not Use List, a list of abbreviations that should never be used in documentation.[158]

**Table 2.8** Financial and Quality Perspectives

| Topic | Financial Perspective | Quality Perspective |
|---|---|---|
| Outcomes | Margins | Mortality, functional status |
| Readmissions | Reimbursement penalty | Transitions of care |
| Risk management | Case mix index | Severity of illness |
| Staffing | Payroll/productivity | Staff-to-bed ratios |
| Bad debt | Unpaid % by payer | Medically underserved |
| Value basis | Payment | Care delivery |

Healthcare leaders may find that a different vocabulary used across clinical and financial disciplines can impede the intent and understanding of a conversation. While the topic of discussion may be understood, the details may not. In a discussion about what measures best reflect organizational performance in a topic of discussion, varying perspectives could lead to inconsistent actions.

## Reframe Positive Outcomes

Research suggests that the human brain has a bias toward remembering negative events, sometimes clouding how people think and behave.[159] This can be especially challenging in healthcare quality where reporting oftentimes focuses on negative findings (i.e., mortality and morbidity, never events, failure mode analyses, near misses, and outliers). Positive psychology suggests that the brain has the capacity to filter the lens through which an issue is viewed and impact business outcomes.[160] Drawing on best practices in communication from healthcare and other industries, presentations, reports, and key messages, the healthcare quality professional can reframe the message to the audience to encourage a positive lens. Leveraging competencies discussed in the *Health Data Analytics* and *Quality Leadership and Integration* sections, the healthcare quality professional can influence accountability for innovative ideas, positive actions, and healthy quality behaviors. Achor's TED Talk, "The Happy Secret to Better Work," on positive psychology suggests that if the lens can be changed, then the educational and business outcomes are changed at the same time.[160]

## Storytelling

Storytelling is a powerful means of communication. It existed long before written human history as a means of entertaining, providing safety, sharing traditions, and passing down knowledge and morals from one generation to the next. Stories are told through words, pictures, photography, videos, and, today, social media. Stories contain wisdom, teach, give knowledge about how to act, and encourage motivation to act.

In healthcare, stories take on new meaning. For example, narrative medicine uses a patient-centered approach to understand suffering, disability, ailment, and personhood in the practice of medicine and care for the patient holistically.[161] Every patient has a story that extends before, during, and after the parameters of the current illness. The role of the healthcare quality professional is to present the collective patient story and motivate multiple stakeholders to take an action that improves the value of care for the patient, population, and organization.

There are many resources available for building and improving storytelling capabilities including podcasts, blogs, and websites, TED Talks, and books.[162–165] Leveraging this body of knowledge informs a three-part framework for storytelling in healthcare quality that appeals to the intellect with data (analysis), engages the emotions with real-life stories that inform and inspire (relevance), and builds on a foundation of credibility and confidence (trust).

### Analysis

Analysis is the foundation for the story of healthcare quality. How the foundation is built requires creating clarity for your audience. The role of a healthcare quality professional is to find and tell the story in a way that is meaningful to stakeholders who can make a difference. Analytics—spreadsheets, dashboards, public data, star ratings, patient charts—appeals to the intellect of your audience (i.e., logical, factual arguments). In Aristotle's persuasion principles, the *Art of Rhetoric*, this is Logos.[166] The quality professional needs to communicate measure results so that they resonate with a disparate set of stakeholders from frontline caregivers to health leaders and executives.

### Presenting Best Practices

The goal of storytelling is to take complex ideas and make them relatable to the audience. Once the data are collected, analysis is done, and relevance and trust are established, the information must be conveyed to stakeholders in a meaningful way that facilitates rational, repeatable, defensible decision making.

Eighty-two seconds into the launch of the space shuttle Columbia in 2003, a piece of foam struck the shuttle's wing. To help NASA officials assess the damage while the shuttle was still in flight, Boeing engineers prepared three reports containing a total of 28 Microsoft PowerPoint slides explaining the debris impact. The conclusion by NASA officials was the shuttle was safe and no further action needed.[167] Unfortunately, that was not the case. Tufte, a Yale professor and leading expert on visualization of data, was brought on by NASA to participate in the accident review board. He famously analyzed the slides used to assess the damage and concluded that the presentation misled the audience.[168] In his book, *Beautiful Evidence*, Tufte devotes an entire chapter to the consequences of the misuse of PowerPoint including lack of clarity, misleading bullets, too much clutter, and the like.[169]

In the world of business communication, PowerPoint became the industry standard for presentations. While the tool itself is effective, how the message is presented and perceived can influence the decisions that are made and lend credibility to the healthcare quality professional's role as a trusted advisor. An informal survey in 2020 of 14 healthcare business leaders suggests key barriers to creating effective presentations.[170] The barriers are consistent with many of Tufte's recommendations (**Table 2.9**).

### Visualizing Data

Reports are simply a record of the findings of the data aggregation from which the analysis can be formed. Reports can be produced in many forms from Microsoft Excel or Microsoft Word to dashboards to interactive visualization. They serve to inform the user about the results of the quality measure calculations and the associated attributes and should be accurate and clearly defined. To make the quality report impactful, it needs to hold the user's attention, clearly direct the user to the salient points that need to be made, and be actionable. Reports should be designed to appeal to the reader at first glance, point to what information is important, and have easy-to-find points of interest.[171] When designing paper-based reports (i.e., printed Excel, Word, or PDF documents, these tips are useful; **Table 2.10**).

Business intelligence and data visualization tools enable the organization to configure reports into dashboards that enable stakeholder-specific, self-service analysis. Many organizations have developed BI standards for how a dashboard should be structured including color, font, drill paths, logo placement, etc.

**Table 2.9** Key Barriers to Creating Effective Presentations

| Issue | Discussion | Resolution |
|---|---|---|
| Dense and cluttered slides | It is tempting to put a lot of data on the slide, but when slides are overly dense, it is difficult for the audience to focus on a key message. Too many concepts at one time can be confusing. | ■ Use a balance of white space.<br>■ Limit the number of levels (second level, third level, fourth level, fifth level bullets).<br>■ Keep one concept per slide.<br>■ In the 16:9 format, use no more than four images (graphs, tables, etc.); and no more than two images in the 4:3 format. |
| Reading the slides | The audience can read the slides for themselves; reading the slide may indicate too much content. | ■ Use the bullets as a reminder of the additional detail to be discussed.<br>■ If it is necessary to have detailed sentences on the slide, a supplementation document may be warranted. |
| Font type and size | Admitting that a slide is an "eye chart" suggests that it is unreadable and cannot be consumed by the audience. | ■ Use a font size of at least 16 points.<br>■ When showing a dashboard or report with a lot of data, crop out the important points and make the image larger. |
| Graphics | Over- and underuse of graphics can be detrimental to the presentation. | ■ If used well, graphics appeal to visual learners.<br>■ Do not overuse animation and transitions—it can be distracting, and if viewers are using Zoom, there can be delays and choppy transitions.<br>■ Make sure the pictures are relevant to the topic; use a picture to tee up a discussion and back it up by pertinent points.<br>■ Make sure the graphics can be easily read. |
| Color and design | Poor color choices, or dark fonts on dark background, asymmetry, mix and match fonts, mix of lower- and uppercase fonts from slide to slide appears to lack professionalism needed to persuade the audience. | ■ Healthcare organizations typically use a branded PowerPoint template designed by the marketing department.<br>■ Adhering to the style guide lends professionalism to the presentation. |
| Time management | Too many slides to review in the time allotted; rushing through slides and running out of time for audience questions is disrespectful. | ■ Anticipate an average of 3 minutes per slide to assess the amount of content that will be shared.<br>■ Add a buffer to the time frame (i.e., for a 1-hour presentation plan for 45 minutes of content).<br>■ Always finish five minutes early in case your audience members need to get to another meeting. |
| Set the objective | Presentation objectives can be either informing, educating, or selling (i.e., they need to make a go/no go decision—do not skip around or talk ahead). | ■ State up front what the audience should learn, think, or do at the end of the presentation. |
| Spelling and grammar | Misspelled words and poor use of grammar will distract the audience from the key message. | ■ Always spell/grammar check<br>■ If time allows, have a colleague review the content. |

When designing dashboards, the healthcare quality professional should consider applying the same principles used in journalism—the inverted pyramid, which is illustrated in **Figure 2.17**.

The inverted pyramid, which has its roots in the 1800s and the telegraph, divides content into three categories: the lead, the body, and the tail.[172] The lead is the most important or relevant and is at the top.

Like a news story headline, in the context of dashboards, this would include the most significant information such as high-level indicators with directional value of the outcome (i.e., how close the metric is to expected and which direction it is going). The body, or supporting information, is in the middle. This would include trends and comparison data supportive of the top level (i.e., reminiscent of the old newspaper

**Table 2.10** **Preparing Audience-Relatable Reports**

| Attributes of the Report | Description |
|---|---|
| Has a clear purpose | Include title, report criteria such as cohort, time frame, exclusions, exceptions, and so on. Add comments to ensure the reader understands the intent of the report and why they should care. |
| Appears easy to read | Consider design elements such as layout, font type, size, and color. |
| Contains visuals that reinforce the content | Visuals should reflect the subject matter of your content. |
| Is easy to navigate and pick up the main points | Guide the user through the report with consistent navigation signals. |
| Has charts and graphs that are easy to understand | Keep the layout clean and uncluttered. |
| Uses consistent and meaningful color | Use color sparingly to pick out important patterns. |

Data from Agency for Healthcare Research and Quality. Six tips for making a quality report appealing and easy to skim. Page last reviewed October 2019. Accessed January 11, 2022. https://www.ahrq.gov/talkingquality /resources/design/general-tips/index.html

vernacular "above the fold"). The tail is background and is in the details at the bottom. An example of the inverted pyramid follows in **Figure 2.18**.

For more on reporting, see the *Health Data Analytics* section.

### Relevance

Analytics must be supported by relevant, real-life situations that support the data and reinforce the need to act. Aristotle calls this "pathos," persuading the audience by appealing to their emotions. Wang, a global ethnographer, calls it the "human narrative," the human insights missing from big data.[173] Once conclusions are drawn from the analysis, it is important to assess the human component to determine factors that do not present in the data. Consider the observations or questions in **Table 2.11** to analyze cost contributors.

Interviews with physicians, nurses, and other caregivers and focus groups with patients and community leaders can yield knowledge beyond the data and impact the magnitude and urgency of decisions that need to be made.

### Trust

The third component of the storytelling framework is trust. Aristotle calls this "ethos"—appealing to ethics, morals, and character to inspire trust in the

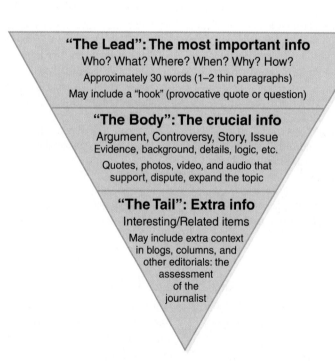

**Figure 2.17** Inverted Pyramid for Organizing Writing

Reproduced from NSCC and Rosemary Martinelli. Tools and tactics for the PR toolbox (Chapter 9). In: *The Evolving World of Public Relations: Beyond the Press Release*. NSCC; 2021. Accessed January 12, 2022. https://pressbooks.nscc.ca/evolvingpr/chapter/chapter-9-tools-and-tactics-for-the-pr-toolbox/#return -footnote-149-2

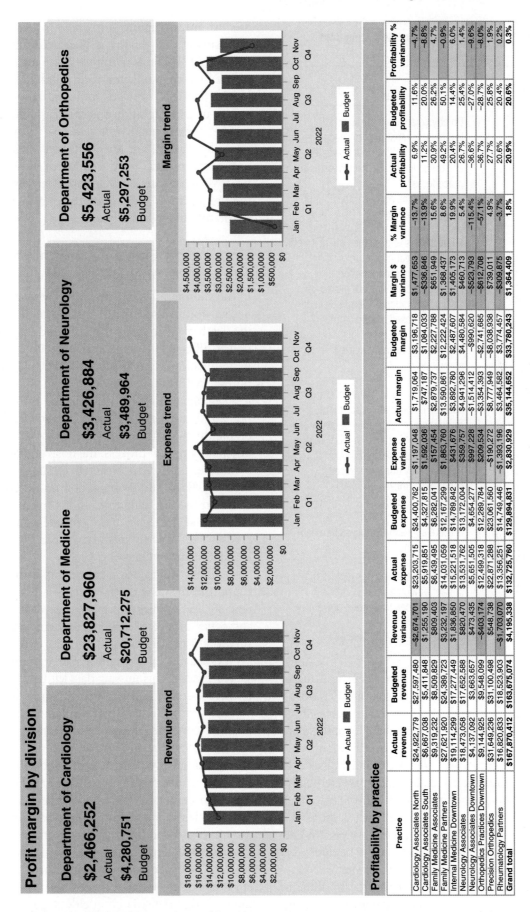

**Profit margin by division**

**Department of Cardiology**
$2,466,252
Actual
$4,280,751
Budget

**Department of Medicine**
$23,827,960
Actual
$20,712,275
Budget

**Department of Neurology**
$3,426,884
Actual
$3,489,964
Budget

**Department of Orthopedics**
$5,423,556
Actual
$5,297,253
Budget

Revenue trend · Expense trend · Margin trend

**Profitability by practice**

| Practice | Actual revenue | Budgeted revenue | Revenue variance | Actual expense | Budgeted expense | Expense variance | Actual margin | Budgeted margin | Margin $ variance | % Margin variance | Actual profitability | Budgeted profitability | Profitability % variance |
|---|---|---|---|---|---|---|---|---|---|---|---|---|---|
| Cardiology Associates North | $24,922,779 | $27,597,480 | −$2,674,701 | $23,203,715 | $24,400,762 | −$1,197,048 | $1,719,064 | $3,196,718 | $1,477,653 | −13.7% | 6.9% | 11.6% | −4.7% |
| Cardiology Associates South | $6,667,038 | $5,411,848 | $1,255,190 | $5,919,851 | $4,327,815 | $1,592,036 | $747,187 | $1,084,033 | −$336,846 | −13.9% | 11.2% | 20.0% | −8.8% |
| Family Medicine Associates | $9,319,232 | $8,509,829 | $809,403 | $6,439,495 | $6,282,041 | $157,454 | $2,879,737 | $2,227,788 | $651,949 | 15.6% | 30.9% | 26.2% | 4.7% |
| Family Medicine Partners | $27,621,920 | $24,389,723 | $3,232,197 | $14,031,059 | $12,167,299 | $1,863,760 | $13,590,861 | $12,222,424 | $1,368,437 | 8.6% | 49.2% | 50.1% | −0.9% |
| Internal Medicine Downtown | $19,114,299 | $17,277,449 | $1,836,850 | $15,221,518 | $14,789,842 | $431,676 | $3,892,780 | $2,487,607 | $1,405,173 | 19.9% | 20.4% | 14.4% | 6.0% |
| Neurology Associates | $18,473,058 | $17,652,588 | $820,470 | $13,531,762 | $13,172,004 | $359,757 | $4,941,296 | $4,480,584 | $460,713 | 5.4% | 26.7% | 25.4% | 1.4% |
| Neurology Associates Downtown | $4,137,092 | $3,663,657 | $473,435 | $5,651,505 | $4,654,277 | $997,228 | −$1,514,412 | −$990,620 | −$523,793 | −115.4% | −36.6% | −27.0% | −9.6% |
| Orthopedics Practices Downtown | $9,144,925 | $9,548,099 | −$403,174 | $12,499,318 | $12,289,784 | $209,534 | −$3,354,393 | −$2,741,685 | −$612,708 | −57.1% | −36.7% | −28.7% | −8.0% |
| Precision Orthopedics | $31,649,236 | $31,100,498 | $548,738 | $22,871,288 | $23,061,560 | −$190,272 | $8,777,949 | $8,038,938 | $739,011 | 4.9% | 27.7% | 25.8% | 1.9% |
| Rheumatology Partners | $16,820,833 | $18,523,903 | −$1,703,070 | $13,356,251 | $14,749,446 | −$1,393,196 | $3,464,582 | $3,774,457 | −$309,875 | −3.7% | 20.6% | 20.4% | 0.2% |
| **Grand total** | **$167,870,412** | **$163,675,074** | **$4,195,338** | **$132,725,760** | **$129,894,831** | **$2,830,929** | **$35,144,652** | **$33,780,243** | **$1,364,409** | **1.8%** | **20.9%** | **20.6%** | **0.3%** |

**Figure 2.18** Dashboard Example Using Inverted Pyramid

**Table 2.11** Considerations When Analyzing Cost Contributors

| Contributors to Cost | Questions to Answer |
|---|---|
| Physician decisions | ▪ Do physicians have product loyalties or sensitivity to specific products or vendors, for example, implants, diagnostic, and therapeutic procedures?<br>▪ Are physicians aware of the cost of drugs and implants? |
| Patient contribution | ▪ What SDOHs impact the patient's well-being and health outcomes?<br>▪ Are there other markers for comorbid conditions not picked up by the *International Classification of Diseases*–based risk adjustment?<br>▪ Are patients in a medically underserved or marginalized community? |
| Process variation | ▪ Do delays occur in high-traffic areas, such as emergency department throughput, or start time delays in the operating room? Are there backups in the intensive care unit?<br>▪ Does surgery duration exceed scheduled time?<br>▪ How do delays impact overtime and fatigue?<br>▪ Is there appropriate access to rehab/skilled nursing? |
| Unexpected outcomes | ▪ Are there increased risk factors that impact outcomes?<br>▪ Is there missed or delayed preventive care?<br>▪ Is there patient compliance? |

audience. While credibility and trust are used many times interchangeably, there is a subtle difference—credibility comes from the head, and trust comes from the heart.[174] Credibility requires reliability and expertise. Attributes like educational qualifications and subject matter expertise, references, and polish and confidence in presentation skills encompass credibility. Trust, on the other hand, must be earned and has much in common with character. It is the belief in the likelihood that a person will behave in certain ways.[175] While credibility suggests that if a task needs to be done, the owner *can* do it, trust suggests that the owner *will* do it.

The Quality Leadership and Integration dimension of NAHQ's competency framework exemplifies how to turn credibility into trust. The healthcare quality professional's role to direct the quality infrastructure provides instant credibility by assuring that quality is measured and managed. Presenting findings supported by evidence, augmented by human factors, and validated by industry knowledge that protects confidentiality earns audience trust. Engaging in interprofessional teamwork, the healthcare quality professional provides objective information, not for blame but for learning and improvement. Leading the audience through a logical process of analysis creates opportunities to advance the organization and elevate the quality professional to the role of trusted advisor.

### Enhancing Equity Through Analysis, Relevance, and Trust

In the summer of 2020, the city of Minneapolis, Minnesota, found itself in the middle of riots following the death of George Floyd at the hands of Minneapolis police officers. In neighboring St. Paul, HealthPartners Regions Hospital found itself in its own social unrest. With the diverse population of the Twin Cities, Regions had always made health equity a priority, but 2020 cast light on the need for increased focus on eliminating disparities in care. As part of its ongoing quality review process, the hospital's health equity committee found that, although the top box scores for their HCAHPS survey suggested no difference when stratified by race, language, and ethnicity, the experience of case managers and interpreters suggested otherwise. The "top box" is the most positive response to HCAHPS Survey items.

*Analysis.* At Regions, a partnership with the decision support team was a crucial success factor. The integration of race, ethnicity, and language data with clinical and experience data helped them identify a disparity in survey return rates, with communities of color returning surveys at a much lower rate despite oversampling by the survey vendor. This missing data left many populations underrepresented and their voices unheard.

*Relevance.* Rather than seek more surveys, the hospital convened focus groups among the diverse communities focusing first on its birth center, where 60% of patients who deliver are people of color and 25% need interpreters for their care. For example, the birth center partnered with the Hmong Health Care Professionals Coalition to learn more about the childbirth preferences of Hmong women. They learned that for centuries, Hmong women have adhered to a specific diet of chicken soup after delivery that was not offered by the hospital. After working with dietitians, Hmong elders, patients, and the resident Hmong chef at Regions, this became a special component of the childbirth experience.

*Trust.* Using real-life experience augmented the missing data and created an atmosphere of trust and credibility among the healthcare leaders, staff, patients, and community. In turn, patient and employee experiences improved, marking not only better scores but greater community partnership (S. Van Dyke, personal communication, December 2021). For a video summary of this story, see *Online Resources* at the end of the section.

Key points to sharing organizational performance results are listed in **Box 2.10**.

---

### Box 2.10 Key Points: Sharing Performance Results

- The healthcare quality professional must engage in effective communication to prevent information overload and help stakeholders with diverse responsibilities and mental models drive to consensus.
- Building a common vocabulary across clinical and financial disciplines can minimize misunderstandings about quality measures that lead to inconsistent actions.
- Use storytelling to present the collective patient story and motivate multiple stakeholders to take an action that improves the value of care for the patient, population, and organization.
- Transparency of quality, patient experience, and price enables patients to be a partner with the provider in decisions about their own care and treatment, producing better quality.
- Effective presentation skills and use of presentation tools are a must for the healthcare quality professional to convey meaning and drive credibility.

---

## Summary

As the cost of healthcare skyrockets, the need to share accountability for the value of the healthcare dollar implicates all stakeholders—providers, payers, suppliers, and patients. Reimbursement has become increasingly tied to clinical outcomes and processes, compelling the healthcare quality professional to take a central role in the analysis, review, interpretation, and communication of quality measures and participation in value-based programs. This section lays a foundation for an end-to-end strategy for managing quality review and accountability with value in mind.

Current and emerging payment models drive new relevance to quality metrics and their impact on revenue. Trends in healthcare payment reform lean toward value-based care with varying degrees of financial risk for the outcome of the patient as defined by quality metrics. It is imperative that the negotiation of new payment contracts include the healthcare quality professional to ensure that measures are relevant to and achievable by the organization because how quality metrics are defined within the contract has a direct impact on revenue.

While the relationship of cost and quality is complex, healthcare organizations need to have visibility to the cost of care and the impact of quality on that cost when negotiating a payment contract. Measuring the intersection of cost and quality helps to quantify and prioritize quality improvement initiatives and communicate the organization's performance through the lenses of both the provider and the payer. Organizational systems and processes need to leverage both quality management and cost analysis tools to align stakeholders to focus on key opportunities to improve.

Building a business case for quality requires an understanding of the potential impact of new payment contracts on revenue and how quality metrics impact the incentives or penalties that may be incurred by the organization. The healthcare quality professional is in a unique position to advise leadership on the types of tools that are needed to measure quality and model the impact of quality on each payment contract.

Participation in external forums to gain expertise about payment reform and its impact on quality, as well as providing input to measure development enables the healthcare quality professional to provide critical information for the strategic direction of the organization. Instilling a culture of collaboration across the organization begins with leadership and is bolstered by the expertise of the quality professional to implement strategies and tactics to support compliance with regulations, standards, and policies relevant to the types of measure requirements used in payment contracts. Utilizing tools for data acquisition activities, data management, measure calculation, and reporting, including stakeholder collaboration to interpret specifications for electronic measures reporting are key tactics for ensuring high reliability of quality measures. Building a strategic competency around presentation, communication, and transparency of quality measures empowers the healthcare quality professional to guide the organization through internal and external reporting initiatives, identify priorities for improvement, and equip clinicians with knowledge about their own performance.

This section, combined with others in *HQ Solutions,* prepares the healthcare quality professional to achieve the aim of value-based programs—better health outcomes, reduced expense, enhanced patient experience, and joy in work.

# References

1. Centers for Medicare & Medicaid Services. Office of the Actuary releases 2019 national health expenditures. Published December 16, 2020. Accessed November 1, 2021. https://www.cms.gov/newsroom/press-releases/cms-office-actuary-releases-2019-national-health-expenditures

2. Peterson Center on Healthcare Kaiser Family Foundation. How does health spending in the U.S. compare to other countries? Published December 23, 2020. Accessed October 28, 2021. https://www.healthsystemtracker.org/chart-collection/health-spending-u-s-compare-countries/

3. Mercado, SE. NAHQ's perspective on healthcare quality as business strategy, *J Healthc Qual.* 2020;42(2):65. doi:10.1097/JHQ.0000000000000250

4. Congress.gov. U.S. health care coverage and spending (congress.gov). Updated January 26, 2021. Accessed November 12, 2021. https://crsreports.congress.gov/product/pdf/IF/IF10830

5. Makary M, Daniel M. Medical error—the third leading cause of death in the US. *BMJ.* 2016;353:i2139.

6. Shrank W, Rogstad T, Parekh N. Waste in the US health care system: estimated costs and potential for savings. *JAMA.* 2019;322(15):1501-1509. doi:10.1001/jama.2019.13978

7. Health Payer Intelligence. Strategies to improve payer–provider relationship, data quality. Published November 4, 2019. Accessed January 5, 2022. https://healthpayerintelligence.com/news/strategies-to-improve-payer-provider-relationship-data-quality

8. The Advisory Board. Addressing the needs of your rising-risk patients. Updated February 1, 2018. Accessed January 6, 2022. https://www.advisory.com/topics/high-risk-patient-management/2018/02/addressing-the-needs-of-your-rising-risk-patients

9. Health Payer Intelligence. Using technology to close care gaps, improve care quality and cost. Published May 13, 2019. Accessed January 6, 2022. https://healthpayerintelligence.com/news/using-technology-to-close-care-gaps-improve-care-quality-and-cost

10. KaufmanHall. National hospital flash report. Published November 2021. Accessed December 21, 2021. https://www.kaufmanhall.com/sites/default/files/2021-11/nov.-2021-national-hospital-flash-report_final.pdf

11. Akinleye DD, McNutt LA, Lazariu V, McLaughlin CC. Correlation between hospital finances and quality and safety of patient care. *PLoS One.* 2019;14(8):e0219124. doi:10.1371/journal.pone.0219124

12. Agency for Healthcare Research and Quality. Estimating the additional hospital inpatient cost and mortality associated with selected hospital-acquired conditions. Rockville, MD: Agency for Healthcare Research and Quality. Content last reviewed November 2017. Accessed December 14, 2021. https://www.ahrq.gov/hai/pfp/haccost2017.html

13. Centers for Medicare & Medicaid Services. Hospital-Acquired Condition Reduction Program. https://www.cms.gov/Medicare/Medicare-Fee-for-Service-Payment/AcuteInpatientPPS/HAC-Reduction-Program.html

14. Weiner-Lastinger LM, Pattabiraman V, Konnor RY, et al. The impact of coronavirus disease 2019 (COVID-19) on healthcare-associated infections in 2020: a summary of data reported to the National Healthcare Safety Network. *Infect Control Hosp Epidemiol.* 2021;43(1):1-14. doi:10.1017/ice.2021.362

15. Hajjaj FM, Salek MS, Basra MK, Finlay AY. Non-clinical influences on clinical decision-making: a major challenge to evidence-based practice. *J R Soc Med.* 2010;103(5):178-187. doi:10.1258/jrsm.2010.100104

16. Wasterlain AS, Melamed E, Bello R, Karia R, Capo JT, Science of Variation Group. The effect of price on surgeons' choice of implants: a randomized controlled survey. *J Hand Surg Am.* 2017;42(8):593-601.e6. doi:10.1016/j.jhsa.2017.05.005

17. RevCycleIntelligence. Giving providers hospital cost accounting data will lower costs. Published July 5, 2018. Accessed December 23, 2021. https://revcycleintelligence.com/news/giving-providers-hospital-cost-accounting-data-will-lower-costs

18. Definitive Healthcare. Current procedural terminology (CPT). Accessed January 12, 2022. https://www.definitivehc.com/resources/glossary/current-procedural-terminology

19. Shah A, Course S. Building the business case for quality improvement: a framework for evaluating return on investment. *Future Healthc J.* 2018;5(2):132-137.

20. American Hospital Association. Evolving care models: Aligning care delivery to emerging payment models. Published 2019. Accessed November 8, 2021. https://www.aha.org/system/files/media/file/2019/04/MarketInsights_CareModelsReport.pdf

21. Geyman J. COVID-19 has revealed America's broken health care system: what can we learn? *Int J Health Serv.* 2021;51(2): 188-194. doi:10.1177/0020731420985640

22. Centers for Disease Control and Prevention. Introduction to COVID-19 racial and ethnic health disparities. Updated December 10, 2020. Accessed December 20, 2021. https://www.cdc.gov/coronavirus/2019-ncov/community/health-equity/racial-ethnic-disparities/index.html

23. Bradywood A, Leming-Lee TS, Watters R, Blackmore C. Implementing screening for social determinants of health using the Core 5 screening tool. *BMJ Open Qual.* 2021;10(3):e001362. doi:10.1136/bmjoq-2021-001362

24. Agency for Healthcare Quality and Research. Estimating the additional hospital inpatient cost and mortality associated with selected hospital-acquired conditions. Published November 2017. Accessed December 17, 2021. https://www.ahrq.gov/hai/pfp/haccost2017-results.html

25. Robert Wood Johnson Foundation. Medicaid's role in addressing social determinants of health. Published February 1, 2019. Accessed December 20, 2021. https://www.rwjf.org/en/library/research/2019/02/medicaid-s-role-in-addressing-social-determinants-of-health.html

26. Centers for Medicare & Medicaid Services. Medicare inpatient prospective payment system. Updated December 11, 2020. Accessed December 20, 2021. https://www.ahd.com/ip_ipps08.html#:~:text=The%20Medicare%20Inpatient%20Prospective%20Payment%20System%20%28IPPS%29%20was,paid%20a%20pre-determined%20rate%20for%20each%20Medicare%20admission

27. Very Well Health. Diagnostic related grouping and how it works. Updated November 25, 2020. Accessed December 20, 2021. https://www.verywellhealth.com/drg-101-what-is-a-drg-how-does-it-work-3916755#citation-7

28. Mercado S. The profession of healthcare quality focuses on improving healthcare by improving workforce competencies for quality and safety. *J Healthc Qual.* 2021;43(5):261-262. doi:10.1097/JHQ.0000000000000315

29. National Association of Health Care Quality. NAHQ's healthcare quality competency framework. Accessed December 20, 2021. https://nahq.org/nahq-intelligence/competency-framework/

30. Institute for Healthcare Improvement. Improvement tip: "quality" is not department. Published April 2021. Updated with comments May 5, 2018. Accessed December 20, 2021.

http://www.ihi.org/resources/Pages/ImprovementStories/ImprovementTipQualityIsNotaDepartment.aspx#:~:text=Quality%20is%20not%20a%20program%20or%20a%20project%3B,Director%20is%20basically%20the%20coach%2C%20facilitator%20and%20cheerleader

31. Aetna. Better health at lower costs: why we need value-based care now. Published March 2019. Accessed December 17, 2021. https://www.aetna.com/employers-organizations/resources/value-based-care.html

32. Agency for Healthcare Research and Quality. Comparative health system performance initiative. AHRQ Pub. No. 16(17)-0040-EF; 2016. Accessed January 11, 2022. https://www.ahrq.gov/sites/default/files/wysiwyg/chsp/chsp-fact-sheet-0717.pdf

33. Heeringa J, Mutti A, Furukawa MF, Lechner A, Maurer KA, Rich E. Horizontal and vertical integration of health care providers: a framework for understanding various provider organizational structures. *Int J Integr Care*. 2020;20(1):2. doi:10.5334/ijic.4635

34. HealthScape Advisors. *Value-based contracting: How to think like a payer.* Published 2018. Accessed January 6, 2022. https://www.healthscape.com/wp-content/uploads/2018/03/Value-Based-Contracting-How-to-Think-Like-a-Payer.pdf

35. Healthcare.gov. Affordable Care Act (ACA). Published June 21, 2013. Accessed November 1, 2021. https://www.healthcare.gov/glossary/affordable-care-act/

36. Centers for Medicare & Medicaid Services. Value-based programs. Modified December 1, 2021. Accessed January 4, 2022. https://www.cms.gov/Medicare/Quality-Initiatives-Patient-Assessment-Instruments/Value-Based-Programs/Value-Based-Programs

37. Crook HL, Saunders RS, Roiland R, Higgins A, McClellan MB. A decade of value-based payment: lessons learned and implications for the Center for Medicare and Medicaid Innovation, Part 1. *Health Affairs* [blog], June 9, 2021. doi:10.1377/forefront.20210607.656313

38. World Economic Forum. Value in healthcare laying the foundation for health system transformation: moving beyond fee-for-service at the Centers for Medicare and Medicaid Services; 2017:22. Accessed January 4, 2022. https://www3.weforum.org/docs/WEF_Insight_Report_Value_Healthcare_Laying_Foundation.pdf

39. Centers for Medicare & Medicaid Services. Innovation center strategy refresh. Published 2021. Accessed January 4, 2022. https://innovation.cms.gov/strategic-direction-whitepaper

40. Kaiser Family Foundation. 2020 employer health benefits survey. Published October 2020. Accessed November 18, 2021. https://www.kff.org/report-section/ehbs-2020-summary-of-findings/

41. Vogenberg FR, Santilli J. Key trends in healthcare for 2020 and beyond. *Am Health Drug Benefits*. 2019;12(7):348-350. Accessed January 11, 2022. https://www.ncbi.nlm.nih.gov/pmc/articles/PMC6996619/

42. Call K, McAlpine D, Garcia C, et al. Barriers to care in an ethnically diverse publicly insured population: is health care reform enough? *Med Care*. 2014;52:720-727. doi:10.1097/MLR.0000000000000172

43. Berchick ER, Hood E, Barnett JC. Health insurance coverage in the United States; 2017. Published September 2018. Accessed November 9, 2021. https://www.census.gov/content/dam/Census/library/publications/2018/demo/p60-264.pdf

44. Ramesh T, Gee E; Center for American Progress. Rural hospital closures reduce access to emergency care. Published September 9, 2019. Accessed November 9, 2021. www.americanprogress.org/issues/healthcare/reports/2019/09/09/474001/rural-hospital-closures-reduce-access-emergency-care/

45. Malone T, Pink G, Holmes, M. Decline in inpatient volume at rural hospitals. *J Rural Health*. 2021;37(2):347-352. doi:10.1111/jrh.12553

46. Abuzeineh M, Muzaale AD, Crews DC, et al. Telemedicine in the care of kidney transplant recipients with coronavirus disease 2019: Case reports. *Transplant Proc*. 2020;52:2620-2625. doi:10.1016/j.transproceed.2020.07.009

47. Centers for Disease Control and Prevention. Trends in the use of telehealth during the emergency of the COVID-19 pandemic—United States, January-March 2020. *MMWR Morb Mortal Wkly Rep*. 2020;69(43):1595-1599. Accessed January 11, 2022. https://www.cdc.gov/mmwr/volumes/69/wr/mm6943a3.htm

48. InstaMed. Consumer healthcare payments survey 2020. Published 2020. Accessed November 12, 2021. https://www.instamed.com/white-papers/trends-in-healthcare-payments-annual-report/

49. Centers for Medicare & Medicaid Services. CMS announces comprehensive strategy to enhance hospital capacity amid COVID-19 surge. Published Nov 25, 2020. Accessed November 12, 2021. https://www.cms.gov/newsroom/press-releases/cms-announces-comprehensive-strategy-enhance-hospital-capacity-amid-covid-19-surge

50. World Health Organization. Social determinants of health; 2022. Accessed November 12, 2021. https://www.who.int/health-topics/social-determinants-of-health#tab=tab_1

51. Reese EC, Healthcare Financial Management Association (HFMA). COVID-19 magnifies impact of SDOH on U.S. healthcare system. Published January 22, 2021. Accessed January 4, 2022. https://www.hfma.org/topics/financial-sustainability/article/covid-19-magnifies-impact-of-sdoh-on-u-s--healthcare-system.html

52. CMS Innovation Center. Health care payment learning and action network. Updated June 21, 2021. Accessed December 14, 2021. https://innovation.cms.gov/innovation-models/health-care-payment-learning-and-action-network

53. Sokol E. RevCycleIntelligence. Healthcare reimbursement still largely fee-for-service driven. Published March 26, 2020. Accessed December 14, 2021. https://revcycleintelligence.com/news/healthcare-reimbursement-still-largely-fee-for-service-driven

54. American Hospital Association. Evolving care models: aligning care delivery to emerging payment models. Published 2019. Accessed November 8, 2021. https://www.aha.org/system/files/media/file/2019/04/MarketInsights_CareModelsReport.pdf

55. National Quality Forum. Home page. Accessed November 12, 2021. https://www.qualityforum.org/Home.aspx

56. National Association for Healthcare Quality. About NAHQ. Accessed November 12, 2021. https://nahq.org/about-nahq/

57. Institute for Healthcare Improvement. About IHI. Accessed November 12, 2021. http://www.ihi.org/about/Pages/default.aspx

58. Stiefel M, Nolan K. *A Guide to Measuring the Triple Aim: Population Health, Experience of Care, and Per Capita Cost. IHI Innovation Series white paper*. Cambridge, MA: Institute for Healthcare Improvement; 2012. Available at www.IHI.org

59. Healthcare Financial Management Association. About us. Accessed November 12, 2021. https://www.hfma.org/about-hfma.html

60. Healthcare Financial Management Association. Improving value in health care: foundational strategies. Accessed

November 12, 2021. https://www.hfma.org/industry-initiatives/the-value-project.html

61. Healthcare Financial Management Association. Research and trends. Accessed November 12, 2021. https://www.hfma.org/industry-initiatives/research-trends.html

62. National Association of ACOs. Welcome. Accessed December 21, 2021. https://www.naacos.com/

63. Center for Improvement in Healthcare Quality. About our organization; 2022. Accessed January 12, 2022. https://cihq.org/about_our_organization.asp

64. American Nurses Credentialing Center. ANCC Magnet Recognition program. Accessed November 17, 2021. https://www.nursingworld.org/organizational-programs/magnet/

65. American Nurses Credentialing Center. ANCC Pathway to Excellence Program. Accessed November 17, 2021. https://www.nursingworld.org/organizational-programs/pathway/

66. Pennsylvania Health Care Cost Containment Council. Hospital performance report—2020 data. Published December 16, 2021. Accessed December 22, 2021. https://www.phc4.org/reports/hpr/20/

67. Khetrapal S, Bhatia R. Impact of COVID-19 pandemic on health system & sustainable development goal 3. *Indian J Med Res*. 2020;151(5):395-399. doi:10.4103/ijmr.IJMR_1920_20

68. Centers for Medicare & Medicaid Services. COVID-19 emergency declaration blanket waivers for health care providers. Updated May 21, 2021. Accessed December 23, 2021. https://www.cms.gov/files/document/covid-19-emergency-declaration-waivers.pdf

69. Shrank WH, Rogstad TL, Parekh N. Waste in the US health care system: estimated costs and potential for savings. *JAMA*. 2019;322(15):1501-1509. doi:10.1001/jama.2019.13978

70. Healthcare Financial Management Association. Reducing clinical variation to drive success in value-based care (Part 1). Published March 16, 2019. Accessed December 23, 2021. https://www.hfma.org/topics/operations-management/article/reducing-clinical-variation-to-drive-success-in-value-based-care0.html

71. 3M US. Hospital inpatients classified by admission, severity of illness and risk of mortality. Published September 20, 2021. Accessed December 10, 2021. https://www.3m.com/3M/en_US/health-information-systems-us/drive-value-based-care/patient-classification-methodologies/apr-drgs/

72. McKenna P, Heslin SM, Viccellio P, Mallon WK, Hernandez C, Morley EJ. Emergency department and hospital crowding: causes, consequences, and cures. *Clin Exp Emerg Med*. 2019;6(3):189-195. Published online July 12, 2019. Accessed December 10, 2021. https://www.ceemjournal.org/journal/view.php?doi=10.15441/ceem.18.022

73. OR Management News. Rosenthal T. What is a minute worth in the OR? Published June 6, 2018. Accessed December 10, 2021. https://www.ormanagement.net/Clinical-News/Article/06-18/What-Is-a-Minute-Worth-in-the-OR-/48791

74. Cheng H, Clymer JW, Po-Han Chen B, et al. Prolonged operative duration is associated with complications: a systematic review and meta-analysis. *J Surg Res*. 2018;229:134-144. doi:10.1016/j.jss.2018.03.022

75. Centers for Medicare & Medicaid Services. Explore & download Medicare provider data. Accessed December 22, 2021. https://data.cms.gov/provider-data/

76. Centers for Medicare & Medicaid Services. Hospital Value Based Purchasing (HVBP) Program FY 2019—2027 measures. Accessed November 23, 2021. https://qualitynet.cms.gov/inpatient/hvbp/measures

77. Centers for Medicare & Medicaid Services. Performance standards: Hospital Value-Based Purchasing (HVBP) Program. Accessed November 23, 2021. https://qualitynet.cms.gov/inpatient/hvbp/performance

78. Centers for Medicare & Medicaid Services. Payment: Hospital Value-Based Purchasing (HVBP) Program. Accessed November 23, 2021. https://qualitynet.cms.gov/inpatient/hvbp/payment

79. Centers for Medicare & Medicaid Services. Hospital price transparency. Updated December 1, 2021. Accessed December 22, 2021. https://www.cms.gov/hospital-price-transparency

80. *Federal Register*. Medicare and Medicaid programs: CY 2020 hospital outpatient PPS policy changes and payment rates and ambulatory surgical center payment system policy changes and payment rates; price transparency requirements for hospitals to make standard charges public; 45 CFR §180.50. Published November 27, 2019. Accessed December 21, 2021. https://www.federalregister.gov/documents/2019/11/27/2019-24931/medicare-and-medicaid-programs-cy-2020-hospital-outpatient-pps-policy-changes-and-payment-rates-and#p-1010

81. *Federal Register*. Medicare and Medicaid programs: CY 2020 hospital outpatient PPS policy changes and payment rates and ambulatory surgical center payment system policy changes and payment rates; price transparency requirements for hospitals to make standard charges public; 45 CFR §180.60. Published November 27, 2019. Accessed December 21, 2021. https://www.federalregister.gov/documents/2019/11/27/2019-24931/medicare-and-medicaid-programs-cy-2020-hospital-outpatient-pps-policy-changes-and-payment-rates-and#p-1010

82. American Medical Association. What is information blocking? Part 1. Published May 1, 2020. Accessed December 21, 2021. https://www.ama-assn.org/system/files/2021-01/information-blocking-part-1.pdf

83. CHIME Public Policy. Overview of three types of actors eligible for penalties under information blocking final rule. Rule published April 24, 2020. Accessed December 21, 2021. https://chimecentral.org/wp-content/uploads/2020/05/ONC-Rule-Definitions-Cheat-sheet-Final-Rule-FINAL.pdf

84. Congress.gov. 21st Century Cures Act; Sec. 4004:144. Published December 13, 2016. Accessed December 21, 2021. https://www.congress.gov/114/plaws/publ255/PLAW-114publ255.pdf

85. The Joint Commission. What are the key elements needed to meet the ongoing professional practice evaluation (OPPE) requirements? Updated November 18, 2021. Accessed November 5, 2021. https://www.jointcommission.org/standards/standard-faqs/critical-access-hospital/medical-staff-ms/000001500/

86. Swing SR. The ACGME outcome project: retrospective and prospective. *Med Teach*. 2007;29(7):648-654. doi:10.1080/01421590701392903

87. Data USA. Physician assistants. Accessed November 5, 2021. https://datausa.io/profile/soc/physician-assistants

88. American Association of Nurse Practitioners. Nurse practitioner fact sheet. Updated May 20, 2021. Accessed November 5, 2021. https://www.aanp.org/about/all-about-nps/np-fact-sheet

89. Healthcare Financial Management Association (HFMA). Advanced practice providers optimize efficiency and improve financial performance. Published January 15, 2019. Accessed November 5, 2021. https://www.hfma.org/topics/trends/62811.html

90. The Joint Commission. Credentialing and privileging—requirements for physician assistants and advanced practice

registered nurses. Published May 12, 2017. Updated November 29, 2021. Accessed December 12, 2021. https://www.jointcommission.org/standards/standard-faqs/critical-access-hospital/medical-staff-ms/000002124/

91. Campanella P, Vukovic V, Parente P, et al. The impact of public reporting on clinical outcomes: a systematic review and meta-analysis. *BMC Health Serv Res*. 2016;16:296. doi:10.1186/s12913-016-1543-y

92. The Leapfrog Group. About. Accessed January 19, 2017. http://www.leapfroggroup.org/about

93. Healthgrades. About. Accessed January 11, 2022. https://www.healthgrades.com/about/

94. Fung CH, Lim YW, Mattke S, Damberg C, Shekelle PG. Systematic review: the evidence that publishing patient care performance data improves quality of care. *Ann Intern Med*. 2008;148(2):111-123. doi:10.7326/0003-4819-148-2-200801150-00006

95. Centers for Medicare & Medicaid Services. Quality measures. Updated December 1, 2021. Accessed December 17, 2021. https://www.cms.gov/Medicare/Quality-Initiatives-Patient-Assessment-Instruments/QualityMeasures#:~:text=CMS%20uses%20quality%20measures%20in%20its%20various%20quality,one%20or%20more%20quality%20goals%20for%20health%20care

96. Centers for Medicare & Medicaid Services. Measures management system. Updated December 1, 2021. Accessed December 17, 2021. https://www.cms.gov/Medicare/Quality-Initiatives-Patient-Assessment-Instruments/MMS/MMS-Content-Page

97. Centers for Medicare & Medicaid Services. Measure inventory tool. Updated June 30, 2021. Accessed December 17, 2021. https://cmit.cms.gov/CMIT_public/ListMeasures

98. Centers for Medicare & Medicaid Services. Hospital Readmissions Reduction Program (HRRP). Modified December 1, 2021. Accessed January 5, 2022. https://www.cms.gov/Medicare/Medicare-Fee-for-Service-Payment/AcuteInpatientPPS/Readmissions-Reduction-Program

99. Kaiser Health News. Medicare punishes 2,499 hospitals for high readmissions. Published October 28, 2021. Accessed January 5, 2022. https://khn.org/news/article/hospital-readmission-rates-medicare-penalties/

100. Centers for Medicare & Medicaid Services. Hospital-Acquired Condition Reduction Program. Updated December 1, 2021. Accessed January 5, 2022. https://www.cms.gov/Medicare/Medicare-Fee-for-Service-Payment/AcuteInpatientPPS/HAC-Reduction-Program

101. AAPC. What is MACRA? Last reviewed December 29, 2020. Accessed December 7, 2021. https://www.aapc.com/macra/macra.aspx

102. Centers for Medicare & Medicaid Services. Quality measures: traditional MIPS requirements. Accessed December 3, 2021. https://qpp.cms.gov/mips/quality-requirements

103. Centers for Medicare & Medicaid Services. 2021 annual call for quality measures fact sheet. Published February 8, 2021. Accessed December 7, 2021. https://www.cms.gov/files/document/mips-call-quality-measures-overview-fact-sheet-2021.pdf

104. Centers for Medicare & Medicaid Services. Merit-based incentive payment system (MIPS) 2021 quality performance category quick start guide: traditional MIPS. Updated August 26, 2021. Accessed December 7, 2021. https://qpp-cm-prod-content.s3.amazonaws.com/uploads/1294/2021%20MIPS%20Quality%20Quick%20Start%20Guide.pdf

105. Centers for Medicare & Medicaid Services. Accountable care organizations (ACOs): general information. Updated June 4, 2021. Accessed November 23, 2021. https://innovation.cms.gov/innovation-models/aco

106. Centers for Medicare & Medicaid Services. Quality measurement methodology and resources: Medicare Shared Savings Program. Updated December 2020. Accessed November 23, 2021. https://www.cms.gov/files/document/2020-quality-measurement-methodology-and-resources.pdf

107. MDInteractive. The APM performance pathway—preparing your ACO for success. Published January 21, 2021. Accessed January 5, 2022. https://mdinteractive.com/mips-blog/apm-performance-pathway-preparing-your-aco-success

108. Hoque DME, Kumari V, Hoque M, Ruseckaite R, Romero L, Evans SM. Impact of clinical registries on quality of patient care and clinical outcomes: a systematic review. *PLoS ONE*. 2017;12(9):e0183667. Accessed December 7, 2021. doi:10.1371/journal.pone.0183667

109. Gliklich RE, Dreyer NA, Leavy MB. *Registries for Evaluating Patient Outcomes: A User's Guide*. 3rd ed. Rockville, MD: Agency for Healthcare Research and Quality, 2014. Accessed January 12, 2022. https://effectivehealthcare.ahrq.gov/sites/default/files/pdf/registries-guide-3rd-edition_research.pdf

110. National Cancer Institute. SEER Program: what is a cancer registry? Accessed December 8, 2021. https://seer.cancer.gov/registries/cancer_registry/index.html

111. National Institutes of Health. List of registries. Reviewed December 20, 2021. Accessed December 21, 2021. https://www.nih.gov/health-information/nih-clinical-research-trials-you/list-registries

112. Centers for Medicare & Medicaid Services. Measures management system: a brief overview. Published October 2018. Accessed December 8, 2021. https://www.cms.gov/Medicare/Quality-Initiatives-Patient-Assessment-Instruments/MMS/Downloads/A-Brief-Overview-of-Qualified-Clinical-Data-Registries.pdf

113. Centers for Medicare & Medicaid Services (CMS). 2021 qualified clinical data registry (QCDR) fact sheet. Accessed December 8, 2021. https://scorh.net/wp-content/uploads/2020/07/CMS-2021-MIPS-QCDR-Self-Nomination-Fact-Sheet.pdf

114. American College of Radiology. MIPS qualified clinical data registry. Accessed December 8, 2021. https://www.acr.org/Practice-Management-Quality-Informatics/Registries/Qualified-Clinical-Data-Registry

115. Agency for Healthcare Research and Quality. A profile. Published July 2014. Updated March 2018. Accessed November 23, 2021. https://www.ahrq.gov/cpi/about/profile/index.html

116. Agency for Healthcare Research and Quality. Healthcare cost and utilization project (HCUP). Updated December 21, 2021. Accessed December 29, 2021. https://www.hcup-us.ahrq.gov/

117. Agency for Healthcare Research and Quality. AHRQuality Indicators. Content last reviewed July 2018. Accessed November 23, 2021. https://www.ahrq.gov/cpi/about/otherwebsites/qualityindicators.ahrq.gov/qualityindicators.html

118. Agency for Healthcare Research and Quality. Get to know the AHRQ quality indicators. Updated (indicator changes) February 17, 2021. Accessed November 23, 2021. https://qualityindicators.ahrq.gov/Default.aspx

119. Agency for Healthcare Research and Quality. AHRQ QI software. Updated July 20, 2021. Accessed December 21, 2021. https://qualityindicators.ahrq.gov/Software/Default.aspx

120. National Committee for Quality Assurance. About NCQA. Accessed November 23, 2021. https://www.ncqa.org/about-ncqa/

121. National Committee for Quality Assurance. HEDIS and performance measurement. Accessed November 23, 2021. https://www.ncqa.org/hedis/

122. National Committee for Quality Assurance. NCQA's health plan report cards. Updated ratings September 2021. Accessed November 23, 2021. https://reportcards.ncqa.org/health-plans

123. Centers for Medicare & Medicaid Services. HCAHPS survey instructions. Published December 2021. Accessed December 8,2021. https://hcahpsonline.org/globalassets/hcahps/survey-instruments/mail/effective-december-1-2021-and-forward-discharges/2021_survey-instruments_english_mail_updateda.pdf

124. Centers for Medicare & Medicaid Services. HCAHPS: patients' perspectives of care survey. Updated December 1, 2021. Accessed December 8, 2021. https://www.cms.gov/Medicare/Quality-Initiatives-Patient-Assessment-Instruments/HospitalQualityInits/HospitalHCAHPS

125. Agency for Healthcare Research and Quality. CAHPS clinician & group adult survey 3.1. Published fall 2020. Accessed December 8, 2021. https://www.ahrq.gov/sites/default/files/wysiwyg/cahps/surveys-guidance/cg/adult-english-cg-3-1-2351a.pdf

126. Centers for Medicare & Medicaid Services. Electronic clinical quality measures basics. Page last modified December 1, 2021. Accessed December 21, 2021. https://www.cms.gov/Regulations-and-Guidance/Legislation/EHRIncentivePrograms/ClinicalQualityMeasures

127. The Office of the National Coordinator for Health Information Technology. What is an electronic health record (EHR)? Accessed December 21, 2021. https://www.healthit.gov/faq/what-electronic-health-record-ehr#:~:text=An%20electronic%20health%20record%20%28EHR%29%20is%20a%20digital,information%20available%20instantly%20and%20securely%20to%20authorized%20users

128. University of Illinois at Chicago. What is clinical Informatics? Informatics. Accessed December 21, 2021. https://pathology.uic.edu/what-is-clinical-informatics/

129. Centers for Medicare & Medicaid Services. Medicare and Medicaid promoting interoperability program basics. Page last modified November 1, 2021. Accessed November 22, 2021. https://www.cms.gov/Regulations-and-Guidance/Legislation/EHRIncentivePrograms/Basics

130. The Office of the National Coordinator for Health Information Technology. Accessed November 22, 2021. https://www.healthit.gov/

131. The Office of the National Coordinator for Health Information Technology. 2015 edition. Content reviewed October 4, 2021. Accessed November 22, 2021. https://www.healthit.gov/topic/certification-ehrs/2015-edition

132. The Office of the National Coordinator for Health Information Technology. 2015 edition cures update—base electronic health record (EHR) definition. Content last reviewed December 9, 2021. Accessed November 11, 2021. https://www.healthit.gov/topic/certification-ehrs/2015-edition-test-method/2015-edition-cures-update-base-electronic-health-record-definition#:~:text=2015%20Edition%20Cures%20Update%20Base%20EHR%20Definition%20%E2%80%93,%281%29%20%28C%20...%20%203%20more%20rows%20

133. MDinteractive. Merit based incentive payment system (MIPS)—what is MIPS? Accessed November 22, 2021. https://mdinteractive.com/MIPS#:~:text=The%20 4%20scorable%20MIPS%20categories%20in%20 2021%20are%3A,%2825%25%20of%20score%29%20 Improvement%20Activities%20%2815%25%20of%20score%29

134. Practice Builders. Tips: are you spending enough on your healthcare marketing budget? Posted September 6, 2018. Accessed November 5, 2021. https://www.practicebuilders.com/blog/are-you-spending-enough-on-your-healthcare-marketing-budget/

135. Purcarea VL. The impact of marketing strategies in healthcare systems. *J Med Life.* 2019;12(2):93-96. doi:10.25122/jml-2019-1003

136. Techopedia. Data management. Updated April 17, 2017. Accessed January 7, 2022. https://www.techopedia.com/definition/5422/data-management

137. United States Government Accountability Office. *Data Governance: Agencies Made Progress in Establishing Governance, but Need to Address Key Milestones.* GAO-21-152 December 2020; 6. Accessed July 7, 2022. https://www.gao.gov/assets/gao-21-152.pdf

138. Raghupathi W, Raghupathi V. Big data analytics in healthcare: promise and potential. *Health Inf Sci Syst.* 2014;2:3. doi:10.1186/2047-2501-2-3

139. Centers for Medicare & Medicaid Services. Hospital Readmission Reduction Program: payment reduction methodology. Accessed January 12, 2022. https://qualitynet.cms.gov/inpatient/hrrp/methodology

140. Centers for Medicare & Medicaid Services. Hospital Readmission Reduction Program: reporting. Accessed January 12, 2022. https://qualitynet.cms.gov/inpatient/hrrp/reports

141. Centers for Medicare & Medicaid Services. Medicare billing form CMS-1450 and the 837I booklet. Published March 2021. Accessed December 8, 2021. https://www.cms.gov/Outreach-and-Education/Medicare-Learning-Network-MLN/MLNProducts/Downloads/837I-FormCMS-1450-ICN006926.pdf

142. Agency for Healthcare Research and Quality. Databases used for hospital quality measures. Content last reviewed June 2016. Accessed December 8, 2021. https://www.ahrq.gov/talkingquality/measures/setting/hospitals/databases.html

143. U.S. Department of Health & Human Services. HITECH Act enforcement interim final rule. Content last reviewed June 16, 2017. Accessed December 8, 2021. https://www.hhs.gov/hipaa/for-professionals/special-topics/hitech-act-enforcement-interim-final-rule/index.html

144. Centers for Disease Control and Prevention. FastStats—electronic medical records. Accessed December 8, 2021. https://www.cdc.gov/nchs/fastats/electronic-medical-records.htm

145. Office of the National Coordinator for Health Information Technology. Hospitals participating in the CMS EHR incentive programs: health IT quick stat #45. Published August 2017. Accessed December 8, 2021. https://www.healthit.gov/data/quickstats/hospitals-participating-cms-ehr-incentive-programs

146. Centers for Medicare & Medicaid Services. HCAHPS: Patients' Perspectives of Care Survey. Last modified December 1, 2021. Accessed December 8, 2021. https://www.cms.gov/Medicare/Quality-Initiatives-Patient-Assessment-Instruments/HospitalQualityInits/HospitalHCAHPS

147. Health Measures. Intro to PROMIS. https://www.healthmeasures.net/explore-measurement-systems/promis/intro-to-promis

148. Centers for Medicare & Medicaid Services. Meaningful Measures 2.0: moving from measure reduction to modernization. Page last modified March 31, 2021. Accessed December 20, 2021. https://www.cms.gov/meaningful-measures-20-moving-measure-reduction-modernization

149. National Library of Medicine. PROMIS: clinical outcomes assessment. Last reviewed January 29, 2019. Accessed December 20, 2021. https://commonfund.nih.gov/promis/index

150. The Joint Commission. Measures. Accessed November 12, 2021. https://www.jointcommission.org/measurement/measures/

151. Gazelle Consulting. HIPAA technical vs. physical vs. administrative safeguards. Published July 15, 2019. Accessed November 12, 2021. https://gazelleconsulting.org/hipaa-technical-vs-physical-vs-administrative-safeguards/

152. Centers for Medicare & Medicaid Services. CMS coverage email updates Listserv. Page last modified December 1, 2021. Accessed December 21, 2021. https://www.cms.gov/Medicare/Coverage/InfoExchange/listserv

153. Centers for Medicare & Medicaid Services (CMS). CMSHHSgov—YouTube. Accessed December 1, 2021. https://www.youtube.com/user/CMSHHSgov/search?app=desktop&query=specify+your+measures

154. The Joint Commission. Quality measurement webinars & videos. Accessed December 21, 2021. https://www.jointcommission.org/measurement/quality-measurement-webinars-and-videos/

155. Levitin DJ. *The Organized Mind: Thinking Straight in the Age of Information Overload*. New York, NY. Random House; 2016.

156. Left brain–right brain. *Psychol Today*; n.d. Accessed January 12, 2022. https://www.psychologytoday.com/us/basics/left-brain-right-brain

157. My American Nurse. Financial terms 101. Published April 19, 2017. Accessed December 15, 2021. https://www.myamericannurse.com/financial-terms-101/

158. The Joint Commission. Do not use list. Published April 11, 2016. Updated November 18, 2021. Accessed December 15, 2021. https://www.jointcommission.org/resources/news-and-multimedia/fact-sheets/facts-about-do-not-use-list/

159. Positive Psychology. What is the negativity bias and how can it be overcome? Published December 14, 2021. Accessed December 15, 2021. https://positivepsychology.com/3-steps-negativity-bias/

160. Achor S. The happy secret to better work [video]. Published May 2011. Accessed December 15, 2021. https://www.ted.com/talks/shawn_achor_the_happy_secret_to_better_work?language=en

161. Muneeb A, Jawaid H, Khalid N, Mian A. The art of healing through narrative medicine in clinical practice: a reflection. *Perm J*. 2017;21:17-013. Accessed December 8, 2021. doi:10.7812/TPP/17-013

162. Feedspot.com. Best 80 storytelling podcasts you must follow in 2021. Published December 22, 2021. Accessed December 24, 2021. https://blog.feedspot.com/storytelling_podcasts/?_src=search

163. Feedspot.com. Top 25 storytelling blogs and websites to follow in 2021. Published December 21, 2021. Accessed December 24, 2021. https://blog.feedspot.com/storytelling_blogs/?_src=search

164. TED Talks. Storytelling [playlist]. Latest published November 2021. Accessed December 8, 2021. https://www.ted.com/topics/storytelling

165. Up Journey. The 18 best books on storytelling (to read in 2021). Published February 23, 2021. Accessed December 8, 2021. https://upjourney.com/

166. The Secret Professor. Aristotle and the rhetoric triangle. Accessed December 8, 2021. https://thesecretprofessor.com/aristotle-rhetoric-triangle/

167. NASA. Report of Columbia accident investigation board; vol. I. Published August 26, 2003. Accessed November 12, 2021. https://www.nasa.gov/columbia/home/CAIB_Vol1.html

168. Edward Tufte forum: PowerPoint does rocket science—and better techniques for technical reports. Published 2005. Accessed November 12, 2021. https://www.edwardtufte.com/bboard/q-and-a-fetch-msg?msg_id=0001yB&topic_id=1

169. Tufte E. *Beautiful Evidence*. Cheshire, CT: Graphics Press, LLC; 2017.

170. Bulger D. *The storyteller's playbook: a guide to making quality memorable*. On-demand presentation; 2021; NAHQNext.

171. Agency for Healthcare Research and Quality. Six tips for making a quality report appealing and easy to skim. Content last reviewed October 2019. Accessed December 10, 2021. https://www.ahrq.gov/talkingquality/resources/design/general-tips/index.html

172. Sisence. Dashboard design best practices—4 key principles. Published August 7, 2019. Accessed November 10, 2021. https://www.sisense.com/blog/4-design-principles-creating-better-dashboards/

173. Wang T. The human insights missing from big data [video]. Published July 19, 2017. Accessed November 10, 2021. https://www.bing.com/videos/search?q=tricia+wang+ted+talk&&view=detail&mid=5CF61958B3D4401137C25CF61958B3D4401137C2&&FORM=VDRVRV

174. Chief Executive Group. The critical difference between credibility and trust. Published December 18, 2019. Accessed December 10, 2021. https://chiefexecutive.net/the-critical-difference-between-credibility-and-trust/

175. What is trust? *Psychol Today*. Published October 9, 2018. Accessed December 10, 2021. https://www.psychologytoday.com/us/blog/hot-thought/201810/what-is-trust

## Suggested Readings

American Hospital Association, Center for Health Innovation. Evolving care models: aligning care delivery to emerging payment models. Accessed March 26, 2022. https://www.aha.org/center/emerging-issues/market-insights/evolving-care-models/aligning-care-delivery-emerging-payment-models

Boylan MR, Suchman KI, Korolikova H, Slover JD, Bosco JA. Association of Magnet nursing status with hospital performance on nationwide quality metrics. *J Healthc Qual*. 2019;41(4):189-194. doi:10.1097/JHQ.0000000000000202

Center for Medicare & Medicaid Innovation. Innovation strategy refresh; 2021. Accessed March 25, 2022. https://innovation.cms.gov/strategic-direction-whitepaper.

Centers for Medicare & Medicaid Services. Quality measures: how they are developed, used, & maintained; your guide to what goes into building quality measures and what happens after they are built; 2021. Accessed March 25, 2022. https://www.cms.gov/files/document/quality-measures-how-they-are-developed-used-maintained.pdf

Crook HL, Zheng J, Bleser WK, Whitaker RG, Masand J, Saunders RS. How are payment reforms addressing social determinants of health? Policy implications and next steps. Accessed March 25, 2022. https://www.milbank.org/wp-content/uploads/2021/02/Duke-SDOH-and-VBP-Issue-Brief_v3-1.pdf#:~:text=The%20movement%20toward%20value-based%20care%20provides%20a%20significant,payment%20to%20encourage%20and%20promote%20addressing%20social%20needs

Dai M, Peterson LE, Phillips RL. Quality changes among primary care clinicians participating in the transforming clinical practice initiative. *J Healthc Qual.* 2021;43(4):e64-e69. doi:10.1097/JHQ.0000000000000287

Hasan MM, Alam NE, Wang X, Zepeda ED, Young JG. Hospital readmissions to nonindex hospitals: patterns and determinants following the Medicare readmission reduction penalty program. *J Healthc Qual.* 2020;42(1):e10-e17. doi:10.1097/JHQ.0000000000000199

Heath C, Heath D. *Made to Stick: Why Some Ideas Survive and Others Die.* New York, NY: Random House; 2007.

Hong YR, Kates F, Song SJ, Lee N, Duncan RP, Marlow NM. Benchmarking implications: analysis of Medicare accountable care organizations spending level and quality

of care. *J Healthc Qual.* 2018;40(6):344-353. doi:10.1097/JHQ.0000000000000123

Johnson JK, Miller SH, Horowitz SD; ACGME. Systems-based practice: improving the safety and quality of patient care by recognizing and improving the systems in which we work. Accessed March 25, 2022. https://www.ahrq.gov/downloads/pub/advances2/vol2/Advances-Johnson_90.pdf#:~:text=Systems-based%20practice%20can%20be%20thought%20of%20as%20an,ourselves%20to%20document%2C%20assess%2C%20and%20improve%20our%20practice.%E2%80%9D2

Lassen T, Revere L, Hailemariam D, Hogan PJ, Hernandez ED. Bundled payment programs in joint replacement care hold promise for improving patient outcomes? *J Healthc Qual.* 2020;42(2):83-90. doi:10.1097/JHQ.0000000000000238

Modica C. The value transformation framework: an approach to value-based care in federally qualified health centers. *J Healthc Qual.* 2020;42(2):106-112. doi:10.1097/JHQ.0000000000000239

Soltoff S, Koenig L, Demehin AA, Foster NE, Vaz C. Identifying poor-performing hospitals in the Medicare hospital-acquired condition reduction program: an assessment of reliability. *J Healthc Qual.* 2018;40(6):377-383. doi:10.1097/JHQ.0000000000000128

Spaulding A, Hamadi H, Martinez L, Martin T, Purnell JM, Zhao M. Hospital value-based purchasing and trauma-certified hospital performance. *J Healthc Qual.* 2019;41(1):39-48. doi:10.1097/JHQ.0000000000000147

World Economic Forum in collaboration with The Boston Consulting Group (BCG). Value in healthcare laying the foundation for health system transformation. Accessed March 25, 2022. https://www3.weforum.org/docs/WEF_Insight_Report_Value_Healthcare_Laying_Foundation.pdf

# Online Resources

## Agency for Healthcare Research and Quality

- **AHRQ QI Software**

  https://qualityindicators.ahrq.gov/Software/Default.aspx

## CareDash

https://www.caredash.com/

## Centers for Medicare & Medicaid Services

- **Hospital Consumer Assessment of Healthcare Providers and Systems (HCAHPS)**

  https://hcahpsonline.org/en/

- **Measures Inventory Tool**

  https://cmit.cms.gov/CMIT_public/ListMeasures

- **Medicare Provider Data**

  https://data.cms.gov/provider-data/

- **YouTube Channel**

  https://www.youtube.com/user/CMSHHSgov

## DocSpot

https://www.docspot.com/

## Healthgrades

https://www.healthgrades.com/

## Kaiser Family Foundation

- **Look Up Your Hospital: Is It Being Penalized by Medicare?**

  https://khn.org/news/hospital-penalties/?penalty=readmission

## International Classification of Diseases (ICD)

https://icd.who.int/en

## Regions Hospital

- **Regions Hospital to Offer a Taste of Home to New Hmong Moms**

  https://www.youtube.com/watch?app=desktop&v=AGLvtnsn0qc

*University of North Carolina Cecil G. Sheps Center for Health Services Research*

- **Rural Hospital Closures**

  https://www.shepscenter.unc.edu/programs-projects/rural-health/rural-hospital-closures/

*The Joint Commission*

- **Quality Measurement Webinars and Videos**

  https://www.jointcommission.org/measurement/quality-measurement-webinars-and-videos/

*WebMD*

  https://doctor.webmd.com/

*ZocDoc*

  https://www.zocdoc.com/

# SECTION 3

# Regulatory and Accreditation

Luc R. Pelletier and Christy L. Beaudin

## SECTION CONTENTS

# Introduction

Compliance with laws, regulations, and accreditation standards is vital to the success of any organization. And a vital role of the healthcare quality professional is advising on myriad requirements and helping their organization attain and sustain compliance. This includes ensuring an infrastructure for safety, quality, and performance improvement programs supports continuous readiness and understanding the nuances of regulations or standards applicable to the healthcare setting. This section will address how to

- promote awareness of local and national statutory and regulatory requirements within the organization;
- develop, deploy, and support processes for evaluating, monitoring, and improving compliance with state and federal requirements;
- evaluate appropriate accreditation, certification, and recognition options; and
- maintain survey or accreditation readiness.

Through leadership commitment, individual accountability, organizational assessment, and robust survey procedures, the healthcare quality professional can promote the adoption and/or adherence to approaches to meet and exceed locally and nationally recognized regulatory and accreditation quality and safety standards.

# Laws and Regulations

There are differences between laws and regulations and how they impact the work of the healthcare quality professional.[1]

- *Federal laws.* These are bills passed by both houses of Congress and signed by the U.S. president, passed over the president's veto, or allowed to become law without the president's signature. Individual laws, also called Acts, are arranged by subject in the United States Code. Regulations are rules made by executive departments and agencies and are arranged by subject in the *Code of Federal Regulations (CFR)*.
- *Federal rules and regulations.* The *CFR* is a codification of the general and permanent rules published in the *Federal Register* by the executive departments and agencies of the federal government. The *Federal Register* is published every business day by the National Archives and Records Administration. It contains federal agency regulations; proposed rules and notices; and executive orders, proclamations, and other presidential documents.
- *State-specific laws and regulations.* There are healthcare laws and regulations that govern healthcare practices at the state level. Typically, state laws and regulations supersede federal laws and regulations if more stringent including licensure, privacy of medical records, durable power of attorney, certificate of need, and mandated healthcare coverage.
- *Quasi-regulatory.* Accreditation agencies are differentiated from federal and state regulatory and lawmaking entities but are recognized as quasi-regulatory. Accreditation "sets standards that are considered optimal and achievable, more rigorous than the minimum standards of licensure, and with a stated intent to foster a culture of improvement."[2(p2)] Accreditation may be considered voluntary but is frequently required to participate in third-party payer programs such as Medicare, Medicaid, and health plans. For example, The Joint Commission (TJC) enforces standards that meet the federal conditions of participation. "Deeming" authority is granted to TJC by the Centers for Medicare & Medicaid Services (CMS). If the healthcare organization receives "deemed status" after being surveyed by TJC, it would not be subject to the Medicare survey and certification process.

Laws, regulations, and accreditation/certification standards are dynamic and ever changing. This requires organizations to maintain an infrastructure and dedicated resources to sustain performance and ensure compliance, which is important for maintaining an organization's public reputation for providing safe, effective, reliable, and person-centered care. Healthcare is not a unique industry in this regard; other industries are also highly regulated (e.g., the airline industry). Like these other industries, there is an opportunity for staff to have specialized knowledge and skill sets focusing on regulatory and accreditation compliance. Titles of these professionals may vary, but large organizations often have personnel titles or department names, such as standards and compliance, regulatory affairs, accreditation and regulatory readiness, or licensing. Other organizations might use an integrated approach in which the quality or administration departments and operational leaders assume these responsibilities. Alternatively, organizations may outsource or purchase consultation services in this area.

Healthcare quality professionals are responsible for supporting the organization in ensuring ongoing compliance with laws and regulations pertaining to business operations. This includes working with federal, state, and/or local regulatory agencies on specific requirements for relevant business lines. For example, requirements for an outpatient medical practice are different from those for an outpatient ambulatory surgery center, a critical access hospital, a comprehensive medical rehabilitation hospital, a hospice organization, or a freestanding acute psychiatric hospital. General acute care hospitals have different requirements than medical homes, disease management programs, home infusion therapy providers, or accountable care organizations.

## Federal Laws and Regulations

The healthcare industry is regulated by all levels of government—federal, state, and local—presenting challenges for healthcare organizations and quality professionals, such as being confident that they possess an understanding of regulatory requirements. A simple Internet search on "healthcare regulation" yields about 420 million citations—an overwhelming place to start. Healthcare regulations create circumstances in which healthcare quality professionals spend inordinate amounts of time responding to changing rules concurrently with demonstrating compliance with complex existing rules. For example, according to the American Hospital Association, health systems, hospitals, and post-acute providers must comply with 629 discrete regulatory requirements across nine domains:

1. Quality reporting
2. New models of care/value-based payment models
3. Meaningful use of medical records
4. Hospital conditions of participation
5. Program integrity
6. Fraud and abuse
7. Privacy and security
8. Post-acute care
9. Billing and coverage verification requirements[3]

Further, providers spend nearly $39 billion per year solely on administrative activities related to regulatory compliance; this amounts to 59 full-time employees dedicated to regulatory compliance for an average size hospital.[3] In a dynamic marketplace, organizations are driven to expand and refine the services offered to meet the needs of the community. This creates an ongoing need for healthcare quality professionals to research and interpret regulations that are applicable to the organization's new or unique situation.

Although there are federal laws and regulations significantly impacting healthcare organizations, healthcare quality professionals will want to become familiar with the following foundational federal laws and regulations:

- *Emergency Medical Treatment and Active Labor Act (EMTALA).* EMTALA was enacted by Congress in 1986 as part of the Consolidated Omnibus Budget Reconciliation Act of 1985 (42 U.S.C. §1395dd). Referred to as the "anti-dumping" law, it was designed to prevent hospitals from transferring uninsured or Medicaid patients to public hospitals without, at a minimum, providing a medical screening examination to ensure they were stable for transfer. Any hospital participating in Medicare and offering emergency services must provide a medical screening examination when a request is made for examination or treatment for an emergency medical condition, including active labor, regardless of an individual's ability to pay. The hospital is then required to provide stabilizing treatment for patients with emergency medical conditions. If a hospital is unable to stabilize a patient within its capability, or if the patient requests, an appropriate transfer should be implemented.[4]
- *Clinical Laboratory Improvement Amendments (CLIA).* In 1988, Congress passed CLIA, which established quality standards for all laboratories (regardless of where the test was performed) to ensure the accuracy, reliability, and timeliness of patient test results. There are different certificates that can be issued (e.g., Certificate of Waiver, Certificate for Provider-Performed Microscopy Procedures, Certificate of Registration, Certificate of Compliance, and Certificate of Accreditation). CLIA regulations are stratified based on the complexity of the test method: waived complexity; moderate complexity, including the subcategory of provider-performed microscopy; and high complexity. The regulations specify quality standards for laboratories performing moderate- and/or high-complexity tests and require waived laboratories to enroll in CLIA and follow manufacturers instructions.[5]
- *Health Insurance Portability and Accountability Act (HIPAA) of 1996.* HIPAA is a federal law that created national standards to protect sensitive patient health information from being disclosed without the patient's consent or knowledge. The U.S. Department of Health & Human Services (HHS) issued the HIPAA Privacy Rule to implement the requirements of HIPAA. The HIPAA Security Rule protects a subset of information covered by the Privacy Rule and sets rules about who can have access to protected health information.[6]
- *Health Information Technology for Economic and Clinical Health (HITECH) Act.* Initiated in 2009, this law promotes the adoption and meaningful

use of health information technology.[7] HITECH, in concert with HIPAA, has helped safeguard patient privacy with the electronic transmission of health information, especially in the era of COVID, where telehealth became an alternative to face-to-face healthcare encounters.

- *Patient Safety and Quality Improvement Act of 2005 (PSQIA).* Signed into law in 2005 and implemented in 2009, PSQIA was a response to the initial Institute of Medicine (now the National Academy of Medicine) report, *To Err Is Human: Building a Safer Health System.* The law created a framework for patient safety organizations that identified and reduced risks to patient safety; reporting and analysis of data related to near miss and patient safety events; and maintaining a culture of safety that included anonymous reporting and confidentiality and legal protections for reporters.[8]

- *Patient Protection and Affordable Care Act (PPACA or ACA).* The ACA was signed into law in 2010, putting in place comprehensive U.S. health insurance reforms that greatly impact accountability (Public Law, 111–148, PPACA). The intent of the ACA was to transform and modernize the American healthcare system. The Act created new programs and payment models with goals of rewarding value and quality. These models include accountable care organization models, medical home models focused on primary care, and new models of bundling payments for episodes of care. In these alternate payment models (APMs), healthcare providers are accountable for the quality and cost of the care they deliver to patients and have a financial incentive to coordinate care for their patients—who are therefore more likely to receive evidence-based, team-based care. The start of 2017 saw a strong push, under a new president and federal administration, to repeal the ACA. In 2021, the Supreme Court upheld the ACA.[9] Healthcare quality professionals are encouraged to monitor the impact of federal governmental action on the ACA and the resultant impact on their respective healthcare organizations.

- *Medicare Access and CHIP (Children's Health Insurance Program) Reauthorization Act Quality Payment Program.* This Act was signed into law in 2015, and a final rule was issued in late 2016. The Act impacts the way providers are reimbursed through a merit-based incentive payment system and alternate payment model, collectively referred to as the Quality Payment Program. Healthcare quality professionals are encouraged to refer to the most up-to-date CMS information as elements of this law continue to go into effect. While this Act provides an incentive for providers working together, the Physician Self-Referral Law (i.e., the Stark law), prohibits physicians from referring patients to receive designated health services payable by Medicare or Medicaid from entities with which the physician or an immediate family member has a financial relationship, unless an exception applies.

- *21st Century Cures Act.* The Cures Act became Public Law No. 114-255 in December 2016. The intent was to improve the flow and exchange of electronic health information, including advancing interoperability, prohibiting information blocking, and enhancing the usability, accessibility, and privacy and security of health information technology (IT). The Act also clarified HIPAA privacy rules and supporting substance use and mental health services. The Cures Act defined *interoperability* as the ability to exchange and use electronic health information without special effort on the part of the user and as not constituting information blocking.

## Federal Agencies

There are federal agencies with which the healthcare quality professional interfaces. A huge government agency, the U.S. Department of Health & Human Services (HHS) has 11 operating divisions, including eight agencies in the U.S. Public Health Service and three human services agencies. These divisions administer a wide variety of health and human services and conduct life-saving research for the nation, protecting and serving all Americans. HHS's mission is "to enhance the health and well-being of all Americans, by providing for effective health and human services and by fostering sound, sustained advances in the sciences underlying medicine, public health, and social services for individuals, families, and communities, including seniors and individuals with disabilities."[10(¶1)] It works to accomplish its mission through the individual and collaborative efforts of the operating divisions and staff divisions within the office of the secretary. The primary goal of the office is to provide leadership, direction, and policy and management guidance to the department. HHS is working to integrate strategic planning, performance measurement and management, enterprise risk management, and evaluation into its management approach (**Figure 3.1**).

HHS works closely with state and local governments, and because many HHS-funded services are provided by state or county agencies, or through

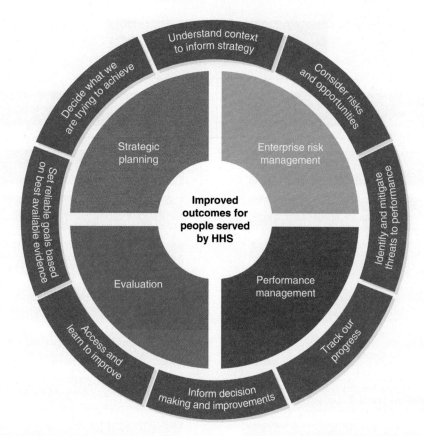

**Figure 3.1** HHS Strategy Integration (2018–2022)

Reproduced from U.S. Department of Health & Human Services. Overview: HHS Strategic Plan, FY 2018–2022. 2021. Accessed December 13, 2021. https://www.hhs.gov/about/strategic-plan/overview/index.html

private sector grantees, it may be difficult for healthcare professionals to distinguish between the federal role in regulation versus the role as an insurer, and the state role acting on behalf of the federal programs. **Figure 3.2** shows the organizational structure for the HHS. Several of the HHS agencies are described next.[11]

- *Administration for Children & Families (ACF).* Promotes the economic and social well-being of families, children, individuals, and communities through a range of educational and supportive programs in partnership with states, tribes, and community organizations. As a division of HHS, ACF encourages strong, healthy, supportive communities to provide a positive impact on quality of life and the development of children.

- *Administration for Community Living (ACL).* Brought together the Administration on Aging, the Administration of Developmental Disabilities, and Office on Disabilities upon its founding in 2012. ACL increases access to community support and resources for the unique needs of older Americans and people with disabilities by funding services and supports provided primarily by networks of community-based organizations, and with investments in research, education, and innovation.

- *Agency for Healthcare Research and Quality (AHRQ).* Produces evidence to make healthcare safer, of higher quality, more accessible, equitable, and affordable, and it works within HHS and with other partners to make sure that the evidence is understood and used. AHRQ accomplishes its mission by focusing on three core competencies— health systems research, practice improvement, and data and analytics.

- *Agency for Toxic Substances and Disease Registry (ATSDR).* Prevents exposure to toxic substances and the adverse health effects and diminished quality of life associated with exposure to hazardous substances from waste sites, unplanned releases, and other sources of environmental pollution.

- *Centers for Disease Control and Prevention (CDC).* Works 24/7 to protect America from threats to health, safety, and health security, both from foreign sources and in the United States. Whether diseases start at home or abroad; are chronic or acute, curable, or preventable; or are the result of human error or deliberate attack, CDC fights disease and supports communities and citizens to do the same. CDC increases the health security of the United States.[12]

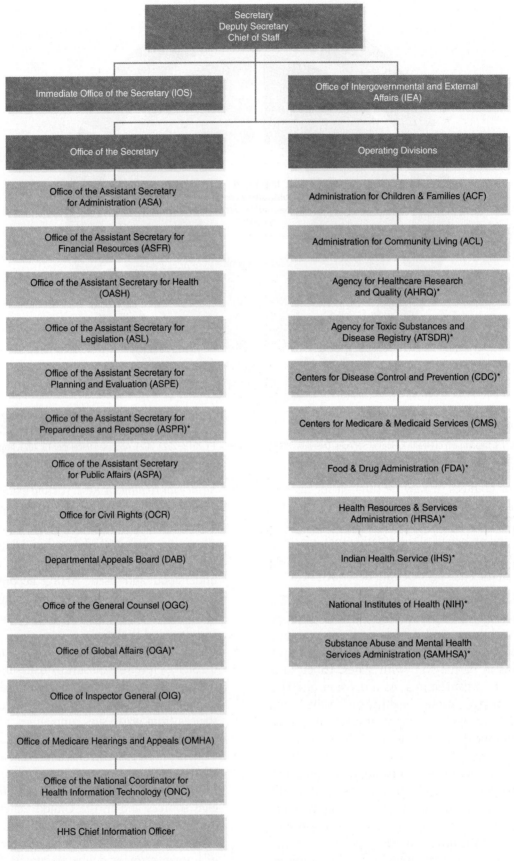

* Components of the Public Health Service.

**Figure 3.2** HHS Organizational Chart

Reproduced from U.S. Department of Health & Human Services. HHS organization chart. n.d. Accessed December 13, 2021. https://www.hhs.gov/about/agencies/orgchart/index.html

- *Centers for Medicare & Medicaid Services (CMS).* Combines the oversight of the Medicare program, the federal portion of the Medicaid program and State Children's Health Insurance Program, the health insurance marketplace, and related quality assurance activities.[13]
- *Food & Drug Administration (FDA).* Protects the public health by ensuring the safety, efficacy, and security of human and veterinary drugs, biological products, and medical devices; and by ensuring the safety of our nation's food supply, cosmetics, and products that emit radiation. FDA also plays a significant role in the nation's counterterrorism capability. FDA fulfills this responsibility by ensuring the security of the food supply and by fostering development of medical products to respond to deliberate and naturally emerging public health threats.[14]
- *Health Resources & Services Administration (HRSA).* Provides equitable healthcare to people who are geographically isolated and economically or medically vulnerable. HRSA's programs also support health infrastructure, including through training of health professionals and distributing them where they are needed most, providing financial support to healthcare providers, and advancing health.[15]
- *Indian Health Service (IHS).* Responsible for providing federal health services to American Indians and Alaska Natives. IHS is the principal federal health center provider and health advocate for Indian people, and its goal is to raise their health status to the highest possible level.[16]
- *National Institutes of Health (NIH).* Comprises the U.S. medical research agency—making important discoveries that improve health and save lives.[17] NIH supports biomedical and behavioral research with the United States and abroad, conducts research in its own laboratories and clinics, trains promising young researchers, and promotes collecting and sharing medical knowledge.
- *Office of Inspector General (OIG).* Stands at the forefront of the efforts since 1976 to fight fraud, waste, and abuse and to improve the efficiency of Medicare, Medicaid, and more than 100 other HHS programs. OIG is the largest inspector general's office in the federal government, with most of the resources going toward the oversight of Medicare and Medicaid. OIG's mission in protecting the most vulnerable is to "provide objective oversight to promote the economy, efficiency, effectiveness, and integrity of HHS programs, as well as the health and welfare of the people they serve"[18(¶1)] The five most important federal fraud and abuse laws that apply to physicians are the False Claims Act, the Anti-Kickback Statute, the Physician Self-Referral Law (called the "Stark law"), the exclusion authorities, and the Civil Monetary Penalties Law.
- *Substance Abuse and Mental Health Services Administration (SAMHSA).* Leads public health efforts to advance behavioral health in the United States. SAMHSA's mission is to reduce the impact of substance abuse and mental illness on America's communities.[19]

Leadership for the HHS operating divisions is divided into geographic regional offices; these are the offices with which healthcare quality professionals work directly in addition to state-level agencies.[20] Healthcare quality professionals may be involved with one or more HHS operating divisions depending on the segment of healthcare where they are employed (**Table 3.1**). However, most will become familiar with several key divisions, including CMS, CDC, FDA, and AHRQ. Up-to-date information is available on each agency's respective websites.

The federal government plays a role in directing laws and regulations for *managed care*, which is "a health care delivery system organized to manage cost, utilization, and quality."[21(¶1)] Health plans pay the cost of medical care. Healthcare quality professionals working with health plans will want to understand the regulations specific to their situation in the state where business is conducted and healthcare delivery occurs. The federal government regulates managed care and other health plans sponsored by the private sector. However, the states regulate the business of insurance, which includes managed care organizations (MCOs) such as health maintenance organizations (HMOs) that offer managed care policies to individuals, employers, or other purchasers. To add to the complexity, if a private sector employer sponsors a plan that is not purchased from an MCO (e.g., the plan is self-insured), then the plan is regulated solely by the federal government. If that employer contracts with an MCO to provide managed care services to employees, then the regulation depends on who bears the risk: if it is the MCO, the plan is regulated by the state; if the risk is borne to any degree by the employer, then the plan is subject to federal law only.

This complex division of regulatory responsibilities between the federal and state governments resulted from provisions of several federal laws and subsequent decisions of federal courts. The Employee Retirement Income Security Act of 1974 preempted the states from regulating health plans

**Table 3.1** U.S. Department of Health & Human Services Regional Offices

| Region | Geographic Area |
|---|---|
| Region 1: Boston | Connecticut, Maine, Massachusetts, New Hampshire, Rhode Island, Vermont |
| Region 2: New York | New Jersey, New York, Puerto Rico, the Virgin Islands |
| Region 3: Philadelphia | Delaware, District of Columbia, Maryland, Pennsylvania, Virginia, West Virginia |
| Region 4: Atlanta | Alabama, Florida, Georgia, Kentucky, Mississippi, North Carolina, South Carolina, Tennessee |
| Region 5: Chicago | Illinois, Indiana, Michigan, Minnesota, Ohio, Wisconsin |
| Region 6: Dallas | Arkansas, Louisiana, New Mexico, Oklahoma, Texas |
| Region 7: Kansas City | Iowa, Kansas, Missouri, Nebraska |
| Region 8: Denver | Colorado, Montana, North Dakota, South Dakota, Utah, Wyoming |
| Region 9: San Francisco | Arizona, California, Hawaii, Nevada, American Samoa, Commonwealth of the Northern Mariana Islands, Federated States of Micronesia, Guam, Marshall Islands, Republic of Palau |
| Region 10: Seattle | Alaska, Idaho, Oregon, Washington |

Reproduced from U.S. Department of Health & Human Services. HHS regional offices. 2021. Accessed November 16, 2021. https://www.hhs.gov/about/agencies/iea/regional-offices/index.html

of private sector employers but left to the states the regulation of the business of insurance. Although the HMO Act of 1973 established certain federal standards for HMOs that elected to operate under federal law, almost all other regulatory authority over the business of health insurance remained with the states. This deferral to state regulation of insurers was altered in 1996 with the passage of HIPAA (P.L. 104-191), which applied federal minimum requirements to state-regulated insurers as well as to employer-sponsored plans, including managed care plans.

Managed care regulations vary state by state, although there are many state laws and regulations based on the National Association of Insurance Commissioners HMO Model Act. The Commissioners published model laws on quality assessment and improvement, provider credentialing, network adequacy, grievance procedures, and standards for utilization review.[22]

## Federal Role in Quality

The Social Security Act mandated the establishment of minimum health and safety standards that must be met by providers and suppliers participating in the Medicare and Medicaid programs.[23] In 1935, the Social Security Act was signed by President Franklin D. Roosevelt to provide benefits for retirees and the unemployed. This was amended in 1965, signed by President Lyndon B. Johnson, to create the Medicare and Medicaid programs.

As a federal insurance program, Medicare provides a wide range of benefits for most people 65 years and older, Social Security beneficiaries younger than 65 years who are entitled to disability benefits, and individuals needing renal dialysis or renal transplantation. Care is rendered by providers and suppliers participating in the Medicare program, which entitles them to receive reimbursement from Medicare. In Medicare terminology, *providers* include patient care institutions, such as hospitals, critical access hospitals, hospices, nursing homes, and home health agencies. *Suppliers* are agencies for diagnosis and therapy rather than sustained patient care, such as laboratories, clinics, and ambulatory surgery centers. Providers and suppliers are subject to federal healthcare quality standards; thus, the federal government plays a large role in setting quality standards and oversight of compliance to these standards for Medicare beneficiaries.

CMS developed conditions of participation (CoP) and conditions for coverage (CfC) that healthcare organizations must meet to participate in the Medicare and Medicaid programs and receive reimbursement for services. These standards are the foundation for improving quality and protecting the health and safety of beneficiaries. CoP and CfC apply to all types of healthcare organizations like comprehensive outpatient rehabilitation facilities, federally qualified health centers, home health agencies, intermediate care facilities for individuals with intellectual disabilities, and programs of all-inclusive care for the elderly.

Although each program's CoP or CfC will be different, the table of contents from the hospital program (**Table 3.2**; U.S. Government Publishing Office)[24] provides an example to gain insight into the kinds of regulations found in the CoP and how they are organized.[25] These federal quality standards are organized in state operations manuals (SOMs) as conditions, with subsidiary standards under each condition.[26] There are individual sets of conditions or requirements for each type of provider or supplier subject

**Table 3.2** Hospital Conditions of Participation Table of Contents

**Subpart A: General Provisions**

§482.1 Basis and scope.
§482.2 Provision of emergency services by nonparticipating hospitals.

**Subpart B: Administration**

§482.11 Condition of participation: Compliance with federal, state, and local laws.
§482.12 Condition of participation: Governing body.
§482.13 Condition of participation: Patient's rights.

**Subpart C: Basic Hospital Functions**

§482.21 Condition of participation: Quality assessment and performance improvement program.
§482.22 Condition of participation: Medical staff.
§482.23 Condition of participation: Nursing services.
§482.24 Condition of participation: Medical record services.
§482.25 Condition of participation: Pharmaceutical services.
§482.26 Condition of participation: Radiologic services.
§482.27 Condition of participation: Laboratory services.
§482.28 Condition of participation: Food and dietetic services.
§482.30 Condition of participation: Utilization review.
§482.41 Condition of participation: Physical environment.
§482.42 Condition of participation: Infection control.
§482.43 Condition of participation: Discharge planning.
§482.45 Condition of participation: Organ, tissue, and eye procurement.

**Subpart D: Optional Hospital Services**

§482.51 Condition of participation: Surgical services.
§482.52 Condition of participation: Anesthesia services.
§482.53 Condition of participation: Nuclear medicine services.
§482.54 Condition of participation: Outpatient services.
§482.55 Condition of participation: Emergency services.
§482.56 Condition of participation: Rehabilitation services.
§482.57 Condition of participation: Respiratory care services.
§482.58 Special requirements for hospital providers of long-term care services (swing beds).

**Subpart E: Requirements for Specialty Hospitals**

§482.60 Special provisions applying to psychiatric hospitals.
§482.61 Condition of participation: Special medical record requirements for psychiatric hospitals.
§482.62 Condition of participation: Special staff requirements for psychiatric hospitals.
§482.68 Special requirements for transplant centers.
§482.68 Definitions.

Reproduced from U.S. Government Publishing Office. Code of Federal Regulations: Title 42—Public Health. Chapter IV—Centers for Medicare & Medicaid Services, Department of Health & Human Services. Subchapter G—Standards and certification: Part 482—Conditions of participation for hospitals. 2015. Accessed November 16, 2021. https://www.gpo.gov/fdsys/pkg/CFR-2015-title42-vol5/xml/CFR-2015-title42-vol5-part482.xml to certification. The condition or requirement in the SOMs is expressed in a summary paragraph, which describes the quality or result of operations to which all the subsidiary standards are directed.

The HHS secretary delegates to CMS regional offices the authority for ensuring healthcare providers and suppliers participating in the Medicare, Medicaid, and CLIA programs meet applicable federal requirements. CMS regional offices use state health agencies to determine whether healthcare entities meet federal standards. This process is called certification.

State and local agencies with agreements under section 1864(a) of the Act perform the following functions:

- Survey and make recommendations regarding the organization or providers' ability to meet the Medicare CoP or requirements.
- Conduct validation surveys of deemed status facilities, providers, and suppliers.
- Perform other surveys and carry out other appropriate activities and certify their findings to CMS.
- Make recommendations regarding the effective dates of provider agreements and supplier approvals in accordance with §489.13.[27]

State agencies that evaluate healthcare entities against federal regulations are usually the same agencies responsible for state licensing; however, they are reimbursed with federal funds for this work. There are also provisions for CMS-approved accreditation bodies to determine if healthcare entities meet the Medicare CoP. These providers are referred to as "deemed status" providers for participation, also known as the "deeming process." Therefore, CMS-certified healthcare entities can receive a visit from federal, state, or accreditation agencies to evaluate federal standards for certification or recertification, for compliance investigations, or as part of random validation programs to confirm accreditation or state survey findings as valid and reliable. CMS-approved accrediting organizations for various programs include but may not be limited to Accreditation Association for Ambulatory Health Care, Accreditation Commission for Health Care, American Association for Accreditation of Ambulatory Surgery Facilities, Center for Improvement in Healthcare Quality, DNV–Healthcare, National Association of Boards of Pharmacy, The Compliance Team, The Joint Commission, and Utilization Review Accreditation Commission.[28] To ensure evaluations are done in a consistent manner by these agencies, the SOMs are published and available publicly on the Internet. Healthcare quality professionals are encouraged to search for the relevant SOMs and review them

for further guidance in preparing an organization for on-site surveys. They include very explicit survey methods and processes as well as specific interpretive guidance for determining if an organization meets a standard.

The survey process varies depending on the services under review and may vary slightly depending on individual state resources, such as the staff or disciplines available to conduct surveys. During a survey, healthcare professional surveyors determine if each standard is met by conducting document reviews; interviewing staff, leaders, and patients; and observing routine procedures and patient care. After a CMS survey, the state agency (acting as a CMS surveyor) prepares a certification report for the CMS regional office and sends the healthcare organization a statement of deficiencies. The healthcare organization needs to respond to CMS with a plan of correction for each cited deficiency. Once the plan of correction is accepted by CMS, it is ultimately made available publicly through the Freedom of Information Act. Even though an organization may fail to comply with one or more of the subsidiary standards during any given survey, it cannot participate in Medicare unless it meets every condition. If the healthcare organization does not come into compliance with all conditions within the period accepted as reasonable by CMS, it is certified as noncompliant, and a termination process begins for the Medicare and Medicaid programs. Termination means the healthcare entity cannot receive federal reimbursement for services, which typically represents a financial loss for organizations.

Healthcare quality professionals are familiar with the National Practitioner Data Bank (NPDB), which is a federal data bank created because of the Medicare and Medicaid Patient and Program Protection Act of 1987 to serve as a repository of information about healthcare providers in the United States.[29] NPDB was designed to protect program beneficiaries from unfit healthcare practitioners and required reporting of adverse licensure, hospital privilege, and professional society actions against physicians and dentists related to quality of care. In addition, NPDB tracks malpractice payments made for all healthcare practitioners.

The passage of HIPAA in 1996 led to the creation of the Healthcare Integrity and Protection Data Bank (HIPDB). HIPDB served as a tracking system to alert users that a comprehensive review of the practitioner, provider, or supplier's past actions may be prudent. It was suggested that HIPDB's information be used in combination with information from other sources in making determinations on employment, affiliation, certification, or licensure. Section 6403 of the ACA authorized the secretary of HHS to cease the operation of HIPDB and to consolidate the operation of HIPDB with NPDB. The goal was to eliminate duplication between NPDB and HIPDB. In May 2013, NPDB and HIPDB merged into one database—NPDB.[30] This data bank was established with strict confidentiality protections; the HHS Office of Inspector General has the authority to impose civil money penalties on those who violate the confidentiality provisions.[31]

NPDB authorizes the government to collect information concerning sanctions taken by state licensing authorities and entities against healthcare practitioners. In 1990, Congress amended the law by broadening the language to include any negative action or finding by these authorities, not just sanctions. Intended to improve the quality of healthcare, this law encourages state licensing boards, hospitals, professional societies, and healthcare organizations to identify and discipline those who engage in unprofessional behavior, to report medical malpractice payments, and to restrict the ability of incompetent physicians, dentists, and other healthcare practitioners to move between states without disclosure or discovery of their previous history. Examples of adverse actions include revocation or alteration to licensure, clinical privileges, and professional society membership, as well as exclusions from Medicare and Medicaid. Government peer-review organizations and private accreditation organizations are required to report negative actions taken against healthcare practitioners or organizations.

## Federal Resources

Finding information about federal regulations is progressively easier because the government invested in publicly available electronic databases accessed through the Internet. Healthcare quality professionals are encouraged to take advantage of the Internet in seeking the most up-to-date federal regulations through the review of information posted on official governmental sites. The *Federal Register* is the official daily publication for rules, proposed rules, and notices of federal agencies and organizations, as well as presidential executive orders. *CFR* is the codification of these rules published in the *Federal Register*, which is divided into 50 titles that represent broad areas subject to federal regulation. It is updated by amendments that appear daily in the *Federal Register*. Each volume of the *CFR* is updated once each calendar year.

Twice a year, federal agencies publish a new edition of the *Unified Agenda of Regulatory and Deregulatory Actions*.[32] This agenda can be very helpful for healthcare quality professionals to understand the direction for selected federal agencies in the coming year. As an example, the HHS plan provides not only the annual priorities for the fiscal year as an overview but also the detailed information about each of the priorities (whether the priority is an unfunded mandate, legal authority, statement of need, legal basis, alternative, cost and benefit, risk, timetable, and contact information). These documents are useful communication tools for healthcare quality professionals to understand future directions for regulations.

The process to change regulations can be slow and frustrating, resulting in outdated regulations. There are many challenges to keeping evidence-based regulatory standards current.[33] Federal, state, and local government regulators must provide due process to those affected by their actions—this provides the healthcare industry the opportunity to review proposed changes with any known supporting evidence and to provide written feedback or testimony prior to changes in the regulation. Individuals, members of professional associations, and healthcare associations like NAHQ can comment on proposed regulations.

## State Laws and Regulations

State governments maintain state health departments that operate licensing programs for healthcare providers and organizations. Licensing requires organizations, providers, and practitioners to meet legal requirements to practice or provide services. In addition to providing licensing services, these departments usually operate enforcement programs for both state licensing requirements and federal certification requirements. In some states, local governments, such as counties and municipalities, can also have their own health departments (which may be branches of the state health department). Licensure for practitioners may be the responsibility of state health departments or separate entities accountable for disciplinary investigations and actions.

State regulations vary greatly in content, detail, and organization of regulations. This requires regulatory professionals to possess state-specific knowledge to guide organizations within the given state. Corporate healthcare entities that operate in multiple states depend on regulatory and quality professionals who play a critical role to navigate requirements within each state.

State healthcare surveys appear much like federal surveys and likely have the same personnel performing the survey. State regulators survey health-care organizations for licensure, for enforcement of regulations, and in response to complaints made to the agency by consumers of the healthcare service, their family members, or concerned staff. Licensure visits may be routine inspections within defined time periods or may be random, unannounced visits conducted based on the resources available to the state agency. State laws may dictate reporting requirements of licensed organizations for serious reportable or adverse events, and the law may require the state agency to investigate certain self-reports within a given time frame. Discretion on how the agencies respond to and investigate complaints may be allowed, based on the nature of the complaint and the severity of the allegation.

As with federal surveys, state agencies provide organizations with deficiency reports and require written responses (corrective actions) within a defined period. If organizations are not able to become compliant with state regulations, they risk loss of both licensure within the state and the ability to provide healthcare services. In addition, states report their actions to CMS and accrediting bodies that may initiate their own investigations. Reports of investigations and the organization's response to citations may also become public information or released upon request. Healthcare quality professionals are encouraged to become familiar with relevant state healthcare regulations impacting their practice setting. Most state regulatory agencies post an abundance of relevant information on the Internet.

## Private Quasi-Regulators

Although regulation is primarily a government role, there are also private organizations that serve as quasi-regulators in healthcare. Field provides a rich historical perspective on regulation in healthcare, as well as an introduction to private regulators.[34] The American Medical Association (AMA) may be the most well-known organization. AMA sponsored creation of organizations with oversight roles for the medical profession to supplement government regulators, such as organizations that accredit medical schools, administer licensure examinations, and certify specialists. State medical boards, for example, use privately administered examinations in granting medical licenses, and the Medicare program relies on specialty certification as an indicator of physician quality. **Box 3.1** identifies key points of laws and regulations.

---

### Box 3.1  Key Points: Laws and Regulations

- Develop a process to receive, review, and communicate updates within the organization since laws and regulations continuously change.
- Become familiar with federal HHS agencies and *State Operations Manuals*.
- CMS-certified healthcare entities may receive a visit from federal, state, or accreditation agencies to evaluate compliance with federal standards.
- Adopting a continuous compliance strategy ensures alignment with federal and state regulations, accreditation standards, and contractual obligations.

---

# Accreditation, Certification, and Recognition

*Accreditation* and *certification* are terms used in many industries in the United States, including healthcare. The terms are often used incorrectly or interchangeably, which may create confusion.

- *Accreditation* may be defined as an official authorization or approval, or recognition of conforming to standards. Accreditation is voluntary and granted by private sector organizations (trade associations, professional societies, or independent businesses).
- *Certification* is the recognition of meeting standards and qualifications within a field. Certification can be provided by either private-sector organizations or government agencies.
- *Recognition* programs empower employers, health plans, patients, and consumers to make informed healthcare decisions based on quality. Participation in a National Committee for Quality Assurance (NCQA) Recognition Program, as an example, demonstrates compliance with guidelines and standards that support quality healthcare delivery and evidence-based practices and clinical protocols (e.g., Diabetes Recognition Program, Patient-Centered Medical Home Recognition Program).

In healthcare, accreditation commonly refers to a process reviewing an entire organization's operations (e.g., ambulatory surgery center), whereas certification commonly refers to a review of part of the organization's operations or care for a specific population or competency (e.g., sepsis). Certification may also be a reference to an individual's competency (e.g., ambulatory care nursing) or the determination of an organization's eligibility to participate in a government program.

Federal certification requirements are found across the healthcare continuum. For example, a federal certification requirement is CMS regulations for all laboratory testing performed on humans through CLIA.[35] All clinical laboratories must be certified to receive Medicare or Medicaid payments. CLIA maintains a list of CMS-approved accrediting organizations that may perform laboratory inspections, whose requirements are deemed as being equivalent to or more stringent than CMS requirements (CMS accepts the accrediting organization's inspection in lieu of its own inspection). Another federal certification requirement is found in the Mammography Quality Standards Act (MQSA) as amended by the Mammography Quality Standards Reauthorization Acts of 1998 and 2004, which requires that all facilities providing mammography must be certified by FDA.[36] To become certified, a facility must be accredited by FDA-designated accrediting bodies. As of October 1, 2021, there are over 8700 mammography facilities certified.[37]

## Value of Accreditation

Although many hospitals and many health plans are accredited, accreditation is not uniformly adopted across all segments of the healthcare industry. Home care and hospice agencies, among the fastest growing segments of the continuum, may also be accredited. Nursing home accreditation continues to evolve. A study comparing accredited and nonaccredited nursing homes confirmed previous findings that demonstrate a consistent pattern of superior performance among accredited nursing homes.[38] There are not the same

financial incentives to seek accreditation since legislation does not authorize deemed status in Medicare or Medicaid for private accrediting bodies to substitute for government oversight. CMS (for Medicare and Medicaid) and the states (for Medicaid) have regulatory standards and government survey and certification programs to enforce nursing home regulations. In the primary care setting, an increased focus is placed on attainment of patient-centered medical home recognition or certification. Recognition signifies that patient treatment is coordinated through a primary care provider who ensures the patient receives the necessary care when and where needed and in a manner that the patient can understand.[39,40]

As the healthcare industry faces ongoing pressure for cost containment, questions surface as to the value of accreditation in relation to the cost. Literature continues to grow about the benefits of accreditation, which include improved accountability and transparency.[41,42] One of the most extensive reviews of accreditation value is a literature review published by Accreditation Canada, which summarizes literature findings on the value and impact of healthcare accreditation.[43] This information may be helpful to articulating the value proposition and business case for quality and safety. The review includes results and conclusions from research, gray literature, and experience-based articles. Accreditation is an integral part of healthcare services in more than 70 countries, as either a voluntary or government-mandated requirement. See **Table 3.3** for a summary of cited benefits of accreditation with expanded discussion of several below.

**Table 3.3** Benefits of Accreditation, Certification, and Recognition Programs

**Better Care**
- Improves patient's health
- Improves organization's reputation among end users and stakeholders
- Enhances consumer awareness and perception of quality care as well as overall satisfaction level
- Provides a framework to improve operational effectiveness and advance positive health outcomes

**Organizational Effectiveness**
- Promotes a quality and safety culture
- Increases the healthcare organization's compliance with quality and safety
- Demonstrates credibility and a commitment to quality and accountability
- Supports the efficient and effective use of resources in healthcare services
- Sustains improvements in quality and organizational performance
- Promotes the sharing of policies, procedures, and best practices among healthcare organizations

*(continues)*

**Table 3.3** **Benefits of Accreditation, Certification, and Recognition Programs** *(continued)*

- Provides healthcare organizations with a well-defined vision for sustainable quality improvement
- Enhances the organization's understanding of the continuum of care
- Stimulates sustainable quality improvement efforts
- Continuously raises the bar regarding quality improvement structure, process, and outcomes
- Leads to the improvement of internal practices (e.g., reliability of laboratory testing)
- Identifies areas for additional funding for healthcare organizations and provides a platform for negotiating this funding

**Workforce**

- Ensures an acceptable level of quality among healthcare providers
- Promotes capacity building, professional development, and organizational learning
- Decreases variances in practice among healthcare providers and decision makers
- Improves communication and collaboration internally and with external stakeholders
- Enables ongoing self-analysis of performance in relation to standards
- Strengthens interprofessional team effectiveness
- Provides an opportunity for team building and improves staff understanding of coworkers' jobs and responsibilities
- Promotes an understanding of how each person's job contributes to the organization's mission and services
- Contributes to increased job satisfaction among physicians, nurses, and other providers

**Risk Management**

- Decreases liability costs
- Mitigates the risk of adverse events

Modified from Nicklin W. The value and impact of health care accreditation: A literature review. Accreditation Canada. 2013. Accessed November 11, 2021. https://www.aventa.org/pdfs/valueimpactaccreditation.pdf

## External Credibility

Consistent with the historical view in the United States, accreditation is cited as improving an organization's reputation among end users and enhancing awareness and perception of quality care. It is also cited as improving communication and collaboration internally and with external stakeholders. All of this is thought to demonstrate credibility and a commitment to quality, accountability, and transparency, which are hallmarks of ongoing healthcare reform.

## Improved Quality

Accreditation provides an evidence-based framework for organizations to improve the patient experience, engagement, and outcomes. The improved outcomes may result from accreditation, which provides a framework to create and implement systems and processes to improve operational effectiveness. Accreditation is also cited as providing healthcare organizations with a well-defined vision for sustainable, highly reliable quality improvement initiatives. This vision and framework enable organizations to sustain improvements in quality and organizational performance,

enable ongoing self-analysis of performance in relation to standards, and ensure an acceptable level of quality among healthcare providers. These quality improvements are realized as the accreditation process achieves the following:

- Increases the healthcare organization's compliance with quality and safety standards
- Decreases variance in practice among healthcare providers and decision makers by standardizing core processes
- Codifies organizational policies and procedures
- Continuously raises the bar regarding quality improvement initiatives, policies, and processes

## Organizational Learning

Accreditation is cited as promoting capacity building, professional development, and organizational learning. The accreditation process itself could highlight practices that were working well and may have a spillover effect, whereby the accreditation of one service helps to improve the performance of others. This fosters *systemness*—"the ability to implement system-oriented approaches."[44(912)] Accreditation is also cited as enhancing an organization's understanding of equity, the care continuum, social determinants of health, trauma-informed care, and the wholeness of the individual. Healthcare industry benefits are also realized through sharing policies, procedures, and best practices among accredited healthcare organizations.

## Staff Effectiveness

Accreditation is cited as contributing to the effectiveness of the organization's staff in the following ways: strengthening interprofessional team effectiveness; promoting an understanding of how each person's job contributes to the healthcare organization's mission and services; providing a team-building opportunity for staff and improving their understanding of their coworkers' functions; and contributing to increased job satisfaction among physicians, nurses, and other providers (and the acknowledgment of moral distress and burnout in the workforce). Recently highlighted is the focus on joy in work, engagement, well-being, and resilience in response to the global COVID-19 pandemic.

## Reduced Costs

Accreditation is cited as decreasing liability costs and mitigating the risk of adverse events, which would ultimately reduce costs as well. Standardization leads to less variation and ultimately fewer defects and less waste. Accreditation could also impact costs by helping to identify an organization's areas that need additional funding and then providing a platform for negotiating for this funding.

# Accreditation, Certification, and Recognition Programs

There are usually several ways an organization fulfills mandatory external validation requirements. The healthcare quality professional is typically responsible for ensuring that the organization meets expectations for all mandatory external regulatory and accreditation programs. As a change agent and innovator, the healthcare quality professional needs to understand the various options available to meet these requirements. In addition, there might be several options for attaining optional disease-specific and specialty certifications from one or more different accrediting or certifying bodies.

Depending on the size, scope, and complexity of the organization, the responsibility of meeting these expectations may belong solely to the healthcare quality professional, or it may be shared with other department or service leaders (chief nursing officer, chief operating officer, chief quality officer, etc.). The nature and scope of external requirements typically depend upon the type of organization, the specific services provided, and the state-specific regulatory requirements that are usually tied to licensure. Healthcare quality professionals may be asked to take the lead in quantifying the specific accreditation and certification-related costs, both external (directly related to the accreditation agency) and internal (related to the staff, time, and resources required to meet accreditation standards and achieve compliance).

**Box 3.2** outlines key points in accreditation and certification.

---

### Box 3.2 Key Points: Accreditation and Certification

- Healthcare quality professionals
  - typically take the lead in quantifying specific accreditation and certification-related costs and develop the business case for quality and safety; and
  - must be familiar with reporting for adverse events/ serious reportable events for their respective state department of health.
- Many accreditation and certification organizations provide tools or resources to help consumers understand or evaluate compliance with elements of performance.
- The accreditation process may highlight practices working well and may have a spillover effect, which fosters systemness—the ability to implement system-oriented approaches.

---

Accreditation agencies continue to evolve and grow, and they now represent a significant segment of the healthcare industry. Not only has the number of organizations that offer services increased, but the services provided have also expanded to be more accessible. Agencies no longer offer one program as their single service line but offer diversified products across the healthcare continuum, representing payers and providers with their accreditation, certification, and recognition programs (e.g., the recent additions of home infusion therapy and advanced telehealth programs; **Table 3.4**).

Most accreditation agencies provide applications, templates, and tools, as well as associated education or consultation programs to assist organizations with survey readiness activities. Healthcare quality professionals are encouraged to explore agency websites to learn specific information about agencies that accredit or certify their organizations. Survey cycles vary by accrediting agency and by healthcare sector. Many of the organizations provide tools or resources on their

**Table 3.4**  **Accreditation, Certification, and Recognition Programs**

| Organization | Program Type |
|---|---|
| Accreditation Association for Ambulatory Health Care (AAAHC) | *Accreditation*<br>Ambulatory surgery center, primary care provider, health plan, international healthcare provider |
| Accreditation Commission for Health Care, Inc. (ACHC) (includes Health Facilities Accreditation Program) | *Accreditation*<br>Ambulatory surgery center, critical access hospital, end stage renal disease facilities, home health agency, hospice, hospital, assisted living, behavioral health, clinical laboratory, compounding pharmacy, dentistry, home infusion therapy, office-based surgery, pharmacy, private duty, renal dialysis, and sleep<br>*Certification*<br>Joint replacement, lithotripsy, stroke and wound care |
| American Association for Accreditation of Ambulatory Surgery Facilities (AAAASF) | *Accreditation*<br>Outpatient (surgical, procedural, oral maxillofacial pediatric dentistry), Medicare programs (surgical/ambulatory surgery center, physical therapy, rural health clinics), international programs (surgical, physical therapy, dental) |
| American College of Surgeons (ACS) | *Accreditation*<br>Commission on Cancer, Metabolic and Bariatric Surgery Accreditation and Quality Improvement Program and National Accreditation Program for Breast Centers<br>*Verification*<br>Children's surgery, geriatric surgery, and pediatric surgery |
| CARF International (CARF) | *Accreditation*<br>Aging services, behavioral health, continuing care retirement communities, child and youth services, employment and community services, medical rehabilitation, opioid treatment programs, and vision rehabilitation services |
| Community Health Accreditation Program (CHAP) | *Accreditation*<br>Home health, hospice, home care, palliative care, home infusion therapy, pharmacy |
| DNV—Healthcare | *Accreditation*<br>Critical access hospital, hospital, psychiatric hospital<br>*Certification*<br>Cardiac Center of Excellence, chest pain, extracorporeal, heart failure, ventricular assistive device facility; infection prevention; sterile processing; stroke care; Orthopaedic Center of Excellence, foot and ankle surgery, hip and knee replacement, shoulder and spine surgery; and palliative care |
| National Association of Boards of Pharmacy (NABP) | *Pharmacy Accreditation*<br>Community; compounding; digital; durable medical equipment, prosthetics/orthotics, and supplies (DMEPOS); home infusion; specialty<br>*Distributor Accreditation*<br>Drug, over-the-counter medical devices<br>*Inspections*<br>Verified Pharmacy Program, supply chain |
| National Committee for Quality Assurance (NCQA) | *Accreditation*<br>Health plans, disease management, case management, credentialing, health equity, long-term services and supports, managed behavioral healthcare organizations, and population health<br>*Certification*<br>Credentials verification organizations, health information products, health IT/data collection, and physician and hospital quality<br>*Recognition*<br>Diabetes, heart/stroke, patient-centered specialty care, and patient-centered medical homes |

*(continues)*

**Table 3.4** Accreditation, Certification, and Recognition Programs *(continued)*

| Organization | Program Type |
|---|---|
| The Compliance Team | *Accreditation*<br>Durable medical equipment, prosthetics, orthotics and supplies, rural health clinics, patient-centered medical homes<br>*Certification*<br>Testing, immunization |
| The Joint Commission (TJC) | *Accreditation*<br>Ambulatory care, assisted living community, behavioral health care, critical access hospitals, home care, hospitals, laboratory services, nursing care centers, office-based surgery<br>*Certification*<br>Specialty services such as cardiac, stroke, palliative care, total hip and total knee replacement, behavioral health home, community-based palliative care, healthcare staffing, integrated care, patient blood management, perinatal care, and patient-centered medical homes (ambulatory care, hospitals, and critical access hospitals) |
| URAC | *Accreditation*<br>Pharmacy, patient care management, administrative management, digital health and telehealth, health plans, mental health and substance use parity |

*Note*: Summary table intended to illustrate a sample of organizations and different programs available. The types of accreditation and certification are subject to change.
Data from www.aaahc.org; www.achc.org; www.aaaasf.org; www.carf.org; www.chapinc.org; www.cihq.org; www.dnvglhealthcare.com; https://nabp.pharmacy; www.ncqa.org; https://ndacommission.com/contact/; www.thecomplianceteam.org; www.jointcommission.org; www.urac.org

websites to help consumers understand or evaluate compliance or quality of care when considering the services of an organization. Healthcare providers and other organizations may also find assessment, gap analysis, quality improvement plan, or evaluation tools made available by these agencies instrumental in their effort to improve the quality and safety of care across the healthcare industry. Descriptions of several agencies follow.

## Association for the Advancement of Blood & Biotherapies

Association for the Advancement of Blood & Biotherapies accreditation is granted for collection, processing, testing, distribution, and administration of blood and blood components; hematopoietic progenitor cell activities; cord blood activities; perioperative activities; relationship testing activities; and immunohematology reference laboratories.

## Accreditation Association for Ambulatory Health Care

The Accreditation Association for Ambulatory Health Care (AAAHC) is a private, not-for-profit organization formed in 1979. Its standards advance and promote patient safety, quality care, and value for ambulatory healthcare through peer-based accreditation processes, education, and research. AAAHC accredits ambulatory healthcare settings including ambulatory healthcare clinics, ambulatory surgery centers, birthing centers, office-based surgery centers, community health centers, medical home practices, MCOs, Indian health centers, military healthcare facilities, and others. In 2019, AAAHC introduced a learning management system, 1095 Learn, to support its accreditation program, built upon a "1095 Strong, quality every day" philosophy that promotes continuous readiness.[45]

## Accreditation Commission for Health Care

In existence since 1985, the Accreditation Commission for Health Care (ACHC) began offering accreditation services nationally in 1996. The Health Facilities Accreditation Program (HFAP) was acquired by ACHC in 2020. As a brand within ACHC, HFAP provides additional offerings such as accreditation programs for ambulatory specialty care (office-based surgery), non-deemed accreditation, and specialty certification for four levels of stroke care, laser, and lithotripsy services, inpatient and outpatient joint replacement, and wound care.[46]

ACHC has deeming authority for home health, hospice, renal dialysis, home infusion therapy, and DMEPOS. The merger now offers expanded services, adding programs with CMS deeming authority for hospitals, ambulatory surgery centers, clinical laboratories, and critical access hospitals. Since 2013, ACHC and DNV Healthcare have partnered to provide a single-source accreditation solution for hospitals and health systems with ancillary services.

## American College of Radiology

Since 1987, the American College of Radiology has accredited more than 39,000 facilities in 10 different imaging modalities. The American College of Radiology offers accreditation programs in computed tomography, magnetic resonance imaging, breast magnetic resonance imaging, breast ultrasound, mammography, nuclear medicine and positron emission tomography, stereotactic breast biopsy, ultrasound, and radiation oncology practice.

## American College of Surgeons

The American College of Surgeons (ACS) is a scientific and educational association of surgeons that was founded in 1913 to improve the quality of care for the surgical patient by setting consensus-driven standards. The ACS Committee on Trauma implements programs that support injury prevention and ensure optimal outcomes through advocacy, education, best practice creation, outcome assessment, and continuous quality improvement.[47]

## College of American Pathologists

The College of American Pathologists (CAP) Laboratory Accreditation Program accredits a variety of laboratory settings from complex university medical centers to physician office laboratories. It covers a complete array of disciplines and testing procedures. CMS granted the CAP Laboratory Accreditation Program deeming authority. It is also recognized by TJC and can be used to meet many state certification requirements. CAP provides laboratory accreditation to forensic drug-testing facilities, biorepository facilities, and reproductive laboratories, in collaboration with the American Society for Reproductive Medicine. Twenty-one discipline-specific accreditation checklists contain CAP program requirements,

developed on more than 50 years of insight and pathology expertise.[48]

## Commission of Office Laboratory Accreditation

Completing the Commission of Office Laboratory Accreditation (COLA) program demonstrates that a clinical laboratory is following CLIA. It accredits different types of laboratories, such as physicians' offices, community hospitals, mobile clinics, Veterans Health Administration, and Department of Defense. In addition, COLA is recognized by TJC and is approved by CMS to accredit laboratories for certain specialties such as cannabis, chemistry, genetic testing, hematology, microbiology, immunology, and immunohematology/transfusion services.

## CARF International

CARF International (CARF) assists service providers to demonstrate and improve outcomes while meeting internationally recognized standards. CARF has surveyed hundreds of thousands of providers throughout North and South America, Europe, Africa, and Asia since it was founded as an independent, nonprofit accreditor in 1966. Accreditation programs are offered across the healthcare continuum. CARF provides an online provider search tool and resources for consumers.

## Community Health Accreditation Partner

The Community Health Accreditation Partner (CHAP) is an independent, not-for-profit, accrediting body for home and community-based healthcare organizations. Created in 1965 as a joint venture between the American Public Health Association and the National League for Nursing, CHAP was the first accrediting body for home and community-based healthcare organizations in the United States. Through deeming authority granted by CMS, CHAP has the regulatory authority to survey agencies providing home health, hospice, home medical equipment services, home care, pharmacy, and home infusion therapy to determine if they meet the Medicare CoP and CMS Quality Standards. They also provide palliative care certification.

## DNV Healthcare

The National Integrated Accreditation for Healthcare Organizations (NIAHO) requirements combine hospital accreditation with ISO 9001. The core of

DNV hospital accreditation in the United States and internationally is the NIAHO standards platform, created by DNV in 2008 for U.S. hospitals. DNV's platform is that accreditation is not an inspection but rather a catalyst for quality and patient safety, proposing to change the culture of accreditation based on empowerment, not fear.[49] The organization follows a collaborative approach to help healthcare providers identify, assess, and manage risk while ensuring sustainable business practices. DNV's NIAHO assesses both Medicare CoP and ISO 9001 standards for the formation and implementation of quality and performance improvement systems. DNV formed an alliance with ACHC to meet an organization's ancillary accreditation needs. ACHC has Medicare deeming authority for home health, hospice, and DMEPOS, and additional services include pharmacy, private duty, behavioral health, convenient care clinics, and sleep.

## The Joint Commission

For 70 years, TJC has been an independent, not-for-profit organization that accredits and certifies 22,000 healthcare organizations and programs in the United States. TJC accreditation and certification is recognized nationwide as a symbol of quality (via The Gold Seal of Approval) that reflects an organization's commitment to meeting certain performance standards. TJC accredits different types of healthcare organizations,[50] and Joint Commission International accredits facilities globally.

## National Association of Boards of Pharmacy

The National Association of Boards of Pharmacy (NABP) is the independent, international, and impartial association that assists its member boards in protecting the public health. Initially established to assist the state boards of pharmacy in creating uniform education and licensure standards, NABP now supports patient and prescription drug safety through examinations that assess pharmacist competency, pharmacist licensure transfer and verification services, and various pharmacy accreditation programs.[51]

## National Committee for Quality Assurance

Founded in 1990, the National Committee for Quality Assurance (NCQA) is a private, not-for-profit organization that accredits and/or certifies healthcare organizations. NCQA screens, trains, and certifies organizations that collect or audit data for health plans and providers.

## National Dialysis Accreditation Commission

The National Dialysis Accreditation Commission is the only accreditation organization in the United States formed by dialysis experts with the exclusive focus of serving the dialysis community. It was the first dialysis accreditation organization in the country to apply for and receive approval from CMS for deeming authority for Medicare certification.[52]

## The Compliance Team

The Compliance Team is a nationally recognized healthcare accreditation organization with deeming authority from CMS for home infusion therapy and rural health clinics. The Compliance Team's proprietary accreditation status is known as Exemplary Provider Accreditation, awarded to those healthcare providers who demonstrate outstanding patient care practices and Safety-Honesty-Caring quality standards.[53] They offer a range of other accreditation services (DMEPOS, patient-centered medical home, etc.).

## URAC

Formerly known as the Utilization Review Accreditation Commission, URAC accredits many types of healthcare organizations depending on the specific functions they carry out with a portfolio of programs that spans the healthcare industry. URAC accreditation, certification, and designation addresses administrative management (e.g., provider-based population health), digital health and telehealth (e.g., health websites), health plans (e.g., marketplace, Medicare Advantage, and dental), mental health and substance use disorder parity, pharmacy (e.g., community, infusion, and mail service), and patient care management (e.g., independent review organizations).

# Accreditation and Certification Terms and Concepts

Before moving into the discussion about continuous readiness, terms and concepts associated with accreditation, certification, and survey processes are explained. This serves as context for understanding the overall accreditation and certification processes that will be addressed in the remainder of this section.

## Requirements

Accreditation agencies have requirements that must be met to seek initial accreditation or reaccreditation. They cover key areas such as the following:

- Quality improvement
- Population health
- Network management
- Utilization management
- Credentialing and recredentialing
- Rights and responsibilities
- Benefits and services

Each accreditation agency usually directs applicants to have a consultative call with program experts before desired survey start dates. There are standards and tools that must be purchased, and a gap analysis is recommended to compare the standards to an organization's policies, procedures, processes, and practices. An online survey application is required, as is submission of other support documents.

## Standards

Like regulatory requirements, accreditation and certification standards are published and available to organizations that are applying for review or considering pursuit of accreditation or certification. A standard is a statement about performance expectations, structures, processes, and outcomes that must be in place. These standards are developed based on evidence for practice, expert opinion and consensus, or research. Accrediting agencies wishing to provide CMS deemed status are preapproved by CMS to assure their minimum standards meet or exceed the CoP or CfC. The requirements or standards that are not tied to CMS requirements evolve over time with industry knowledge and technology and are more responsive to changes than government regulations. Standards may focus on the infrastructure of the organization, the processes of care delivery, or the outcomes of the care delivery system.

## Standards Compliance

Organizations must be able to demonstrate that they are following or adhering to all the elements outlined in the standard. Some accrediting agencies will include elements of performance as part of their standards to provide further guidance to the organization to ensure that the organization is meeting the expectation. Compliance may be demonstrated in a variety of ways and is not limited to survey processes through regulatory or accrediting agency visits or surveys. However, on-site surveys conducted by accrediting agency surveyors are the most visible mechanisms for demonstrating compliance as part of the accreditation process. Some healthcare organizations consult with experts in the field to conduct mock surveys to identify gaps in compliance to ensure readiness for the official on-site or virtual survey.

## Application

Accreditation cycles begin with an application requesting an initial or follow-up review or reaccreditation. The accrediting agency reviews the application to determine the scope of the review by evaluating the size and scope of the organization and services to be reviewed. It is critical that healthcare quality professionals and other organizational leaders address all elements of the application. In accordance with the requirements of HIPAA Privacy Rule and Security Rule and modified by HITECH provisions of the American Recovery and Reinvestment Act of 2009, a healthcare organization and the accrediting agency sign a business associate agreement before the organization's survey can begin. A business associate agreement outlines the access, use, and disclosure of any patient-protected health information between the accrediting agency and the healthcare organization.

## Costs

Accreditation comes at significant cost to an organization. Not only are staff resources required to maintain compliance and continuous readiness, but fees are also associated with the accreditation process. Online and hard copy accreditation or certification standards and online applications are typically provided for a fee. Fees often are on a sliding scale, reflecting the size and complexity of the organization. Organizational fees also include education and support to the leadership team and healthcare quality professional. Education fees outside of the organizational fee may be required to support accreditation and regulatory functions (e.g., conferences and webinars provided by professional associations to review new standards and tactics for meeting them).

For on-site surveys, the number of surveyor hours or days required for the review affects pricing. There are often annual participation fees as well. Costs for survey preparation, hosting the survey team for the on-site survey process, intracycle monitoring, and fees assessed for the regular survey cycle are also factors considered as organizations choose an accreditation agency. Because these fees can be substantial, they must also be included in operating budgets. Revisits to verify implementation of plans of correction and complaint surveys add additional costs. All these costs should be included in any return-on-investment cost analysis.

## Review Cycle

The review cycle varies with each accreditation agency and by healthcare sector and type of accreditation or certification. However, many are two- or three-year cycles. For example, psychiatric hospitals are accredited by DNV Healthcare for a three-year period, subject to annual survey to verify continuing compliance with NIAHO and other requirements.

## Intracycle Requirements

For accreditation to be part of the organization's ongoing process for continuous readiness, accreditation agencies may require intracycle activities to confirm sustained compliance. Requirements for a periodic self-assessment or performance review between surveys may require submission of data and reports to the agency or for public reporting or attestations of process completion.

## Performance Measures

Performance measures are a required element of accreditation and certification and are publicly reported. Measures may be developed by the review organization, by professional organizations through consensus, or through national organizations such as the National Quality Forum (NQF). NQF was created in 1999 by a coalition of public- and private-sector leaders after the President's Advisory Commission on Consumer Protection and Quality in the Healthcare Industry identified the need for an organization to promote and ensure patient protections and healthcare quality through measurement and public reporting. As of 2021, about 300 NQF-endorsed measures are used in more than 20 federal public reporting and pay-for-performance programs as well as in private-sector and state programs and are often used by accreditation agencies to judge quality.[54] About 30%

of NQF-endorsed measures have been developed by professional/specialty societies.

Performance measurement may be an ongoing review for accreditation, with quarterly or annual performance ratings sometimes included on public websites. For example, in the hospital industry, TJC was one of the first accreditation agencies to include on its public website not only the organization's accreditation status, but also comparative performance with respect to national patient safety goals and national quality improvement goals (e.g., emergency department throughput measures, venous thromboembolism, immunization). NCQA reports its accreditation decisions on its public website. It includes plan-specific information about performance on the Healthcare Effectiveness and Data Information Set (HEDIS), including 90 measures grouped into the following six domains:

1. Effectiveness of care
2. Access/availability of care
3. Experience of care
4. Utilization and risk-adjusted utilization
5. Health plan descriptive information
6. Measures reported using electronic clinical data systems[55]

HEDIS is designed to provide purchasers and consumers with the information they need to reliably compare the performance of health plans. HEDIS and Consumer Assessment of Healthcare Providers and Systems survey results are included in Quality Compass, an interactive, web-based comparison tool that allows users to view plan results and benchmark information. See *Performance and Process Improvement*, *Health Data Analytics*, and *Quality Review and Accountability* for more information on performance measures.

## Reportable Events

Some state agencies and accrediting organizations require or strongly encourage healthcare organizations to report serious events, which are then known as "serious reportable events." For example, under Washington state law (Chapter 70.56 RCW; 246-302 WAC), hospitals, psychiatric hospitals, child birthing centers, Department of Corrections medical facilities, and ambulatory surgical facilities are required to report adverse events/SREs to the Washington State Department of Health. In Washington, the list includes 29 NQF-endorsed SREs, which are adverse events that are of concern to both the public and healthcare professionals and providers; clearly identifiable and measurable, and thus feasible to include in a reporting system; and of a nature such that the risk of occurrence is significantly influenced by the policies and procedures of the healthcare facility. Facilities are required to conduct a root cause analysis and send the findings to the state. Reported events are posted quarterly on the Department of Health website for public review.[56]

TJC adopted a formal sentinel event policy in 1996 to help hospitals that experience serious adverse events improve safety and learn from those sentinel events. *Sentinel events* include "a patient safety event (not primarily related to the natural course of the [patient's] illness or underlying condition that reaches a [patient] and results in death, severe harm [regardless of duration of harm], or permanent harm [regardless of severity of harm])."[57(¶4)] An event can also be considered sentinel if the event signaled the need for immediate investigation and response.[57] Each accredited organization is strongly encouraged, but not required, to self-report sentinel events to TJC. Healthcare quality professionals work with organizational leaders to develop policies and procedures for the reporting of SREs internally and externally. More on this topic can be found in the *Leadership and Accountability* and *Patient Safety* sections.

# Continuous Readiness

The goal of continuous readiness programs is to break crisis-management cycles and just-in-time (or just-too-late) cultures to provide continuous safe, high-quality patient care and sustained compliance with regulations, standards, evidence-based practices, and professional standards. Benefits to continuous readiness include increased likelihood that the organization is meeting expectations for consumer-centric and safe care as well as a safe environment on a consistent, daily basis. Key components of successful continuous readiness programs include leadership commitment, management accountability, and compliance oversight. Continuous survey readiness includes organizational assessment, survey readiness oversight, requirements and standards oversight, and leading the survey process (preparation, survey outcomes, and postsurvey activities).

## Leadership Commitment

The expectation and support for continuous readiness must come from the C-Suite. It is then up to the healthcare quality professional to translate the expectation into action. To understand the role of leadership in creating a culture of continuous readiness, it is useful to first examine the concept. *Culture* is the tacit social order of an organization that shapes attitudes and behaviors in wide-ranging and durable ways. It fosters an organization's capacity to thrive and can evolve flexibly and autonomously in response to changing opportunities and demands.[58] *Continuous readiness* is the state of being organizationally prepared by "proactively maintaining a safe healthcare environment conducive to high-quality patient care. It essentially means having staff at all levels doing the right things for the right reasons because they understand those reasons."[59(¶1)] The outcome of these activities is continuous *compliance*, whereby the organization commits to an active, ongoing process to ensure that legal, ethical, and professional standards are met by consistently applying fundamental compliance principles (e.g., implementing and maintaining written policies, procedures, and standards of conduct; conducting effective training, education, and simulation; developing effective lines of communication; and conducting internal monitoring and auditing).[60]

Drawing on these definitions, one sees that a culture of continuous readiness is an attitude and value demonstrated throughout the organization in goals and practices that yield an uninterrupted state of mental preparedness by demonstrating that staff throughout the organization are immediately physically ready or available to demonstrate compliance. Given the current healthcare environment and public expectations for safe patient care, discrete survey readiness is not a central focus in this definition. This is because each patient, rather than each survey, deserves continuous care and service that meets regulatory and accreditation requirements—every day.

Leadership commitment to continuous readiness must be in place for programs to be successful and sustained. Leaders must be willing to change their organization's culture to one of readiness, which requires the leaders to commit to personal change and create an environment where the values, ways of thinking, managerial styles, paradigms, and approaches to problem solving support a culture of readiness. Leaders must be patient and persistent to see this transformation through by defining what readiness looks like within their organization, aligning staff with that vision, and inspiring staff despite obstacles that will surface.

To commit, leaders must understand the business case for compliance and the costs of noncompliance. Costs may be known from previous ramp-up activities or noncompliance situations, or there may be potential costs from adverse media attention and loss of business. With the expanding culture of transparency and public reporting of performance measures, organizations are subject to scrutiny from a variety of perspectives once media attention is drawn to them. In this era of social media influence, negative press can have immediate consequences (e.g., reports of ransomware attacks that lead some patients to seek services elsewhere). The business case for continuous readiness also includes the impact of ramp-up activities and crisis compliance management. Staff and managers can experience frustration and burnout with crisis compliance management and seek employment elsewhere, thus depleting organizations of experienced employees and of those who possess crucial institutional memory.

Leaders must include continuous readiness within organizational strategic priorities to change the culture. Continuous readiness must be part of the operational budgeting process and key leadership activities, as well as a foremost topic that leaders inquire about in routine discussions with staff and managers during rounding, briefings, and huddles. Leaders also must be willing to hold managers accountable for readiness responsibilities. Staying on the pulse of employee fatigue and resilience during pandemics and disasters is essential, such as the recent long-term COVID-19 pandemic. This will affect how employees respond to requests to participate in regulatory or accreditation readiness activities. Surveyors are interested in how organizations adapt their core processes during events that disrupt business operations. For example, the frontline staff developed innovations as a response to crisis levels of patients that occurred at times during the pandemic. The response by leadership and staff to the surge should be highlighted during introductory remarks by leadership during an accreditation visit.

## Management Accountability

The management team plays a central role in continuous readiness activities. Compliance is evaluated by what happens at the point of care delivery, for which managers are accountable. Policies and procedures need to be aligned with the most current standards and regulations to provide the guidance and structure for those providing or supporting care delivery. Current practice and policies must be aligned to achieve compliance. It is the manager's role to determine when practice and policies are inconsistent, understand root causes of variance, and take corrective action required for either policy adjustments or staff behavior adjustments.

Managers are also responsible for ensuring that individuals within their span of control are held accountable to regulatory and accreditation expectations. Managers evaluate individuals while they are doing their work to ensure that key process and policy expectations are always met. Individuals need to be held answerable for their performance, and the manager's role is to provide coaching, feedback, and positive reinforcement for behavior that meets policy expectations, as well as escalating to progressive discipline within a just culture framework, as appropriate. Managers also bear in mind how the COVID-19 pandemic, or a response to any local disaster that resulted in changes in practice and operations, has affected their workforce resilience and productivity.

Healthcare quality professionals in leadership roles cannot be the lone voices requiring compliance in complex organizations. The management team provides operational oversight within an organization and is the key to ensuring continuous compliance within its areas of accountability. Healthcare quality professionals must provide the program structure and education to help managers understand the requirements. New managers have steep learning curves to understand not only their departmental operations but also functional interrelations associated with regulatory and accreditation requirements on systemness. As managers learn to juggle operations, fiscal accountabilities, staffing, and the patient experience (satisfaction and engagement), they must also incorporate sustained compliance into their busy, unpredictable days. Unfortunately, it may be easier to allocate time to the faces and duties of the given day rather than to proactive readiness responsibilities. Thus, the culture of the organization and the leaders' strategic priorities will be determining factors in the success of continuous readiness programs. Day-to-day surveillance of quality and safety can be woven into the fabric of care delivery through short briefings, huddles, and rounding.

## Compliance Oversight

Healthcare is a highly regulated industry with an increasingly challenging business environment. Every organization needs a compliance program and/or enterprise risk management program that is both effective and sustainable. The program is an intentional, formalized effort to prevent, detect, and respond to business conduct that is inconsistent with federal and state laws and with an organization's values. Reliable practices within the healthcare industry are paramount since most providers receive significant financial support from the government through such programs as Medicare and Medicaid. The federal OIG helps healthcare providers such as hospitals and physicians comply with relevant federal healthcare laws and regulations; OIG creates compliance resources. OIG compliance documents include special fraud alerts, advisory bulletins, podcasts, videos, brochures, and papers providing guidance on compliance with federal healthcare program standards. OIG also issues advisory opinions, which cover the application of the federal anti-kickback statute and other fraud and abuse authorities to the requesting party's existing or proposed business arrangement. States also maintain some form of an OIG with statutory authority that works closely with federal, state, and local law enforcement agencies to detect, prevent, investigate, and prosecute any fraudulent, abusive, or wasteful activity involving the state Medicaid programs. The state's OIG conducts audits and investigations and may terminate providers who are in violation of federal and state statutes, rules, and regulations.

The federal OIG developed a series of voluntary compliance program guidance documents directed at various segments of the healthcare industry, such as hospitals, nursing homes, third-party billers, and durable medical equipment suppliers, to encourage the development and use of internal controls to monitor adherence to applicable statutes, regulations, and program requirements.[61] At a minimum, healthcare organizations should develop and deploy a compliance program that encompasses the evolving requirements as they pertain to clinical risk, operational risk, patient safety, and workforce safety.

The ACA mandates compliance programs for Medicare and Medicaid providers. Although the law speaks specifically to individual and small-group practices, the intent is for all healthcare professionals to implement a compliance program in their offices/practices. Although a compliance program is not a guarantee that fraud, defects, waste, abuse, or inefficiency will not occur; OIG and CMS believe that the implementation of a good compliance program will aid in better business practices. The ACA has seven fundamental elements for an effective compliance program.

1. Implementing written policies, procedures, and standards of conduct
2. Designating a compliance officer and a compliance committee
3. Conducting effective training and education
4. Developing effective lines of communication
5. Conducting internal monitoring and auditing
6. Enforcing standards through well-publicized disciplinary guidelines
7. Responding promptly to detected offenses and undertaking corrective action

The compliance program should also outline functions, including

- the roles of and relationships between the organization's audit, compliance, and legal departments;
- the mechanism and process for issue reporting within an organization;
- the approach to identifying legal, regulatory, and accreditation risks; and
- methods of encouraging enterprise-wide accountability for achievement of compliance goals and objectives.[62]

A continuous readiness philosophy can be built into the compliance program, which can serve as the formal plan to stay abreast of the ever-changing regulatory landscape and operating environment. The readiness plan may involve periodic updates from informed staff who possess an understanding of the dynamic regulatory environment. This will ensure compliance with the requirements of governmental, regulatory, and accreditation agencies and supporting quality assessment and improvement programs throughout the organization. Healthcare quality professionals might find becoming a member of national and state industry associations is helpful for staying on top of the myriad of legislative and accreditation changes to remain in compliance with emerging trends.

# Continuous Survey Readiness

Organizational leaders and healthcare quality professionals set the approach to ensuring compliance with external standards and regulations. Full compliance involves ensuring that leaders, staff, and physicians across the organization are meeting all elements of the standards and regulations on a consistent basis, not only at the time of survey; they must maintain continuous survey readiness (CSR).

## Organizational Assessment

A comprehensive organizational assessment includes evaluating organizational compliance and technology, tools, and strategies (checklists, work plans and tracers). Periodic and ongoing self-assessment is a cornerstone of CSR programs. The ability to evaluate the state of compliance with key regulatory and accreditation requirements is a critical step in this process. Accreditation and regulatory requirements cover a broad scope, including clinical practice, service quality, documentation, patient experience and engagement, quality assessment, performance and process improvement, patient safety, and management of adverse or serious reportable events. In the just-in-time preparation model, compliance is not sustained but fluctuates in response to known survey cycles—compliance improves immediately before a survey and gradually declines after each survey. The goal of CSR programs is the opposite—sustained compliance. To do this, an organization must evaluate its compliance state on a regular basis and maintain an infrastructure that sustains the effort.

With an annual self-assessment, organizations plan for a thorough assessment, often at the beginning of the budget planning cycle for the new fiscal year, with the results used to drive a compliance work plan with adequate resources for the upcoming fiscal year. Resources are dedicated for the review, whether conducted internally or by an external consultant, because time is required for content experts to conduct actual reviews and document their findings. In this model, an assessment is completed and presented to leadership and quality, safety, and performance improvement oversight committees, and often to the governing body as part of the annual quality plan or annual budget presentation. Ideally, the outcome of the assessment is formatted in a report that includes a gap analysis related to specific standards, with findings and recommendations written in a manner that facilitates corrective action planning with key department leaders identified as responsible for each action with specific timelines for milestone actions leading to full compliance.

With an ongoing assessment, organizations plan for a thorough assessment during the year, often dividing the workload into smaller monthly activities. Although some organizations will dedicate individuals or departments to CSR through the designation of specific roles for annual and ongoing self-assessment, action planning, and overall accreditation activity management, not all organizations are able to do this. The advantage of an ongoing assessment is that the assessment can be resourced and integrated into operational activities and reported over an ongoing (but defined) period, allowing for action plan development, implementation, and monitoring throughout the year. A disadvantage of this model is that it requires focused project management with sufficient coordination to ensure completion of the entire assessment and to ensure monitoring and oversight of required corrective actions. There is a risk of not completing the entire assessment; it may be difficult for the organization to have a snapshot of compliance to accurately understand performance.

Regardless of how the organization is staffed or structured to support ongoing self-assessment, as the assessment components are completed, findings are presented to leadership and oversight committees. Presentation to the organization's governing body, as appropriate, can be periodically delivered as a summary of the assessment components, rather than a single completed report. This type of report is also most useful when in the format of a gap analysis related to specific standards, with findings and recommendations written in a manner that facilitates rapid corrective action planning. Once the findings are presented, corrective action plans must be developed and monitored on an ongoing basis. Monitoring schedules, however, is more complex because it must incorporate scheduled assessments to be completed as well as follow-up activities on those already completed. Assigning accountability is critical in any action planning activity.

Many organizations find that a minimum of monthly status reports is required on assessment components and the corrective actions to provide the oversight necessary to achieve compliance. Less frequent status reports (e.g., quarterly) are not recommended because there is a high risk that the organization will not be aware of slippage soon enough to take appropriate action.

Accrediting organizations publish reports summarizing top deficiencies reports and tips for compliance. For example, CHAP provides a report on top 10 infusion therapy deficiencies, where the number one deficiency is review of medication and supplies. Tips for compliance include "Performing regular audits to ensure documentation of coordination of care regarding medication regimen, equipment and supplies between nursing and pharmacy staff is present."[63(¶1)] ACHC's annual common deficiencies report found that most of its findings in 2020 were not repeat deficiencies and there was a low volume of deficiencies found in the emergency department.[64]

## Survey Readiness Oversight

CSR is the goal, and since most surveys are unannounced, the CSR model is ideal. Healthcare quality professionals may hold a role with primary responsibility for survey readiness oversight. One effective way of providing survey readiness oversight is through the formation of interdepartmental and interprofessional work groups or ongoing committees representing the full scope of services included in the anticipated survey(s) whose composition will vary depending on the type of organization and services provided (e.g., ambulatory care center, hospital, managed care organization, long-term care facility, home health agency). Some organizations create work groups for related clusters of accreditation standards and others have a single multidisciplinary group to evaluate readiness on the standards across the entire organization. At a minimum, each work group consists of the healthcare quality professional and appropriate departmental representatives with sufficient knowledge to identify gaps in compliance and the authority to modify organizational practices and processes to become compliant with current and emerging expectations.

Departments consistently requiring representation include nursing, medical staff, pharmacy, plant operations, environmental services, and infection control. Membership on these work groups will further depend on the size and scope of the organization as well as the scope of the individual work group (when more than one work group is formed). In a hospital setting, other members might include the safety officer, risk manager, and director of health information and analytics. In an MCO, additional members might include a customer relations representative, physician relations or medical staff coordinator, network coordinator, information systems or data analytics representative, and benefits administrator. Medical staff play a significant role and bear the responsibility of accountability for compliance and performance improvement; however, it may be challenging to schedule time for their participation in planning activities and to clear their schedules when the actual survey process commences. Medical staff participation requires constant communication as new standards and requirements become available.

The frequency with which survey readiness groups meet will vary depending on the outcome of ongoing self-assessments, gap analyses, and available resources to complete identified tasks. Accrediting agencies like TJC offer resources to support readiness efforts. As an example, TJC developed the Survey Analysis for Evaluating Risk (SAFER) Matrix to provide healthcare organizations with the information they need to prioritize resources and focus corrective action plans in areas that are most in need of compliance activities and interventions. Each requirement for improvement (RFI) is noted within the final report that is plotted on the SAFER Matrix according to the likelihood the RFI could cause harm to patient(s), staff, and/or visitor(s), as well as the scope at which the RFI was observed. As the risk level of an RFI increases, the placement of the standard and [element of performance] EP moves from the bottom left corner (lowest risk level) to the upper right (highest risk level).[65(94)]

**Figure 3.3** shows the SAFER Matrix, which can be used by the organization to identify potential for widespread quality initiatives and better organize survey findings by level of potential patient impact.

If the oversight and planning personnel perform this work in a continuous fashion and the organization embraces the CSR culture, any last-minute rush and accompanying stress will be lessened as the survey window approaches. Publications and commercial and accreditor education programs are available with suggested checklists to assist with survey preparation. The most important element, however, is a coordinated, ongoing effort to show evidence to meet the intent of the regulations or standards.

Organizations that are not far along in the journey to high reliability may employ just-in-time regulatory or accreditation readiness models, which come with great financial and personnel costs. When organizations use just-in-time programs with ramp-up activities in the months prior to anticipated surveys, tremendous additional resources are required to demonstrate regulation or standard compliance. Extra staff, consultants, external resources, or extra time are required for self-assessments or gap analyses; for corrective actions to assure compliance; for meetings to discuss policy revision approvals; and for frontline staff education on policy revisions, operational process improvements, and expected survey procedures.

These organizations experience tremendous relief when surveys are completed and may commit to a vision that the next two- to three-year cycle will be different. However, organizational memory can be short, personnel changes may occur, and competing priorities may replace the vision of CSR. Organizations that experience unplanned surveys with numerous citations may also experience a crisis-management cycle, which requires tremendous unplanned additional resources. Compliance issues can be costly to organizations in terms of financial outlays for corrections, public reputation damage that leads to further financial losses in competitive markets, and staff turnover, as the work environment may no longer be healthy. Many organizations started to embrace a CSR approach when on-site surveys became unannounced. Some work to embed CSR into the quality and safety structure and culture of the organization.

One strategy as part of the ongoing organizational assessment process is just-in-time staff education. As areas of opportunity are identified and addressed, staff are reminded of regulatory and accreditation expectations in an educational and coaching manner. Wherever possible, the healthcare quality professional relates the specific desired behavior as

## SAFER Matrix

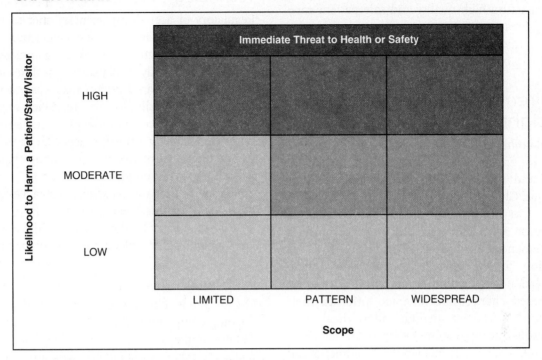

## Placement of RFI on *SAFER* Matrix and Follow-Up Activity

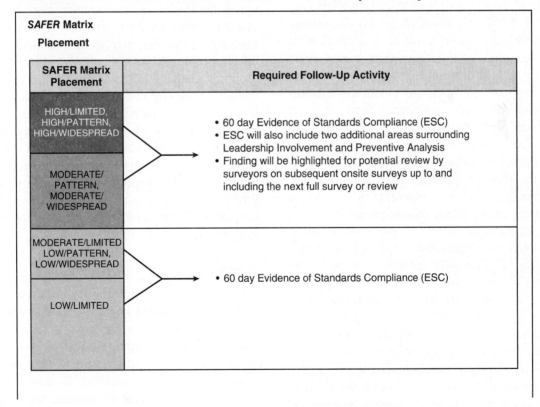

**Figure 3.3** SAFER Matrix

expected in the regulation or accreditation standard to the impact on high-quality and safe patient care. CSR programs require solid organization-wide education programs with staff participation from all levels within an organization.

## Requirements and Standards Oversight

A critical component of a CSR program is a defined process to ensure the organization is aware of changes and places an emphasis in standards or regulations. Changes may be in the form of additions, deletions, or clarifications. Most regulatory or accreditation agencies define processes for changes in requirements and standards. This usually involves notification to the affected organizations; there is a period during which comments or feedback on proposed changes are accepted prior to their publication. Comment periods allow healthcare organizations the opportunity to provide feedback on proposed changes in regulations. Comments can be submitted individually or as an organization. Once official changes are released, clarifications may be found in frequently asked questions documents as well. Healthcare quality professionals check with the agencies and organizations that survey their facilities to understand the relative frequency with which changes are made; the process for assimilating public feedback and comments from affected organizations; and the notification process to the affected organizations, including the medium (e.g., email, paper letter, website announcements) and to whom in the affected organization's communications are directed (e.g., the chief executive officer versus the regulatory or healthcare quality professional).

Once changes are identified, gap analyses must be completed to understand implications to the organization. Operational leaders and oversight committees will need guidance as to the scope and urgency of required changes. It is helpful to create a notification list of individuals within the organization who receive communications related to standards. These communications are most effective when they are put into context for the recipient. For example, the communication can include a description of the change, the agency making the change, actions required on the part of the various stakeholders within the organization (leadership, managers, employees), risk assessment of the change, identification of resources required (if any) to implement the change, and deadlines associated with required actions.

## Technology, Tools, and Strategies

Regulatory or accrediting agencies offer tools to help organizations manage self-assessment activities. Access to information such as easy-to-use automated checklists may be readily available on the Internet. Additional computer-based project management programs designed specifically for the identified regulations, accreditation, or certification programs also may be purchased directly from the agencies or from third-party entrepreneurs. External consulting organizations will also provide educational programs or tools for evaluation or preparation activities on a fee-for-service basis. Many of these checklists can also be programmed for easy data entry by the reviewer at the point of service (on an iPad or tablet computer, for example).

## Checklists

Organizations develop checklists to help monitor ongoing compliance as well as day-of-survey activity. As an example, a survey readiness tool for department managers serves as standard work for managers to use when rounding in their departments. The content is developed to meet accreditation expectations and organizational circumstances. A hospital survey readiness document may include clinical rounding, infection control, patient safety, and environmental rounding elements. Clinical rounding elements may include a review of restraint records, high-risk-for-fall lists, care plans, pain assessment/reassessment, and care transition documentation. Infection control elements may include items such as direct observation of hand hygiene, linen cart coverings, dirty and clean utility room observations, and cleaning procedures. Environmental elements for review may include fire procedures, location of fire extinguishers, medical gas storage, and staff identification badges.

## Work Plans

Organizations are encouraged to develop specific work plans to outline key activities that need to take place to support the survey process. For example, a work plan for an unannounced survey would include key activities that need to occur when a survey team shows up at the organization. In addition to each action, key responsible individuals including alternates are identified (including contact information).

## Tracers

A key part of many on-site surveys and survey self-assessment processes is the tracer methodology. The tracer methodology follows the experience of care, treatment, or services for several patients through the organization's entire healthcare delivery process. During surveys or self-assessment processes, tracers allow surveyors and staff or consultants to identify performance issues in one or more steps of the process or interfaces between processes. The types of tracers used by various accrediting and regulatory agencies during the on-site survey are as follows:

- *Individual tracer activity.* These tracers are designed to trace the care experiences that a patient had while at an organization. It is a way to analyze the organization's system of providing care, treatment, or services using actual patients as the framework for assessing standards compliance. Patients selected for these tracers will likely be those in high-risk areas or whose diagnosis, age, or type of services received may enable the best in-depth evaluation of the organization's processes and practices.
- *System tracer activity.* This activity includes an interactive session with relevant staff members in tracing one specific system or process within the organization, based on information from individual tracers. Although individual tracers follow a patient through their course of care, the system tracer evaluates the system or process, including the integration of related processes, and the coordination and communication among disciplines and departments in those processes. Examples of topics evaluated by system tracers during accreditation surveys include data management, infection control, and medication management.
- *Accreditation program–specific tracers.* The goal of these tracers is to identify risk points and safety concerns within different levels and types of care, treatment, or services. Program-specific tracers focus on important issues relevant to the organization, such as clinical services offered and high-risk, high-volume patient populations.[66]

## Staff Education

Healthcare quality professionals must develop effective and efficient education and training that target defined levels within the organization:

- Leadership must receive information to prioritize resources for readiness, to model required changes in behavior, and to speak to key leadership and other relevant standards when surveyors visit their facilities.
- Managers must have information related to care delivery requirements and structure or process requirements, as well as required documentation that must be immediately available to surveyors. Managers need to participate in staff education programs, often becoming the staff educator after train-the-trainer programs.
- Frontline staff must receive information to comply with standards and regulations related to direct care delivery, which will be found in policies, procedures, and competencies related to their work. There will also be documentation requirements they must understand and integrate into their practice, such as specific care documentation, equipment checks for maintenance or performance within defined parameters (e.g., test results or calibration), communication documentation with transitions in care, or required education and training that must be documented.

Effective education plans must target defined departments within an organization but must also acknowledge interprofessional interdependencies. For example, key messages for large care delivery departments such as nursing may be different from key messages for smaller ancillary departments or specialty departments. If programs are not designed specifically for an intended audience, participants may believe most of the material applies to another department or may be unable to apply the message or relevance to its own department.

Education departments can help organizations design targeted programs and provide the structure for delivery. Because CSR is ongoing, a variety of approaches and learning methods are used, including the following:

- Face-to-face education
- Virtual, asynchronous educational offerings
- Rounds of work areas with environment assessment and staff knowledge assessment (also, briefings and huddles)
- Question and answer tools (daily, weekly, and monthly frequently asked questions)
- Online and hard copy resource books of current common standards
- Self-assessment tools to identify gaps in comparison to standards and education and other action plans to address the gaps
- Visual tools or cognitive aids such as posters on safety goals or performance improvement models
- Content experts to respond one-on-one to questions or interpretation of standards
- Unit or department champions who are well versed in standards/requirements
- Mock surveys to assess compliance with standards in an ongoing manner

- Quality and safety expositions
- Tools for tracer activities
- Just-in-time training

Successful CSR education programs are the outcome of creative education modalities that reach staff and leaders alike and effectively impart key messages and reinforce them across the organization. Social media technologies can be used if they meet privacy requirements. Healthcare quality professionals must be creative in developing effective ongoing programs because the workforce is constantly changing as healthcare staff change roles or organizations. Although healthcare quality professionals work to maintain a continuous state of readiness for survey activity, education calendars are planned as part of a cohesive program. Creating an ongoing series will be more effective than a sporadic offering of seemingly unrelated topics. Educational programs may best be long-range programs designed around multiyear survey cycles.

The coordination required to achieve favorable accreditation or certification status or successful regulatory licensing or certifications must be delegated to those individuals with the most knowledge about healthcare quality, regulations, and standards interpretation and implementation. This coordination role can be delegated to a leader or manager within the quality area or to a designated role in larger organizations or health systems, such as a director of accreditation and regulatory readiness. Important preparation tasks for organizations to complete are generally outlined in survey manuals and can be planned for each anticipated survey.

Formal plans are recommended, with multiple staff and leaders familiar with the process. The organization's general survey procedure planning will likely include the components described in the following section. **Table 3.5** provides additional examples of survey readiness activities to prepare for anticipated surveys.

## Table 3.5 Examples of Survey Readiness Activities

- Clarify vacation and planned time off expectations of key staff and leaders based on known survey windows.

- Assign survey roles for key staff duties such as command center operators, space planners, surveyor escorts, runners, scribes, sweep teams, moderators, and IT support personnel. Determine both a primary and a backup person for each role and provide an overview of expectations for the role in advance.
  - An escort's primary function is to remain with the surveyor always so the surveyor is not unattended. Escorts develop a relationship with an individual surveyor and should be consistent throughout the survey, unless there is not a good match with the surveyor's personality. Escorts should be matched to surveyors with similar skill sets, for example, a physician with a physician or a nurse with a nurse. In some organizations, executives such as the chief executive officer (CEO) or chief operating officer (COO), chief nursing officer (CNO), and chief medical officer (CMO) will serve as escorts to demonstrate the organization's commitment to the accreditation process.
  - Runners are responsible for contacting the command center to provide a brief report of activity, surveyor location, and specific surveyor requests.
  - Scribes are responsible for documenting the activities of the surveyor, taking notes, and keeping information organized.
  - Sweep teams are groups of individuals who round in advance of the surveyors to answer questions that staff may have and ensure compliance with standards.
  - If using virtual technology, assign a moderator to ensure staff are getting on and off calls in a timely way; also, this person can monitor comments made by participants in the chat function.
  - Have IT support available for technology issues (e.g., face-to-face or virtual surveys).

- Determine if confidentiality releases, security codes, access cards, or additional name badges will be needed, and be sure both scribes and escorts have access to all required clinical areas.

- Update organizational charts that can be attached to the phone lists to facilitate location of key staff during a survey.

- Update lists of phone numbers and create distribution lists for survey communications that include the organization's most common communication methods (email, cell phones, walkie-talkies) to facilitate rapid communication during the survey. Set up a digital messaging structure when text pager or phone systems are unavailable.

- Review previous regulatory or accreditation survey reports and the respective corrective action plans to evaluate sustained compliance.

- Ensure that the most current licenses, certificates, and required signage are posted.

- Assemble required documents to ensure easy access to the most current versions.

*(continues)*

**Table 3.5** **Examples of Survey Readiness Activities** *(continued)*

- Review policies and procedures to ensure all are current.

- Test systems to quickly produce required lists of patients, residents, or clients including scheduled procedures or visits.

- Sweep care areas and departments for outdated policies, procedures, guidelines, order sets, forms, and privilege binders.

- Prepare surveyor orientation materials for documentation reviews for medical records that introduce electronic records or components of hybrid electronic and paper systems.

- Conduct medical record reviews of open records to ensure records are compliant for vulnerable topics. If paper records are in use and a record has been thinned, ensure the appropriate information is included in the new volume and that the previous volumes are available if requested.

- Audit the human resources file system to ensure access to the complete human resources file is readily available on site and that required documentation for education and training is available.

- Check education materials and brochures to ensure availability in the common languages for the populations served by the organization.

- Check that required postings are present (e.g., patient/client rights and responsibilities, posting about the survey visit).

- Monitor the environment to ensure that it is clean and compliant with applicable environmental, fire, and life safety codes.

- If the organization is spread out over a large geographic area, determine whether drivers or shuttles are needed to take surveyors to distant clinical areas. If employees are using their own vehicles, be sure vehicles are clean inside and out.

- Determine surveyor parking plans. Designated spaces close to the main entrance can be identified once a survey has begun. Parking vouchers may be provided. There may also need to be reserved parking spaces for employees driving surveyors or those coming in during the day for key interviews.

- Prepare packets to be given to surveyors upon arrival. The packets should include a map of the facility, a facility contact list with phone numbers, an organizational chart for the senior leadership team, parking information, and guest ID badges, if required. Information or brochures on local area restaurants and attractions also may be appreciated after the survey if the team has traveled to the survey location.

# Leading the Survey Process

Survey procedures are planned based on what is expected with anticipated surveys. Healthcare quality professionals may have the responsibility to develop and manage survey procedures for the organization because they serve as internal experts and consultants. An accreditation or regulatory site visit requires organization and preparation and is the culmination of CSR activities. **Table 3.6** lists the components of a visit for presurvey activities, on-site survey activities, and postsurvey activities.

## Survey Duration

The length of the survey is dependent on the type of survey, the size of the organization, the number of surveyors, and the complexity of services offered. Certification surveys for small programs can be as few as one surveyor for one day; accreditation surveys for large organizations can be as large as five surveyors or more for five days or more. CMS validation surveys at large organizations can involve as many as 20 or more surveyors for two weeks or longer, depending on the programs being evaluated, previous survey findings, corrective action plans, and on current findings.

## Surveyors

On-site accreditation surveys are completed by professionals from within the field of review. In addition to document review (reports, data, management plans, risk assessments, evaluations, etc.), which may take place in advance of the on-site review, interviews with staff, patients, and providers are a normal part of a survey. Organizations typically are informed of the names of the surveyors and their backgrounds prior to the survey. Healthcare quality professionals typically work with clinical departments in developing guides for interacting with surveyors. Surveyors may ask staff about the following:

**Table 3.6** **Possible Activities for a Survey Conducted by The Joint Commission**

| Activity | Tasks |
|---|---|
| **Presurvey activities** | <ul><li>Start 12 months after the last onsite survey if already accredited; new applicant processes will vary</li><li>Addressing and hardwiring opportunities from the last survey</li><li>Top deficiencies reviewed</li><li>Maintaining improvements of corrective action plans</li><li>Keeping staff apprised of key standards and regulations and changes</li><li>Conducting self-assessment compliance gap analyses</li><li>Executing educational programs for building skills related to regulatory, accreditation, or performance and quality improvement</li><li>Activities to prepare staff and leadership for anticipated survey activities (expos, huddles, rounding)</li><li>Verifying that survey planning documents are current and relevant</li><li>Conduct a mock survey</li></ul> |
| **Space planning and hosting** | <ul><li>Establishing a surveyor workroom</li><li>Establishing a command center</li><li>Designating other conference rooms and arranging for virtual set-ups for surveyor meetings with staff</li><li>Documentation preparation</li><li>Arranging for IT and equipment support</li><li>Arranging for food and beverage service</li></ul> |
| **On-site survey** | <ul><li>Assign escorts and scribes</li><li>Assign central point of contact</li><li>Plan for arrival of surveyors</li><li>Welcome the surveyor(s)</li><li>Obtain photo identification</li><li>Assemble individuals and teams (use the phone tree)</li><li>Organizational notification</li><li>Post flyers with words to this effect: "XYZ organization would like to welcome XXX (accreditation organization) to our facility today."</li><li>Establish survey command centers</li><li>Determine who will be the survey coordinator in charge</li><li>Define staff roles and track key information</li><li>Make sure IT support is available</li><li>Plan for other considerations:<ul><li>Office supplies: chart pads, easels, grease boards, clipboards, projectors, etc.</li><li>Communications equipment: phones and scanning/facsimile lines</li><li>Computers and/or access to IT systems and electronic medical records</li><li>A tracking system for surveyor requests</li><li>The following key documents for easy access:<ul><li>Current organizational charts</li><li>Program descriptions</li><li>Plans for the provision of care</li><li>Governing body structures</li><li>Professional staff bylaws</li><li>Copies of licenses</li><li>Governing body minutes</li><li>Key quality and administrative reports</li></ul></li></ul></li></ul> |
| **Identification of deficiencies using Survey Analysis for Evaluating Risk (SAFER) Matrix** | <ul><li>Compare areas of noncompliance at an aggregate level to evidence of standard compliance</li><li>Require organizational follow-up activity and corrective action within 60 days</li><li>Identify immediate threats to life</li><li>Identify incidents of immediate jeopardy: a mechanism to escalate crisis survey issues immediately</li><li>Note that such a deficiency will automatically result in a condition-level deficiency under the applicable Medicare Condition(s) of Participation</li></ul> |

*(continues)*

**Table 3.6** Possible Activities for a Survey Conducted by The Joint Commission *(continued)*

| Activity | Tasks |
|---|---|
| **Survey exit conferences** | ▪ Surveyors summarize the findings and deficiencies that will be cited and disclose anticipated next steps in the survey process<br>▪ Organization conducts its own debriefing as soon as possible to evaluate the survey process<br>▪ Evaluate how the organization managed the survey process<br>▪ Decide whether to accept or dispute the outcome<br>▪ Senior leaders (CEO or COO, CNO, CMO) consider a special communication to the organization's staff to share survey outcome appreciation |
| **Postsurvey activities** | ▪ Sustain compliance, especially opportunities for improvement identified in the survey<br>▪ Develop correction action plans for<br> • the topic or standard cited,<br> • compliance issues for correction,<br> • planned actions,<br> • the target deadline for completion, and<br> • the name of the person accountable for the action.<br>▪ Effective staff recognition:<br> • Personal words of thanks<br> • Notes of appreciation<br> • Public acknowledgment in committees |

Data from Brown DS. Regulation, accreditation, and continuous readiness. In: Pelletier LR, Beaudin CL, eds. *Q Solutions: Essential Resources for the Healthcare Quality Professional*. 3rd ed. Chicago, IL: National Association for Healthcare Quality; 2012; Center for Improvement in Healthcare Quality. Accreditation policies for acute care hospitals. Effective January 2021. Accessed November 16, 2021. http://www.cihq.org/home.asp; Centers for Medicare & Medicaid Services. State operations manual: Appendix Q: Guidelines for determining immediate jeopardy. Published 2019. Accessed November 16, 2021. https://www.cms.gov/Regulations-and-guidance/Guidance/Manuals/downloads/som107ap_q_immedjeopardy.pdf; The Joint Commission. SAFER Matrix scoring process. Published 2021. Accessed November 16, 2021. https://www.jointcommission.org/resources/news-and-multimedia/fact-sheets/facts-about-safer-matrix-scoring-process/; and The Joint Commission. Survey analysis for evaluating risk (SAFER). n. d. Accessed November 16, 2021. https://www.jointcommission.org/-/media/tjc/documents/accred-and-cert/safer-matrix/safer-infographic.pdf

- Organization processes that support or may be a barrier to the individual served/patient/resident care, treatment, and services
- Communications and coordination with other licensed independent practitioners (hospitalists, consulting physicians, and primary care practitioners)
- Discharge planning or other care transitions-related resources and processes available through the organization
- Awareness of roles and responsibilities related to the environment of care, including prevention of and response to incidents and reporting of adverse events that occurred
- The education or information they have been provided on antimicrobial resistance and the organization's antimicrobial stewardship program
- In ambulatory care, as applicable to the organization's services, the surveyor may select a patient receiving care, treatment, or services related to the organization's annual antimicrobial stewardship goal and discuss antimicrobial stewardship guidelines the organization is using

and provider training and education about appropriate prescribing practices
- Pain assessment, pain management, and safe opioid prescribing initiatives, when applicable, and resources made available by the organization; the prescription drug monitoring database and criteria for accessing it, when applicable
- Awareness of and participation in a safety culture assessment; and awareness of assessment results and action plans developed
- Reporting near misses/close calls as well as actual errors; awareness of any organization processes to look at these occurrences[67(p44-45)]

## Observations and Summation

Depending on the healthcare services under review, on-site surveys will also encompass observations of routine care delivery and the associated medical record documentation (electronic and supplemental hard copy), staff performing procedures, and visits to home care patients. Most reviews conclude with a summation conference by the survey team to inform leadership of compliance findings and concerns.

## Accreditation Decision

Following review of all the data and evidence sources, an accreditation decision is determined for the organization. The decision usually includes an overall assessment of the organization or service that reflects a full accreditation decision, or a decision with limitations or restrictions that the organization must resolve within a designated time frame.

## Deficiencies and Findings

Depending on the number and scope of deficiencies cited, follow-up surveys may be part of the accreditation decision. Cited deficiencies or requirements for improvement must be corrected and documentation submitted to the reviewing organization within predetermined time frames. The organization's leaders often receive in-depth information that can be used internally to prioritize performance improvement activities to enhance care quality and patient safety, with the implicit expectation that the organization will use this feedback in its continuous quality, safety, and performance improvement programs.

The accreditation decision is shared with external stakeholders such as consumers, patients, purchasers, and government agencies that require accreditation or certification for participation. The level of detail shared outside the accreditation agency ranges from a simple list of organizations that were successful (with no indication of organizations that failed) to detailed information on performance.

## Survey Outcomes

Most accreditation organizations improve the timeliness of processes that result in an accreditation or certification decision. Some organizations use proprietary software that captures surveyor observations and translates observations into an overall survey decision outcome, whereas others provide written reports back to the accrediting organization where further internal review occurs before a final survey outcome decision is made. Individual accreditation agencies have procedures for disputing survey outcome decisions, and healthcare quality professionals are familiar with processes available to challenge or dispute findings both during and after the on-site survey. Artificial intelligence and machine learning are evolving to better assist organizations in their preparation and after-visit activities. For example, TJC is using an artificial intelligence technology called "Machine Learning for Survey Consistency."[68] Through this technology, artificial intelligence is used to correctly identify standards and elements of performance in scoring an accreditation survey or certification review. This ensures consistency and accuracy of survey findings.

## Postsurvey Activities

Follow-up on the corrective action plan drives many activities such as educational programming. When deficiencies are cited or even suspected from a survey, the organization designs and implements corrective actions immediately in anticipation of the final report. Final reports can be delayed when they require a state agency to submit a report to a federal agency for final approval of the survey decisions or if accreditation agencies wish a review of challenging findings by their central office. When the report is delayed, it may be difficult to remember the details of the survey citation or leadership attention may be on new matters, making corrective action planning more difficult. Even with delayed reports, a short deadline (e.g., 10 days) may be given to submit corrective actions. Survey findings form the basis for future leadership oversight on appropriate committee and leadership meeting agendas.

**Box 3.3** reiterates organizational approaches to continuous survey readiness.

---

**Box 3.3  Key Points: Organizational Approaches to Continuous Survey Readiness**

- Continuous readiness is an attitude valued throughout the organization.
- Using a just-in-time approach requires tremendous additional resources to demonstrate compliance with laws, regulations, and/or accreditation standards.
- Compliance should be evaluated on a regular basis to achieve a state of continuous readiness.
- Day-to-day surveillance of quality and safety can be woven into the fabric of care delivery through briefings, huddles, and rounding.
- Clear accountability should be assigned for any action planning activity.

---

## Summary

This section began with a description of various federal and state regulations that guide operations and practice in healthcare. Important federal regulations and various regulatory and accrediting agencies are described. Recent changes in the healthcare reimbursement landscape make the role of the healthcare quality professional even more critical as value, translated in part through compliance with regulations, accreditation, highly reliable care, and service delivery, becomes the focus for true healthcare transformation. Armed with resources, knowledge, principles, tools, and techniques, the healthcare quality professional is an invaluable change agent in the healthcare enterprise. Agility is a key leadership attribute. Through leadership, management, education, training and communication, the healthcare quality professional ensures that processes and practices are current, evidence based, and effective in providing essential, safe, equitable healthcare services.

# References

1. U.S. Senate. Laws and regulations. Accessed December 5, 2021. https://www.senate.gov/reference/reference_index_subjects/Laws_and_Regulations_vrd.htm

2. Mate KS, Rooney AL, Supachutikul A, Gyani G. Accreditation as a path to achieving universal quality health coverage. *Global Health.* 2014;10(68):1-8.

3. American Hospital Association. Regulatory overload: assessing the regulatory burden on health systems, hospitals and post-acute care providers. Published October 2017. Accessed November 16, 2021. https://www.aha.org/sites/default/files/regulatory-overload-report.pdf

4. Centers for Medicare & Medicaid Services. Emergency Medical Treatment & Labor Act (EMTALA). Published March 4, 2021. Accessed November 16, 2021. www.cms.gov/Regulations-and-Guidance/Legislation/EMTALA/index.html?redirect=/EMTALA

5. Centers for Medicare & Medicaid Services. Clinical Laboratory Improvement Amendments (CLIA). Published November 16, 2021. Accessed November 22, 2021. https://www.cms.gov/regulations-and-guidance/legislation/clia?redirect=/clia

6. Centers for Medicare & Medicaid Services, Office of Civil Rights. HIPAA for professionals. Published May 17, 2021. Accessed November 16, 2021. https://www.hhs.gov/hipaa/for-professionals/index.html

7. U.S. Department of Health & Human Services. HITECH act enforcement interim final rule. Published June 16, 2017. Accessed November 16, 2021. https://www.hhs.gov/hipaa/for-professionals/special-topics/hitech-act-enforcement-interim-final-rule/index.html

8. U.S. Department of Health & Human Services. Patient Safety and Quality Improvement Act of 2005. Published June 16, 2017. Accessed November 16, 2021. https://www.hhs.gov/hipaa/for-professionals/patient-safety/statute-and-rule/index.html

9. Supreme Court of the United States. *California v. Texas.* Published June 17, 2021. Accessed November 20, 2021. https://www.supremecourt.gov/opinions/20pdf/19-840_6jfm.pdf

10. U.S. Department of Health & Human Services. Introduction: about HHS. Published February 28, 2018. Accessed November 20, 2021. https://www.hhs.gov/about/strategic-plan/introduction/index.html

11. U.S. Department of Health & Human Services. HHS agencies & offices. Published October 27, 2015. Accessed November 20, 2021. https://www.hhs.gov/about/agencies/hhs-agencies-and-offices/index.html

12. Centers for Disease Control and Prevention. About CDC 24/7: mission, role and pledge. Published May 13, 2019. Accessed December 1, 2021. https://www.cdc.gov/about/organization/mission.htm

13. Centers for Medicare & Medicaid Services. About us. Accessed November 17, 2021. https://www.cms.gov/About-CMS/About-CMS.html

14. U.S. Food & Drug Administration. What we do. Published March 28, 2018. Accessed December 1, 2021. https://www.fda.gov/about-fda/what-we-do

15. Health Resources & Services Administration. About HRSA. Published November 2021. Accessed December 1, 2021. https://www.hrsa.gov/about/index.html

16. Indian Health Service. About IHS. Accessed December 1, 2021. https://www.ihs.gov/aboutihs/

17. National Institutes of Health. Who we are. Accessed December 1, 2021. https://www.nih.gov/about-nih/who-we-are

18. Office of Inspector General. About OIG. Accessed December 18, 2021. https://oig.hhs.gov/about-oig/

19. Substance Abuse and Mental Health Services Administration. About us. Published September 17, 2021. Accessed December 1, 2021. https://www.samhsa.gov/about-us

20. U.S. Department of Health & Human Services. Regional offices. Accessed November 16, 2021. https://www.hhs.gov/about/agencies/iea/regional-offices/index.html

21. Medicaid.gov. Managed care. Accessed November 17, 2021. https://www.medicaid.gov/medicaid/managed-care/index.html

22. National Association of Insurance Commissioners. NAIC model laws; 2021. Accessed November 20, 2021. https://content.naic.org/cipr_topics/topic_naic_model_laws.htm

23. Centers for Medicare & Medicaid Services. Regulations & guidance. Accessed November 17, 2021. www.cms.hhs.gov/Regulations-and-Guidance/Regulations-and-Guidance.html

24. U.S. Government Publishing Office. "Conditions of participation for hospitals," Title 42 *Code of Federal Regulations,* Pt 482. 2015 ed. Accessed November 16, 2021. https://www.gpo.gov/fdsys/pkg/CFR-2015-title42-vol5/xml/CFR-2015-title42-vol5-part482.xml

25. National Archives and Records Administration. "Conditions of participation for hospitals," Title 42 *Code of Federal Regulations,* Pt 482. 2021 ed. Accessed November 17, 2021. http://www.ecfr.gov/cgi-bin/text-idx?tpl=/ecfrbrowse/Title42/42tab_02.tpl

26. Centers for Medicare & Medicaid Services. State operations manual: Appendix A—survey protocol, regulations and interpretive guidelines for hospitals. Revised February 21, 2020. Accessed November 17, 2021. https://www.cms.gov/Regulations-and-Guidance/Guidance/Manuals/downloads/som107ap_a_hospitals.pdf

27. All Titles. "General provisions," Title 42 *Customs Mobile,* Pt 488, subpt A. 2021 ed. Accessed November 17, 2021. https://www.customsmobile.com/regulations/expand/

title42_chapterIV_part488_subpartA_section488.7#title42_chapterIV_part488_subpartA_section488.10

28. Centers for Medicare & Medicaid Services. CMS approved accrediting organizations contacts for prospective clients, Centers for Medicare & Medicaid Services, 2020. Accessed December 5, 2021. https://www.hhs.gov/guidance/document/cms-approved-accrediting-organizations-contacts-prospective-clients

29. U.S. Department of Health & Human Services, Health Resources & Services Administration. National Practitioner Data Bank. Accessed November 17, 2021. https://www.npdb.hrsa.gov/

30. U.S. Department of Health & Human Services, Health Resources and Services Administration. *NPDB Guidebook*. Rockville, MD: U.S. Department of Health & Human Services; 2018. Accessed November 17, 2021. https://www.npdb.hrsa.gov/resources/aboutGuidebooks.jsp

31. U.S. Department of Health & Human Services, Health Resources and Services Administration. *NPDB Guidebook: General Information: Civil Money Penalties*. Rockville, MD: U.S. Department of Health & Human Services; 2018. Accessed November 20, 2021. https://www.npdb.hrsa.gov/guidebook/AGeneralInformation.jsp

32. Office of Information and Regulatory Affairs. Spring 2021 unified agenda of regulatory and deregulatory actions. Accessed November 17, 2021. https://www.reginfo.gov/public/do/eAgendaMain

33. Conway P, Berwick D. Improving the rules for hospital participation in Medicare and Medicaid. *JAMA*. 2011;306(20):2256-2257. doi:10.1001/jama.2011.1611

34. Field RI. *Healthcare Regulation in America: Complexity, Confrontation and Compromise*. New York, NY: Oxford University Press; 2007.

35. Centers for Medicare & Medicaid Services. FY 2015 Report to Congress (RTC): review of Medicare's program oversight of accrediting organizations (AOs) and the Clinical Laboratory Improvement Amendments of 1988 (CLIA) Validation Program. Published January 29, 2016. Accessed November 17, 2021. https://www.cms.gov/Medicare/Provider-Enrollment-and-Certification/SurveyCertificationGenInfo/Downloads/Survey-and-Cert-Letter-16-07.pdf

36. U.S. Food & Drug Administration. Radiation-emitting products: Mammography Quality Standards Act and Program. Published October 1, 2021. Accessed November 17, 2021. https://www.fda.gov/radiation-emitting-products/mammography-quality-standards-act-and-program

37. U.S. Food & Drug Administration. MSQA insights: 2021 scorecard statistics. Published November 1, 2021. Accessed November 20, 2021. https://www.fda.gov/radiation-emitting-products/mqsa-insights/2021-scorecard-statistics#oct

38. Williams SC, Morton DJ, Braun BI, Longo BA, Baker DW. Comparing public quality ratings for accredited and nonaccredited nursing homes. *JAMDA*. 2017;18:24-29. doi:10:1016/j.jamda.2016.07.025

39. American College of Physicians. What is the patient-centered medical home? Accessed November 17, 2021. https://www.acponline.org/practice-resources/business/payment/models/pcmh/understanding/what-pcmh

40. Park J, Dowling, NM. Do nurse practitioner-led medical homes differ from physician-led medical homes? *Nurs Outlook*. 2020;68(5):601-610. doi:10.1016/j.outlook.2020.05.010

41. Centers for Disease Control and Prevention. Benefits & impacts of accreditation. Accessed November 16, 2021. https://www.cdc.gov/publichealthgateway/accreditation/benefits.html

42. Hussein M, Pavlova M, Ghalwash M, et al. The impact of hospital accreditation on the quality of healthcare: a systematic literature review. *BMC Health Serv Res*. 2021;1057. doi:10.1186/s12913-021-07097-6

43. Accreditation Canada. The value and impact of health care accreditation: a literature review. Published October 2013. Accessed November 16, 2021. https://www.aventa.org/pdfs/valueimpactaccreditation.pdf

44. Hut N. Amid the COVID-19 pandemic, research finds hospital organizations looking to capitalize on the benefits of systemness. Published April 30, 2021. Accessed November 22, 2021. https://www.hfma.org/topics/news/2021/04/amid-the-covid-19-pandemic--research-finds-hospital-organization.html

45. Accreditation Association for Ambulatory Health Care. 1095 strong journey. Accessed November 22, 2021. https://www.aaahc.org/1095-strong-journey/

46. Health Facilities Accreditation Program. HFAP joins ACHC. Published October 20, 2020. Accessed November 24, 2021. https://www.hfap.org/wp-content/uploads/2020/10/Merger-Announcement-Press-Release-FINAL-10-20-20.pdf

47. American College of Surgeons. Quality programs. Accessed November 22, 2021. https://www.facs.org/quality-programs

48. College of American Pathologists. Accreditation checklists. Accessed November 22, 2021. https://www.cap.org/laboratory-improvement/accreditation/accreditation-checklists

49. DNV Healthcare USA. Our approach: healthcare. Accessed November 24, 2021. https://www.dnv.us/assurance/healthcare/index.html

50. The Joint Commission. Facts about The Joint Commission. Accessed November 17, 2021. www.jointcommission.org/facts_about_the_joint_commission

51. National Association of Boards of Pharmacy. About. Published 2020. Accessed December 1, 2021. https://nabp.pharmacy/about/

52. National Dialysis Accreditation Commission. About. Accessed December 1, 2021. https://ndacommission.com/company/

53. The Compliance Team. About The Compliance Team. Accessed December 1, 2021. https://thecomplianceteam.org/about-us/exemplary-provider-accreditation/

54. National Quality Forum. NQF's work in quality measurement. Accessed November 20, 2021. https://www.qualityforum.org/about_nqf/work_in_quality_measurement/

55. NCQA. HEDIS and performance measurement. Accessed November 20, 2021. https://www.ncqa.org/hedis/

56. Washington State Department of Health. Adverse events. Accessed November 20, 2021. https://www.doh.wa.gov/ForPublicHealthandHealthcareProviders/HealthcareProfessionsandFacilities/PatientCareResources/AdverseEvents#heading28531

57. The Joint Commission. Sentinel event definition, policy revised. Published July 21, 2021. Accessed December 12, 2021. https://www.jointcommission.org/resources/news-and-multimedia/newsletters/newsletters/joint-commission-online/july-21-2021/sentinel-event-definition-policy-revised/

58. Groysberg B, Lee J, Price J, Yo-Jud Cheng J. The leader's guide to corporate culture: how to manage the eight critical elements of organizational life. *Harv Bus Rev*. January–February 2018. Accessed April 18, 2022. https://hbr.org/2018/01/the-leaders-guide-to-corporate-culture

59. Stymiest DL. Continuous compliance: maintaining a constant state of regulatory readiness. ASHE Health Facilities. May 1, 2011. Accessed April 18, 2022. https://www.hfmmagazine.com/articles/787-continuous-compliance

60. Health Care Fraud and Enforcement Action Team, Office of Inspector General. *Health Care Compliance Program Tips.* n.d. Accessed April 18, 2022. https://oig.hhs.gov/documents/provider-compliance-training/945/Compliance101tips508.pdf

61. U.S. Department of Health & Human Services Office of Inspector General. Compliance. Accessed December 13, 2021. https://oig.hhs.gov/compliance/

62. U.S. Department of Health & Human Services. *Practical Guidance for Health Care Governing Boards on Compliance Oversight.* April 2015. Accessed May 15, 2022. https://www.hhs.gov/guidance/document/practical-guidance-health-care-governing-boards-compliance-oversight

63. CHAP. Top 10 infusion therapy nursing deficiencies. Published April 23, 2021. Accessed November 28, 2021. https://chapinc.org/wp-content/uploads/2021/04/Top-Ten-Infusion-Therapy-Nursing-Deficiencies-Handout-4-23-21.pdf

64. Morse S. Accreditation quality review shows common deficiencies in hospitals, ambulatory care centers and labs. *Healthcare Finance.* Published October 6, 2021. Accessed November 28, 2021. https://www.healthcarefinancenews.com/news/accreditation-quality-review-shows-common-deficiencies-hospitals-ambulatory-surgery-centers-and

65. The Joint Commission. *Survey Analysis for Evaluating Risk (SAFER).* Accessed December 5, 2021. https://www.jointcommission.org/-/media/tjc/documents/accred-and-cert/safer-matrix/safer-infographic.pdf?db=web&hash=69AB3EB96FE743C26C8F3D75C9FFB466&hash=69AB3EB96FE743C26C8F3D75C9FFB466#:~:text=The%20Joint%20Commission%20has%20developed,of%20compliance%20activities%20and%20interventions

66. The Joint Commission. Tracer methodology. Accessed November 28, 2021. https://www.jointcommission.org/resources/news-and-multimedia/fact-sheets/facts-about-tracer-methodology/

67. The Joint Commission. All accreditation programs survey activity guide: January 2021. Published January 20, 2021. Accessed December 1, 2021. https://www.jointcommission.org/-/media/tjc/documents/accred-and-cert/survey-process-and-survey-activity-guide/2021/2021-all-programs-organization-sag.pdf

68. The Joint Commission. Using technology to improve consistency of survey findings. Published May 11, 2021. Accessed November 17, 2021. https://www.jointcommission.org/resources/news-and-multimedia/blogs/dateline-tjc/2021/05/utilizing-technology-to-improve-consistency-of-survey-findings/

## Suggested Readings

Boylan MR, Suchman KI, Korolikova H, Slover JD, Bosco JA. Association of Magnet nursing status with hospital performance on nationwide quality metrics. *J Healthc Qual.* 2019;41(4):189-194. doi:10.1097/JHQ.0000000000000202

Bracewell N, Winchester DE. Accreditation in health care: does it make any difference to patient outcomes? *BMJ Qual Saf.* 2021;30:845-847. doi:10.1136/bmjqs-2020-012533

Greenfield D, Usman I, O'Connor E, Conlan N, Wilson H. An appraisal of healthcare accreditation agencies and programs: similarities, differences, challenges and opportunities. *Int J Qual Health Care.* 2021;33(4). doi:10.1093/intqhc/mzab150

Iannello J, Levitt MP, Poetter, D, et al. Improving inpatient tobacco treatment measures: outcomes through standardized treatment, care coordination, and electronic health record optimization. *J Health Qual.* 2021;43(1):48-58. doi:10.1097/JHQ.0000000000000251

Khadjesari Z. Regulation and accreditation of addictive behaviour applications: navigating the landscape. *Addiction.* 2021;116(12):3276-3283. doi:10.1111/add.15484

Nair S, Chen J. Improving quality of care in federally qualified health centers through ambulatory care accreditation. *J Healthc Qual.* 2018;40(5):301-309. doi:10.1097/JHQ.0000000000000105

Schultz OA, Shi L, Lee M. Assessing the efficacy of certificate of need laws through total joint arthroplasty. *J Healthc Qual.* 2021;43(1):e1-e7. doi:10.1097/JHQ.0000000000000286

## Online Resources

### Accreditation Association for Ambulatory Health Care (AAAHC)

www.aaahc.org

### Accreditation Commission for Health Care, Inc. (ACHC)

www.achc.org

### Agency for Healthcare Research and Quality (AHRQ)

www.ahrq.gov

### American College of Radiology (ACR)

www.ACRAccreditation.org

### American College of Surgeons (ACS)

www.facs.org

### Association for the Advancement of Blood & Biotherapies (AABB)

www.aabb.org

### CARF International

www.carf.org

### Centers for Disease Control and Prevention

www.cdc.gov

### Centers for Medicare & Medicaid Services

www.cms.gov

*Clinical Laboratory Improvement Amendments*

www.cms.hhs.gov/clia

*Code of Federal Regulations*

https://www.ecfr.gov/

*College of American Pathologists (CAP)*

www.cap.org

*Commission of Office Laboratory Accreditation (COLA)*

www.cola.org

*Community Health Accreditation Partner (CHAP)*

www.chapinc.org

*DNV GL Healthcare*

https://www.dnv.us/assurance/healthcare/ac.html

*Emergency Medical Treatment and Active Labor Act*

www.cms.gov/EMTALA

*Federal Register*

www.federalregister.gov

*Health Insurance Portability and Accountability Act*

www.hhs.gov/ocr/privacy

*Institute for Healthcare Improvement*

www.ihi.org

*The Joint Commission (TJC)*

www.jointcommission.org

*National Committee for Quality Assurance (NCQA)*

www.ncqa.org

*National Quality Forum: Field Guide to NQF Resources*

http://www.qualityforum.org/Field_Guide/

*Occupational Safety and Health Administration*

www.osha.gov

*U.S. Department of Health & Human Services*

www.hhs.gov

*U.S. Food & Drug Administration*

www.fda.gov

*URAC*

www.urac.org

# Patient Safety

Christy L. Beaudin and Luc R. Pelletier

## SECTION CONTENTS

# Introduction

The duty of any healthcare professional is to work with others to provide safe care, treatment, and services using current evidence-based principles, practices, and tools. This section offers a comprehensive overview of safety principles and practices relevant to healthcare delivery across the continuum of care. The safety imperative is discussed and various patient safety programs described. Patient safety culture approaches and systems thinking principles are examined with a review of practical tools for assessment, planning, implementation, and evaluation that healthcare quality professionals can use in daily practice.

The successful integration of safety concepts and practices results from leadership commitment and the healthcare workforce understanding about what works and what does not in healthcare structure and processes. A culture of safety thrives in a learning organization with effective leadership, an engaged and intentional healthcare workforce, and activated patients. See the *Performance and Process Improvement* and *Quality Leadership and Integration* sections for more information about frameworks and tools used in quality, safety, and performance improvement.

*Note: Patient safety* is used throughout this section. The term *patient* represents any label for the user of healthcare services across the continuum such as a patient, client, resident, consumer, customer, stakeholder, recipient, or partner.

# The Patient Safety Imperative

Eliminating errors and reducing harm are imperative to deliver on the promise of care delivery, treatment, and services in a safe environment free of errors and harm. In the seminal Institute of Medicine (IOM) report, *Crossing the Quality Chasm: A New Health System for the 21st Century,* the Committee on Quality of Health Care in America stated healthcare frequently harms and routinely fails to deliver its potential benefits. It was noted that the American healthcare delivery system needed fundamental change.[1(p1)] In addition, it concluded healthcare was not being provided with the best scientific knowledge. The IOM report suggested an agenda for "crossing the chasm" by changing the healthcare delivery system. Its agenda includes the following components:

- All healthcare constituencies (e.g., purchasers, healthcare professionals, regulators, and consumers) can commit to a national statement of purpose for the healthcare system, setting six aims for improvement to raise the quality of care to unprecedented levels.
- Clinicians, patients, and healthcare organizations need to adopt a new set of principles to guide the redesign of care processes.
- Through the U.S. Department of Health & Human Services (HHS), a set of priorities must be identified to focus initial efforts, provide resources to stimulate innovation, and initiate the change process.
- Healthcare organizations need to design and implement more effective support processes to make change in the delivery of care possible.

Fostering and rewarding improvement in the context of ever-expanding knowledge and rapid change is accomplished by creating an infrastructure that supports evidence-based practice, uses information technology (IT), aligns incentives with outcomes, and prepares the workforce to better provide care, treatment, and services. There are many evolving safety challenges related to telehealth, nursing homes, home-based care, health information technology, and the delivery of behavioral, primary, and prenatal healthcare services to vulnerable persons living in rural and urban communities. The sections that follow detail and describe key components that support the work of the healthcare quality professional.

# Concepts, Principles, and Practices

Patient safety reflects science, encompasses practices and interventions, and aims to reduce the occurrence of preventable events. It requires intention, vigilance, perseverance, and trust to build a culture of safety. These are important as one considers the person and the healthcare delivery system. Patient safety and quality improvement are intertwined. Different techniques can be used to assess and improve performance with the findings used to inform change. "It is important to adopt various process-improvement techniques to identify inefficiencies, ineffective care, and preventable errors, and influence changes associated with systems."[2(p3-1)]

**Box 4.1** lists the key points for the patient safety imperative and concepts.

## Concepts

Understanding and integrating safety concepts is important to the work of the healthcare quality professional responsible for leading and informing patient safety activities in an organization. Through the work of various government, quasi-government, and voluntary groups, different definitions of *patient safety* emerged that address the prevention of errors and the reduction of harm, such as the following:

- The "freedom from accidental injury due to medical care or medical errors."[3(p4)]
- A concept that is "indistinguishable from the delivery of quality health care,"[4(p5)] in a culture of safety where ". . . caregivers are encouraged to report medical errors, 'near misses,' or adverse events, where they can be discussed in an atmosphere of trust and mutual respect without fear of blame or retribution."[5(p195)]
- The "freedom from accidental or preventable injuries produced by medical care. Thus, practices or interventions that improve patient safety are those that reduce the occurrence of preventable adverse events."[6(¶1)]
- "A discipline in the health care sector that applies safety science methods toward the goal of achieving a trustworthy system of health care delivery. It is also an attribute of health care systems; it minimizes the incidence and impact of, and maximizes recovery from, adverse events."[7(p6)]
- "The prevention and mitigation of harm caused by errors of omission or commission that are associated with healthcare, and involving the establishment of operational systems and processes that minimize the likelihood of errors and maximize the likelihood of intercepting them when they occur."[8]

- A public health issue. It is "a framework of organized activities that creates cultures, processes, procedures, behaviors, technologies and environments in health care that consistently and sustainably lower risks, reduce the occurrence of avoidable harm, make error less likely and reduce the impact when it does occur."[9(¶1)]

From these definitions, one can quickly recognize the myriad of patient safety issues across the continuum of care that could be encountered, and demand attention as part of the healthcare quality professional's body of work (e.g., hazards and patient complexities in behavioral health environments or outpatient settings). Some issues may be less obvious but just as serious. Some issues are experienced by most types of healthcare organizations. However, there are issues unique to the setting where care, treatment, and services are provided. The healthcare quality professional will want to be familiar with these to direct patient safety activities in their setting and help define what patient safety means in the organization. **Table 4.1** offers examples of the kinds of safety concerns that the healthcare quality professional might encounter in different healthcare settings. Race/ethnic disparities and emergency/pandemic preparedness and response topped some of the industry's lists.

## Systems Thinking

Human error is inevitable, even among the most conscientious professionals who practice the highest standards of care. Human error happens when "there is general agreement that the individual should have done other than what they did, and in the course of that conduct inadvertently causes or could cause an undesirable outcome, the individual is labeled as having committed an error."[10(p6)] Identification and reporting of human error events are critical to an organization's efforts to continuously improve patient safety and contribute to a robust learning environment. Likewise, healthcare leaders have a duty to recognize the inevitability of human error, design systems that make such error less likely, and avoid punitive reactions to honest errors. Pham and colleagues offer that incident reporting systems can help the organization identify local system hazards, bolster the patient safety culture, and share lessons learned within and across organizations.[11] Incident reporting, however, should not be the only component of an enterprise-wide patient safety program.

**Table 4.1** **Patient Safety Concerns Across the Continuum of Care**

| Organization Type | Safety Concerns | |
|---|---|---|
| Any healthcare organization | *Safety Culture*<br>■ Low vaccination coverage and disease resurgence<br>■ Patient identification<br>■ Workplace safety and reporting<br>■ Work/stress burnout<br>■ Staffing shortages<br>■ Standardizing safety efforts<br>■ Trauma from workplace violence<br>■ Just culture (fair and blame-free)<br>■ Failure to embrace a culture of safety<br>■ Incivility/bullying<br>*Care and Treatment*<br>■ Racial and ethnic disparities/health equity<br>■ Supply chain interruptions<br>■ Telehealth and workflow challenges<br>■ Improvised use of medical devices<br>■ Inadequate monitoring for respiratory depression in patients on opioids<br>■ Inadequate test result reporting and follow-up<br>■ Peripheral vascular harm<br>■ Moving, transferring, and lifting patients<br>■ Workplace aggression from patients and visitors<br>■ Missed and delayed diagnoses<br>■ Medical supply shortages<br>■ Surgical mistakes<br>■ Wrong patient<br>■ Pressure ulcers<br>■ Death<br>■ Unexpected additional care<br>■ Severe temporary harm<br>■ Patient identification errors<br>■ Care coordination and transitions (within facility, between facilities, to the community)<br>■ Delay in treatment<br>■ Falls<br>■ Inadequate management of behavioral health issues<br>■ Radiation errors<br>■ Readmissions<br>■ Sepsis<br>■ Leaving/terminating treatment against medical advice<br>■ Unsafe injection practices | *Medication Related*<br>■ Adverse drug events<br>■ Drug shortages<br>■ Medication errors (includes those related to pounds and kilograms)<br>■ Methotrexate therapy<br>■ Look-alike, sound-alike medications<br>*Infection Prevention and Control*<br>■ Antibiotic resistance<br>■ Healthcare-associated infections<br>■ Pandemic preparedness<br>■ Risk from aerosol-generating procedures<br>■ Inadequate antimicrobial stewardship<br>■ Superbugs<br>*Environmental Safety*<br>■ Emergency preparedness and response<br>■ Exposure to workplace hazards<br>■ Facility safety<br>*Health Information*<br>■ Vulnerability in third-party software components—cybersecurity<br>■ Managing medical devices with emergency use authorization<br>■ Fatal medication errors<br>■ Rapid adoption of telehealth<br>■ Artificial intelligence (AI) applications for diagnostic imaging<br>■ Remote operation of medical devices<br>■ Insufficient quality assurance of 3D printed medical devices<br>■ Patient safety event/data transparency<br>■ Disclosure of private or confidential health information<br>■ Data integrity<br>■ Unrecognized patient deterioration<br>■ Electronic health record (EHR) system training<br>■ EHR system support and communication<br>■ EHR patient safety and quality issues<br>■ EHR and workflow/work process (e.g., alert fatigue)<br>■ Health IT configurations and organizational workflow that do not support each other<br>■ Misuse of universal serial bus ports, causing devices to malfunction | |
| Acute care—general medical | ■ Antibiotic resistance<br>■ Diagnostic errors<br>■ Healthcare-acquired infections<br>■ Medication errors<br>■ Handoffs<br>■ Patient identification<br>■ Trauma from workplace violence<br>■ Inadequate cleaning of flexible endoscopes<br>■ Missed alarms/alarm fatigue | ■ Drug shortages<br>■ Inadequate surveillance of monitored patients<br>■ Inappropriate patient ventilation<br>■ Test results reporting errors | |

*(continues)*

**Table 4.1** **Patient Safety Concerns Across the Continuum of Care** *(continued)*

| Organization Type | Safety Concerns | |
|---|---|---|
| Acute care—general surgical | <ul><li>Antibiotic resistance</li><li>Insufficient training of clinicians in operating room technology</li><li>Operative/postoperative complications</li><li>Patient identification</li><li>Wrong patient, wrong site, wrong procedure</li><li>Trauma from workplace violence</li><li>Unintended retention of a foreign body</li><li>Reprocessing issues</li><li>Failure to effectively monitor postoperative patients for opioid-induced respiratory depression</li></ul> | <ul><li>Gamma camera mechanical failures</li><li>Healthcare-acquired infections</li><li>Sepsis</li><li>Test results reporting errors</li><li>Unintentional retained objects during surgery even with correct count</li><li>Team communication</li></ul> |
| Acute care—pediatric | <ul><li>Death</li><li>Medication errors</li><li>Patient identification</li><li>Trauma from workplace violence</li><li>Inadequate management of behavioral health issues</li><li>Test results reporting errors</li></ul> | <ul><li>Catheter-associated urinary tract infections</li><li>Central-line–associated bloodstream infections</li><li>Falls</li><li>Peripheral IV infiltrations and extravasations</li><li>Pressure injuries</li><li>Readmissions</li><li>Surgical site infections</li><li>Unplanned extubations</li><li>Ventilator-associated pneumonia</li><li>Venous thromboembolism</li></ul> |
| Acute care—psychiatric | <ul><li>Access</li><li>Antibiotic resistance</li><li>Elopement</li><li>Healthcare-acquired infections</li><li>Medication errors</li></ul> | <ul><li>Patient identification</li><li>Suicide attempt/successful suicide</li><li>Trauma from workplace violence</li><li>Workforce shortages</li></ul> |
| Nursing home/long-term care | *Safety Culture*<ul><li>Communication openness</li><li>Compliance with procedures</li><li>Handoffs</li><li>Nonpunitive response to mistakes</li><li>Organizational learning</li><li>Staffing</li><li>Training and skills</li><li>Teamwork</li><li>Trauma from workplace violence</li></ul> | *Care and Treatment*<ul><li>Antibiotic resistance</li><li>Delirium</li><li>Falls</li><li>Healthcare-associated infections</li><li>Medication errors</li><li>Pressure ulcer reduction</li><li>Pain management (including palliative)</li><li>Missed alarms; alarm hazards; alarm fatigue</li><li>Workplace aggression from residents/visitors</li></ul> |
| Ambulatory care/surgery centers | *Safety Culture*<ul><li>Burnout</li><li>Communication about patient information</li><li>Communication openness</li><li>Staffing, work pressure, and pace</li><li>Teamwork</li><li>Staff training</li><li>Response to mistakes</li><li>Incivility/bullying</li></ul> | <ul><li>Organizational learning—continuous improvement</li><li>Management support for patient safety</li></ul>*Care and Treatment*<ul><li>Antibiotic resistance</li><li>Communication in the surgery/procedure room</li><li>Coordination of care</li><li>Care transitions</li><li>Diagnostic errors (missed and delayed)</li><li>Medication errors</li><li>Surgical mistakes</li></ul> |

*(continues)*

**Table 4.1** **Patient Safety Concerns Across the Continuum of Care** *(continued)*

| Organization Type | Safety Concerns | |
| --- | --- | --- |
| Primary care | <ul><li>Antibiotic resistance</li><li>Diagnostic errors and test results (missed or delayed)</li><li>Care coordination</li><li>Communication and information flow processes</li><li>Delays in proper treatment or preventive services</li></ul> | <ul><li>Medication errors (inappropriate and overprescribing)</li><li>Mistakes in surgery</li><li>Patient identification</li><li>Inadequate management of behavioral health issues</li></ul> |
| Home health | <ul><li>Aggression/violence</li><li>Antibiotic resistance</li><li>Falls</li><li>Mismatch of physical space, equipment, and supplies</li><li>Home oxygen fires</li><li>Medication errors</li></ul> | <ul><li>Patient identification</li><li>Caregiver's health and well-being neglected by self and others</li><li>Lack of preparation, training, and support of caregivers</li><li>Needlestick and sharps injuries</li></ul> |

Data from Agency for Healthcare Research and Quality. Improving health information technology patient safety: a resource list for users of the AHRQ health information technology item set. Published 2019. Accessed December 7, 2021. https://www.ahrq.gov/sites/default/files /wysiwyg/sops/quality-patient-safety/patientsafetyculture/healthitresourcelist.pdf; Agency for Healthcare Research and Quality. Improving patient safety in ambulatory surgery centers: a resource list for users of the AHRQ Ambulatory Surgery Center Survey on Patient Safety Culture. Published 2019. Accessed December 7, 2021. https://www.ahrq.gov/sites/default/files/wysiwyg/sops/surveys/asc/asc-resource-list.pdf; Agency for Healthcare Research and Quality. Improving patient safety in nursing homes: a resource list for users of the AHRQ Nursing Home Survey on Patient Safety Culture. Published 2019. Accessed December 7, 2021. https://www.ahrq.gov/sites/default/files/wysiwyg/sops/surveys/nursing-home-resource-list.pdf; Agency for Healthcare Research and Quality. Improving workplace safety in hospitals: a resource list for users of the AHRQ workplace safety supplemental items. Published 2021. Accessed December 7, 2021. https://www.ahrq.gov/sites/default/files/wysiwyg/sops/surveys/hospital/workplace-safety /workplace_safety_resource_list.pdf; Agency for Healthcare Research and Quality. PSNet: Ambulatory care safety. Published 2019. Accessed December 8, 2021. https://psnet.ahrq.gov/primer/ambulatory-care-safety; Agency for Healthcare Research and Quality. PSNet: Long-term care and patient safety. Published 2019. Accessed December 7, 2021. https://psnet.ahrq.gov/primer/long-term-care-and-patient-safety; Agency for Healthcare Research and Quality. PSNet: Patient safety in primary care. Published 2020. Accessed December 8, 2021. https://psnet.ahrq.gov/perspective/patient-safety-primary-care; American Health Information Management Association. Patient identification remains advocacy priority for 2021. Published 2021. Accessed December 8, 2021. https://journal.ahima.org/patient-identification-remains-advocacy-priority-for-2021/; Carbajal E, Masson G, Bean M. 10 top patient safety issues for 2021. *Becker's Clinical Leadership & Infection Control*. Published 2020. Accessed December 7, 2021. https://www.beckershospitalreview.com/patient-safety-outcomes/10-top-patient-safety-issues-for-2021.html; Children's Hospital Association Solutions for Patient Safety. SPS prevention bundles. Published 2021. Accessed December 7, 2021. https://www.solutionsforpatientsafety.org/wp-content/uploads/SPS-Prevention-Bundles_NOV-2021-1.pdf; Dzubak J. Top 5 patient safety concerns. Published 2017. Accessed December 7, 2021. https://ohnurses.org/top-5-patient-safety-concerns/; ECRI Institute. Executive brief: top 10 patient safety concerns for healthcare organizations 2021. Published 2021. Accessed December 7, 2021. https://assets.ecri.org/PDF/White-Papers-and-Reports/ECRI_Top10_Patient-Safety-Concerns_2021_v2.pdf; ECRI Institute. Executive brief: top 10 health technology hazards for 2021. Published 2021. Accessed December 7, 2021. https://assets.ecri.org/PDF/Solutions/Device-Evaluations/ECRI-Top10Hazards_2021_EB.pdf; Ellenbecker CH, Samia L, Cushman MJ, Alster K. Patient safety and quality in home health care. In: Hughes RG, ed. *Patient Safety and Quality: An Evidence-Based Handbook for Nurses*. Rockville, MD: Agency for Healthcare Research and Quality; 2008: chapter 13. Accessed December 8, 2021. https://www.ncbi.nlm.nih.gov/books/NBK2631/; The Joint Commission. 2022 Behavioral health care and human services national patient safety goals. Published 2021. Accessed December 8, 2021. https://www.jointcommission.org/-/media/tjc/documents/standards/national-patient-safety-goals/2022/simple_2022-bhc-npsg-goals-101921.pdf; The Joint Commission. 2022 Home care national patient safety goals. Published 2021. Accessed December 8, 2021. https://www.jointcommission.org/-/media/tjc/documents/standards/national-patient-safety-goals/2022/simple_2022-ome-npsg-goals-101921.pdf; The Joint Commission. 2022 Hospital national patient safety goals. Published 2021. Accessed December 8, 2021. https://www.jointcommission.org/-/media/tjc/documents/standards/national-patient-safety-goals/2022/simple_2022-hap-npsg-goals-101921.pdf; The Joint Commission. 2022 Office-based surgery national patient safety goals. Published 2021. Accessed December 8, 2021. https://www.jointcommission.org/-/media/tjc/documents/standards/national-patient-safety-goals/2022/simple_2022-obs-npsg-goals-101921.pdf; The Joint Commission. Sentinel event data released for first six months of 2021. Published 2021. Accessed December 8, 2021. https://www.jointcommission.org/resources/news-and-multimedia/newsletters/newsletters/joint-commission-online/sept-29-2021/sentinel-event-data-released-for-first-six-months-of-2021/#:~:text=The%20 summary%20data%20of%20sentinel%20event%20statistics%20for,patient%E2%80%99s%20death.%2024%25%20led%20to%20unexpected%20 additional%20care; National Academies of Science, Engineering, and Medicine. Improving diagnosis in health care. Published 2015. Accessed December 8, 2021. http://www.nationalacademies.org/hmd/reports/2015/improving-diagnosis-in-healthcare; National Institute for Occupational Safety and Health (NIOSH). NIOSH fast facts: injury data. Published 2019. Accessed December 8, 2021. https://www.cdc.gov/niosh/topics/violence/fastfacts.html; and National Institute for Occupational Safety and Health (NIOSH). NIOSH training and education: online workplace violence prevention courses for nurses. Published 2021. Accessed December 8, 2021. https://www.cdc.gov/niosh/topics/violence/training.html; World Health Organization. Patient safety: key facts. Accessed April 9, 2022. https://www.who.int/news-room/fact-sheets/detail/patient-safety

A safety management system is a proactive, collaborative process to find and fix workplace hazards before employees are injured or become ill. Almost all successful systems include six core elements:

1. Management leadership
2. Employee participation
3. Hazard identification and assessment
4. Hazard prevention and control
5. Education and training
6. Program evaluation and improvement

Many healthcare organizations already have these elements in place to comply with accreditation requirements for patient safety, and some have adopted a related set of high reliability organization concepts. It is a natural fit to extend the same principles to employee safety.

A formal patient safety program is part of system design. The program considers the following:

- Mission, vision, core values, and goals of the organization
- Interrelationships between and among functions, departments, and disciplines
- Acknowledging differences in the patient safety mindset
- Silos that might exist for overlapping, duplicative, or misaligned goals and objectives
- Forming cross-departmental (interprofessional) teams for collaboration
- Identifying where processes can be streamlined to improve organizational or system effectiveness

The written program and plan incorporate the patient safety goals and objectives. It describes how efforts are coordinated to support organization-wide assessment, evaluation, and improvement of interrelated processes. Different aspects of the plan can include the following:

- Governance and leadership
- Goals and objectives
- Planning, designing, and redesigning safe processes
- Culture of safety
- Reduction of preventable errors (e.g., identifying and mitigating risks and hazards, adverse events, sentinel events, and peer review processes)
- Adherence to evidence-based clinical practice guidelines
- Patient, family, and caregiver engagement
- Measurement, monitoring, and evaluating program effectiveness and success
- Transparency and dissemination of results across the organization

The healthcare quality professional can guide the organization in determining which performance improvement methodology can be adopted proactively and retrospectively. An organization also can look to build the skills of those working on improving patient safety, such as avowing common pitfalls when conducting a root cause analysis (RCA)[12] and developing strong harm reduction actions that are sustainable.

## Harm Reduction

The IOM report, *To Err Is Human: Building a Safer Health System*, and its subsequent reports, garnered the attention of providers, payers, and consumers by illustrating the direct relationship between quality of care and patient outcomes.[3] Further, Becher and Chassin pointed out the experience of patient harm as the result of three types of quality issues: underuse, overuse, and misuse of health services.[13] Underuse occurs when patients do not receive beneficial health services. For instance, only 30.5% (or 16.1 million people) with any mental illness perceived an unmet need for mental health services.[14] Overuse occurs when patients undergo treatment or procedures from which they do not benefit (e.g., X-rays performed on patients with back pain are unnecessary). Misuse occurs when patients receive appropriate medical services provided poorly, adding to the risk for preventable complications.

Underuse, overuse, and misuse are considered waste, and waste is costly. Berwick and Hackbarth believe the best healthcare reform and cost reduction strategy is to eliminate waste.[15] In 2011, they identified six categories where considerable costs are represented by waste. Total waste cost of the United States was $558 billion to $1263 billion. Shrank and colleagues updated these estimates in 2019; they reported that 25% of the $3.6 trillion healthcare market ($760 billion to $935 billion) is potentially wasteful.[16] These are examples of waste related to harm reduction:

- *Failures of care delivery.* Waste from poor execution or lack of best practice adoption resulting in injuries and poor outcomes ($102.4 billion to $165.7 billion).
- *Failures of care coordination.* Waste related to fragmented care resulting in complications, readmissions, declines in functional status, and increased dependency of the chronically ill ($27.2 billion to $78.2 billion).
- *Overtreatment or low-value care.* Waste from rendering care that is not useful ($75.7 billion to $101.2 billion).[16(p1501)]

Other domains identified as healthcare waste include:

- *Pricing failure*. Waste as prices migrate far from those expected in well-functioning markets ($230.7 billion to 240.5 billion).
- *Fraud and abuse*. Waste that results from fraudsters who issue fake bills and run scams ($58.5 billion to $83.9 billion).
- *Administrative complexity*. Waste resulting from government, accreditation agencies, payers, and others create inefficient or misguided rules ($265.6 billion).[16(pp1501-1502)]

Further, Dietz and colleagues predicted that one-third of healthcare costs—amounting to $1.4 trillion—is attributable to defects in healthcare.[17]

## Human Factors

*Human factors* are "the application of knowledge about human capabilities (physical, sensory, emotional, and intellectual) and limitations to the design and development of tools, devices, systems, environments, and organizations . . ."[18(p1)] A basic premise of human factors engineering is that well-designed systems capitalize on human capabilities and compensate for human limitations. Human factors engineering "takes into account human strengths and limitations in the design of interactive systems that involve people, tools and technology, and work environments to ensure safety, effectiveness and ease of use."[19(¶3)]

Human factors associated with healthcare personnel and patient safety are complex. Employee attitudes, motivation, physical and psychological health, education, training, and cognitive functioning can influence the likelihood of an error or accident. In healthcare, 85% of errors are the result of systems issues, and 15% are attributable to human factors.[20] According to the Institute for Healthcare Improvement (IHI), reliability is key in making systems and processes safer. Their four foundational principles for making systems and processes more reliable include standardization, simplification, reduction of autonomy, and highlighting deviations from practice.[21] Causes for human error are important in system design and redesign. Examples of human factors found to contribute to errors include the following:

- Human interaction with machines[22]
- Workload leading to errors and mistakes in providing the best care for patients, when there are not enough staff to handle the workload or work hours are inadequate[23]
- Disruptive behavior of healthcare personnel that undermines a culture of patient safety[24]
- Fatigue and stress leading to less than expected performance[25]

Any improvement efforts focused on eliminating errors requires a just culture, detailed analysis of the care delivery process, human factors influencing processes of care, and the resources to bring about sustained system change.

Drawing from many other disciplines such as anatomy, physiology, physics, biomechanics, and ergonomics, IHI defines human factors as "the study of all the factors that make it easier to do the work in the right way."[26(¶1)] The science applied to healthcare fosters these principles in designed work processes:

- Simplify to take steps out of a process.
- Standardize to remove variation and promote predictability and consistency.
- Use forcing functions and constraints that makes it impossible to do a task incorrectly and creates a hard stop that cannot be passed unless actions are changed. Check, restrict, or compel to avoid or perform an action.
- Use redundancies such as double-checking someone's work.
- Avoid reliance on memory by using tools such as checklists.[27]
- Take advantage of habits and patterns to perform consistently (habit) and in a recognizable way (pattern).
- Promote effective team functioning (e.g., teamwork and communication).
- Automate and use technology carefully.[26]

## High Reliability

Healthcare organizations and systems are working toward becoming highly reliable. To become a high-reliability industry, healthcare "needs a radical cultural transformation, like the one that has taken place in aviation over the past thirty years . . . If aviation could do it, health care can too."[28(p7)] Adopting high-reliability principles and practices helps the healthcare organization strive for a near-zero-defect culture. As Reason offers, "Perhaps the most important distinguishing feature of high reliability organizations is their collective preoccupation with the possibility of failure. They expect to make errors and train their workforce to recognize and recover them."[29(p770)]

*High-reliability organizations* (HROs) are "organizations with systems in place that are exceptionally consistent in accomplishing their goals and avoiding catastrophic errors."[30,31(p298)] Five key concepts frame and impact the HRO. They include the following:

1. *Sensitivity to operations*. Preserving constant awareness and vigilance by leaders and staff about the state of the systems and processes affecting patient

care. This awareness is central to noting risks and preventing them. The healthcare quality professional should apply situational awareness and carefully designed change management processes.

2. *Reluctance to simplify.* Simple processes are good, but simplistic explanations for why things work or fail are risky. Avoiding overly simple explanations of failure (unqualified staff, inadequate training, communication failure, etc.) is essential to understand the true reasons patients are placed at risk. The healthcare quality professional should promote solid root cause analysis practices.

3. *Preoccupation with failure.* When near misses occur, these are viewed as evidence of systems to improve for reduction of potential harm to patients. Rather than viewing near misses as proof the system has effective safeguards, they are viewed as symptomatic of areas in need of more attention. The healthcare quality professional should pay attention to close calls and near misses (being lucky versus being good) and focus more on failures than on successes.

4. *Deference to expertise.* If leaders and supervisors are not willing to listen and respond to the insights of staff who know how processes work and the risks patients face, high reliability in the organization's safety culture may not be possible. They should listen to the experts on the frontlines (e.g., authority follows expertise).

5. *Resilience.* Leaders and staff need to be trained and prepared to know how to respond when system failures do occur. Resources are continually devoted to identification of stress, corrective action plans, and training.[32-34(p1)]

These concepts lead to mindfulness, an important component of reliability, which keep HROs at a high level of vigilance.[32(p7)] Chassin and Loeb propose organizations use *robust process improvement*, "a combination of Lean, Six Sigma, and change management" as a new set of tools to achieve high reliability and maintain patient safety.[35(p481)] These can achieve outcomes such as decreased morbidity and mortality through the application of replicable and scalable patient safety interventions. Many organizations now use the Lean practice of system redesign with a focus on the human factors in their patient safety programs. By acting mindfully, an HRO organizes itself so the unexpected is noticed and stopped from advancing.

Using these principles, the healthcare quality professional can work with others in the organization to create a mindful infrastructure that prevents harm from happening, reduces the damage produced by unexpected events, and promotes reliable performance. See the *Performance and Process Improvement* section for more information on Lean and Six Sigma and the *Quality Leadership and Integration* section for more information on change management.

Marx has been working with high reliability in the context of a just culture and offered that "it is through the lessons of our everyday errors that we can design our work environment."[36(p3)] High reliability is dependent on making good choices and becoming less error prone and more error tolerant. Marx works from a model-based approach to managing risk (proactive or anticipatory) instead of an event-driven approach (reactive). The focus on highly reliable outcomes derives from a core set of principles[37] that include the following:

- Zero is not possible.
- There is no such thing as an HRO; there are only organizations that are highly reliable around those things they value.
- Humans are not inherently rule followers—they are threat and hazards avoiders.
- There is a preoccupation with risk. Faulty equipment and fallible human beings can still produce great results.
- Strive to be three human errors away from harm with robust system design.
- It is about system design and choices and managing the right things.
- Doing less is often the better path—adopt smart designs that are often less extensive.

An example of system design and redesign is the Lean Healthcare program developed and deployed by Hagg and colleagues for different initiatives.[38] The program strategy enabled the robust implementation of quality and performance improvement initiatives including clinical practice bundles. See **Figure 4.1** for techniques and methodologies used. The program applied Lean and systems engineering methodologies and was structured to sustain improvements in process effectiveness and patient outcomes. The idea is to build sustainable programs, because when change is frequent or not sustained, the result is often accompanied by increased staff fatigue, a more stressful work environment, and increased costs.[38(p1)]

Different projects were successfully implemented affecting patient safety such as emergency department patient flow, surgical flow, medication delivery process redesign, intensive care unit (ICU) length-of-stay reduction (including ventilator-associated pneumonia/glycemic control bundles), central-line and methicillin-resistant *Streptococcus aureus* bundles, and patient fall reduction. Mitigating risk by using proven techniques contributes to high reliability—whether it

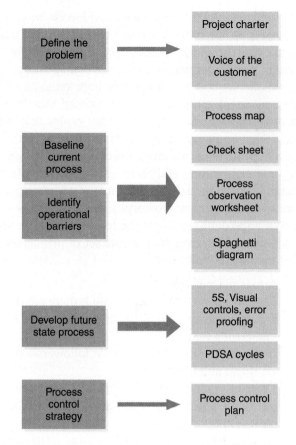

**Figure 4.1** Lean Healthcare System Redesign Approach; Plan-Do-Study-Act

Reproduced from Hagg HW, Workman-Germann J, Flanagan ME, Doebbeling BN. Implementation of systems redesign: approaches to spread and sustain adoption. In: Henriksen K, Battles JB, Keyes MA, Grad ML, eds. *Advances in Patient Safety: New Directions and Alternative Approaches* (Vol. 2: Culture and Redesign). Agency for Healthcare Research and Quality; 2008. Techniques and methodologies utilized within the Lean Healthcare Program (Figure 1).

is the behavior of the organization or the outcomes that result from the organization's processes.

Another example of system design for infection prevention and control is the journey to zero that includes innovative strategies to eradicate healthcare-associated infections (HAIs) through a process of laying the foundation to prioritize (sizing the internal infection burden), crafting a multipronged strategy (establishing frontline awareness and minimizing pathogen opportunity), and ensuring sustainable success and promoting long-term gains.[39(pp18-19)] Hand hygiene is an example of where the principles of high reliability bring promise. To get to zero HAIs, The Joint Commission Center for Transforming Healthcare developed its *Hand Hygiene Targeted Solutions Tool* to manage change so hand hygiene practices can be sustained using principles of leadership, safety culture, and performance improvement.[40] Many organizations use this tool to increase the frequency of hand hygiene practices.

**Box 4.2** outlines patient safety principles and practices.

# Leadership

The provision of care, treatment, or services across the continuum is composed of various elements including assessing, planning, providing, and coordinating care to address patient needs. This section synthesizes current knowledge related to patient safety, preventing errors, and reducing harm across the continuum of care. Strategic and operational components of developing a patient safety program are presented.

To build an organization's safety culture means tackling the most important patient safety issues facing healthcare organizations today, which include the following:

- Working within the context of economic and sociopolitical challenges
- Adopting and sustaining a culture of safety
- Identifying organizational champions
- Deploying and sustaining patient safety strategies
- Determining key drivers for patient safety programs
- Sustaining the gains of implementing safety innovations
- Ensuring the adoption of current and evolving safety-related technologies

There are many aspects of patient safety that are important, such as leadership and the mindful integration of safety concepts into an organization's vision, mission, strategic plan, core values, goals, and objectives. Whereas "do no harm" was previously an individual responsibility, a paradigm shift makes safety a system priority.[1(p67)]

When patient harm occurs, the cause is frequently traced to flaws in the system of care. Adopting systems thinking requires a healthcare organization to think beyond the person and beyond blame. Whereas individual behavior can result in an error, looking at health delivery from a systems perspective enables the organization to identify and manage errors differently. Using a systems approach, the conditions under which an individual works and the complexity of the process are the foci. By recognizing human and process variability in a systemic way, leadership and healthcare personnel can work together to avert errors or mitigate their effects. The Framework for Safer Health Care offers one way to organize contextual factors and threats to safety along the continuum of care (**Figure 4.2**).

National pressures mount, and new expectations emerge for healthcare leaders. These come from government agencies (e.g., the Centers for Medicare & Medicaid Services [CMS]), public reporting groups (e.g., The Leapfrog Group and *U.S. News & World Report*), accreditation agencies (e.g., The Joint Commission and the Accreditation Council for Graduate Medical Education), and third-party payers. Third-party payers are using the practice of nonpayment for certain reasonably preventable conditions (e.g., pressure ulcers) and serious preventable events (e.g., leaving a sponge in a patient during surgery). Leaders drive change and improvement in patient safety practices that address these pressures and expectations. A *patient safety practice* is "a type of process or structure whose application reduces the probability of adverse events resulting from exposure to the healthcare system across a range of diseases and procedures."[41(p13)] Applicability of various safety practices is dependent upon many factors, including the healthcare setting, the populations served, high-risk processes, volume-driven practices, and previous performance data. Organizations can use quality tools such as a prioritization matrix to select safety standards relevant to populations served. See **Table 4.2** for examples of safety practices.

Leadership works with others in the organization to prioritize needs, select practices for improvement, allocate resources to successfully implement patient safety practices, and ensure commitment to interventions and improvement are sustained over time. The governing board and medical leadership participate in the analysis and prioritization process. Patient safety practices are integrated into the organization's strategic direction. Goals that are both realistic and aspirational are developed. Various national organizations employ consensus-driven processes to identify patient safety practices to be adopted by healthcare organizations. Because there is now an abundance of consensus-driven standards, healthcare quality professionals can look to the vetted work of others to develop their own safety practices.

As part of its duties, the governing body or board of directors holds accountability for quality of care and patient safety. The heightened attention to public reporting affects this responsibility. Quality oversight is recognized more clearly as a core fiduciary duty, which is the highest standard of care. A fiduciary duty is not just financial health and reputation. Accountability for quality and safety cannot be fully delegated to the medical staff and executive leadership. A purpose- and

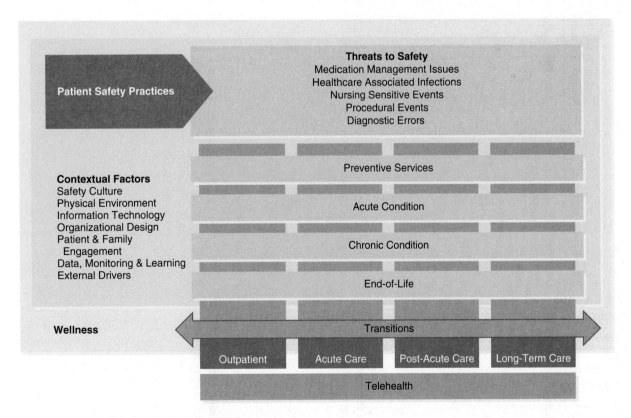

**Figure 4.2** Framework for Making Healthcare Safer

Reproduced from Agency for Healthcare Research and Quality. *Making Healthcare Safer III: Executive Summary*. Author; 2020. https://www.ahrq.gov/research/findings/making-healthcare-safer/mhs3/exe-summary.html

**Table 4.2** Patient Safety Practices

| Patient Safety Practice | Key Safety Outcomes | Studies/Systematic Reviews (Number) | Settings | Key Takeaways/Points |
|---|---|---|---|---|
| **Diagnostic error:** Peer review | ▪ Diagnostic errors<br>▪ Diagnostic discrepancy rates | 14 studies; 2 systematic reviews | Inpatient and outpatient (radiology and pathology) | ▪ Lack of evidence to show that traditional random peer review and feedback mechanisms improve diagnostic quality over time or prevent diagnostic errors from reaching the patient.<br>▪ Nonrandom peer review appears to be more effective at identifying diagnostic errors than random peer review.<br>▪ When nonrandom peer review is conducted prospectively, there is an opportunity to identify and remediate the diagnostic error before it reaches the patient. |
| **Failure to rescue:** Rapid response teams (RRTs) | ▪ Hospital mortality<br>▪ Cardiac arrest rate<br>▪ ICU transfer rate | 4 studies; 3 systematic reviews; 3 meta-analyses | Acute care hospitals | ▪ Inconclusive evidence as to whether RRT implementation is associated with decreased overall hospital mortality or ICU transfer rates.<br>▪ Moderate evidence that decreased non-ICU cardiac arrest rates are associated with implementation of RRTs.<br>▪ Recognition of the benefits of RRT implementation often takes a long time. |
| ***Clostridium difficile:*** Antimicrobial stewardship | ▪ *Clostridium difficile* infection (CDI) rates<br>▪ Amount of prescribed high-risk antimicrobials | 17 studies; 3 meta-analyses; 2 systematic reviews | Inpatient (hospitals and long-term care facilities/nursing homes) | ▪ Most studies showed reductions in CDI following a period of antimicrobial stewardship (both statistically significant and statistically nonsignificant reductions). In the reviewed studies, significant reductions in CDI were associated with higher baseline CDI rates/outbreaks, antimicrobial stewardship programs (ASPs) developed specifically to reduce CDI (as opposed to ASPs focused on other clinical and microbiological outcomes), and ASPs that included restrictions of high-risk antimicrobials and/or a preauthorization component.<br>▪ ASPs require staffing, technological resources, and provider buy-in. |

*(continues)*

(continued)

**Table 4.2** Patient Safety Practices

| Patient Safety Practice | Key Safety Outcomes | Studies/Systematic Reviews (Number) | Settings | Key Takeaways/Points |
|---|---|---|---|---|
| **Controlling multidrug-resistant organisms (MDROs) and preventing MDRO-related infections:** Surveillance for controlling MDROs | ■ MDRO acquisition (MRSA, CRE, VRE, MDR-GNB) ■ MDRO infection (including HAIs) ■ Results reporting completeness and accuracy ■ Compliance with other patient safety practices (PSPs) (such as contact precautions) | 20 studies; 2 systematic reviews; 1 meta-analysis | Hospitals (including intensive care, neonatal intensive care, hematology/oncology, and general care units) | ■ Targeted active surveillance performs as well as universal active surveillance for many MDROs and uses fewer resources. In places where universal active surveillance is already in place, screening for other MRDOs using the same sample may be cost-effective, due to shared risk factors. ■ Consensus exists for screening high-risk patients (those with a history of MDROs or risk factors associated with MDRO colonization/infection) on admission, but any screening approach will require compliance with infection prevention protocols when a positive culture result is found. ■ Surveillance may improve compliance with other PSPs when it is part of a multi-component intervention, but more research is needed on the mechanisms and circumstances of this association, as it can be confounded by the co-implementation of other, bundled practices. |
| **Diabetic agents:** Diabetes protocol for reducing hypoglycemia | ■ Incidence of hypoglycemia ■ Frequency of hypoglycemia ■ Length of stay ■ Blood glucose levels | 11 studies | Emergency department (ED), ICU | ■ Although glycemic outcomes usually improved, a statistically significant difference was rare. ■ Implementation of study protocols were usually implemented by nurses. |
| **Reducing adverse drug events in older adults:** Using the screening tool of older persons' potentially inappropriate prescriptions (STOPP) criteria | ■ Prescribing ■ Potentially inappropriate medications/prescriptions ■ Adverse drug reaction incidence | 14 studies | Primary healthcare center, geriatric psychiatry admission unit, acute care admission, long-term care, nursing homes, geriatric outpatient clinics | ■ STOPP criteria specifically target older adults to reduce avoidable adverse drug events. ■ STOPP criteria are particularly effective when combined with another tool. ■ Implementation of the STOPP criteria was led by either a pharmacist or physician. ■ Studies showed improved prescribing appropriateness but no statistically significant differences in admission or inpatient death rates. |

(continues)

**Table 4.2** Patient Safety Practices *(continued)*

| Patient Safety Practice | Key Safety Outcomes | Studies/Systematic Reviews (Number) | Settings | Key Takeaways/Points |
|---|---|---|---|---|
| **Opioids:** Medication-assisted treatment (MAT) initiation | ▪ Opioid dependence<br>▪ Illicit drug use<br>▪ Treatment retention rates | 25 studies; 1 systematic review | ED, community practice, clinic for the homeless, primary care clinics, outpatient substance use disorder treatment center, federally qualified health center (FQHC) | ▪ MAT can be initiated and provided safely in a variety of healthcare settings.<br>▪ Initiation of MAT in the ED, primary care setting, or outpatient clinics may result in faster access to care and longer retention or adherence to treatment.<br>▪ Most studies were focused on one component of MAT, the initiation of medications, in a few specific settings. |
| **Alarm fatigue:** Safety culture | ▪ Number of alarms<br>▪ Noise level | 10 studies | Hospitals; ICUs; progressive care unit; neonatal intensive care unit; or telemetry, step-down, transplant cardiology, surgical, or surgical orthopedic units | ▪ Current literature on this PSP is primarily quality improvement initiatives and case studies; higher quality studies could help to better understand the impact of implementing elements of safety culture to address alarm fatigue. |
| **Venous thromboembolism (VTE):** Use of aspirin for VTE prophylaxis | ▪ Deep vein thrombosis<br>▪ Pulmonary embolism<br>▪ Operative site bleeding and other major bleeding | 27 studies; 6 systematic reviews | Hospitals, postsurgical care, tertiary care orthopedic referral centers; countries included USA, UK, China, Canada, and Korea | ▪ Use of aspirin following major orthopedic surgery was generally found to be of similar effectiveness as other agents.<br>▪ An overwhelming majority of studies concluded that aspirin has a lower bleeding risk rate than other pharmacologic agents, which, combined with its lower cost, makes it an appealing option for VTE prophylaxis, particularly in low-risk patients.<br>▪ More prospective RCTs are needed to directly compare the effectiveness of aspirin to other prophylactic methods across patient risk levels. |

*(continues)*

**Table 4.2** Patient Safety Practices  *(continued)*

| Patient Safety Practice | Key Safety Outcomes | Studies/Systematic Reviews (Number) | Settings | Key Takeaways/Points |
|---|---|---|---|---|
| **Cross-cutting factors:** Patient and family engagement (PFE) | ▪ Patient and provider perception and attitude to PFE | 1 study; 2 systematic reviews | Hospital | ▪ Studies revealed a lack of understanding about the effects of PFE on patient safety among healthcare providers, patients, and families.<br>▪ PFE implemented through an educational intervention was linked to positive perceptions and attitudes about PFE among healthcare providers.<br>▪ More studies are needed to measure the direct outcomes of patient and family engagement. |
| **Cross-cutting factors:** Cultural competency | ▪ Preventable hospital readmissions<br>▪ Medication adherence<br>▪ LOS<br>▪ Advance care planning and informed consent | 7 studies; 4 systematic reviews | Inpatient, outpatient, and home health | ▪ Most of the small group of reviewed studies found language services were associated with improved patient safety.<br>▪ Need for studies that explore associations between a range of cultural competency interventions and patient safety outcomes.<br>▪ Interventions that are framed around cultural competency and aim to improve patient health and indicators of health have mostly positive outcomes. |
| **Cross-cutting factors:** Monitoring, audit, and feedback | NA | 28 studies; 3 systematic reviews; 1 nonsystematic review | All settings included in searches | ▪ Audit with feedback is a somewhat common strategy for improving compliance with patient safety processes.<br>▪ Audit and feedback appear to be most effective when both written and verbal feedback are used.<br>▪ Studies show more significant improvements when performance was lower at baseline.<br>▪ Research on audit and feedback predominantly focuses on process improvement, and more research is needed to measure the impact of audit and feedback on patient outcomes. |

*(continues)*

**Table 4.2** Patient Safety Practices

*(continued)*

| Patient Safety Practice | Key Safety Outcomes | Studies/Systematic Reviews (Number) | Settings | Key Takeaways/Points |
|---|---|---|---|---|
| Team simulation | ▪ Adverse outcome score<br>▪ Use of teamwork skills<br>▪ Confidence in emergencies<br>▪ Decision-making<br>▪ Workload management | 6 studies; 3 systematic reviews; 1 meta-analysis | Tertiary care medical center, teaching hospital, Veterans Administration facility | ▪ Participants were more confident in their ability to handle emergencies following simulation training.<br>▪ Participants demonstrated greater teamwork skills following simulation training, with some longer-term sustainment reported.<br>▪ Improved neonatal outcomes and a reduction of postpartum hemorrhage cases were associated with the simulation interventions. |
| Simulation-based medical education for residents and fellows | ▪ Complication rates<br>▪ Frequency and time of successful procedures | 5 studies; 3 systematic reviews; 1 meta-analysis | Teaching hospital, tertiary teaching hospital | ▪ Simulation-based medical education curriculums were associated with decreased complication rates, fewer errors, reduced central-line–associated bloodstream infection rates, improved pain management of patients, and a lower proportion of adverse events across studies.<br>▪ Cost savings were associated with reductions in central-line infections, overnight hospital days, or additional hospital days.<br>▪ Improved procedural skills were reported for participants, such as increased rates of successful first attempts to intubate patients, fewer needle passes for central venous catheter insertion, and increased compliance with recommended guidelines and protocols. |

Data from Shekelle PG, Wachter RM, Pronovost PJ, et al. *Making Health Care Safer II: An Updated Critical Analysis of the Evidence for Patient Safety Practices. Comparative Effectiveness Review No. 211.* (Prepared by the Southern California-RAND Evidence-based Practice Center under Contract No. 290-2007-10062-I.) Rockville, MD: Agency for Healthcare Research and Quality. AHRQ publication 13-E001-EF. Published March 2013. Accessed April 9, 2022. www.ahrq.gov/research/findings/evidence-based-reports/ptsafetyuptp.html

values-driven board, in partnership with executive leadership and medical staff, set performance expectations to elimination of harm while mitigating risks.

Quality and safety contribute to financial stability and offer capital opportunities for growing healthcare organizations. As decisions are made about bond ratings, agencies such as Standard & Poor's and Moody's Investors Service stress the importance of the healthcare leader's attention to clinical quality outcomes and safety:

> From a credit perspective, a not-for-profit hospital's focus on a quality agenda can translate into improved ratings through increased volume and market share, operational efficiencies, better rates from commercial payers, and improved financial performance. Like many strategies, [Moody's] recognize[s] that realizing financial returns from a quality strategy may require large capital costs and incurred operating losses in the short term. However, over the long term, a hospital's focus on quality will be viewed as a credit positive if greater patient demand and financial improvements materialize. Many not-for-profit hospitals are launching strategies to improve evidence-based clinical outcomes and patient safety, which we view as the two key facets of a strategy aimed at improving quality. The effort to improve quality is a major component of most hospitals' mission to provide the best patient care possible.[42(p1)]

These perspectives are critical to the conversations about the business case for quality and safety.

When providing quality care and reducing harm as part of an organization's strategy, the board, executives, and medical staff can conduct continual, transparent, and data-informed deliberations about capital and human resource investments. In doing so, they can consider harm and its impact on the bottom line. This criticality was underscored by a Moody's report on for-profit and not-for-profit hospital performance whereby

> technological innovation in healthcare would likely lead to lower patient volumes at both for-profit and not-for-profit hospitals. However, for hospitals at the forefront of healthcare technology, the benefits of innovation will outweigh the reduction in volumes. Telemedicine and remote monitoring, particularly for high-risk populations, will reduce emergency room visits and inpatient admissions because they will improve preventative care. These technologies will also reduce hospital visits by making it clearer when

a patient can be effectively managed at home (e.g., heart-burn vs heart attack). Further, advances in medical technologies and minimally invasive surgeries will also lead to more procedures being done in lower-cost settings, such as physician offices or ambulatory service centers, rather than in hospitals . . . Technological improvements in medical equipment, handheld devices, and electronic health records will also reduce medical errors, which are costly in many ways (including payment penalties, higher insurance and litigation costs).[43(p4)]

Investments in technology that reduce medical errors or that lead to more effective care management also contribute to the hospital or healthcare system's financial stability and growth.

Patient safety must be integrated by leadership into strategic planning. Grossbart highlights six guidelines all boards can consider in their effort to improve quality and reduce harm:

1. Emphasize quality and patient safety goals.
2. Leverage National Quality Forum (NQF)–endorsed measures.
3. Use benchmarking and risk adjustment to select targets.
4. Access data beyond the electronic health record.
5. Provide data and information for multiple organizational levels.
6. Develop a board-specific measurement and presentation strategy.[44]

Furthermore, the American Society for Health Care Risk Management (ASHRM) proposes that both risk appetite and risk capa\city be considered by boards in evaluating risk in pursuing various business objectives. ASHRM cites that a risk-aware culture encompasses these characteristics:

- Quantifies the potential variability of inputs and outputs when evaluating and prioritizing competing projects, initiatives, and strategic directions.
- Identifies the sources of such variability, known as key risk indicators.
- Measures the anticipated consequences—positive and negative—of such variability through the use of key performance indicators.
- Sets risk tolerances to establish the limits of acceptable performance.
- Develops mitigation strategies to lessen the impact of and/or reduce the likelihood of negative consequences.
- Develops contingency plans to deal with negative consequences if mitigation strategies fail or are not available.[45]

As a result of an innovation process, IHI found this to be the current state of board work and education in health system quality[46]:

- Governance of quality is primarily focused on safety.
- Governance of quality is organization centric, with limited focus on population or community health.
- Core processes for governance of quality are variable.
- A clear, consistent framework for governance of health system quality is needed.
- A call to action to raise expectations and improve support for board governance of health system quality is needed.

IHI proposed core components of quality from the patient's perspective, which can drive board oversight (**Figure 4.3**).

With the convergence of clinical care, safety priorities, and economic stability, board member interest will increase over time and create opportunities for healthcare quality professionals to educate organizational leaders on the importance of attending to patient safety. "Board oversight of quality and patient safety rests on the directors' ability to obtain, process, and interpret information; assess current performance; and set strategic direction using a range of metrics tailored to local circumstances."[47(p754)]

Over 100 consensus standards with a focus on patient safety are endorsed by NQF. The first of the 34 endorsed practices are leadership structures and systems.[48] This safe practice for leadership provides an overview of the leadership structures and systems deemed critical to the organization-wide awareness of patient safety performance gaps, direct accountability of leaders for those gaps, and adequate investment in performance improvement abilities, along with the actions necessary to ensure safe care of every patient served.[48] A comprehensive discussion of change and innovation can be found in the *Performance and Process Improvement* section. Also see the *Quality Leadership and Integration* section for more information about leadership, quality improvement, and strategy.

## Safety Culture

The current era of patient safety ushered in thinking such as achieving zero defects, pursuing perfection, and transforming healthcare.[49-51] This thinking influences how organizations create the strategy for culture of safety goals and objectives. Although everyone in the healthcare enterprise is responsible for quality and safety, an organization's leadership must emphasize safety as a core component of the organization's culture, its ongoing strategy planning, and its quality and performance

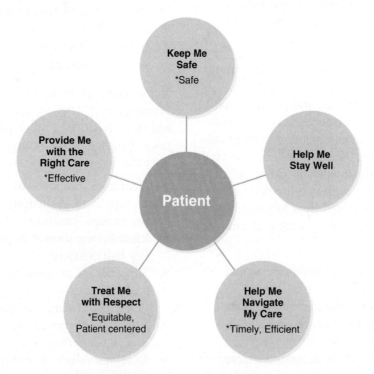

*IOM STEEP dimensions of quality: Safe, Timely, Effective, Efficient, Equitable, and Patient centered

**Figure 4.3** Core Components of Quality from the Patient's Perspective

Daley Ullem E, Gandhi TK, Mate K, Whittington J, Renton M, Huebner J. *Framework for Effective Board Governance of Health System Quality*. IHI white paper. Boston, MA: Institute for Healthcare Improvement; 2018: 11. Accessed April 9, 2022. http://www.ihi.org/resources/Pages/IHIWhitePapers/Framework-Effective-Board-Governance-Health-System-Quality.aspx improvement program. Designing an organizational structure for patient safety is like designing a house:

> Like the physical structure of a house, organizational structure identifies and distinguishes the individual parts of an organization and ties these pieces together to define an integrated whole. Organizational structure differs from the physical structure of a house, however, in that it encompasses more than inanimate characteristics of walls, doors, and windows. Organizational structure includes the interaction patterns that link people to people and people to work, and unlike a house, structural dimensions of organizations frequently change and evolve.[52(p399)]

In creating the organizational structure, leadership should not be preoccupied with failure but recognize that their "leadership is the critical element in a successful patient safety program and is non-delegable."[53(p1)] Leadership works to ensure that patient safety is supported by a strong but flexible foundation with straight walls, working doors, and opaque windows. The Joint Commission explained that the role of leadership is essential in developing the safety culture and described 11 tenets that help an organization achieve and sustain a safety culture.[54] See **Figure 4.4** for a description of these tenets.

The readiness of an organization needs to be assessed for the implementation of patient safety practices. This may typically start at the strategic planning stage with the mission and vision statements, core values, and strategic goals. Reason suggested that different safety culture elements be considered:

- *Informed culture.* Culture in which everyone is clear about acceptable and unacceptable actions. Being informed is supported by the availability of safety data that is actively disseminated.
- *Reporting culture.* Errant behaviors can be reported without fear of punishment or blame.
- *Learning culture.* An organization can learn from its mistakes and make changes.
- *Flexible culture.* The organization and the people in it can adapt effectively to changing demands.
- *Just culture.* Errors and unsafe acts are not punished if the error was unintentional. Those who act recklessly or take deliberate and unjustifiable risks may still be subject to disciplinary action.[55,56]

Healthcare organizations committed to a just culture identify and correct the systems or processes of care contributing to the medical error, adverse events, near miss, or close call—they do not assign blame. It is important that the organization is clear about terms used for identifying, investigating, reporting, and disclosing safety events. Errors, adverse events, preventable adverse events, and sentinel events are described as follows:

- *Medical error.* An error is defined as the failure of a planned action to be completed as intended or the use of a wrong plan to achieve an aim. Errors can include problems in practice, products, procedures, and systems.[57]
- *Adverse event.* An injury caused by something that happened in the delivery of medical care rather than by the underlying disease or condition of the patient. How adverse events might be categorized could be determined by setting (e.g., hospital, skilled nursing facility). Adverse events are sometimes further categorized as follows:
  - *Preventable adverse events.* Those that occurred due to error or failure to prevent error or system design flaw.
  - *Ameliorable adverse events.* Events that, while not preventable, could have been less harmful if care had been different.
  - *Adverse events due to negligence.* Those that occurred due to care that falls below the standards expected of clinicians in the community.[58]
- *Sentinel event.* A patient safety event (not primarily related to the natural course of the [patient's] illness or underlying condition that reaches a [patient] and results in death, severe harm (regardless of duration of harm), or permanent harm (regardless of severity of harm). An event can also be considered sentinel if the event signaled the need for immediate investigation and response.[59]
- *Severe harm.* An event or condition that reaches the individual, resulting in life-threatening bodily injury (including pain or disfigurement) that interferes with or results in loss of functional ability or quality of life that requires continuous physiological monitoring or a surgery, invasive procedure, or treatment to resolve the condition.
- *Permanent harm.* An event or condition that reaches the individual, resulting in any level of harm that permanently alters and/or affects an individual's baseline.[59]

Close calls and near misses are those that never reached a patient, may have reached a patient, or reached a patient with no serious harm. Near misses and close calls may be recognized and defined as follows:

- An event, situation, or error that took place but was captured before reaching the patient.[60]
- An act of commission or omission that had the potential to harm a patient but did not occur due to a planned/unplanned recovery or corrective action and timely intervention.[61,62]

# 11 Tenets of a Safety Culture

## Definition of Safety Culture

Safety culture is the sum of what an organization is and does in the pursuit of safety. The Patient Safety Systems (PS) chapter of The Joint Commission accreditation manuals defines safety culture as the product of individual and group beliefs, values, attitudes, perceptions, competencies, and patterns of behavior that determine the organization's commitment to quality and patient safety.

1 Apply a transparent, nonpunitive approach to reporting and learning from adverse events, close calls and unsafe conditions.

2 Use clear, just, and transparent risk-based processes for recognizing and distinguishing human errors and system errors from unsafe, blameworthy actions.

3 CEOs and all leaders adopt and model appropriate behaviors and champion efforts to eradicate intimidating behaviors.

4 Policies support safety culture and the reporting of adverse events, close calls and unsafe conditions. These policies are enforced and communicated to all team members.

5 Recognize care team members who report adverse events and close calls, who identify unsafe conditions, or who have good suggestions for safety improvements. Share these "free lessons" with all team members (i.e., feedback loop).

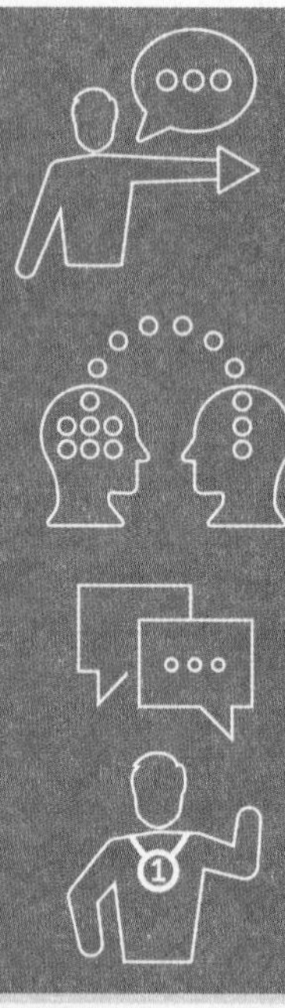

6 Determine an organizational baseline measure on safety culture performance using a validated tool.

7 Analyze safety culture survey results from across the organization to find opportunities for quality and safety improvement.

8 Use information from safety assessments and/or surveys to develop and implement unit-based quality and safety improvement initiatives designed to improve the culture of safety.

9 Embed safety culture team training into quality improvement projects and organizational processes to strengthen safety systems.

10 Proactively assess system strengths and vulnerabilities, and prioritize them for enhancement or improvement.

11 Repeat organizational assessment of safety culture every 18 to 24 months to review progress and sustain improvement.

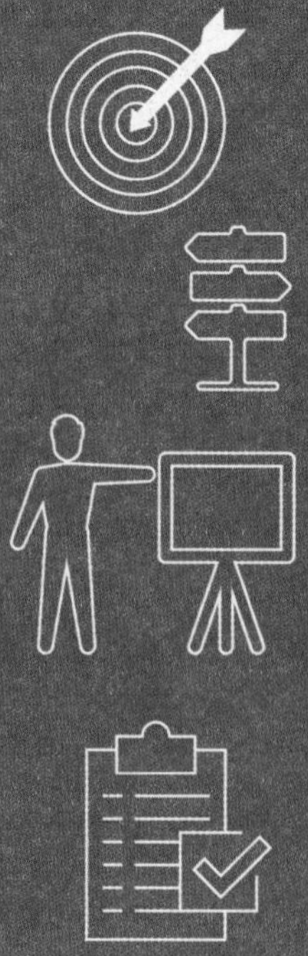

See Sentinel Event Alert Issue 57, "The essential role of leadership in developing a safety culture," for more information, resources and references.

**Figure 4.4** 11 Tenets of a Safety Culture

Reproduced from The Joint Commission. Sentinel event alert 57: the essential role of leadership in developing a safety culture. Published 2018. Accessed December 6, 2021. https://www.jointcommission.org/-/media/tjc/documents/resources/patient-safety-topics/sentinel-event/sentinel_events_11_tenets_of_a_safety_culture_infographic_2018pdf.pdf?db=web&hash=CDA432A1C6BB6F9C6DD3529291AA7364&hash=CDA432A1C6BB6F9C6DD3529291AA7364.

- An event or situation that did not produce patient harm due to either chance or capture before reaching the patient or if it did reach the patient, a timely and robust intervention occurred with no subsequent patient harm.[63]
- An error of commission or omission that could have harmed the patient but serious harm did not occur due to chance, prevention, or mitigation.[64]

By understanding errors and feeling protected by a nonpunitive culture, more healthcare professionals will report errors, near misses, and close calls. This, in turn, will improve patient safety through identification and resolution of systems issues, and lessons will be learned.[65] In a just culture, there is awareness throughout the organization that medical errors are inevitable—humans make errors, and systems can be flawed. Just culture is defined as "organizational accountability for the systems they've designed and employee accountability for the choices they make."[66] Just culture can make the system safer by recognizing that competent professionals make mistakes. It also acknowledges that even competent professionals develop unhealthy norms (shortcuts or routine rule violations); nevertheless, this culture has zero tolerance for reckless behavior. It distinguishes between three behaviors: human error (e.g., slips), at-risk behavior (e.g., taking shortcuts), and reckless behavior (e.g., ignoring required safety steps).[67,68] Three principles of a just culture are described here:

1. Just culture is not an effort to reduce personal accountability and discipline. It is a way to emphasize the importance of learning from mistakes, near misses, and close calls to reduce future preventable errors.
2. An individual is accountable to the system, and the greatest error is to not report a mistake. Doing so prevents the system and others from learning.
3. Policies discouraging any healthcare provider from self-reporting errors are at odds with the goals of a fair and just culture. Even those errors that do not result in harm or injury are reported and serve as learning opportunities.

Success occurs when everyone in a healthcare organization serves as a safety advocate regardless of their position or role. Providers and consumers will feel safe and supported when they report medical errors or near misses and voice concerns about patient safety.

How are the human/emotional aspects associated with patient safety balanced with how the system reflects and responds to those human emotions? In building a safety culture, Botwinick and colleagues[53] noted when leaders begin asking *What happened?* instead of *Who made the error?* the culture within their healthcare institutions begins to change. In this more nurturing culture, *What's wrong with you?* is replaced with *What happened to you?*

As leaders think about accountability and action, they can foster and reward improvement for the spread of best practices, knowledge, and adoption of value-based interventions and innovations in program design and redesign. Measures of success should align with the incentives for the improvement of patient safety. Rogers's work on disseminating innovations is also applicable to the widespread adoption of safety practices.[69] See **Table 4.3** for elements of leadership structures and systems.

Disclosing errors to patients and families is becoming more common practice in healthcare organizations across the country, especially in the aftermath of the Josie King incident in Maryland (see more in *Patient-Centered Care* later in this section). Disclosure is an important part of error discovery in contrast to tactics of the past, which sprang from fear and blame.[70] A just culture supports the disclosure of successes and failures. Healthcare quality professionals typically are involved in the investigation of errors and work with quality management, enterprise risk management (ERM), and legal professionals to determine a course of action. **Table 4.4** outlines NQF consensus standards regarding the disclosure of error or injury to consumers.

Conway and colleagues highlight the respectful management of adverse events. The aims of this group's work were to

- encourage and help every organization to develop a clinical crisis management plan before they need to use it;
- provide an approach to integrating this plan into the organizational culture of quality and safety with a focus on patient- and family-centered care and fair and just treatment for staff; and
- provide organizations with a concise, practical resource to inform their efforts when a serious adverse event occurs in the absence of a clinical crisis management plan and/or culture of quality and safety.[71(p4)]

Organizations can look for ways to encourage reporting using innovations such as the Good Catch programs in Pennsylvania. The PA Patient Safety Authority, through its reporting initiatives, has saved 2800 lives, realized $160 million in savings, and educated 60,000 employees; 3 million reports have been entered into its safety reporting system over 12 years.[72] As an example, one hospital reported that staff nearly failed to rescue a patient who had suffered a heart attack and had mistakenly been designated as

**Table 4.3** Elements of NQF Leadership Structures and Systems

| **Awareness Structures and Systems** | **Accountability Structures and Systems** |
|---|---|
| Awareness structures and systems provide leaders with continuous information about potential risks, hazards, and performance gaps that may contribute to patient safety issues. These structures and systems include (a) identification of risks and hazards; (b) culture management, feedback, and intervention; (c) direct patient input; and (d) governance board and senior management briefings and meetings. | Accountability structures and systems enable leaders to establish direct accountability to the governing body, senior management, mid-level management, physician leaders, and frontline staff. Included in these structures and systems are (a) the patient safety program, (b) the patient safety officer, (c) direct organization-wide leadership accountability, (d) an interdisciplinary patient safety committee, and (e) external reporting activities. |
| **Structures and Systems-Driving Ability** | **Action Structures and Systems** |
| Structures and systems-driving ability allows leaders to assess the capacity, resources, and competence necessary to implement change in the culture and in patient safety performance. This ability includes (a) patient safety budgets, (b) people systems, (c) quality systems, and (d) technical systems. | Action structures and systems enable leaders to take direct and appropriate action. These structures and systems include (a) quality and performance improvement programs; (b) regular actions of governance, including confirmation of values, basic teamwork training, and governance board competence in patient safety; (c) regular actions of senior administrative leadership, including commitment of time to patient safety; culture measurement, feedback, and interventions; basic teamwork training and team interventions; and identification and mitigation of risks and hazards; (d) regular actions of unit, service line, departmental and mid-level management leaders; and (e) regular actions with respect to independent medical leaders. |

Data from the National Quality Forum (NQF). *Safe Practices for Better Healthcare–2010 Update: A Consensus Report*. Washington, DC: NQF; 2010. https://www.qualityforum.org/publications/2010/04/safe_practices_for_better_healthcare_%E2%80%93_2010_update.aspx

do not resuscitate with a yellow wristband. A nurse had placed this wristband on the patient because yellow signified a restricted extremity (do not use this arm for drawing blood) at a facility where she previously worked. Another clinician identified the mistake and rescued the patient. As a result of this close call report, Pennsylvania adopted a standardized system for color-coded wristbands, and, subsequently, 41 states and the U.S. military have adopted standardized colors.[73(p4)] Good catch or near miss programs encourage clinicians to report situations in which patients are at risk and potentially lifesaving actions are warranted.

## Safety Program

Healthcare quality professionals work collaboratively with others to improve compliance with standards set forth by The Joint Commission's National Patient Safety Goals, Leapfrog safe practices, NQF-endorsed measures, and federal government–vetted measures (e.g., AHRQ, National Health Safety Network). Standards and resources for patient safety practices include recommendations to improve accuracy in patient identification, effectiveness of communication among caregivers, precautions when using high-alert medications, and surgery safeguards in various settings.[74] Proposed solutions to improving patient safety range from making electronic health information

readily available to providers and consumers to inviting patients to make decisions collaboratively with their care providers.[75,76]

When thinking about meeting or exceeding standards, part of the healthcare quality professional's work is to identify what interventions to use and their effects—some small things can lead to big and sustainable change. There are important resources to consider, such as systems for collecting reliable and valid data, selecting measures that provide the information for evaluation, and focusing on relevant high-volume problem-prone areas such as safe medication practices. As healthcare quality professionals aim to improve safety for the patient, organization, or system of care, they might consider the following for launching routine monitoring and evaluation of activities and specific projects:

- Establishing the plan to evaluate the actual impact on health outcomes, quality of care, and patient safety due to the effort (patient, healthcare personnel, clinical workflow, other relevant indicators)
- Feasibility, usability, and possibilities when identifying the target population and/or problem to be addressed
- Clearly defining the quantifiable impact of the effort (e.g., number of incidents, rates of occurrence) and who is affected (e.g., patients, clinicians, department, unit)

**Table 4.4** Consensus Standards Related to Disclosure of Error or Injury

**Safe Practice 7: Disclosure**

Following serious unanticipated outcomes, including those that are clearly caused by systems failures, the patient and, as appropriate, the family should receive timely, transparent, and clear communication concerning what is known about the event.

**Applicable Clinical Care Settings**

This practice is applicable to Centers for Medicare & Medicaid Services care settings, to include ambulatory settings, ambulatory surgical centers, emergency rooms, dialysis facilities, home care, home health services/agencies, hospice, inpatient service/hospitals, outpatient hospitals, and skilled nursing facilities.

■ The types of serious unanticipated outcomes addressed by this practice include, at a minimum, sentinel events, serious reportable events, and any other unanticipated outcomes involving harm that require the provision of substantial additional care (such as diagnostic tests, therapeutic interventions, or increased length of stay) or that cause the loss of limb or function lasting seven days or longer.

■ Organizations must have formal processes in place for disclosing unanticipated outcomes, reporting events to those responsible for patient safety, including external organizations where applicable, and identifying and mitigating risks and hazards.

■ The governance and administrative leadership should ensure that such information is systematically used for performance improvement by the organization. Policies and procedures should incorporate continuous quality improvement techniques and provide for annual reviews and updates. Adherence to the practice and participation with the support system is expected and may be considered as part of credentialing.

■ Communication with patients, their families, and caregivers should include or be characterized by the following:
  - The facts—an explicit statement about what happened that includes an explanation of the implications of the unanticipated outcome for the patient's future health, an explanation of why the event occurred, and information about measures taken for its preventability
  - Empathic communication of the facts, a skill that should be developed and practiced in healthcare organizations
  - An explicit and empathic expression of regret that the outcome was not as expected (e.g., "I am sorry this has happened.")
  - A commitment to investigate and as possible prevent future occurrences by collecting the facts about the event and providing them to the organization's patient safety leaders, including those in governance positions
  - Feedback of the results of the investigation, including whether or not it resulted from an error or systems failure, provided in sufficient detail to support informed decision making by the patient
  - Timeliness—an initial conversation with the patient and/or family within 24 hours, whenever possible; early and subsequent follow-up conversations, to maintain the relationship and to provide information as it becomes available
  - An apology from the patient's licensed independent practitioner (LIP) and/or an administrative leader if the investigation reveals the adverse outcome clearly was caused by unambiguous errors or systems failures
  - Emotional support for patients and their families provided by trained caregivers

■ A disclosure and improvement support system to provide the following to caregivers and staff:
  - Emotional support for caregivers and administrators involved in such events provided by trained caregivers in the immediate post event period that may extend for weeks afterward
  - Education and skill building regarding the concepts, tools, and resources that produce *optimal* results from this practice, centered on systems improvement rather than blame, and with a special emphasis on creating a just culture
  - 24-hour availability of advisory support to caregivers and staff to facilitate rapid responses to serious unanticipated outcomes, including the provision of just-in-time coaching and emotional support
  - Education of caregivers regarding the importance and technique of disclosure to care teams of error or adverse events as they happen

■ Healthcare organizations should implement a procedure to ensure and document that all LIPs are provided with a detailed description of the organization's program for responding to adverse events, including the full disclosure of error(s) that may have caused or contributed to patient harm. This is done with the expectation that the healthcare organizations and/or the LIPs will provide this information to their individual medical malpractice liability carriers if they are provided liability coverage from entities outside of the organization. All new employees should also receive this information.

■ A process should be in place to consider providing information to a patient safety organization that would provide a patient safety evaluation program to protect privileged and confidential information.

■ A process should be in place to consider early remediation and the waiving of billing for care services provided during the care episode and for subsequent treatment if the event was due to unambiguous systems failures or human error.

- Determining appropriate tools to use (e.g., RCA, failure mode and effects analysis [FMEA], other Lean tools)
- Identifying mechanisms to share results and efforts resulting in improved safety (e.g., board reports, enterprise-wide communications, patient materials)

As part of developing the patient safety plan, healthcare organizations can conduct a thorough analysis of where patients and healthcare personnel are at risk for errors. In doing so, systems and processes can be hardwired. The organization should actively engage employees in analyzing processes to ensure the organization achieves desired outcomes. It should look for the differences in mindsets and close the gap by removing silos. Cross-functional objectives will promote collaboration in developing the plan.

Patient safety plans are often integrated in quality or performance improvement program plans. These are five components of an effective patient safety system:

1. Monitoring of progress and maintenance of vigilance
2. Knowledge of the epidemiology of patient safety risks and hazards
3. Development of effective practices and tools
4. Building infrastructure for effective practices
5. Achieving broader adoption of effective practices[77(p4)]

An exemplar shown here is the University of California, Los Angeles (UCLA) Health System. The UCLA Health System's Performance Improvement & Patient Safety Plan goals include the following:

- Achieve a patient safety conscious environment throughout the facility.
- Improve the reporting of medical errors by establishing a policy focusing on corrective actions through staff education for those reporting their errors, rather than punitive or disciplinary actions.
- Implement [a] confidential electronic event reporting process that includes documentation of follow-up and reporting processes.
- Expand the implementation of evidence-based practices.
- Monitor hospital-wide indicators for established areas of focus.
- Reduce the number of medication errors.
- Monitor patient safety indicators related to an area's specific "Scope of Service."
- Conduct a proactive risk assessment utilizing the FMEA methodology.
- Monitor and improve areas identified through patient satisfaction surveys.
- Review the governance of medication management and conduct a[n] FMEA and assess the patient safety and alignment of processes with a culture of safety.[78(p6)]

When deploying the plan, various statistical process control and quality improvement tools can be used in patient safety initiatives. Statistical process control techniques and performance improvement tools are applicable to the deployment of patient safety practices throughout a healthcare enterprise. The healthcare quality professional serves an essential role in helping the organization determine if a safety issue in an organization is an infrequent event or endemic. Prioritizing functions should be utilized as part of the safety program.

## Risk Management

In the 1970s, risk management (RM) was the initial reaction to continually increasing litigation. However, as litigation continued to rise, RM assumed a more proactive role in reducing the incidents of unsafe care. Today, healthcare organizations focus on maintaining good and defined standards of practice within clinical and administrative systems to identify hazards posing risks to patients, assess the risks associated with healthcare hazards against the intended benefit, and eliminate (mitigate) or reduce risks to patients.[79] **Table 4.5** summarizes how approaches and processes of healthcare risk management have evolved.

Risk management is the process of making and carrying out decisions that will minimize the adverse effects of accidental losses. Whereas the traditional evolution demonstrates a strong focus on clinical healthcare risk management, the concept of enterprise risk management has become more popular in expanding the focus of risks that affect the entire organization or system, not just clinical operations. "*Enterprise risk management* (ERM) in health care promotes a comprehensive framework for making risk management decisions which maximize value protection and creation by managing risk and uncertainty and their connections to total value."[80(p5)] The major categories of risk in ERM include the following:

- Operational: risks resulting from inadequate or failed internal processes, or systems that affect business operations
- Clinical/patient safety: risks associated with the delivery of care to patients, residents, and other healthcare customers
- Strategic: risks associated with the focus and direction of the organization
- Financial: decisions that affect the financial sustainability of the organization, access to capital or external financial ratings through business relationships or the timing and recognition of revenue and expenses

**Table 4.5** Evolution of Risk Management

| Past | Present |
|---|---|
| Number one goal: protect financial resources and reputation. | Number one goal: improve patient safety and minimize risk of harm to patients through better understanding of systemic factors that limit caregivers' ability to provide safe care. |
| Paper occurrence form required for reporting. | Variety of methods to report: paper form, electronic form, telephone call, anonymous reporting, person-to-person reporting. |
| Investigate only the serious occurrences. | Encourage reporting of near misses, and investigate and discuss the potential root causes for any incident, regardless of severity. |
| Interview staff one-on-one when there is an adverse incident. | Hold root cause analysis meetings with the entire team of caregivers. Identify human and system factors that contributed to the event. |
| Information from investigation kept confidential. | Develop corrective action, share it with the patient safety committee and others in the organization who need to know. |
| Blame and train. | Perform a criticality analysis and determine the root cause of the near miss or the adverse occurrence. Identify human and system factors. |
| Talk to the patient or patient's family only if necessary and be vague about findings. | Advise the physician or other caregiver to speak directly with the patient and/or family. Talk with them about any unexpected outcomes and errors. Share steps taken to make the environment safe for the next patient. |
| Work with department involved to develop corrective action. | Work with the team and the organization's leadership to develop a patient safety improvement plan. |
| Assume that action is taken to correct the problem that occurred, notice only when it happens again that no action was taken. | Monitor the patient safety improvement plan to determine that changes are initiated and that the changes made a difference. |
| Keep patients in the dark about risk management and occurrence reporting. | Establish ongoing patient safety education; publish patient safety bulletins that address specific patient safety issues and the organization's approach to managing them; provide an opportunity for patients to identify methods of improving patient safety and to share them with administration; disclose errors. |

Reproduced from Kuhn AM, Youngberg BJ. The need for risk management to evolve to assure a culture of safety. *Qual Saf Health Care*. 2002;11:158-162. With permission from BMJ Publishing Group Ltd. http://dx.doi.org/10.1136/qhc.11.2.158

- Human capital: risks associated with the organization's workforce, including employee selection, retention, turnover, staffing, absenteeism, etc.
- Legal and regulatory: risks associated with failure to identify manage or monitor legal, regulatory, and statutory mandates on a local, state, and federal level
- Technology: risks associated with machines, hardware, equipment, devices, wearable technologies, and tools, but also includes techniques, systems, and methods of the organization
- Hazard: risks related to assets and their value related to natural exposure and business interruption (logistics/supply chain, facility management, plant age, parking, valuables, construction/ renovation, earthquakes, windstorms, tornadoes, floods, fires, and pandemics[80(p11)]

The American Society for Health Care Risk Management adopted five guiding principles for an ERM framework:

1. Governance & Culture: exercises board oversight; establishes operating structures; defines desired culture; demonstrates commitment to core values; attracts, develops, and retains capable individuals
2. Strategy & Objective Setting: analyzes business context, defines risk appetite, evaluates alternative strategies, and formulates business objectives

3. Performance: identifies risk, assesses severity of risk, prioritizes risk, implements risk responses, develops portfolio view
4. Review & Revision: assesses substantial change, reviews risk and performance, pursues improvement in ERM
5. Information, Communication, & Reporting: leverages information and technology, communicates risk information, reports on risk, culture, and performance[80(p5)]

Effective strategies for proactively reducing errors and ensuring patient safety require an integrated and coordinated approach to synthesizing knowledge and experience. Staff members are encouraged to learn about errors and permit internal reporting of information without blame. There are interdependencies and intersections between healthcare quality and RM. Healthcare quality professionals work in tandem with enterprise ERM to

- improve the effectiveness and efficiency of the organization's processes and operations through consistent identification of risks (threats) to the enterprise;
- identify, evaluate, and prioritize areas of risk affecting the operations of the organization;
- assess whether the identified risks are caused by internal (controllable) or external (uncontrollable) factors;
- develop and propose comprehensive strategies to minimize risks;
- establish action plans to address problems when identified; and
- maintain a periodic evaluation of feedback to monitor the progress of strategies and actions.

The goal of ERM in any organization is to protect from financial losses, which may arise because of the risks to which it is exposed. A healthcare risk manager must consider such things as regulatory compliance, safety management, credentialing, client–provider relations, publicity and media coverage, and, most importantly, patient care. In this way, ERM and patient safety are closely aligned.

Key to ERM program management is the risk manager. This position is an important asset to the organization and is typically charged with functions related to risk identification, risk assessment and evaluation, and application of techniques to reduce risks. Duties vary widely by organization, but the basic ERM functions are as follows:

- Risk identification, assessment, planning, mitigation, and evaluation
- Maintenance and monitoring of effective incident reporting and occurrence screen programs

- Clinical and administrative responsibilities, such as regulatory compliance, policy review, credentialing, contract review, internal and external reporting, and education
- Collaboration and communication with the environmental safety officer, patient safety officer, and quality officer (although not optimal, in some organizations these are the same position)
- Collaboration with the financial officer on insurance and other risk financing methods
- Collaboration and communication with legal representatives for claims management

The risk manager is often charged with developing and deploying the ERM plan to align patient safety efforts so RM activities are not siloed. It is helpful for risk managers to also have some experience and knowledge in these areas: clinical knowledge because they must review care and provide guidance to clinical providers of care; knowledge of healthcare law and thorough understanding of the legal system because review is necessary of defense counsel work and legal documents; knowledge about the insurance industry because risk managers help make decisions about various insurance coverages, such as hospital professional liability, general liability, and workers' compensation.

A healthcare organization typically has a formal, written plan explaining its ERM philosophy. Often the ERM plan is integrated with the quality and patient safety plan because the processes are interdependent. Important plan elements include purpose and board statement of support of ERM, scope of the program, authority, and confidentiality assertions, data collection and reporting mechanisms (both internal and external) and integration with quality management and program effectiveness reviews. Within the plan, prevention of risk is often managed by

- program oversight,
- contract review,
- internal and external reporting processes,
- education of staff and providers,
- policy review to protect the organization, and
- informed consent.

Possible causes of losses for organizations related to patient safety include criminal acts by employees, patient harm related to inability of contractors to perform services, clinical treatment by qualified or unqualified staff, falls with injury, and medication errors with harm. An important aspect of ERM is management of claims. **Table 4.6** lists the types of professional liability sources often considered in determining the validity of a claim.

**Table 4.6** Professional Liability Sources

| | |
|---|---|
| Corporate liability | Based on recognition that the organization owes a duty to the patients it serves. |
| Vicarious liability | Indirect responsibility for the acts of another person; *respondeat superior,* which holds the employer responsible for the wrongful acts of its employees. |
| Ostensible agency | Generally, an organization is not liable for injuries sustained by patients because of the actions of an independent contractor. However, the extension of *respondeat superior* to the doctrine of the ostensible agency may extend liability exposure to the organization for acts of nonemployed, independent contractor physicians where no employer–employee relationship exists. |
| *Res ipsa loquitur* | Allows a patient to prove his or her case without needing to establish the standard of care in which there is clear and obvious negligence. |

Organizations can establish mechanisms for reviewing potential incidents of risk and safety concern. All members of the workforce are responsible for identifying, reporting, and documenting RM and potential quality-of-care problems that influence patient safety. Variance or incident reporting is an important component of any patient safety program. Healthcare quality professionals assist organizations in developing and maintaining an incident reporting system. AHRQ describes four key attributes of voluntary patient safety event reporting systems:

1. Institution must have a supportive environment for event reporting to protect the privacy of staff who report occurrences.
2. Reports are received from a broad range of personnel.
3. Summaries of reported events must be disseminated in a timely fashion.
4. A structured mechanism must be in place for reviewing reports and developing action plans.[81(¶2)]

Only a small portion of healthcare errors (10%–20%) is reported. Of the errors reported, 90%–95% result in no harm to the patient.[82] A report of the DHHS Office Inspector General[83] found "most incidents of patient harm were not being reported. Hospital staff did not report 86 percent of events to incident reporting systems, partly because of staff misperceptions about what constitutes patient harm. Of the events experienced by Medicare beneficiaries discharged in October 2008, hospital incident reporting systems captured only an estimated 14 percent."[83(pii)]

Nurse and physician beliefs that reporting near misses is not important, fear of disciplinary actions, and lack of feedback regarding the errors are the major barriers in reporting adverse incidents.[84] Frequent and routine reporting is more likely in organizations with nonpunitive, just cultures. The *AHRQ SOPS Hospital Survey 2.0* showed only 57% of staff feel their mistakes and event reports are not held against them, and 54% believed that when an event is reported on the unit, it felt like the person, not the problem, was being written up.[85(p11)] The top areas for potential improvement in the culture of safety follow in **Table 4.7**.

Risk identification is the first step to determine what risks can affect the achievement of organizational goals. Both formal and informal methods are used, and the risks may be internal or external to the organization. Approaches used include retrospective, concurrent, pre-interventional, and prospective. Approaches in risk identification are aimed to identify the root causes of risks for things that do go wrong (e.g., RCA) and possible modes by which these functions might fail to perform (e.g., FMEA). It may be "easier to identify all the factors that are critical to success, and then work backward to identify the things that can go wrong with each one."[86(p24)]

Once risks are identified, the next step is to conduct a risk assessment to quantify the magnitude or severity of the risks, the exposure through possible results, the frequency of occurrence, the probability of the occurrence, and the time to act. Through this analysis, the organization can determine which RM techniques can be applied to the exposures to mitigate loss, select the best RM technique for the situation, prioritize actions, identify resources needed, identify risk control and risk financing methods, implement the techniques, monitor the effectiveness of the technique, and trend and analyze results. **Table 4.8** shows domains and measures to be considered for possible clinical risk areas based on NQF's portfolio of performance measures for patient safety.

**Table 4.7** SOPS Hospital Survey 2.0: Potential for Improvement

| Areas with Potential for Most Hospitals | 2019 (%) | 2021 (%) |
|---|---|---|
| **Staffing and Work Pace**<br>The extent to which staff indicated there are enough staff to handle the workload, staff work appropriate hours, do not feel rushed, and there is appropriate reliance on temporary, float, or as-needed staff. | 56 | 58 |
| **Handoffs and Transitions**<br>The extent to which important patient care information is transferred across hospital units and during shift changes. | 58 | 64 |

Data from Agency for Healthcare Research and Quality. Pilot test results from the 2019 AHRQ Surveys on Patient Safety Culture (SOPS) Hospital Survey 2.0. Published 2019. Accessed December 8, 2021. https://www.ahrq.gov/sites/default/files/wysiwyg/sops/surveys/hospital/hsops2-pilot-results-parti.pdf; and Agency for Healthcare Research and Quality. SOPS hospital survey 2.0: 2021 user database report. Accessed December 6, 2021. https://www.ahrq.gov/sites/default/files/wysiwyg/sops/surveys/hospital/2021-HSOPS2-Database-Report-Part-I-508.pdf

**Table 4.8** NQF Patient Safety Portfolio and Related Measures

| Topic Area | Measure |
|---|---|
| Falls | ■ Fall Risk Management (FRM) (0035)<br>■ Falls: Screening, Risk-Assessment, and Plan of Care to Prevent Future Falls (0101)<br>■ Patient Fall Rate (0141)<br>■ Falls with Injury (0202)<br>■ Patient Fall (0266)<br>■ Multifactor Fall Risk Assessment Conducted for All Patients Who Can Ambulate (0537)<br>■ Percent of Residents Experiencing One or More Falls with Major Injury (Long Stay) (0674) |
| General safety measures | ■ Patient Burn (0263)<br>■ Wrong Site, Wrong Side, Wrong Patient, Wrong Procedure, Wrong Implant (0267)<br>■ Surgery Patients with Appropriate Hair Removal (0301)<br>■ Accidental Puncture or Laceration Rate (PDI 1) (0344)<br>■ Accidental Puncture or Laceration Rate (PSI 15) (0345)<br>■ Iatrogenic Pneumothorax Rate (PSI 6) (0346)<br>■ Iatrogenic Pneumothorax Rate (PDI 5) (0348)<br>■ Transfusion Reaction Count (PSI 16) (0349)<br>■ Transfusion Reaction Count (PDI 13) (0350)<br>■ Retained Surgical Item or Un-retrieved Device Fragment Count Technical (PDI 03) (0362)<br>■ Retained Surgical Item or Un-retrieved Device Fragment Count (PSI 05) (0363)<br>■ Ambulatory Surgery Patients with Appropriate Method of Hair Removal (0515)<br>■ Patient Safety and Adverse Events (PSI 90) (0531)<br>■ Percent of Residents Who Were Physically Restrained (Long Stay) (0687)<br>■ Percent of Residents Who Lose Too Much Weight (Long-Stay) (0689)<br>■ Proportion of Patients with a Chronic Condition that have a Potentially Avoidable Complication During a Calendar Year (0709)<br>■ Pulmonary Embolism Anticoagulation ≥ 3 Months (0593) |

*(continues)*

**Table 4.8** NQF Patient Safety Portfolio and Related Measures *(continued)*

| Topic Area | Measure |
|---|---|
| Healthcare-associated infections | ▪ National Healthcare Safety Network (NHSN) Catheter-Associated Urinary Tract Infection Outcome Measure (0138)<br>▪ National Healthcare Safety Network (NHSN) Central-Line–Associated Bloodstream Infection Outcome Measure (0139)<br>▪ Percent of Residents with a Urinary Tract Infection (Long-Stay) (0684)<br>▪ Risk Adjusted Urinary Tract Infection Outcome Measure After Surgery (0751)<br>▪ American College of Surgeons-Centers for Disease Control and Prevention (ACS-CDC) Harmonized Procedure Specific Surgical Site Infection (SSI) Outcome Measure (0753)<br>▪ National Healthcare Safety Network (NHSN) Facility-Wide Inpatient Hospital-Onset Methicillin-Resistant *Staphylococcus aureus* (MRSA) Bacteremia Outcome Measure (1716)<br>▪ National Healthcare Safety Network (NHSN) Facility-Wide Inpatient Hospital-Onset *Clostridium Difficile* Infection (CDI) Outcome Measure (1717) |
| Medication safety | ▪ Use of High-Risk Medications in the Elderly (DAE) (0022)<br>▪ Medication Reconciliation (0097)<br>▪ Documentation of Current Medications in the Medical Record (0419)<br>▪ Proportion of Days Covered (PDC): 3 Rates by Therapeutic Category (0541)<br>▪ Care for Older Adults (COA)-Medication Review (0553)<br>▪ INR Monitoring for Individuals on Warfarin (0555)<br>▪ Antipsychotic Use in Children Under 5 Years Old (2337)<br>▪ Annual Monitoring for Patients on Persistent Medications (2371) |
| Mortality | ▪ Death Rate in Low-Mortality Diagnosis Related Groups (PSI 2) (0347)<br>▪ Failure to Rescue In-Hospital Mortality (risk adjusted) (0352)<br>▪ Failure to Rescue 30-Day Mortality (risk adjusted) (0353)<br>▪ Mortality for Selected Conditions (0530) |
| Pressure ulcers | ▪ Pressure Ulcer Rate (PDI 2) (0337)<br>▪ Pressure Ulcer Prevention and Care (0538)<br>▪ Percent of Residents or Patients with Pressure Ulcers That Are New or Worsened (Short-Stay) (0678)<br>▪ Percent of High Risk Residents with Pressure Ulcers (Long Stay) (0679) |
| Venous thromboembolism (VTE) | ▪ Perioperative Care: Venous Thromboembolism (VTE) Prophylaxis (0239)<br>▪ Venous Thromboembolism Prophylaxis (0371)<br>▪ Intensive Care Unit Venous Thromboembolism Prophylaxis (0372)<br>▪ Venous Thromboembolism Patients with Anticoagulation Overlap Therapy (0373)<br>▪ Perioperative Pulmonary Embolism or Deep Vein Thrombosis Rate (PSI 12) (0450)<br>▪ Deep Vein Thrombosis Anticoagulation ≥ 3 Months (0581) |
| Workforce safety | ▪ Skill Mix (Registered Nurse [RN], Licensed Vocational/Practical Nurse [LVN/LPN], Unlicensed Assistive Personnel [UAP], and Contract) (0204)<br>▪ Nursing Hours per Patient Day (0205)<br>▪ Practice Environment Scale-Nursing Work Index (PES-NWI) (composite and five subscales) (0206) |

Reproduced from National Quality Forum. Patient safety 2015: Appendix B: NQF patient safety portfolio and related measures. 2016:110-111. Accessed April 9, 2022. https://www.qualityforum.org/Publications/2016/02/Patient_Safety_2015_Final_Report.aspx

Risk control is usually managed through incident (or variance) reporting, occurrence screening, and claims management. Data that may be useful when trended or analyzed include

- liability and workers' compensation;
- tort claims (duty, breach of duty, causation, and injury);
- malpractice coverage;
- incident reports and occurrence screens;
- review of records using criteria to note variations;
- details of the occurrence;
- records that need more in-depth review;
- confirmation of the variation or absence of an untoward event;
- summary of data with trends; and
- patient complaints.

# Tools and Techniques

Healthcare quality professionals who lead patient safety programs and initiatives know the importance of using the most current evidence-based information to inform design and implementation efforts. Effective tools and strategies for implementation support the advances and improvement understanding of risk factors associated with the different aspects of healthcare that affect the safe delivery of healthcare—health IT, adverse events reporting, risk identification, infection prevention and control, medication safety, physical plant, and environment of care, to name a few. Using evidence-based tools can promote patient-centered care and accelerate positive changes in the patient safety culture. For example, plan-do-study-act may help implement sustainable improvement by using small tests of change. See the *Performance and Process Improvement* and *Health Data Analytics* sections for more information about tools for evaluating and improving quality and safety.

## Proactive Risk Assessment

Risk assessment helps to identify potential problems and barriers, develop protocols for investigating failures, and arrive at potential solutions in the healthcare environment. There are different kinds of risk assessments, such as reactive (the response is reducing damage and speeding recovery) and predictive (identifying the probability of risk based on situational variables).

Proactive risk management involves carefully analyzing a situation or assessing processes to determine the potential risks, identifying drivers of risks to understand the root cause, assessing probability and impact to prioritize risks, and accordingly preparing a contingency plan. "Proactive risk management improves an organization's ability to avoid or manage both existing and emerging risks and helps adapt quickly to unwanted events or crisis. It helps build an understanding required to measure and manage emerging risks which give organizations a better view of tomorrow's risk and how it impacts their business."[87(p2)]

A workflow example is shown in **Figure 4.5**.

There are different tools for proactive risk assessment, and their processes may overlap.

- *Retrospective.* Root cause analysis
- *Prospective.* Failure mode and effects analysis, healthcare failure mode and effect analysis, and probabilistic risk assessment

**Table 4.9** shows examples of a proactive risk assessment conducted by a multihospital group in south-central Washington to examine high-risk processes found in healthcare.

Tools and techniques are further described later in the section. See the *Performance and Process Improvement* section for more information.

## Failure Mode and Effects Analysis

A failure mode and effects analysis (FMEA) can be used to develop safety program activities and provide continuous readiness for external surveys. It is the *before* analysis—a way for staff to proactively pursue quality and safety versus being reactive; to imagine what could go wrong and correct any risk factors before errors occur. FMEA includes review of the following:

- Steps in the process
- Failure modes (What could go wrong?)
- Failure causes (Why would the failure happen?)
- Failure effects (What would be the consequences of each failure?)[26(¶1)]

More information about FMEAs can be found in the *Performance and Process Improvement* section.

## Root Cause Analysis

Organizations developing and maintaining robust healthcare safety programs are committed to the process of ongoing risk identification and prevention. Staff in these organizations are encouraged to identify potential errors and report any near misses or close calls or good catches that occur. Even when an event is not considered reviewable, HROs conduct RCAs on identified risks to prevent similar events in the future.

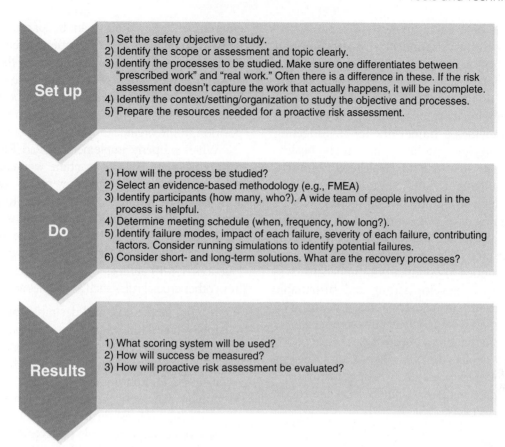

**Set up**
1) Set the safety objective to study.
2) Identify the scope or assessment and topic clearly.
3) Identify the processes to be studied. Make sure one differentiates between "prescribed work" and "real work." Often there is a difference in these. If the risk assessment doesn't capture the work that actually happens, it will be incomplete.
4) Identify the context/setting/organization to study the objective and processes.
5) Prepare the resources needed for a proactive risk assessment.

**Do**
1) How will the process be studied?
2) Select an evidence-based methodology (e.g., FMEA)
3) Identify participants (how many, who?). A wide team of people involved in the process is helpful.
4) Determine meeting schedule (when, frequency, how long?).
5) Identify failure modes, impact of each failure, severity of each failure, contributing factors. Consider running simulations to identify potential failures.
6) Consider short- and long-term solutions. What are the recovery processes?

**Results**
1) What scoring system will be used?
2) How will success be measured?
3) How will proactive risk assessment be evaluated?

**Figure 4.5** Example Workflow for Proactive Risk Assessment

Data from Carayon P, Faye H, Schoofs Hundt A, Tzion Karsh B, Wetterneck TB. Patient safety and proactive risk assessment (Section 12). In: Yih Y, ed. *Handbook of Healthcare Delivery Systems.* Indianapolis, IN: CRC Press; 2011.

**Table 4.9** **Proactive Risk Assessment for Adverse Events**

| Opportunity | Proactive Risk Assessment |
|---|---|
| Event tree analysis of mental health | Assessment performed to understand the risk presented by ED patients with underlying mental health or substance use issues. The study led hospital management to provide training in crisis prevention for staff who might be confronted with similar scenarios. |
| Hazard identification of patient-owned equipment | Following a post surgery hospital incident involving patient-owned equipment, an assessment was completed using a hazard identification checklist. The results led one hospital to bar equipment determined to represent unacceptable potential patient harm. |
| FMEA of interhospital patient transfers | Hospital patients often must be transferred to another community hospital for services (such as diagnostic imaging) and then return. This entails many handoffs and associated patient safety issues. An FMEA was conducted. Process mapping helped the hospitals design a form that includes patient safety–related information and requires staff to check the patient's status. |

Data from Coles G, Fuller B, Nordquist K, Weissenberger S, Anderson L, DuBois B. Three kinds of proactive risk analyses for health care. *Jt Comm J Qual Patient Saf.* 2010;36(8):PAP1-AP3. doi:10.1016/S1553-7250(10)36055-7

RCA is the *after*-event analysis—used to determine the cause of a variation in a process once an event or error occurs. Human, environmental, equipment, policy, and leadership system factors are explored in the analysis. The Oregon Patient Safety Commission developed an exceptional RCA toolkit.[88] It provides a framework for investigating adverse incidents and can be applied in any healthcare setting. The Institute for Healthcare Improvement/National Patient Safety Foundation (NPSF) developed a definitive guide on conducting RCAs.[89] These guidelines have been endorsed by The Joint Commission and other public and private patient safety organizations. The guide provides teams with effective techniques to conduct comprehensive systematic reviews to develop strong and sustainable actions to prevent future occurrence. Asking why five times is another way to determine a root cause.[90] An example is depicted in **Figure 4.6.**

**Figure 4.7** depicts the NPSF Root Cause Analysis and Action (RCA²) Process. RCA is described further in the *Performance and Process Improvement* and *Health Data Analytics* sections.

## Red Rules

Another safety practice—Red Rules—is used by highly reliable industries such as aviation and manufacturing, sparking interest for use in healthcare. "Used within a commitment-based management style as a communication tool to support staff in following safety rules rather than as a disciplinary tool in a control-based environment, Red Rules can be part of a comprehensive strategy to improve patient safety."[91(p137)] Red Rules are those that must be followed to the letter. The most important aspect of a Red Rule is to empower all workers to speak up when a rule is not being followed and to *stop the line* or *safety stop*, regardless of their position in the organization.[92]

When properly implemented, Red Rules foster a culture of safety because frontline workers will know they can stop the line when they notice potential hazards. The most important aspect of a Red Rule is its ability to "empower any worker to speak up when the rule is not being followed and to stop the line, regardless of rank or seniority."[92(¶p2)] The Institute for Safe Medication Practices (ISMP) outlines what differentiates a Red Rule from other crucial rules such as policies and procedures:

- It must be possible and desirable for everyone to follow a Red Rule every time in a process under all circumstances (Red Rules do not contain verbiage such as "except when . . ." or "each breach will be assessed for appropriateness").
- Anyone who notices the breach of the Rule has the authority and responsibility to stop further progress of patient care while protecting the patient or healthcare worker from harm.
- Managers and other leaders (including the board of trustees) always support the work stoppage, immediate rectification of the problem, and addressing the underlying reason for breaking the rule.
- People breaching the Red Rule are given an opportunity to support their behavioral choices and are

---

A patient received the wrong medication.

1) **Why** did the patient receive the wrong medication?

   *The nurse did not complete patient identification.*

2) **Why** did the nurse not complete patient identification?

   *The patient did not have a wristband.*

3) **Why** did the patient not have a wristband?

   *The wristband had been removed for a procedure and not replaced.*

4) **Why** was the wristband not replaced?

   *The printer for the wristbands was not working.*

5) **Why** was the printer not working?

   *The staff needed to support IT had been reduced and was overworked.*

**Figure 4.6** The 5 Whys

Institute for Healthcare Improvement. Patient safety essentials toolkit: 5 whys: finding the root cause of a problem: 3. Published 2019. Accessed April 9, 2022. http://www.ihi.org/resources/Pages/Tools/5-Whys-Finding-the-Root-Cause.aspx

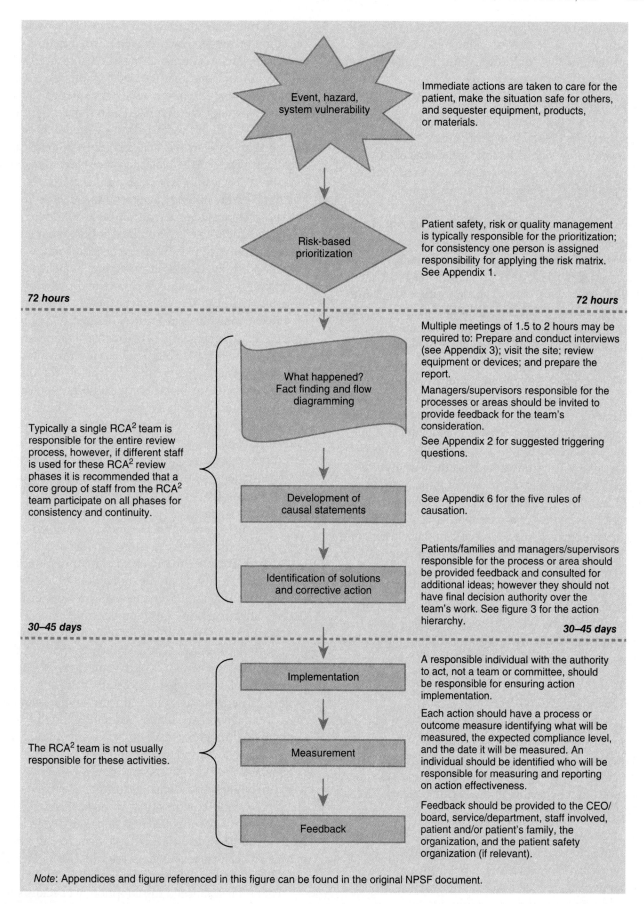

**Event, hazard, system vulnerability**

Immediate actions are taken to care for the patient, make the situation safe for others, and sequester equipment, products, or materials.

**Risk-based prioritization**

Patient safety, risk or quality management is typically responsible for the prioritization; for consistency one person is assigned responsibility for applying the risk matrix. See Appendix 1.

*72 hours*                                                                          *72 hours*

**What happened? Fact finding and flow diagramming**

Multiple meetings of 1.5 to 2 hours may be required to: Prepare and conduct interviews (see Appendix 3); visit the site; review equipment or devices; and prepare the report.

Managers/supervisors responsible for the processes or areas should be invited to provide feedback for the team's consideration.

See Appendix 2 for suggested triggering questions.

Typically a single RCA$^2$ team is responsible for the entire review process, however, if different staff is used for these RCA$^2$ review phases it is recommended that a core group of staff from the RCA$^2$ team participate on all phases for consistency and continuity.

**Development of causal statements**

See Appendix 6 for the five rules of causation.

**Identification of solutions and corrective action**

Patients/families and managers/supervisors responsible for the process or area should be provided feedback and consulted for additional ideas; however they should not have final decision authority over the team's work. See figure 3 for the action hierarchy.

*30–45 days*                                                                          *30–45 days*

**Implementation**

A responsible individual with the authority to act, not a team or committee, should be responsible for ensuring action implementation.

The RCA$^2$ team is not usually responsible for these activities.

**Measurement**

Each action should have a process or outcome measure identifying what will be measured, the expected compliance level, and the date it will be measured. An individual should be identified who will be responsible for measuring and reporting on action effectiveness.

**Feedback**

Feedback should be provided to the CEO/board, service/department, staff involved, patient and/or patient's family, the organization, and the patient safety organization (if relevant).

*Note*: Appendices and figure referenced in this figure can be found in the original NPSF document.

**Figure 4.7** Root Cause Analysis and Action (RCA$^2$) Process

Reproduced from National Patient Safety Foundation. *RCA$^2$: Improving Root Cause Analyses and Actions to Prevent Harm, Version* 2; 2016. Available at ihi.org then judged fairly based on the reasons for breaking the rule, regardless of rank and experience.

- There are few Red Rules, and they must be well understood and memorable.[92(¶7)]

Healthcare scenarios for which Red Rules can be beneficial include patient identification (using two identifiers before administering tests of any kind), sponge-count reconciliation, time-outs before an invasive procedure, timely alarm response, and correct labeling of specimens.

Newer to healthcare quality and safety, there is a mixed reception of Red Rules. Red Rules are part of a just culture although the way they are deployed could impact how they are received by affected personnel. There are circumstances where they are experienced as blaming and punitive, which is not aligned with a just culture. The way that Red Rules are deployed may not support trust and transparency. Jones and O'Connor examined four measures of patient safety culture among two groups of hospitals that completed the AHRQ Hospital Survey on Patient Safety Culture and compared hospitals that did or did not implement Red Rules as a patient safety strategy.[91] The four measures were (1) staff perceptions of safety; (2) frequency of events reported; (3) number of events reported; and (4) staff perceptions of no punitive response. The study found that there were no differences in the four measures between those hospitals that used Red Rules and those that did not. The authors did suggest that Red Rules can be effective as part of a comprehensive strategy to improve patient safety when used within a commitment-based management style.

Red Rules can be used as a communication tool to support staff in following safety rules rather than a disciplinary action. If misused or poorly supported, they will not be effective and may even introduce patient risks if systems and processes are not in place to facilitate adherence to the Red Rule.[92]

## Safety Checklists

A checklist is an algorithmic, evidence-based listing of actions to be performed with the goal of no step being forgotten. Grounded in human factors engineering, checklists can shape the organizational and systematic thinking and behaviors in healthcare delivery. Checklists are found to

- improve communication,
- strengthen adherence with guidelines,
- improve human factors,
- reduce the incidence of adverse events, and
- decrease mortality and morbidity.[93]

Patient safety checklists "allow complex pathways of care to function with high reliability by giving users the opportunity to pause and take stock of their actions before proceeding to the next step."[94(¶1)] Checklists can be developed for internal processes (surgical checklist)[95] or can be consumer focused.[96,97] Surgical checklists are the most commonly used, but other checklists are developed for safe childbirth, trauma care, and Pandemic H1N1 and other patient safety events, such as blood clots and central-line–associated bloodstream infections. The CDC *Antibiotic Stewardship Program Assessment Tool*[98] and the *Clinician Checklist for Outpatient Antibiotic Stewardship*[99] are recommended for facilities and programs to systematically assess the core key elements, actions to ensure optimal antibiotic prescribing, and limiting the overuse and misuse of antibiotics.

Checklists are helpful in preparing, implementing, monitoring, and evaluating workforce and environmental safety. Healthcare services can be directly or indirectly provided to individuals in a variety of settings (e.g., hospitals, clinics, emergency departments, home health, and skilled nursing facilities). There are many health and safety hazards that workers face across the different settings including blood-borne pathogens, potential drug exposures, respiratory hazards, ergonomic hazards, and workplace violence. There are accreditation standards; regulations; and state, federal, and local laws governing workplace safety. Checklists can support an organization's workforce and environmental safety efforts. **Figure 4.8** offers an example for blood-borne pathogens in residential care (page 1 of the checklist).

The benefit of using checklists was cemented with the publication of the Keystone Initiative findings by Pronovost in the *New England Journal of Medicine*. This project focused on the reduction of catheter-related bloodstream infections using a checklist to ensure adherence to infection-control practices— handwashing, using full-barrier precautions during the insertion of central venous catheters, cleaning the skin with chlorhexidine, avoiding the femoral site if possible, and removing unnecessary catheters. This project garnered success by reducing and sustaining rates of catheter-related bloodstream infection that was maintained throughout the 18-month study period.[100]

Gawande advanced thinking about checklists.[101,102] Regimentation of checklists can reduce risk and save lives in complex situations. Healthcare is highly specialized. Couple complexity with specialization, the routine might be overlooked and steps skipped in processes. Consistent use and improvement of checklists may offer healthcare providers a tool to focus less of their efforts on the routine and more on the difficult.

There is resistance to the adoption of checklists in healthcare. Based on work by Treadwell, Lucas, and Tsou,[103(p302)] barriers to implementation can fall into these categories:

| 1. Control of exposure to bloodborne pathogens | | | 29 CFR 1910.1030 |
| --- | --- | --- | --- |
| **Completed** ☐ | **In Progress** ☐ | **Not Started** ☐ | The facility has workplace policies in place to protect employees from occupational exposure to blood and other potentially infectious materials (OPIM). These policies must include:<br>☐ Practicing universal precautions;<br>☐ Using safety engineered needles and sharps;<br>☐ Consideration and documentation of safety engineered sharps on an annual basis, including documented input from non-managerial staff with occupational exposure;<br>☐ Placing contaminated reusable sharps into an appropriate container until they are processed;<br>☐ Using submersible tray, tongs, or other method to avoid reaching by hand into a container of contaminated reusable sharps for cleaning;<br>☐ Washing exposed skin following contact, and washing hands after glove removal;<br>☐ Having eyewash stations located within 10 seconds of where exposure is likely to occur;<br>☐ Having sharps containers as close as possible to the immediate area where sharps are used, and routinely inspecting to ensure that they do not become overfilled;<br>☐ Using personal protective equipment (PPE) whenever exposure is possible. PPE should be provided at no cost to the employees, and should be suitably sized and impervious;<br>☐ Maintaining a sufficient supply of protective gloves, facemasks, face shields, mouthpieces, and gowns necessary for day-to-day operations;<br>☐ Creating and following a housekeeping schedule for cleaning and disinfecting equipment and work surfaces that may become contaminated with blood or OPIM. The schedule should include frequency of activities and the registered disinfectants being used;<br>• If a bleach solution is used as a surface disinfectant, the solution is a 1:10 bleach to water ratio and is made up daily.<br>☐ Eating, drinking, smoking, applying cosmetics or lip balm, and handling contact lenses are prohibited in work areas where there is a reasonable likelihood of occupational exposure;<br>☐ Storing food and drinks only in areas where blood or OPIM are not present;<br>☐ Offering Hepatitis B vaccinations to all employees with exposure to blood or OPIM;<br>☐ Maintaining vaccination and treatment records or declination forms in the employees' medical file in a secure and locked location. |

**Figure 4.8** Controlling Hazards in Residential Care Facilities Checklist: Control of Exposure to Blood-borne Pathogens (29 CFR 1910.1030)

Reproduced from Occupational Safety & Health Consultation Program, Georgia Technical and Research Institute. *Controlling Hazards in Healthcare Facilities: 1. Control of Exposure to Bloodborne Pathogens*. 4th ed., 2. Published 2019. Accessed December 6, 2021. https://oshainfo.gatech.edu/wp-content/uploads/2019/03/Medical%20Facilities%20Checklist.pdf

1. Confusion regarding how to properly use the checklist,
2. pragmatic challenges to efficient workflow,
3. access to resources, and
4. individual beliefs and attitudes.

Healthcare quality professionals can bring knowledge about the benefits of checklists as part of the organization's overall quality management system. Examples of sources include ISO9001:2015 and the Baldrige Excellence Framework. See the *Performance and Process Improvement* section for more discussion on tools for improvement.

**Box 4.3** outlines the uses of risk management and patient safety tools.

---

### Box 4.3  Key Points: Tools and Techniques

- Promote effective risk management strategies through use of safety practices, tools, and technology such as incident reporting, sentinel/adverse event review, RCA, FMEA, and checklists.
- Regimentation of checklists reduces risk and saves lives in complex situations.
- Evaluation and improvement of patient safety require using tools and health information technology for identifying risks and harm reduction.

---

## Infection Prevention and Control

The goal of an infection prevention and control (IPC) program is to identify and reduce the risks of acquiring and transmitting endemic and epidemic infections among patients, employees, physicians, other IPC programs, contractors, volunteers, students, and visitors. This includes both direct patient care and support staff. The three major aspects of the IPC program are surveillance, prevention, and control. The usual responsibilities of the IPC program include

- definitions of healthcare-associated infections (HAIs),
- definitions of data elements,
- the rationale for the surveillance method selected,
- a description of the patient population studied,
- data collection methods,
- quality control procedures for data validation,
- responsibility,
- systems for reporting and follow-up,
- reporting to public health authorities, and
- documentation of employee infections of epidemiologic significance.

The prevention and control methods used in IPC include the following:

- Policies and procedures to protect and prevent infections

- Defined barrier precautions
- Orientation and ongoing education of staff
- Reporting to public health official
- Methods for screening and documentation of epidemiologically significant infections
- Systems for required waste identification
- Use of personal protective equipment and supplies, including the following:
  - Patient care supplies and equipment (e.g., sterile and nonsterile supplies, hand hygiene facilities)
  - Protective apparel
  - Engineering controls
- Precautions used to reduce the risk of infection, including the following:
  - Surveillance
  - Assessment and analysis of infection rates
- Decontamination, high-level disinfection, and sterilization, including the following:
  - Reusable medical equipment
  - Policies and procedures
  - Processes identified:
    - Principles of asepsis
    - Disinfection, sterilization
    - Sanitation of rooms, equipment
    - Selection, use, and cleaning of personal protective equipment
    - Traffic control

The IPC program is based on a risk assessment of the organization. This assessment includes factors such as

- the geographic location of the organization;
- populations within the region or organization and level of risk (e.g., neonates, infants and children, and patients in various ICUs, congregate living facilities; other persons in the home with an infectious or immunocompromised person);
- the volume of patients served and the volume of conditions (e.g., the number of patients with positive human immunodeficiency virus, tuberculosis, and colonized with methicillin-resistant *Staphylococcus aureus*, or other high-consequence infection such as COVID-19);
- the clinical focus of programs (e.g., types of surgeries and invasive procedures, immunocompromised patients such as patients on chemotherapy, and transplant patients);
- the number of employees (often encompasses employee health services); and
- the scope of services provided (e.g., acute, ambulatory, long-term, and home care).

After the risk assessment is completed, priorities are identified and strategies to prevent or mitigate problems are determined. In many healthcare settings, the prevention of HAIs in high-risk units (ICUs, neonatal and pediatric ICUs, transplant units, dialysis units, and surgical units) is a key responsibility. These HAIs must be monitored and analyzed to determine trends and ways to reduce their occurrence. The types of surveillance for IPC programs include total facility, priority directed, targeted, problem oriented, and outbreak response.

The most important factor in monitoring prevention of HAIs is proper hand hygiene. The monitoring of hand hygiene using either the Centers for Disease Control and Prevention or the World Health Organization criteria is a requirement of The Joint Commission and one of its National Patient Safety Goals. Specific monitoring is performed for surgical-site infections and for device-related infections including ventilator-associated pneumonia, central-line–associated bloodstream infections, and catheter-associated urinary tract infections.

Another key role is to identify communicable diseases, control outbreaks when identified in patients, and report specific results to the public health department. One preventive measure for controlling certain outbreaks is immunization programs conducted in collaboration with occupational health staff. These might include vaccination for hepatitis B, influenza, pneumonia, COVID-19, and other viral diseases. The infection preventionist is also responsible for monitoring epidemiologically important and multidrug-resistant organisms such as methicillin-resistant *Staphylococcus aureus, Clostridium difficile,* and vancomycin-resistant *Enterococcus.* As more multidrug-resistant organisms develop, professionals must remain current and be vigilant in monitoring these cases and risk to others.

Tools are being developed for collecting data to monitor these high-risk areas for causing adverse events or harm to patients as well as the availability of a national database for some comparisons. As conditions or areas of concern for quality and patient safety are identified, healthcare quality professionals need to stay informed of new knowledge, trends, and tools to address risk to patients. The models described for specific conditions can be utilized to address key questions about interventions and measures specific to the condition.

## Safe Medication Practices

Medical errors have economic and emotional consequences that are recognized by regulatory requirements for patient safety and error reduction identified in federal, state, and local mandates, standards for practice in accreditation standards (e.g., The Joint Commission, the National Committee for Quality Assurance, and CARF International), and guidance for safe practices using evidence-based guidelines (e.g., NQF and AHRQ Patient Safety Network).

Even though many treatment procedures involve some risk, by far the most common errors occur with the use of medications. The frequency of medication use in the United States is startling. More than four out of five U.S. adults take at least one medication (prescription or over-the-counter drug, vitamin, mineral, or herbal supplement), and almost one-third take at least five different medications. Further, it is estimated that the extra medical costs of treating medication-related injuries amounts to $3.5 billion per year.[104] In healthcare facilities, most errors occur in the prescribing and administration stages of medication therapy. Further, it is estimated that it costs the United States $289 billion per year for medication nonadherence.[105]

As a foundation, a patient safety culture is devoid of blame and uses systematic ways to welcome the reporting of medication errors. Because 85% of errors are the result of system failures and traditionally only 15% are due to human error, the exploration of systems issues is primary to identifying a root cause of error.[20] Both public and private sector organizations that have worked tirelessly to reduce medication errors include ISMP, the ECRI Institute, and the Food & Drug Administration (FDA).

Through a consensus process, NQF endorsed the adoption of safe practices related to medication administration (**Table 4.10**; see also best practices under the Institute for Safe Medication Practices). Other organizations such as The Leapfrog Group have shown support by their endorsements. To improve patient safety and hold the gains, healthcare organizations conduct a thorough analysis of where and how patients are at risk for potential medical errors and hardwire systems and processes to prevent them. Leadership style and climate affect medication practices so the routine administration of culture of safety surveys may prove beneficial to identify opportunities for improvement at the organization and unit levels.[106]

## Technology

Technological solutions can enhance patient safety programs. A *patient safety solution* is defined as "any system design or intervention that has demonstrated the ability to prevent or mitigate patient harm stemming from the processes of health care."[107(p2)] The premise of these solutions is that if processes are standardized and the potential for medical error is reduced by the automation of processes, errors will be mitigated. Clancy proposed a formula for healthcare improvement composed of four health IT elements: (1) connect health records, (2) build smart systems, (3) put the patient at the center of care, and (4) put prevention at the center of treatment.[5] This is illustrated in **Table 4.11**.

**Table 4.10** Safe Practices Related to Medication Administration

| | Practice Statement |
|---|---|
| **Safe Practice 13:** Order Read-back and Abbreviations | Incorporate within the organization a safe, effective communication strategy, structures, and systems to include the following:<br>▪ For verbal or telephone orders or for telephonic reporting of critical test results, verify the complete order or test result by having the person who is receiving the information record and "read back" the complete order or test result.<br>▪ Standardize a list of "Do Not Use" abbreviations, acronyms, symbols, and dose designations that cannot be used throughout the organization. |
| **Safe Practice 16:** Safe Adoption of Computerized Prescriber Order Entry | ▪ Implement a computerized prescriber order entry system built upon the requisite foundation of reengineered evidence-based care, an assurance of healthcare organization staff and independent practitioner readiness, and an integrated information technology infrastructure. |
| **Safe Practice 17:** Medication Reconciliation | ▪ Develop, reconcile, and communicate an accurate medication list throughout the continuum of care. |
| **Safe Practice 18:** Pharmacist Leadership Structures and Systems | ▪ Pharmacy leaders should have an active role on the administrative leadership team that reflects their authority and accountability for medication management systems performance across the organization. |

Reproduced from National Quality Forum. *Safe Practices for Better Healthcare—2010 Update: A Consensus Report.* Abridged version. Washington, DC: NQF; 2010:vii-xi. https://www.qualityforum.org/publications/2010/04/safe_practices_for_better_healthcare_%E2%80%93_2010_update.aspx

**Table 4.11** Information Technology Commonly Used by Healthcare Professionals

| *Direct Care Delivery Technology* | *Patient Assessment, Monitoring, and Surveillance* |
|---|---|
| ▪ Barcoded medication administration<br>▪ Automated medication cabinets<br>▪ Call systems, including emergency call bells<br>▪ Computerized physician/provider order entry<br>▪ Clinical results available at point of care<br>▪ Standardized order sets<br>▪ E-Prescribing | ▪ Telemetry<br>▪ Bedside monitoring<br>▪ Ventilators<br>▪ Video surveillance<br>▪ Pulse oximetry<br>▪ Smart pumps |
| *Indirect Care Delivery Technology* | *Remote Patient Monitoring* |
| ▪ Robotics<br>▪ Radio frequency identification<br>▪ Electronic inventory systems<br>▪ Computerized staffing systems<br>▪ Automated customized patient directives and education | ▪ Telemedicine and telehealth<br>▪ Robotics |
| *Communication with Healthcare Team Members* | *Continuous Learning* |
| ▪ Electronic medical records<br>▪ Documentation at point of care<br>▪ Electronic ordering systems<br>▪ Clinical decision support<br>▪ Communication devices (cell phones, personal digital assistants, interactive voice response systems, paging systems) | ▪ Distance learning<br>▪ Video conferencing<br>▪ Online training (webinars)<br>▪ Simulation |

*(continues)*

**Table 4.11** **Information Technology Commonly Used by Healthcare Professionals** *(continued)*

| *Patient Protective Devices* | *Pattern Identification (to Learn from Errors and Systems; Influences Adverse Events)* |
|---|---|
| ▪ Abduction, elopement or wandering alarms<br>▪ Fall alarms<br>▪ Alerts or results on handheld devices<br>▪ Radio frequency identification | ▪ Electronic medical or health record<br>▪ Workload and staffing data systems<br>▪ Interdisciplinary charting<br>▪ Laboratory, pathology, and radiology results<br>▪ Automated patient safety-related reports |

Modified from Powell-Cope G, Nelson AL, Patterson ES. Patient care technology and safety. In: Hughes RG, ed. *Patient Safety and Quality: An Evidence-Based Handbook for Nurses.* Rockville, MD: Agency for Healthcare Research and Quality; 2008:3. AHRQ publication 08-0043. Accessed December 8, 2021. https://archive.ahrq.gov /professionals/clinicians-providers/resources/nursing/resources/nurseshdbk/nurseshdbk.pdf. Copyright 2008 by Agency for Healthcare Research and Quality.

Health IT holds promise in making healthcare services safer and offers clinical decision support through electronic health records (EHRs). If health IT is to work, the healthcare consumer must be at the center of the healthcare system and be empowered with their personal healthcare data. Often these questions are asked: *Is health IT easy to use? How quickly does it process information? How functional is it?* and *How can it help me?* If health IT is to be effective in the care setting, it needs to be integrated with the patient and clinical workflow and aligned with available resources and the expectations of the end users.

Leadership plays a critical role in the adoption of health IT (EHRs, personal health records, and e-prescribing systems) and ensuring risks associated with health IT are avoided altogether or mitigated. The Joint Commission provides a framework for maintaining a culture of safety vis-à-vis health IT by

1. collective mindfulness focused on identifying, reporting, analyzing, and reducing health IT-related hazardous conditions, close calls, or errors;
2. comprehensive and systematic analysis of each adverse event causing harm to determine if health IT contributed to the event in any way; and
3. shared involvement and responsibility for the safety of health IT among the healthcare organization, clinicians, and vendors/developers.[108(pp2-3)]

EHRs typically include four core components: electronic clinical documentation, results reporting and management, e-prescribing, and clinical decision support. Over time, other functionalities such as bar coding and patient engagement tools were added. As displayed in **Figure 4.9**, creating a framework for measurement complements approaches to safety such as the Singh and Sitting sociotechnical system that can be paired with the elements of an enterprise risk model to ensure that health IT lives outside organizational siloes.[109]

Health IT and interoperable systems are requisites for healthcare delivery in the 21st century. An IOM report examined the state of the art in system safety and opportunities to build safer systems and concluded as the following:

- Safety is an emergent property of a larger system that accounts for not just the software but also how it is used by clinicians.
- The sociotechnical system includes technology (software, hardware), people (clinicians, patients), processes (workflow), organization (capacity, decisions about how health IT is applied, incentives), and the external environment (regulations, public opinion).
- Safer implementation and use of health IT is a complex, dynamic process that requires a shared responsibility between vendors and healthcare organizations.
- Poor user-interface design, poor workflow, and complex data interfaces threaten patient safety.
- Lack of system interoperability is a barrier to improving clinical decisions and patient safety.
- Constant, ongoing commitment to safety—from acquisition to implementation and maintenance—is needed to achieve safer, more effective care.[110(ppS2-S4)]

EHRs have the potential to capture data for purposes of patient safety performance and improvement. However, some say not enough evidence exists to support the link between the EHR and patient safety[111] and may have unintended consequences as follows:

- Workarounds and alarm fatigue such as "delayed response time to alarms, disabled alarms, volumes set to inaudible, parameters limits set to unsafe zones, or alarms paused without a thoughtful consideration of the warning message."[112(pE1),113]
- Incorrect patient matching where some or all data retrieved via health information exchange (HIE) relate to a different (and incorrect) patient. Such

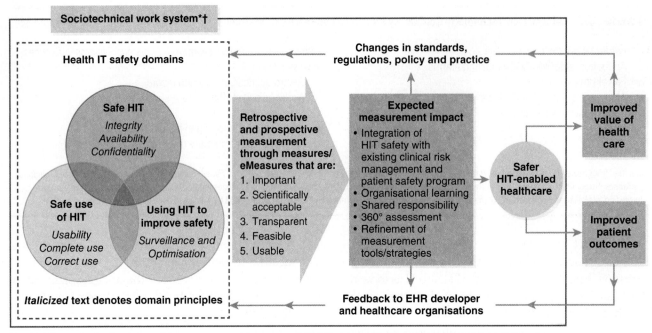

Health information technology safety measurement framework (HITS Framework). *Includes eight technological and non-technological dimensions. †Includes external factors affecting measurement such as payment systems, legal factors, national quality measurement initiatives, accreditation and other policy and regulatory requirements. EHR, electronic health record.

**Figure 4.9** Health Information Technology Safety Measurement Framework

Reproduced from Singh H, Sittig DF. Measuring and improving patient safety through health information technology: the Health IT Safety Framework. *BMJ Qual Saf.* 2016;25:226-232. With permission from BMJ Publishing Group Ltd. doi:10.1136/bmjqs-2015-004486

errors can happen because of flawed matching algorithms used for HIE.

- Data quality issues, such as incomplete patient data, duplicate patient records, or data entry errors, can propagate through HIEs, increasing the potential for adverse safety events.
- Loss of data integrity during transmission. For example, if the HIE process alters the meaning of the data or errors in translation that occur between different systems, reflecting differences in vocabularies. If the HIE degrades EHR or other system performance, critical delays in accessing HIE data can result.[114]

*Artificial intelligence* (AI) and machine learning (a subset of AI) are evolving technologies, referring to "a computer applying human intellectual characteristics to problem solve, namely the ability to reason, make generalizations, and to learn from previous experiences."[115(¶1)] Through machine learning, vast amounts of data can be mined to identify patterns and make decisions. Algorithms are developed from the data and can be used in predictive modeling, "a statistics technique used to predict future behavior or outcomes using historical and current data."[116(p27)] **Table 4.12** provides potential benefits and safety concerns of IT commonly used in healthcare.

As part of national efforts to improve the use of health IT, the Nationwide Health Information Network (NHIN) was established. The NHIN comprises standards, services, and a trust fabric that enables the secure exchange of health information over the Internet. This critical part of the national IT strategy is that health information follows the consumer, is available for clinical decision making, and supports appropriate use of healthcare information beyond direct patient care to public health. A key component of the technology strategy is providing a common platform for HIE across diverse entities, within communities and across the country, helping to achieve the goals of the Health Information Technology for Economic and Clinical Health Act.[117(p4)]

Free, open-source software was developed to support local and national efforts to provide HIE. This kind of information exchange is critical for community-wide patient safety efforts as the NHIN will

- improve the coordination of care information among hospitals, laboratories, physician offices, pharmacies, and other providers;
- ensure appropriate information is available at the time and place of care;
- ensure consumer health information is secure and confidential;

**Table 4.12** Potential Benefits and Safety Concerns of Health IT Components

**Computerized Provider Order Entry (E-Prescribing)**
This is an electronic system that allows providers to record, store, retrieve, and modify orders (e.g., prescriptions, diagnostic testing, treatment, and/or radiology/imaging orders).

*Potential Benefits*
- Large increases in legible orders
- Shorter order turnaround times
- Lower relative risk of medication errors
- Higher percentage of patients who attain their treatment goals

*Safety Concerns*
- Increases relative risk of medication errors
- Increased ordering time
- New opportunities for errors, such as
  - fragmented displays preventing a coherent view of patient medications,
  - inflexible ordering formats generating wrong orders,
  - function separation that facilitates double dosing, and
  - incompatible orders
- Disruptions in workflow

**Clinical Decision Support**
This support monitors and alerts clinicians of patient conditions, prescriptions, and treatment to provide evidence-based clinical suggestions to health professionals at the point of care.

*Potential Benefits*
- Reductions in
  - relative risk of medication errors,
  - risk of toxic drug levels,
  - time to therapeutic stabilization,
  - management errors of resuscitating patients in adult trauma centers, and
  - prescriptions of nonpreferred medications
- Can effectively monitor and alert clinicians of adverse conditions
- Improve long-term treatment and increase the likelihood of achieving treatment goals

*Safety Concerns*
- Rates of detecting drug–drug interactions vary widely among different vendors
- Increases in mortality rate
- High override rate of computer-generated alerts (alert fatigue)

**Bar Coding**
Bar coding can be used to track medications, orders, and other healthcare products. It can also be used to verify patient identification and dosage.

*Potential Benefits*
Significant reductions in relative risk of medication errors associated with
- transcription,
- dispensing, and
- administration errors.

*Safety Concerns*
Introduction of workarounds; for example, clinicians can
- scan medications and patient identification without visually checking to see if the medication, dosing, and patient identification are correct;
- attach patient identification barcodes to another object instead of the patient; and
- scan orders and medications of multiple patients at once instead of doing it each time the medication is dispensed.

**Patient Engagement Tools**
Tools such as patient portals, smartphone applications, email, and interactive kiosks, which enable patients to participate in their healthcare treatment.

*Potential Benefits*
- Reduction in hospitalization rates in children
- Increases in patients' knowledge of treatment and illnesses

*Safety Concerns*
Reliability of data entered by
- patients,
- families,
- friends, or
- unauthorized users.

*(continues)*

**Table 4.12** Potential Benefits and Safety Concerns of Health IT Components *(continued)*

**Artificial Intelligence and Machine Learning**
Computerized systems that include machine learning, natural language processing, rule-based expert systems, physical robots, and robotic automation.

| *Potential Benefits* | *Safety Concerns* |
| --- | --- |
| ▪ Decrease diagnostic errors (i.e., imaging) | ▪ Acceptance of AI into clinical practice |
| ▪ Decrease medical errors | ▪ Limited availability of quality data from which to build and maintain AI applications |
| ▪ Diagnose and treat rare diseases | ▪ Limited effectiveness research on logarithms |
| ▪ Make healthcare accessible and affordable | ▪ Evolving curricula to teach health providers how to use AI |
| ▪ Telehealth: digital health technology | |
| ▪ Savings related to chronic care management | |

Table is not exhaustive but representative of the most common potential benefits and safety concerns. Data from Institute of Medicine, Committee on Patient Safety and Health Information Technology. *Health IT and Patient Safety: Building Safer Systems for Better Care*. National Academies Press; 2012. Copyright 2012 by National Academies Press, with permission; Agyemang-Gyau P. Artificial intelligence in healthcare and the implications for providers. *Online J Nurs Inform*. 2020;25(2). Accessed December 14, 2021. https://www.himss.org/resources/online-journal-nursing-informatics; IBM. Understanding the fundamental value of AI in healthcare. Accessed December 14, 2021. https://www.ibm.com/watson/health/resources/artificial-intelligence-medical-imaging/; and JASON. Artificial intelligence for health and health care. Published 2017. Accessed December 14, 2021. https://www.healthit.gov/sites/default/files/jsr-17-task-002_aiforhealthandhealthcare12122017.pdf

give consumers new capabilities to manage and control their personal health records, as well as provide access to their health information from EHRs and other sources;

• reduce risks from medical errors and support the delivery of appropriate, evidence-based medical care; and

• lower healthcare costs resulting from inefficiencies, medical errors, and incomplete patient information.[118]

Exemplifying this strategy is Maryland's Chesapeake Regional Information System for Our Patients. Begun in 2006, the HIE is composed of hundreds of connected providers, consisting of hospitals, EHRs, pharmacies, payors, health departments, and health centers. Its mission is to "enable and support the healthcare community in Maryland and our region to appropriately and securely share data in order to facilitate care, reduce costs, and improve health outcomes."[119(¶2)] Another example is the Delaware Health Information Network, the first live statewide HIE public–private partnership that includes all hospitals, skilled nursing facilities, and laboratories in the state.[120]

Healthcare quality professionals work with others in the organization to use health IT to mitigate risks, manage care, and reduce preventable harm. As they undertake their work, these professionals should consider the available tools to organize and support initiatives. For example, patient identification-related events present risk for patient care. The partnership for Health IT Patient Safety is a multistakeholder group

working to identify how to optimize health IT for safer care. The partnership currently offers two toolkits—patient identification and cut and paste. The Health IT Safe Practices: The Safe Use of Health IT for Patient Identification toolkit offers a framework of eight safety practice recommendations using IDENTIFY—include, detect, evaluate, normalize, tailor, innovate, follow up, and yield.[121] This model is useful when looking at the independent and interacting effects of behaviors and technology. The partnership descriptions for each practice are shown in **Figure 4.10**.

Also, see the *Health Data Analytics* section for more discussion of health information.

# Evaluating and Improving Patient Safety

Healthcare quality professionals collaborate with other healthcare professionals by evaluating and improving patient safety through public reporting, measurement and improvement, and fostering a culture of safety.

## Public Reporting

Public reporting in healthcare moved from its starting point with voluntary and/or regulatory agency-driven reporting to mandatory and improvement-focused reporting. Beginning with the reporting of mortality rates by CMS in the 1980s, over the decades more public and private sector reporting development has occurred, producing comparable data and science-based methodology. These developments were also

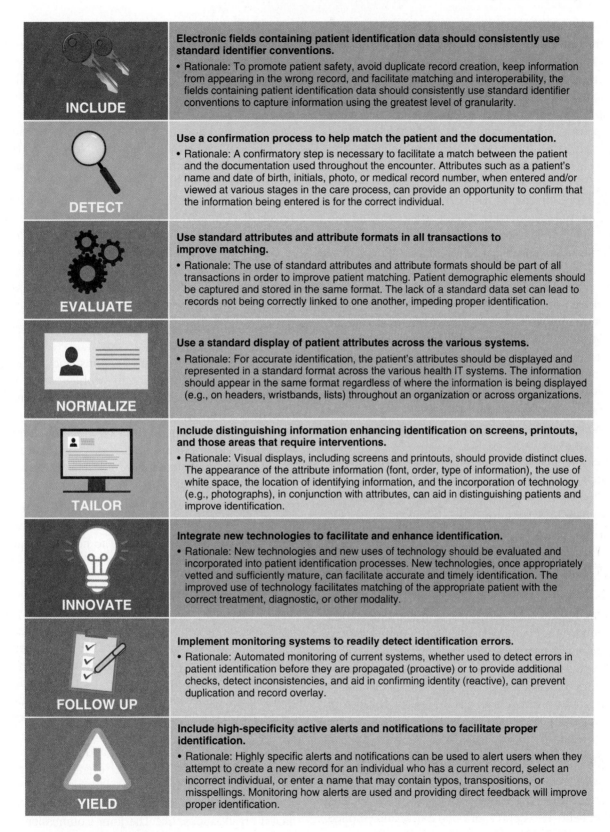

**INCLUDE**

**Electronic fields containing patient identification data should consistently use standard identifier conventions.**

- Rationale: To promote patient safety, avoid duplicate record creation, keep information from appearing in the wrong record, and facilitate matching and interoperability, the fields containing patient identification data should consistently use standard identifier conventions to capture information using the greatest level of granularity.

**DETECT**

**Use a confirmation process to help match the patient and the documentation.**

- Rationale: A confirmatory step is necessary to facilitate a match between the patient and the documentation used throughout the encounter. Attributes such as a patient's name and date of birth, initials, photo, or medical record number, when entered and/or viewed at various stages in the care process, can provide an opportunity to confirm that the information being entered is for the correct individual.

**EVALUATE**

**Use standard attributes and attribute formats in all transactions to improve matching.**

- Rationale: The use of standard attributes and attribute formats should be part of all transactions in order to improve patient matching. Patient demographic elements should be captured and stored in the same format. The lack of a standard data set can lead to records not being correctly linked to one another, impeding proper identification.

**NORMALIZE**

**Use a standard display of patient attributes across the various systems.**

- Rationale: For accurate identification, the patient's attributes should be displayed and represented in a standard format across the various health IT systems. The information should appear in the same format regardless of where the information is being displayed (e.g., on headers, wristbands, lists) throughout an organization or across organizations.

**TAILOR**

**Include distinguishing information enhancing identification on screens, printouts, and those areas that require interventions.**

- Rationale: Visual displays, including screens and printouts, should provide distinct clues. The appearance of the attribute information (font, order, type of information), the use of white space, the location of identifying information, and the incorporation of technology (e.g., photographs), in conjunction with attributes, can aid in distinguishing patients and improve identification.

**INNOVATE**

**Integrate new technologies to facilitate and enhance identification.**

- Rationale: New technologies and new uses of technology should be evaluated and incorporated into patient identification processes. New technologies, once appropriately vetted and sufficiently mature, can facilitate accurate and timely identification. The improved use of technology facilitates matching of the appropriate patient with the correct treatment, diagnostic, or other modality.

**FOLLOW UP**

**Implement monitoring systems to readily detect identification errors.**

- Rationale: Automated monitoring of current systems, whether used to detect errors in patient identification before they are propagated (proactive) or to provide additional checks, detect inconsistencies, and aid in confirming identity (reactive), can prevent duplication and record overlay.

**YIELD**

**Include high-specificity active alerts and notifications to facilitate proper identification.**

- Rationale: Highly specific alerts and notifications can be used to alert users when they attempt to create a new record for an individual who has a current record, select an incorrect individual, or enter a name that may contain typos, transpositions, or misspellings. Monitoring how alerts are used and providing direct feedback will improve proper identification.

**Figure 4.10** Eight Safety Practices for Patient Identification

Reproduced from ECRI Institute for Health IT Patient Safety. Eight safe practice recommendations. Published 2017. Accessed December 6, 2021. https://www.ecri.org/Resources/HIT/Patient%20ID/Recommendations_Patient_ID_Handout.pdf

framed by stakeholder expectations for accountability, transparency, and improvement. Stakeholders include a host of healthcare providers and payers—government at all levels, health plans, hospitals, ambulatory care, long-term care, physicians, and group practices to name a few. Accreditation agencies and private interest groups are stakeholders. Most important, the public and consumer interests and involvement have grown.

As the stakeholder base for public reporting expands and diversifies, Halpern and colleagues suggest that "public reporting should be used to hold systems accountable to their own goals."[122(p32)] In linking quality and patient safety efforts, information should be published on what was learned, recommendations and changes made, and the responsiveness of the institution to patient safety issues. There is no doubt that public reporting offers value related to the allocation of the healthcare dollars, but work is still needed to better understand what value is brought to the consumer in choosing a healthcare provider or health plan.[123]

Twenty-seven states plus the District of Columbia passed legislation or regulation supporting adverse event reporting to a state agency. The laws and regulations intended to raise accountability in healthcare organizations. Public reporting has the potential to improve patient safety through event analysis and by disseminating lessons learned.[124] Eight states use the NQF reportable adverse incident list in their reporting systems; seven states use a modified or partial NQF list, and 12 states use their own non-NQF list.[124(p8)] The effectiveness of reporting systems is not yet fully understood. However, many reporting system administrators experienced an "impact on communication among facilities, provider education, internal agency tracking or trending, and/or implementation of facility processes to address quality of care. Nine states report increased levels of provider and facility transparency and awareness of patient safety because of their reporting systems."[124(p3)]

## Reporting and Tracking

An array of reporting and tracking programs related to patient safety have been deployed by the federal government. The Center for Food Safety and Applied Nutrition (CFSAN) Adverse Event Reporting System (CAERS) is a database containing information on adverse event and product complaints related to foods, dietary supplements, and cosmetics that are submitted to FDA. It is designed to support the safety surveillance program.[125] The Vaccine Adverse Event Reporting System (VAERS) is a national safety surveillance program comanaged by CDC and FDA. The system collects information about adverse events that occur after the administration of vaccines licensed for use in the United States.[126] During the COVID-19 pandemic, they were responsible for collecting information about COVID-19 vaccines during the time they were used under emergency use authorization.

The National Healthcare Safety Network (NHSN) is far reaching in its tracking and reporting for patient safety. Attention to infection prevention and control began to grow as part of the national effort to achieve zero HAIs. Public reporting of infection rates became the "new clinical mandate."[127(p3)] NHSN also plays a leadership role in promoting patient safety by providing a secure, Internet-based safety surveillance system. Through its efforts, it applies quality and safety improvement methods by

- collecting and reporting on national and state-specific standardized infection ratios;
- providing facilities, states, regions, and the nation with data needed to identify problem areas, measure progress of prevention efforts, and ultimately eliminate HAIs; and
- allowing healthcare facilities to track blood safety errors and important healthcare process measures (e.g., healthcare personnel influenza vaccine status and infection-control adherence rates).[128]

In October 2014, CMS began reducing Medicare payments for certain hospitals that ranked in the worst performing quartile with respect to hospital-acquired conditions. The measures reflect a composite of NHSN data and AHRQ patient safety indicators.

Expectations about voluntary and mandatory incident reporting systems at organizational and system levels are still evolving. In 1999, the IOM advocated the use of the incident reporting system. The IOM recommended that "a nationwide mandatory reporting system should be established that provides for the collection of standardized information by governments about adverse events that result in death or serious harm. Reporting should initially be required of hospitals and eventually be required of other institutional and ambulatory care delivery settings."[129(p9)] State-level event reporting systems that focus on adverse events with intent to improve patient safety have increased, but mandates vary. Accreditation organizations, like The Joint Commission, have voluntary and mandatory event reporting.

## Hospital and Outpatient Performance

CMS began its hospital and outpatient rating and reporting systems with Hospital Compare in 2002. This was a joint effort between Medicare and the

Hospital Quality Alliance. Over 10 years, CMS and the Alliance worked together to grow public reporting efforts in a meaningful way and beyond structural measures of quality, including the Hospital Consumer Assessment of Healthcare Providers and Systems (HCAHPS). The Hospital Quality Alliance ceased in 2012 after accomplishing its goals.

With Hospital Compare and HCAHPS serving as both the foundation and experience, CMS continued its development efforts, launching other compare programs for healthcare providers across the continuum of care—Physician Compare, Nursing Home Compare, Home Health Compare, and the like. In 2020, Hospital Compare was consolidated with other CMS Compare sites on the Care Compare site.[130] Consumers and payers can search for quality and safety information on doctors and clinicians, hospitals, nursing homes, home health services, hospice care, inpatient rehabilitation facilities, long-term care hospitals, and dialysis facilities. These programs offer payers and consumers valuable tools for value-based purchasing and selecting providers for personal healthcare services and treatment. Performance on safety measures is available on timely and effective care, complications and deaths, unplanned hospital visits (readmissions), payment, and value of care.

### Health Plan Performance

The National Committee for Quality Assurance (NCQA) develops standards and measures that hold health plans accountable for the care provided to their constituents. Its performance measurement system, the Healthcare Effectiveness Data and Information Set (HEDIS), is one of the most widely used performance measure data sets that is targeted toward health plans, wellness and health promotion, and disease management programs. This tool is used by more than 90% of America's health plans to measure performance on important dimensions of care and service. Because so many plans collect HEDIS data, there is comparability and acceptability by third-party payers. Some patient safety areas addressed by HEDIS include the following:

- Safe and judicious antipsychotic drug use in children and adolescents
- HAIs
- Follow-up after an emergency visit for mental illness, alcohol, and other drug dependence
- Falls risk management

HEDIS is publicly reported with available benchmarks. The results are used by consumers to select the best health plan for their needs by looking at the plan performance and comparing plan performance with other plans.[131] HEDIS reporting is a third-party payer requirement for health plans.

## Measurement and Improvement

Continuous measurement and monitoring can yield important insights about the impact of interventions and improvement projects on patient safety. These insights can be leveraged into the ongoing, sustainable action plan. Gathering and using real-time data will help the organization improve and protect patients from harm. Selected measures may relate to structure, process, outcomes, resource use, or composite of measure attributes. With the proliferation of reliable and valid safety measures, the healthcare quality professional can examine available measures and determine which will be the most meaningful to the organization's internal and external stakeholders.

There is no one single source for safety measures, so the healthcare quality professional can review available measures for the healthcare setting. The most logical place to start is measures from organizations that require certain measures for payment or accreditation. These measures may have been developed and validated by the sponsoring organization (e.g., NCQA and HEDIS) or are endorsed measures that are used by third-party payers or accreditation agencies (e.g., NQF). The following are possible sources of such measures. See *Performance and Process Improvement, Health Data Analytics,* and *Quality Review and Accountability* sections for more information on measures and improvement.

### The Joint Commission

Through its accreditation standards and other activities, The Joint Commission (TJC) strives to help organizations achieve no patient harm. Standards require organizations to gather and analyze the data generated through standardized monitoring. Results are used to inform the goals and objectives of care, treatment, or services, and the outcomes of care, treatment, or services provided to the population served by aggregating and analyzing the data gathered through the standardized monitoring effort. TJC assists healthcare organizations in collecting and reporting performance improvement and accountability data through ORYX® and core measure sets.[132] Results are publicly reported on TJC's Quality Check website.

National Patient Safety Goals (NPSGs) are another way that TJC assists healthcare organizations and programs in the United States through accreditation surveys and continuous readiness. Currently, there are safety goals for ambulatory healthcare, assisted living communities, behavioral healthcare, critical access hospitals, home care, hospitals, laboratories, nursing care centers, and office-based surgery.[133] **Table 4.13** describes examples of current Joint Commission NPSGs for hospitals.

## The Leapfrog Group

The Leapfrog Group is a voluntary initiative that serves to mobilize employer purchasing power to guide America's health industry in adopting giant leaps in patient safety. The group's mission is "to trigger giant leaps forward in the safety, quality and affordability

**Table 4.13** Examples of The Joint Commission National Patient Safety Goals

| Goal 1. Improve the Accuracy of Patient Identification | |
| --- | --- |
| Example | Use at least two patient identifiers to verify a patient's identity upon admission or transfer to another hospital or other care setting and prior to the administration of care. |

| Goal 2. Improve the Effectiveness of Communication Among Caregivers | |
| --- | --- |
| Example | Report critical results of tests on a timely basis by defining who should receive the results; who should receive the results when the ordering provider is not available, what results require timely and reliable communication, when the results should be actively reported to the ordering provider with explicit time frames, how to notify the responsible provider, and how to design, support, and maintain the systems involved (Lippi & Mattiuzzi, 2016). |

| Goal 3. Improve the Safety of Using Medications | |
| --- | --- |
| Example | Maintain and communicate accurate patient medication information through medication reconciliation to avoid inadvertent inconsistencies across transitions in care by reviewing the patient's complete medication regimen at the time of care transitions (e.g., admission, transfer, discharge) (AHRQ, 2019). |

| Goal 7. Reduce the Risk of Healthcare-Associated Infections | |
| --- | --- |
| Example | Comply with current hand hygiene guidelines (e.g., CDC, 2021; or current World Health Organization [WHO] hand hygiene guidelines, 2021). |

| Goal 15. The Hospital Identifies Safety Risks Inherent in Its Patient Population | |
| --- | --- |
| Example | Use a zero suicide approach to identify patients at risk for suicide by screening for suicidal thoughts or behaviors at admission or intake and complete a full risk assessment when a patient screens positive (WICHE, 2017). |

| Universal Protocol for Preventing Wrong-Site, Wrong-Procedure, and Wrong-Person Surgery | |
| --- | --- |
| Example | A time-out is performed before the procedure that includes the confirmation of the correct patient, correct side and site, agreement on the procedure to be performed, correct patient position, availability of needed equipment/supplies/implants, and the presence and review of relevant radiologic images (if applicable) (AORN, 2021). |

Data from Agency for Healthcare Research and Quality. Patient safety primer: medication reconciliation. Published 2019. Accessed December 8, 2021. https://psnet.ahrq.gov/primers/primer/1/medication-reconciliation; Association of periOperative Registered Nursing. National time out day is June 9, 2021. Published 2021. Accessed December 8, 2021. https://aorn.org/timeout/; Centers for Disease Control and Prevention. Hand hygiene in healthcare settings. Published 2019. Accessed December 8, 2021. https://www.cdc.gov/handhygiene/index.html; Lippi G, Mattiuzzi C. Critical laboratory values communication: summary recommendations from available guidelines. *Ann Transl Med.* 2016;4(20):400. doi:10.21037/atm.2016.09.36; The Joint Commission. National patient safety goals. Accessed December 8, 2021. https://www.jointcommission.org/standards/national-patient-safety-goals/; Western Interstate Commission for Higher Education Mental Health Program (WICHE MHP) & Suicide Prevention Resource Center (SPRC). *Suicide Prevention Toolkit for Primary Care Practices: A Guide for Primary Care Providers and Medical Practice Managers.* Rev. ed. Boulder, CO: WICHE MHP & SPRC; 2017. Accessed December 8, 2021. https://sprc.org/settings/primary-care/toolkit; and World Health Organization. Hand hygiene: the evidence for clean hands. Published 2021. Accessed December 8, 2021. https://www.who.int/teams/integrated-health-services/infection-prevention-control/hand-hygiene/guidelines-and-evidence of U.S. healthcare by using transparency to support informed healthcare decisions and promote high-value care."[134(96)] In 2001, Leapfrog launched a hospital survey to collect data on three leaps (computerized physician order entry, ICUs appropriately staffed with intensivists, and ensuring enough surgical volume to safely perform certain high-risk procedures). Initially, participating hospitals were ranked, but in 2012 Leapfrog began assigning A, B, C, D, and F letter grades. Employers and other purchasers as well as health plans and community leaders are using Leapfrog Hospital Survey results and Leapfrog Hospital Safety Grades for payment reform and public reporting.

The Leapfrog Group's safe practices informed the development of 34 NQF-endorsed safety practices. These hospital practices, when implemented, reduce harm. The practices comprise elements related to leadership, care needs, information transfer and communication, medication management, HAIs, and specific care processes. On the Leapfrog Hospital and Ambulatory Care Surveys, 1596 hospitals reported on cesarean sections, 2184 hospitals reported using computerized order entry, and 2228 hospitals and surgery centers reported on their never events policy.[135]

### National Quality Forum

As a leader in patient safety, NQF is recognized as a voluntary consensus standards-setting organization as defined by the Office of Management and Budget. Since 2002, NQF assembled a portfolio of more than 1149 NQF-endorsed measures in use by both the private and public sectors for public reporting and quality improvement. Most notably, NQF does the following:

- *Sets standards.* NQF-endorsed measures are considered the gold standard in healthcare measurement in the United States. Types of measures include composite, cost and resource use, efficiency, outcome, process, and structure.
- *Recommends measures for use in payment and public reporting programs.* The NQF-convened Measure Applications Partnership advises the federal government and private sector payers on the optimal measures for use in specific payment and accountability programs.
- *Advances electronic measurement.* NQF's health IT initiatives are designed to support the complex, but important move toward electronic measurement.
- *Provides information and tools to help healthcare decision makers.* NQF provides reports, tools, events, and information to help physicians and others on the frontlines of changing healthcare.[136]

NQF endorsed over 100 consensus standards with a focus on patient safety.[48] Its consensus-setting efforts support the evaluation of patient safety using standardized performance measurement. NQF also maintains the Quality Positioning System, which helps to select measures that might align with monitoring, reporting, and improvement interests.[137]

## Evaluating the Culture of Safety

How does an organization evaluate its progress and success in achieving a culture of safety? Patients and healthcare providers generally measure safety culture. Safety culture measures reflect teamwork training, executive walk rounds, and establishing unit-based safety teams. These have been associated with improvements in safety culture measures but have not yet linked to lower error rates. "Communication strategies are desirable, which take little time and effort to complete, deliver comprehensive information efficiently, encourage interprofessional collaboration and limit the probability of error."[138(pp1-2)] The standardized communication tool, *SBAR*, is frequently used by providers in healthcare settings to describe a patient's condition and facilitate care.

> "S = Situation (a concise statement of the problem)
> B = Background (pertinent and brief information related to the situation)
> A = Assessment (analysis and considerations of options—what you found/think)
> R = Recommendation (action requested/recommended—what you want)"[139]

An SBAR example is shown in **Table 4.14**.

Surveys are the most common approach to evaluating the safety climate or safety culture. For the purposes of reporting on NQF Safe Practice 2: Culture Measurement, Feedback, and Intervention, hospitals must conduct a culture of safety survey of their employees within the past 24 months. The units surveyed must account for at least 50% of the aggregated care delivered to patients within the facility and include the high-risk patient safety units or departments using a nationally recognized tool that has demonstrated validity, consistency, and reliability. When selecting a survey tool for the organization, the healthcare quality professional should consider the following:

- Alignment of the survey with the setting where the survey will be administered
- Using a valid and reliable, vetted survey
- Using a survey that is supported by evidence from peer-reviewed literature

---

**Table 4.14** Example of SBAR

**Situation**—What is going on with the patient?

*"I am calling about Mrs. Joseph in room 251. Chief complaint is shortness of breath of new onset."*

**Background**—What is the clinical background or context?

*"Patient is a 62-year-old female post-op day one from abdominal surgery. No prior history of cardiac or lung disease."*

**Assessment**—What do I think the problem is?

*"Breath sounds are decreased on the right side with acknowledgement of pain. Would like to rule out pneumothorax."*

**Recommendation and Request**—What would I do to correct it?

*"I feel strongly the patient should be assessed now. Can you come to room 251 now?"*

Reproduced from Agency for Healthcare Research and Quality. *Pocket Guide TeamSTEPPS 2.0: Team Strategies & Tools to Enhance Performance and Patient Safety.* December 2013. Accessed June 18, 2022. https://www.ahrq.gov/teamstepps/instructor/essentials/pocketguide.html#sbar

---

- Respondent burden is minimized; administrative burden is minimized
- Results offer information that is actionable
- Using a survey for which local, state, or national benchmarking data are available[140]

Validated surveys will have well-detailed methodology to assure a successful survey administration. Healthcare quality professionals should consider using a third-party vendor for the survey administration —the vendor can be a safe intermediary for data collection, ensure anonymity of respondents, and work with the organization to achieve higher response rates. Descriptions of more commonly used assessment and survey tools follow.

## University of Texas Safety Attitudes Questionnaire

The *Safety Attitudes Questionnaire* measures caregiver attitudes about six patient safety-related domains, allows organizations to compare themselves to others, prompts interventions to improve safety attitudes, and measures the effectiveness of these interventions. The Safety Attitudes Questionnaire domain scales are teamwork climate, job satisfaction, perceptions of management, safety climate, working conditions, and stress recognition.[141,142] An organization can use the tool to gather baseline data and measure the effectiveness of change and the adoption of patient safety practices. The surveys and psychometric research about the surveys can be accessed through the University of Texas Health Science Center at Houston/McGovern Medical School's Center for Healthcare Quality and Safety.[143]

## Patient Safety Climate in Healthcare Organizations

The *Patient Safety Climate in Healthcare Organizations* survey is designed to assess the healthcare workforce's perception about the culture of safety in their organization. It assesses different aspects of safety including contributions to safety climate from the hospital, work unit, interpersonal, and other. Contributing factors are measured, including engagement, resources, emphasis on patient safety, unit support, and unit-level factors (e.g., safety norms, recognition, support, and collective learning). The fear of shame and fear of blame and punishment subscales are considered interpersonal contributions to safety climate. The provision of safe care is also examined.[144-146]

## AHRQ Surveys on Patient Safety Culture

As part of its goal to support a culture of patient safety and quality improvement in the nation's healthcare system, AHRQ developed its patient safety culture assessment tools for healthcare. In 2004, AHRQ developed and distributed a valid and reliable safety culture survey, the Hospital Survey on Patient Safety Culture, to help hospitals, nursing homes, and ambulatory outpatient medical offices evaluate the culture of safety in their institutions. In 2008, AHRQ released its first benchmarking report based upon an analysis of data from 400 voluntary participating hospitals. Healthcare organizations can use these surveys to track changes in patient safety over time and evaluate the effects of patient safety interventions.[147] The *Hospital Survey Version 2.0 (SOPS Hospital Version 2.0)* was introduced in 2019. Version 2.0 has fewer items and item wording is different than in the 1.0 survey, as are the names of composite measures.

The *Surveys on Patient Safety Culture (SOPS) Hospital Survey 2.0: 2021 User Database Report* is a compilation of the most recent survey findings.[148] Based on data provided voluntarily by hospitals, the report provides results hospitals can use as benchmarks to establish a culture of safety in comparison to similar hospitals or hospital units. The survey evaluates patient safety issues, medical errors, and event reporting. It includes 32 items that measure 10 areas, or composites, of patient safety culture. Each of the 10 composites or areas and their definitions are described in **Table 4.15**.

In 2021, 172 hospitals submitted survey data, representing 87,856 providers and staff respondents from medicine, surgery, and other areas. The results reflected progress in teamwork, management expectations around promoting patient safety, and organizational learning. However, continued potential for improvement in most hospitals was found for patient safety practices, particularly nonpunitive response to reporting, handoffs and transitions, and workload. Areas of strength are shown in **Table 4.16**.

Validated provider surveys from AHRQ's portfolio of surveys on Patient Safety Culture include the following:

- Hospital
- Medical office
- Nursing home
- Community
- Ambulatory surgery center

These surveys ask providers to rate the safety culture in their unit and the whole organization. Annual benchmarking data are available in AHRQ's comprehensive reports.

**Table 4.15**  SOPS Hospital Survey 2.0 Patient Safety Culture Composites Measures and Definitions

| Patient Safety Culture Composite Measure | Definition: The Extent to Which . . . | Number of Items |
|---|---|---|
| Communication about error | Staff are informed when errors occur, discuss ways to prevent errors, and are informed when changes are made. | 3 |
| Communication openness | Staff speak up when they see something unsafe and feel comfortable asking questions. | 3 |
| Handoffs and information exchange | Important patient care information is transferred across hospital units and during shift changes. | 3 |
| Hospital management support for patient safety | Hospital management shows that patient safety is a top priority and provides adequate resources for patient safety. | 3 |
| Organizational learning—continuous improvement | Work processes are regularly reviewed, changes are made to keep mistakes from happening again, and changes are evaluated. | 3 |
| Reporting patient safety events | Mistakes of the following type are reported: (1) mistakes caught and corrected before reaching the patient and (2) mistakes that could have harmed the patient but did not. | 2 |
| Response to error | Staff are treated fairly when they make mistakes and there is a focus on learning from mistakes and supporting staff involved in errors. | 4 |
| Staffing and work pace | There are enough staff to handle the workload, staff work appropriate hours and do not feel rushed, and there is appropriate reliance on temporary, float, or as-needed staff. | 4 |
| Supervisor, manager, or clinical leader support for patient safety | Supervisors, managers, or clinical leaders consider staff suggestions for improving patient safety, do not encourage taking shortcuts, and take action to address patient safety concerns. | 3 |
| Teamwork | Staff work together as an effective team, help each other during busy times, and are respectful. | 3 |

Reproduced from Sorra J, Yount N, Famolaro T, Gray L. *AHRQ Hospital Survey on Patient Safety Culture Version 2.0: User's Guide*. (Prepared by Westat, under Contract No. HHSP233201500026I/HHSP23337004T.) Rockville, MD: Agency for Healthcare Research and Quality; June 2021. AHRQ publication 19(21)-0076. Accessed April 9, 2022. https://www.ahrq.gov/sops/surveys/hospital/index.html

**Table 4.16** SOPS Hospital Survey 2.0: Strengths

| Areas of Strength (Hospitals) | 2019 (%) | 2021 (%) |
|---|---|---|
| *Teamwork Within Units*<br>The extent to which staff members work together as an effective team, help each other during busy times, and are respectful. | 81 | 82 |
| *Supervisor/Manager Expectations and Actions Promoting Patient Safety*<br>The extent to which supervisors, managers, or clinical leaders consider staff suggestions, do not encourage shortcuts, and address patient safety concerns. | 81 | 80 |

Data from Agency for Healthcare Research and Quality. Pilot test results from the 2019 AHRQ Surveys on Patient Safety Culture (SOPS) Hospital Survey 2.0. Published 2019. Accessed December 8, 2021. https://www.ahrq.gov/sites/default/files/wysiwyg/sops/surveys/hospital/hsops2-pilot-results-parti.pdf; and Agency for Healthcare Research and Quality. SOPS Hospital Survey 2.0: 2021 User database report. Published March 2021. Accessed December 6, 2021. https://www.ahrq.gov/sites/default/files/wysiwyg/sops/surveys/hospital/2021-HSOPS2-Database-Report-Part-I-508.pdf

### Medical Group Management Association Practice Profile Survey

When the IOM published *Crossing the Quality Chasm* in 2001, the extent of preventable medical errors was far reaching.[1] Many initiatives focus on inpatient care, and fewer focus on other settings such as ambulatory or nursing home care. The Health Research and Educational Trust—in partnership with the American Hospital Association (AHA), ISMP, and the Medical Group Management Association (MGMA) and its certifying body, the American College of Medical Practice Executives—developed the Physician Practice Patient Safety Assessment for the medical practice setting.[149] Now known as the MGMA Practice Profile Survey, it is an interactive self-assessment tool for evaluating medication safety, handoffs and transitions, surgery and invasive procedures, personnel qualifications and competency, practice management and culture, and patient education and communication. Healthcare quality professionals in ambulatory settings can use the MGMA Practice Profile Survey data, housed in MGMA DataDive, to view benchmarks, create and save reports, compare 5 years of trend data, create visual graphs and charts for presentations, and compare results to better performers.[150] Other MGMA surveys include the Cost and Revenue Survey, Compensation and Production Survey, and Practice Operations Survey.

### Trust, Report, and Improve Organizations

The Joint Commission Center for Transforming Health Care Trust, Report, and Improve Organizations (TRIO) program combines strategic assessments, structured training, robust process improvement, and proven change management methodologies to assist in the development of a fully functional safety culture within health organizations. Per the Center, TRIO accomplishes the following:

- *Conducts in-depth assessments.* Uses structured surveys, focus groups, and comprehensive document review.
- *Identifies unique organizational needs.* Initial assessments identify opportunities within the organization.
- *Conducts training sessions to identify a path forward.* Includes training sessions for small groups of leaders, built on a foundation of trust.
- *Serves as a helping hand along the way.* Provides continual support and counseling to the organization and its leaders.
- *Sustains improvements.* Incorporates a control plan to monitor and measure ongoing sustainment.[151(¶3)]

All staff at accredited hospitals and critical access hospitals can attain access to TRIO through The Joint Commission Center for Transforming Healthcare's website or be granted access through The Joint Commission Connect.

**Box 4.4** outlines key points for evaluating and improving patient safety.

---

**Box 4.4 Key Points: Evaluating and Improving Patient Safety**

- If processes are standardized by automation, the potential for medical error may be reduced.
- Surveys are the most common approach to evaluating the safety climate or safety culture.
- To improve patient safety and hold the gains, the healthcare quality professional should conduct a thorough analysis of potential medical errors and hardwire systems and processes to prevent them.

# Patient Safety and the Learning Organization

It is imperative that a continuous, dynamic learning healthcare system is achieved. This system is one that "provides the best care at lower cost: (1) managing rapidly increasing complexity; (2) achieving greater value in health care; and (3) capturing opportunities from technology, industry, and policy."[152(p8)] How can this be achieved by a learning organization? The infrastructure of a learning organization embraces lifelong learning as a value, and opportunities are continually provided for capacity building, developing core competencies, and seeking patient safety innovations. This includes cultivating good judgment and having the opportunity to use it. A learning organization embraces team learning, shared vision and goals, shared ways of thinking, individual commitment to lifelong learning, and systems thinking.[153] Greater attention is paid to learning that fosters more rapid progress in patient safety, increases organizational capabilities, strengthens a culture of safety, fixes process problems that contribute to patient harm, and produces higher reliability.[154]

Creating the infrastructure for learning can be accomplished in many ways. As summarized by ISMP,[155] these are suggested steps for creating an infrastructure for learning:

- Identifying reliable sources of information about errors and risks
- Establishing a systematic way to review external information about errors and risk
- Bringing outside points of view into an organization from the literature or experts
- Leveraging the learning of other organizations that had high-profile errors (e.g., contributing factors, how the error was addressed)
- Integrating learning into existing processes in the organization (e.g., safety committee, board reports, and unit-level quality teams)

The healthcare quality professional can work with others in the organization to build a sustainable infrastructure that includes a multifaceted learning and organizational development plan for patient safety that is appropriate for the healthcare setting and is reflective of the development needs of personnel. The plan should be competency-based where individual and team clinical and interpersonal skill development will result in performance excellence for safety processes and outcomes. The plan can be supported by evidence-based publications and materials available from national and international organizations who already have developed curricula for teaching patient safety.

IHI and safe and reliable healthcare stress the importance of continuous reflection to assess performance. Learning systems that support reflection work to "identify defects and act on them; they reward proactivity rather than reactivity. Learning and a healthy culture reinforce one another by identifying and resolving clinical, cultural, and operational defects. By effectively applying improvement science, organizations can learn their way into many of the cultural components of the framework."[156(p8)] The intersections between culture and learning in this framework are shown in **Figure 4.11**.

Some organizational examples to use in building infrastructure are shown alphabetically in the following sections and are by no means exhaustive. These resources are evidence-based and include validated tools for improving safety practices. All organizations offer professional development and learning programs, some with nominal or no charge to the user. Key points for organizational learning are listed in **Box 4.5**.

---

### Box 4.5  Key Points: Organizational Learning

- The healthcare quality professional should work with others in the organization to build a sustainable infrastructure with a multifaceted learning and organizational development plan for patient safety.
- The healthcare quality professional should develop an organizational learning plan that is competency based (individual and team) and supported by evidence-based guidelines and practices.
- The healthcare quality professional should embrace team learning, shared vision and goals, shared ways of thinking, individual commitment to lifelong learning, and systems thinking.

---

## Agency for Healthcare Research and Quality

AHRQ offers a portfolio of free continuing education, case studies, curriculum tools, and toolkits for all healthcare settings.[157] AHRQ tools are practical and research based. Healthcare professionals in all settings can use tools to make care safer and improve their communication and teamwork skills. Examples of these tools are the following:

- Communication and Optimal Resolution Toolkit
- Community-Acquired Pneumonia Clinical Decision Support Implementation

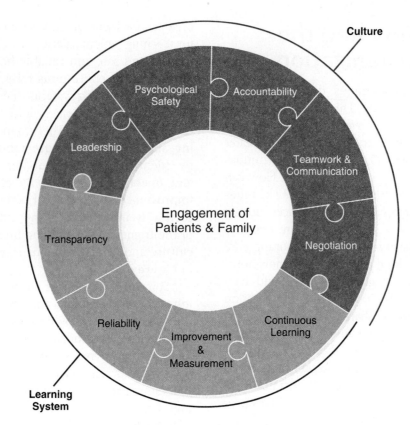

**Figure 4.11** Learning System and Culture Framework

Reprinted with permission from Frankel A, Haraden C, Federico F, Lenoci-Edwards J. *A Framework for Safe, Reliable, and Effective Care*. White paper. Cambridge, MA: Institute for Healthcare Improvement; 2017. Accessed April 9, 2022. www.IHI.org

- EvidenceNOW Tools for Change
- Improving Your Laboratory Testing Process
- SHARE Approach Toolkit for Engaging Patients to Improve Diagnostic Safety
- Toolkit to Improve Antibiotic Use in Long-Term Care
- Toolkit to Improve Safety in Ambulatory Surgery Centers

One of the more widely used programs, Team Strategies and Tools to Enhance Performance and Patient Safety (TeamSTEPPS) is a teamwork system developed by AHRQ and the Department of Defense. TeamSTEPPS 2.0 serves as the core curriculum for training. It is scientifically rooted in more than 20 years of research and lessons from the application of teamwork principles and system error prevention.[158(¶2)] Using tools such as situation, background, assessment, recommendation; huddles; and the two-challenge rule, TeamSTEPPS intends to produce outcomes such as mutual trust, adaptability, and shared mentality.

TeamSTEPPS provides higher quality, safer patient care by increasing team awareness and clarifying team roles and responsibilities.[158(¶3)] It is based on team structure and four teachable, learnable skills: communication, leadership, situation monitoring, and mutual support. **Figure 4.12** shows the framework where there is a two-way dynamic interplay between the four skills and the team-related outcomes. Interaction between the outcomes and skills is the basis of a team striving to deliver safe, quality care and support quality improvement. Encircling the four skills is the team structure of the patient care team, which represents not only the patient and direct caregivers, but also those who play a supportive role within the healthcare delivery system.[159(p4)]

Teams learn about the four competency areas that lead to improved team performance, safer practices, and change in culture:

- *Leadership.* Direct and coordinate, assign tasks, motivate team members, and facilitate optimal performance.
- *Situation monitoring.* Develop common understanding of team environment, apply strategies to monitor teammate performance, and maintain a shared mental model.
- *Mutual support.* Anticipate other team members' needs through accurate knowledge and shift

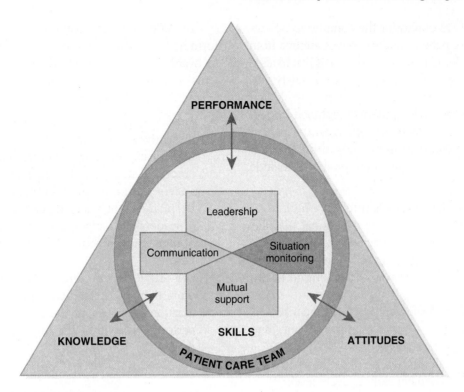

**Figure 4.12** TeamSTEPPS 2.0 Framework

Reproduced from Agency for Healthcare Research and Quality. TeamSTEPPS® 2.0 leadership briefing. Accessed December 20, 2021. https://www.ahrq.gov/teamstepps/about-teamstepps/leadershipbriefing.html

workload to achieve balance during periods of high workload or stress.

- *Communication.* Effectively exchange information among team members, regardless of how it is communicated.

The result will be a higher performing team, where members share a clear vision of the plan and use concise, structured techniques, while maximizing resources for optimal outcomes.

## ECRI Institute

The ECRI Institute (also known as "ECRI") is a non-profit organization dedicated to bringing applied scientific research to improving patient care using the best medical procedures, devices, drugs, and processes. ECRI offers resources by clinical specialty, care setting, and role. This member service organization's clients include hospitals, health systems, public and private payers, U.S. federal and state government agencies, health clinics, patients, policy makers, ministries of health, associations, and accrediting agencies worldwide.

ECRI convened the Partnership for Health IT Patient Safety, which develops and publicly disseminates resources and educational tools that help identify and remediate harm associated with health

IT.[160] FDA/ECRI's *Medical Device Material Safety Summaries: ECRI Reports* are another valuable patient safety resource. The safety summaries provide current knowledge about medical device material performance post-implantation independently investigated by ECRI. It offers updated reviews of the types of problems occurring with medical devices and lessons learned.[161]

## Institute for Healthcare Improvement/National Patient Safety Foundation

Through its Open School, IHI offers quality improvement and patient safety courses based on introductory concepts, intermediate concepts, specialized topics, and project-based learning. IHI offers faculty tools for tracking successful completion of online courses for a nominal fee. The courses specifically related to patient safety include Introduction to Patient Safety; From Error to Harm; Human Factors and Safety; Teamwork and Communication in a Culture of Safety; Responding to Adverse Events; Root Cause and Systems Analysis; Building a Culture of Safety; Partnering to Heal: Teaming Up Against Healthcare-Associated Infections; and Preventing Pressure Ulcers.[162]

NPSF creates resources for the community to create a world where patients and caregivers are free from harm. As a voice for patient safety since 1997, it focuses on patient safety and healthcare workforce safety and disseminates strategies to prevent harm. In March 2017, it merged with IHI to use its combined knowledge and resources to focus and energize the patient safety agenda to build systems of safety across the continuum of care. IHI's patient safety programs include those that do the following:

- Galvanize the safety agenda through a multiorganizational initiative to create a national plan for the prevention of harm in healthcare.
- Engage leadership in change by providing strategic guidance and innovative thinking to health leaders.
- Foster cultures of safety in providing tactical tools to assess, identify areas of improvement, and implement system changes.
- Build skills by offering a range of programs to teach safety and improvement skills at every level.[163]

## Institute for Safe Medication Practices

For over 25 years, ISMP dedicated its efforts to learning about medication errors and understanding system-based causes while promulgating practical recommendations that can help healthcare providers, consumers, and the pharmaceutical industry prevent errors. ISMP is a patient safety organization (PSO) and provides confidential consulting services to healthcare systems to proactively evaluate medication systems or analyze medication-related sentinel events.[164] ISMP initiatives include ISMP Medication Safety Alert![165] newsletters for healthcare professionals, frequent educational programs, and teleconferences on current medication use issues. The organization develops posters, videos, patient brochures, books, and other resources and has valuable medication safety tools such as lists of high-alert drugs and potentially dangerous abbreviations.

## The Joint Commission

TJC accredits organizations across the continuum of care and leverages decades of knowledge and experience to develop and share literature from industry experts and safety scholars from other industries (e.g., nuclear power and air transportation). In addition to developing standards of care, TJC offers conceptual and practical frameworks for patient safety programs, methods, and practices (e.g., safety culture, high reliability, RCA, sentinel events).

In 2008, the Joint Commission Center for Transforming Healthcare was formed to pursue solutions to healthcare's most critical safety and quality problems. Useful resources specific to patient safety are described in the following list:

- *Patient Safety Systems.* This chapter from the *Comprehensive Accreditation Manual* is intended to help inform and educate hospitals about the importance and structure of an integrated patient safety system. Although the information is drawn from hospital patient safety, there is general discussion of leadership, patient safety culture, effective use of data, and proactive risk assessment to prevent harm.[166]
- *Oro 2.0 Resource Library.* This library provides more than 125 references and tools to help organizations learn about the 14 component areas of performance within the high reliability maturity model.[167]

## National Association for Healthcare Quality

The National Association for Healthcare Quality (NAHQ) is solely dedicated to the healthcare quality profession. It is the primary source for healthcare quality education for the healthcare quality professional and has defined the body of knowledge and essential competencies for the healthcare quality professional. Professional development opportunities that relate to patient safety are described in the discussion that follows. NAHQ's Healthcare Quality Competency Framework defines eight areas of competence and applies to all healthcare settings across the continuum of care.[168] The eight areas are quality leadership and integration; performance and process improvement; population health and care transitions; health data analytics; patient safety; regulatory and accreditation; quality review and accountability; and professional engagement.

The Healthcare Quality Competency Framework for patient safety helps healthcare quality professionals cultivate a safe healthcare environment by promoting safe practices, nurturing a just culture and improving processes that detect, mitigate, or prevent harm. Competencies include dimensions to assess patient safety culture, apply safety science principles and methods, identify and report patient safety risks and events, and collaborate to analyze patient safety risks and events. Within each dimension, descriptors are provided for advances and master proficiency levels.

## Occupational Safety and Health Administration

The U.S. Department of Labor's Occupational Safety and Health Administration (OSHA) is an agency that most healthcare professionals will be familiar with no matter where they work in the healthcare continuum. Congress created OSHA via the Occupational Safety and Health Act of 1970 to ensure safe working conditions. The Occupational Safety and Health Act covers most private sector employers and their workers, in addition to some public sector employers and workers in the 50 states and certain territories and jurisdictions under federal authority. OSHA created a suite of resources to help hospitals assess workplace safety needs, implement safety and health management systems, and enhance safe patient handling programs. These resources explore:

- *Understanding the problem.* Hospitals are hazardous workplaces and face unique challenges that contribute to the risk of injury and illness.
- *Safety and health management systems.* A safety and health management system can help build a culture of safety, reduce injuries, and save money.
- *Safe patient handling.* Safe patient handling programs, policies, and equipment can help cost-effectively reduce the biggest cause of workplace injuries.
- *Preventing workplace violence.* A comprehensive prevention program can help address the problem of workplace violence in healthcare facilities.[169]

The agency authorizes OSHA Training Institute Education Centers to deliver occupational safety and health training to the public and private sectors in all industries. There are also many other training resources and learning opportunities offered that will help workers as defined in OSHA standards to receive appropriate safety training related to any potentially hazardous activities. Learn more about OSHA's training resources on its website.

## Patient-Centered Outcomes Research Institute

Established in 2012, the Patient-Centered Outcomes Research Institute (PCORI) has three overarching goals:

1. "Substantially increase the quantity, quality, and timeliness of useful, trustworthy information available to support health decisions;
2. speed the implementation and use of patient-centered outcomes research (PCOR) evidence; and
3. influence clinical and healthcare research funded by others to be more patient-centered."[170(¶8)]

Its research priorities, established as national priorities for health, include:

- Increase evidence for existing interventions and emerging innovations in health—strengthen and expand ongoing clinical effectiveness research focused on both existing interventions and emerging innovations to improve healthcare practice, health outcomes, and health equity.
- Enhance infrastructure to accelerate patient-centered outcomes research—enhance the infrastructure that facilitates patient-centered outcomes research to drive lasting improvements in health and transformation of both the research enterprise and care delivery.
- Advance the science of dissemination, implementation, and health communication—advance the scientific evidence for and the practice of dissemination, implementation, and health communication to accelerate the movement of comparative clinical effectiveness research results into practice.
- Achieve health equity—expand stakeholder engagement, research, and dissemination approaches that lead to continued progress toward achieving health equity in the United States.
- Accelerate progress toward an integrated learning health system—foster actionable, timely, place-based, and transformative improvements in patient-centered experiences, care provision, and ultimately improved health outcomes through collaborative, multisectoral research to support a health system that serves the needs and preferences of individuals.[171(p2)]

## World Health Organization

The World Health Organization's *Patient Safety Curriculum Guide* presents an interprofessional educational approach for healthcare professionals. The guide offers tools and resources on the following topics:

1. What is patient safety
2. Why applying human factors is important for patient safety
3. Understanding systems and the effect of complexity on patient care
4. Being an effective team player
5. Learning from errors to prevent harm
6. Understanding and managing clinical risk
7. Using quality improvement methods to improve care
8. Engaging patients and caregivers
9. Infection prevention and control
10. Patient safety and invasive procedures
11. Improving medication safety[172(p28)]

See WHO facts related to patient safety in **Table 4.17**. Key points for patient safety are listed in **Box 4.6**.

**Table 4.17** Patient Safety: Key Facts

**Medication errors** are a leading cause of injury and avoidable harm in health care systems: globally, the cost associated with medication errors has been estimated at US$ 42 billion annually.

**Health care-associated infections** occur in 7 and 10 out of every 100 hospitalized patients in high-income countries and low- and middle-income countries, respectively.

**Unsafe surgical care procedures** cause complications in up to 25% of patients. Almost 7 million surgical patients suffer significant complications annually, 1 million of whom die during or immediately following surgery.

**Unsafe injections practices** in health care settings can transmit infections, including HIV and hepatitis B and C, and pose direct danger to patients and health care workers; they account for a burden of harm estimated at 9.2 million years of life lost to disability and death worldwide (known as Disability Adjusted Life Years [DALYs]).

**Diagnostic errors** occur in about 5% of adults in outpatient care settings, more than half of which have the potential to cause severe harm. Most people will suffer a diagnostic error in their lifetime.

**Unsafe transfusion practices** expose patients to the risk of adverse transfusion reactions and the transmission of infections. Data on adverse transfusion reactions from a group of 21 countries show an average incidence of 8.7 serious reactions per 100,000 distributed blood components.

**Radiation errors** involve overexposure to radiation and cases of wrong-patient and wrong-site identification. A review of 30 years of published data on safety in radiotherapy estimates that the overall incidence of errors is around 15 per 10,000 treatment courses.

**Sepsis** is frequently not diagnosed early enough to save a patient's life. Because these infections are often resistant to antibiotics, they can rapidly lead to deteriorating clinical conditions, affecting an estimated 31 million people worldwide and causing over 5 million deaths per year.

**Venous thromboembolism (blood clots)** is one of the most common and preventable causes of patient harm, contributing to one third of the complications attributed to hospitalization. Annually, there are an estimated 3.9 million cases in high-income countries and 6 million cases in low- and middle-income countries.

Reproduced from World Health Organization. Patient safety: key facts. Accessed April 9, 2022. https://www.who.int/news-room/fact-sheets/detail/patient-safety

---

**Box 4.6  Key Points: Patient Safety**

- Team STEPPS is based on team structure and four teachable, learnable skills: communication, leadership, situation monitoring, and mutual support.
- The Josie King Foundation offers a patient safety curriculum and offers different tools such as Care Journals, Nurse's Journals, Caregiver's Journals, the Patient Journal App, and *The Josie King Story* DVD.
- The NPSF Checklist for Getting the Right Diagnosis helps patients prepare for appointments with healthcare providers.
- Think Cultural Health features resources for healthcare professionals to learn about CLAS and its implications for safe and effective healthcare delivery.
- To complement learning activities, the healthcare quality professional should consider personal stories such as Frontline Innovators: Patient- and Family-Centered Care (AHRQ); Patient and Family-Centered Care: Partnerships for Quality and Safety (AHA); and Waiting Room (AHRQ).

# Transforming Patient Safety in the 21st Century

The national imperative and patient safety call for action emerged in the first decade of the 21st century. When the Healthcare Research and Quality Act of 1999 was enacted, the call to action was released in IOM's *To Err Is Human: Building a Safer Health System*. In 2000, there was the first National Summit on Medical Errors. Federal actions to reduce medical errors began to appear (e.g., patient safety grants and a national agenda). In 2001, evidence was published about what providers could do to make healthcare safer. By 2007, patient safety indicators were developed, the National Resource Center formed, and the AHRQ Patient Safety Network launched.[173]

In 2008, CMS announced a proposed rule to update payment policies and rates for hospitals under the inpatient prospective payment system. The rule included new additions of hospital-acquired infections for fiscal year 2009, including several conditions identified by NQF as "serious reportable adverse events" (also called "never events"). NQF considers a serious reportable event to be unambiguous, largely, if not entirely, preventable, serious, and any of the following:

- Adverse
- Indicative of a problem in a healthcare setting's safety systems
- Important for public credibility or public accountability
- Of concern to both the public and healthcare professionals and providers

- Clearly identifiable and measurable
- Feasible to include in a reporting system
- Of a nature such that the risk of occurrence is significantly influenced by the policies and procedures of the healthcare organization

The complete list of serious reportable events was updated in 2011 and is shown in **Table 4.18**.[174(pp iii–iv)] Not all categories are applicable to all organization types but generally serious reportable events apply to hospitals, outpatient/office-based surgery centers, ambulatory practice settings/office-based practices, and long-term care/skilled nursing facilities. Each state makes its own determination about which events providers should report. Payers like CMS may withhold payments to hospitals if any of these events occurs in an acute-care facility.

In 2010, the Affordable Care Act legislation required HHS to develop the National Quality Strategy (NQS) "to better meet the promise of providing all Americans with access to healthcare that is safe, effective, and affordable."[175(p2)] The development of the NQS would occur with input from various stakeholders to influence a realistic, achievable strategy. Thus, NQF convened the multistakeholder National Priorities Partnership comprising 48 public and private sector partners to provide input as HHS developed the NQF goals, measures, and strategic opportunities.[175(p2)]

In 2016, the *CMS Quality Strategy* pursued the NQS aims (six aims and the Triple Aim). HHS NQS's aims and priorities outlined in the strategy are displayed as **Figure 4.13**.[175(p11)] The CMS Quality Strategy Goal 1 is to "make care safer by reducing harm caused in the delivery of care."[176(p5)] For this goal, different foundational principles are used to support change and improvement including eliminating disparities, strengthening data structures and systems, enabling local innovations, and fostering learning organizations.[176(pp10-11)] Alternative payment structures promote quality goal attainment as Medicare will increasingly be making payments to providers that are tied to quality or value.

In September 2016, CMS furthered its commitment to patient safety when it awarded $347 million to continue progress toward a safer healthcare system. Awards were made to 16 national, regional, or state hospital associations, quality improvement organizations, and health system organizations for efforts in reducing hospital-acquired conditions and readmissions in the Medicare program. This is only part of broader efforts to transform the healthcare system into one that works better for the American people by delivering better care, spending smartly, and focusing on improved health status.

## National Strategy for Quality Improvement

The *National Strategy for Quality Improvement in Health Care* describes three broad aims of the NQS: better care, healthier people/healthy communities, and affordable care (i.e., the Triple Aim).[177] The NQS also considers six priority areas, one of which is to make care safer. The goals include the following:

- Improve patient, family, and caregiver experience of care related to quality, safety, and access across settings.
- In partnership with patients, families, and caregivers—using a shared decision-making process—develop culturally sensitive and understandable care plans.
- Enable patients and their families and caregivers to navigate, coordinate, and manage their care appropriately and effectively.[175]

The National Priorities Partnership envisions "healthcare that honors each individual patient and family, offering voice, control, choice, skills in self-care, and total transparency, and that can and does adapt to individual and family circumstances, and to differing cultures, languages, and social backgrounds."[178(p17)] The partners vowed to ensure all patients

- provide feedback on the experience of care that healthcare organizations will use to improve care;
- access tools and support systems to the effective navigation and management of care; and
- access information and assistance that enables informed decisions about treatment options.[178(p8)]

Addressing the need to improve the safe delivery of healthcare, Congress passed public and private sector efforts and generated landmark regulations and reports such as the Patient Safety and Quality Improvement Act of 2005, in response to IOM's groundbreaking report, *To Err Is Human*. In consultation with AHRQ, HHS delivered a final report on effective strategies to improve patient safety and reduce medical errors to Congress. Required by the Patient Safety and Quality Improvement Act, the report was made available for public review and comment and for review by the National Academy of Medicine. It outlined several strategies to accelerate progress in improving patient safety, including using analytic approaches in patient safety research, measurement, and practice improvement to monitor risk; implementing evidence-based practices in real-world settings through clinically useful tools

**Table 4.18** The NQF List of 29 Serious Reportable Events

**1. Surgical or Invasive Procedure Events**
1A. Surgery or other invasive procedure performed on the wrong site
1B. Surgery or other invasive procedure performed on the wrong patient
1C. Wrong surgical or other invasive procedure performed on a patient
1D. Unintended retention of a foreign object in a patient after surgery or other invasive procedure
1E. Intraoperative or immediately postoperative/postprocedure death in an American Society of Anesthesiologists Physical Status Classification System Class 1 patient

**2. Product or Device Events**
2A. Patient death or serious injury associated with the use of contaminated drugs, devices, or biologics provided by the healthcare setting
2B. Patient death or serious injury associated with the use or function of a device in patient care, in which the device is used or functions other than as intended
2C. Patient death or serious injury associated with intravascular air embolism that occurs while being cared for in a healthcare setting

**3. Patient Protection Events**
3A. Discharge or release of a patient/resident of any age who is unable to make decisions to anyone other than an authorized person
3B. Patient death or serious injury associated with patient elopement (disappearance)
3C. Patient suicide, attempted suicide, or self-harm that results in serious injury while being cared for in a healthcare setting

**4. Care Management Events**
4A. Patient death or serious injury associated with a medication error (e.g., errors involving the wrong drug, wrong dose, wrong patient, wrong time, wrong rate, wrong preparation, or wrong route of administration)
4B. Patient death or serious injury associated with unsafe administration of blood products
4C. Maternal death or serious injury associated with labor or delivery in a low-risk pregnancy while being cared for in a healthcare setting
4D. Death or serious injury of a neonate associated with labor or delivery in a low-risk pregnancy
4E. Patient death or serious injury associated with a fall while being cared for in a healthcare setting
4F. Any Stage III, Stage IV, and unstageable pressure ulcers acquired after admission/presentation to a healthcare setting
4G. Artificial insemination with the wrong donor sperm or wrong egg
4H. Patient death or serious injury resulting from the irretrievable loss of an irreplaceable biological specimen
4I. Patient death or serious injury resulting from failure to follow up or communicate laboratory, pathology, or radiology test results

**5. Environmental Events**
5A. Patient or staff death or serious injury associated with an electric shock in the course of a patient care process in a healthcare setting
5B. Any incident in which systems designated for oxygen or another gas to be delivered to the patient contain no gas, the wrong gas, or are contaminated by toxic substances
5C. Patient or staff death or serious injury associated with a burn incurred from any source in the course of a patient-care process in a healthcare setting
5D. Patient death or serious injury associated with the use of physical restraints or bedrails while being cared for in a healthcare setting

**6. Radiologic Events**
6A. Death or serious injury of a patient or staff associated with the introduction of a metallic object in the MRI area

**7. Potential Criminal Events**
7A. Any instance of care ordered or provided by someone impersonating a physician, nurse, pharmacist, or other licensed healthcare provider
7B. Abduction of a patient/resident of any age
7C. Sexual abuse/assault on a patient or staff member within or on the grounds of a healthcare setting
7D. Death or serious injury of a patient or staff member resulting from a physical assault (i.e., battery) that occurs within or on the grounds of a healthcare setting

and infrastructure; encouraging the development of learning health systems that integrate continuous learning and improvement in day-to-day operations; and encouraging the use of patient safety strategies outlined in the National Action Plan by the National Steering Committee for Patient Safety.[179]

## Patient Safety Strategies and Quality Improvement

In December 2021, the U.S. Department of Health & Human Services delivered a final report to Congress on effective strategies to improve patient safety and

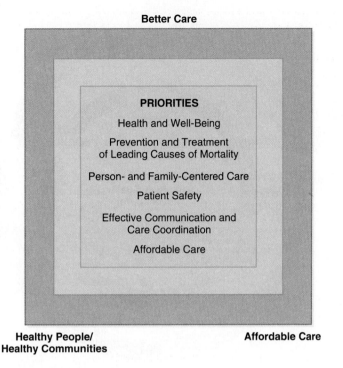

**Figure 4.13** HHS National Quality Strategy Aims and Priorities

Reproduced from National Priorities Partnership. *Input to the Secretary of Health and Human Services on Priorities for the National Quality Strategy*. Washington, DC: National Quality Forum; 2011:11. Copyright 2011, with permission.

reduce medical errors. Required by the Patient Safety Act of 2005, the report was made available for public review and comment and review by the National Academy of Medicine.[180] A learning system framework was used to support the different strategies and initiatives to systematically integrate data with evidence to develop and put into practice new knowledge to improve the quality, safety, and efficiency of care. The work of PSOs and providers under the Patient Safety Act serves as a national learning system for patient safety improvement (**Figure 4.14**).

Other work implemented under the Patient Safety Act immediately upon enactment included operationalizing the network of patient safety databases and creating an inventory of private and public sector patient safety reporting systems to establish an evidence base for developing what are now known as the AHRQ Common Formats for Event Reporting.

## Patient Safety Organizations

At the turn of the 21st century, the IOM sparked national attention to avoidable medical errors. PSOs evolved from public and private sector concerns. The Patient Safety and Quality Improvement Act of 2005 conferred privilege and confidentiality protections for providers who choose to work with PSOs.[181] This promotes shared learning from medical errors and improves patient safety across the nation. To

implement the Patient Safety Act, HHS issued the Patient Safety and Quality Improvement final rule.[182] These authorized the creation of PSOs to improve quality and safety through the collection and analysis of data on patient events.[183] Now many organizations such as NQF, AHRQ, and CMS are working together to ensure the success of the work accomplished by PSOs. As of December 2021, there are 95 active PSOs in 29 states and the District of Columbia currently listed by AHRQ.[184]

With few exceptions, the Act permits any entity to become a federally listed PSO if it can meet the requirements. The requirements include that the entity must submit certain certifications to HHS. The initial and continued listing process is based primarily on self-attestation by the PSO's authorized official. The statutory framework and regulatory approach to PSO listing are designed to minimize burden and maximize protection of the confidential reporting relationship between PSOs and the providers they serve. Patient safety organizations share the goal of improving the quality and safety of healthcare delivery. Eight patient safety activities are carried out by or on behalf of PSOs or healthcare providers, namely,

1. efforts to improve patient safety and the quality of healthcare delivery;
2. collection and analysis of patient safety work product (PSWP);

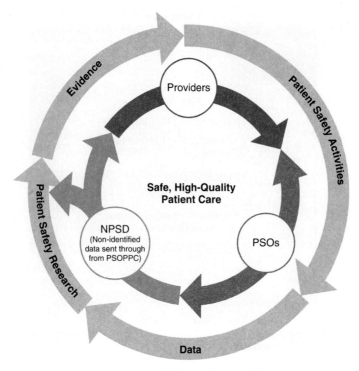

**Figure 4.14** The Patient Safety and Quality Improvement Act of 2005: A National Learning System

*Notes*: NPSD = network of patient safety databases; PSO = patient safety organization; PSOPPC = PSO Privacy Protection Center
Reproduced from *Strategies to Improve Patient Safety: Final Report to Congress Required by the Patient Safety and Quality Improvement Act of 2005*. Rockville, MD: Agency for Healthcare Research and Quality; December 2021. AHRQ publication 22-0009. https://pso.ahrq.gov/sites/default/files/wysiwyg/strategies-improve-patient-safety-final.pdf

3. development and dissemination of information regarding patient safety, such as recommendations, protocols, or information regarding best practices;
4. use of PSWP to encourage a culture of safety and provide feedback and assistance to effectively minimize patient risk;
5. maintenance of procedures to preserve confidentiality with respect to PSWP;
6. provision of appropriate security measures with respect to PSWP;
7. use of qualified staff; and
8. activities related to the operation of a patient safety evaluation system and the provision of feedback to participants in a patient safety evaluation system.[184]

Organizations eligible to become PSOs include public or private entities, for-profit or not-for-profit entities (e.g., ECRI and ISMP), provider entities such as hospital chains, and other entities that establish special components to serve as PSOs. By providing privilege and confidentiality, PSOs create a secure environment in which clinicians and healthcare organizations can collect, aggregate, and analyze data. Privileged information is not subject to disclosure or discovery and cannot be asked about in testimony, thereby permitting more candid discussions about quality of care that may reduce the risks and hazards associated with patient care.

## Outside the Box

Since the IOM started delivering reports on patient safety in 2000, various national organizations, state and federal agencies, accreditation organizations, and professional associations have focused on the identification of safe practices and strategies for organizational or system-wide implementation. In addition, many states established coalitions to promote patient safety. For example, the Connecticut Center for Patient Safety works to "1) Promote patient safety, 2) Improve the quality of health care &, 3) Protect the rights of patients."[185(¶1)] Originally organized by residents who had been harmed by the healthcare system, it provides useful tools and resources for consumers. The Oregon Patient Safety Commission was one of the first legislatively mandated organizations to reduce the risk of serious adverse events occurring in Oregon's healthcare system and encourages a culture of patient safety through patient safety reporting, early discussion and resolution, and quality improvement initiatives. The commission "offers a constructive space for healthcare facilities, providers, and patients to build a culture of safer care."[186(¶2)]

Partnership for Patients: Better Care, Lower Costs is a public–private partnership to help improve the quality, safety, and affordability of healthcare for all Americans. Using as much as $1 billion in new funding provided by the Affordable Care Act and leveraging several ongoing programs, HHS works with a wide variety of public and private partners to achieve the two core goals of this partnership: keep patients from getting injured or sicker in the healthcare system, and help patients heal without complication by improving transitions from acute-care hospitals to other care settings, such as home or a skilled nursing facility. Its mission is to help patients take care into their own hands. The partnership uses Hospital Improvement Innovation Networks (HIINs) that work at the regional, state, national, or hospital system level to sustain and accelerate national progress and momentum toward continued harm reduction in the Medicare program.

Beyond reducing harm caused in hospitals, the Partnership for Patients is an important test of what can occur when the nation acts as one to address a major national health problem. The CMS Innovation Center dedicated more than $500 million to test models of safer care delivery and promote implementation of best practices in patient safety. The Innovation Center "allows the Medicare and Medicaid programs to test models that improve care, lower costs, and better align payment systems to support patient-centered practice."[187(¶1)] In addition, CMS provided $500 million for a community-based care transition program created by the Affordable Care Act to support hospitals and community-based organizations in helping Medicare beneficiaries at high risk for readmission to the hospital to transition safely from the hospital to other care settings. Since 2015, through the Partnership for Patients, 17 hospital engagement networks collaborated to improve patient safety, working with 3500 hospitals, resulting in harm reduction. Since 2016, 16 HIINs worked with 4000 hospitals to further integrate evidence-based safety practices, working with hospitals, providers, and the broader caregiver community, resulting in reductions in all-cause patient harm and readmissions.[177,188]

## The Quadruple Aim

The Triple Aim was introduced by Berwick, Nolan, and Whittington—improving the experience of care, improving the health of populations, and reducing per capita costs of healthcare.[189] Since introduced, thinking about the Triple Aim continues to evolve. A fourth aim—creating a Quadruple Aim—was proposed by Sikka, Morath, and Leape who suggested the added aim of improving the experience of providing care, including workforce engagement and workforce safety.[190] Bodenheimer and Sinsky[191] and more recently Itchhaporia,[192] suggested that the added goal

be improving the work life of healthcare providers, including clinicians and staff.

Organizations such as the AHA continue advancing work in patient safety using the Quadruple Aim to frame principles for practice. The AHA Physician Alliance reaffirmed its commitment to creating safe and highly reliable healthcare organizations to address individual, environmental, and systemic factors that contribute to burnout and to foster resilience and well-being.[193] CMS reframed the aims simply as *better care, smarter spending, healthier people*, as the federal government extends financial support for innovation and efforts continue to improve the healthcare delivery system in the United States. In fact, health outcomes are improving, and adverse events are decreasing as patient safety improves dramatically, thanks in part to the Partnership for Patients. From 2012 to 2015, patient harm fell by 17%, saving 50,000 lives and billions of dollars.[194]

## Patient-Centered Care

Consumers are becoming more engaged in healthcare decision making and are more willing to tell their stories to the public when things do not go right. One of the most poignant stories was the Josie King incident. In 2001, King was 18 months old when she died in a hospital as the result of a cascade of errors including not receiving enough fluids, use of narcotics, and lack of engagement with family members who requested additional assistance due to their concern about Josie's condition. Josie's mother, Sorrel King, later went public with the findings about the breakdowns leading to her daughter's death at a premier medical system in Baltimore, Maryland. The Josie King Foundation was established with the mission to "prevent others from dying or being harmed by medical errors. By uniting healthcare providers and consumers, and funding innovative safety programs, we hope to create a culture of patient safety, together."[195(¶3)]

The Patient Safety Movement Foundation, founded in 2014 by Joe Kiani, is a grassroots collaboration dedicated to eliminating medical errors. Its mission is "focusing to eliminate preventable harm and death in healthcare across the world by creating a sense of urgency and unifying humanity."[196] Its vision is zero preventable deaths by 2030. Its Actionable Patient Safety Solutions provide evidence-based summaries of best practices for the most common safety issues, in language that is easily understood by patients.

Healthcare professionals respect and include patients and families in decision making. They keep the patient and the family at the center of all that they do. Research suggests that clinicians working with patients and their families can contribute to a better understanding of their role and responsibilities related to safety. A Cochrane systematic review including 115 controlled studies representing 34,444 research participants reported that providing patients with decision aids

- improves knowledge regarding their options,
- reduces the decisional conflict,
- increases active role in decision making,
- improves accurate risk perceptions of possible benefits and harms among patients,
- increases the likelihood that choices are more consistent with their informed values, and
- enhances communication between the patient and the clinicians.[197(q15)]

Activated patients—those who manage their own care by having the knowledge, skills, and confidence—are shown to achieve better clinical outcomes.[198]

The healthcare quality professional's role includes support of a person-centered approach in developing safety programs and fostering patient and staff engagement. Safety can be advanced through the consideration of different aspects of clinical excellence such as psychological safety (creating an environment where people are comfortable and have opportunities to raise concerns and questions), leadership (facilitating and monitoring teamwork, improvement, respect, and psychological safety), and transparency (openly sharing data and other information concerning safe, respectful, and reliable care with staff, partners, and families). These and other aspects are shown in the Framework for Clinical Excellence (**Figure 4.15**).

As consumers become more empowered through consumer-directed, value-based healthcare, they will demand more from healthcare organizations. Examples of initiatives to consider in program development for consumer-directed healthcare include the following:

- *Speak Up Program.* TJC empowers consumers by providing educational materials and tools as navigational aids for complex healthcare systems. In 2002, in response to a public outcry regarding unsafe practices, TJC, in collaboration with CMS, launched a national campaign to urge consumers to take an active role in identifying and preventing healthcare errors. The goal of the initiative was to empower consumers to become active, involved, informed, and engaged participants in their care. Speak Up animated videos and posters can be shared with all patients, regardless of their age or reading ability. Animated videos address issues like discrimination, care, antibiotics, doctor's office visits, and surgery.[199]
- *OpenNotes.* Since 2010, this national initiative funded by the Robert Wood Johnson Foundation

and the Commonwealth Fund gives patients access to the visit notes written by their doctors, nurses, or other clinicians. Potential positive effects of using an open medical record include transparency, catching errors in the notes, preventing diagnostic delay, taking medications as prescribed, encouraging patients to speak up, engaging informal caregivers, shared decision making, and enhancing trust. Effective in 2021, all U.S. healthcare systems are required to electronically share clinician's visit notes with patients. This is required as part of the information blocking section of the 21st Century Cures Act (this does not apply to psychotherapy notes and information compiled for use in civil, criminal, or administrative actions).[200,201] OpenNotes has been adopted by facilities and systems of care such as the Department of Veterans Affairs and Geisinger Health Systems. The next generation of OpenNotes is *Our*Notes, which has goals to engage patients (and often their families) more actively in their care and help make visits more focused and efficient for both patients and clinicians by allowing patients to contribute to the visit/encounter note.[202]

What is known is that engagement results in better patient safety outcomes.[203] The healthcare quality professional can work with others in the organization to determine how elements of engagement can be incorporated into strategic intent, the safety plan, and other related activities (e.g., structure to support engagement, needed skills, awareness building, and practices).

One of the six aims of a quality healthcare system is equity. In a perfect world, equitable care does not vary based on a patient's individual characteristics such as sex, gender identity, ethnicity, geographic location, or socioeconomic status. However, disparities exist and include (1) the way healthcare systems are organized and operate; (2) patient attitudes and behaviors; and (3) healthcare provider biases, prejudices, and uncertainty when treating Black people, Indigenous people, and other people of color.[204(pp2-3)] Medical errors can result from ineffective patient–provider communication and the inability of the treating providers to overcome cultural and linguistic barriers. Inequities may result in distrust of healthcare providers and systems.[205] Effective and safe medical treatment depends on good communication between the healthcare team and the patient.

Cultural competence is an important component of patient safety. Full buy-in from the organization's C-suite is essential to the success of any cultural competency or health equity initiative. Lack of cultural

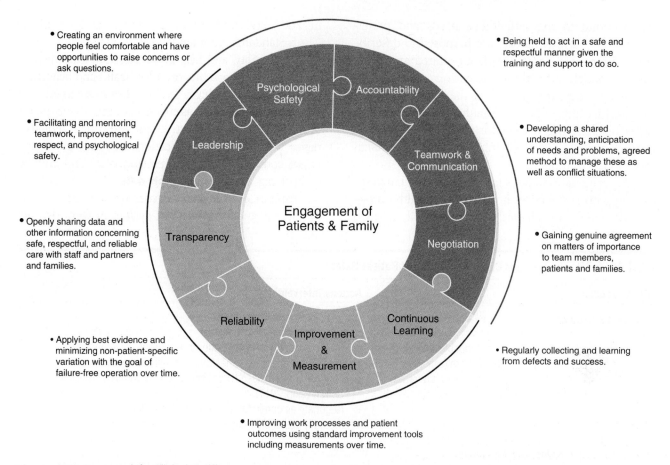

Creating an environment where people feel comfortable and have opportunities to raise concerns or ask questions.

Facilitating and mentoring teamwork, improvement, respect, and psychological safety.

Openly sharing data and other information concerning safe, respectful, and reliable care with staff and partners and families.

Applying best evidence and minimizing non-patient-specific variation with the goal of failure-free operation over time.

Being held to act in a safe and respectful manner given the training and support to do so.

Developing a shared understanding, anticipation of needs and problems, agreed method to manage these as well as conflict situations.

Gaining genuine agreement on matters of importance to team members, patients and families.

Regularly collecting and learning from defects and success.

Improving work processes and patient outcomes using standard improvement tools including measurements over time.

Psychological Safety · Accountability · Leadership · Teamwork & Communication · Transparency · Engagement of Patients & Family · Negotiation · Reliability · Improvement & Measurement · Continuous Learning

**Figure 4.15** Framework for Clinical Excellence

Reprinted from Frankel A, Haraden C, Federico F, Lenoci-Edwards J. A *Framework for Safe, Reliable, and Effective Care*. White paper. Cambridge, MA: Institute for Healthcare Improvement; 2017, with permission. www.IHI.org. © Institute for Healthcare Improvement and Safe and Reliable Healthcare.

humility affects healthcare and patient safety. Action is needed. TJC proposed that improving quality and safety helps address healthcare disparities by taking four actions to ensure health equity:

1. Collect and stratify quality and safety performance data specific to the communities that [the] organization serves and develop communication channels that enable listening and learning.
2. Analyze stratified data and community feedback to identify healthcare disparities and opportunities for improvement.
3. Commit to achieving diversity and inclusion as an important step toward addressing healthcare disparities.
4. Undertake initiatives to rectify healthcare disparities by building sustainable business cases.[206(pp1-4)]

Cross and colleagues defined *cultural competence* as "a set of congruent behaviors, attitudes and policies that come together in a system, agency, or amongst professionals and enables that system, agency and those professionals to work effectively in cross-cultural situations."[207(p iv)] Based on 2018 Census Bureau data, 67.3 million U.S. residents speak a language other than English at home. That translates to 45% of individuals in California, 36% in Texas, and 34% in New Mexico.[208] Patients with low English proficiency (LEP) have increased risk for adverse events. Individuals with LEP have limited access to telehealth,[209] experience higher instances of adverse events involving physical harm (49.1% compared to 29.5% without LEP),[210] and are more likely to have verification of medications disregarded leading to medication errors.[211] Communication is the third most common root cause of sentinel events and unexpected events, which cause death or serious physical or psychological injury.[212]

Because of inequities, individuals across the United States are unable to reach their optimal health potential. Inequities in healthcare are influenced by *social determinants of health*, "non-medical factors that influence health outcomes. They are the conditions in which people are born, grow, live, work and age, and a wider set of forces and systems shaping the conditions of daily life."[213(¶1)] One of the most modifiable factors is culturally and linguistically appropriate services broadly defined as being "about respect and responsiveness: Respect the whole individual and respond to the individual's needs and preferences."[214](¶1) Various models are proposed to describe cultural competence as a patient-centered approach. All the models have these dimensions in common: knowledge (e.g., understanding the meaning of culture and its importance to healthcare delivery), attitudes (e.g., having respect for variations in cultural norms), and skills (e.g., eliciting the patient's explanatory models of illness).[215](p2)

The National Standards for Culturally and Linguistically Appropriate Services in Health and Health Care—the National CLAS Standards—were originally released in 2001 and updated in 2013.[216] The 15 National CLAS Standards are intended to advance health equity, improve quality, and help eliminate healthcare disparities by establishing a blueprint for health and healthcare organizations to achieve equity. These standards are increasingly recognized as effective for improving quality of care, patient safety, effectiveness, and patient centeredness.[216] The standards and actions that an organization might consider to improve patient safety and cultural competency are shown in **Table 4.19**.

Patient-centered care focuses on offering support to patients and their support system in ways that are

**Table 4.19** The National CLAS Standards and Patient Safety

| CLAS Standard | Actions/Interventions |
|---|---|
| **Principal Standard** | |
| 1. Provide effective, equitable, understandable, and respectful quality care and services that are responsive to diverse cultural health beliefs and practices, preferred languages, health literacy, and other communication needs. | ▪ Create a more welcoming, safe, and inclusive environment that contributes to improved healthcare quality for lesbian, gay, bisexual, and transgender patients and their families (The Joint Commission, 2011).<br>▪ Negotiate an understanding within which a safe, effective, and mutually agreeable treatment plan can be implemented. |
| **Governance, Leadership, and Workforce** | |
| 2. Advance and sustain organizational governance and leadership that promotes CLAS and health equity through policy, practices, and allocated resources. | ▪ Ensure diversity to reflect shifting demographics and populations served in the composition of the C-suite executives and board of directors to diversity of thought, experience, and background in the organization's management and boardroom.<br>▪ Create a policy whereby interpreters must be provided to patients and/or family members when obtaining informed consent, having discussions about advance healthcare directives, gathering critical clinical information (e.g., patient's medical history), explaining the plan of care (e.g., procedures), and providing updates on the treatment plan (e.g., discharge planning, care transitions). |
| 3. Recruit, promote, and support a culturally and linguistically diverse governance, leadership, and workforce that are responsive to the population in the service area. | ▪ Advertise for vacancies through targeted publications (e.g., the Institute for Diversity in Healthcare).<br>▪ Develop a board recruitment strategy so the board membership is representative of the community. |
| 4. Educate and train governance, leadership, and the workforce in culturally and linguistically appropriate policies and practices on an ongoing basis. | ▪ Supply clinicians with current information regarding susceptibility of particular racial/ethnic groups to certain diseases and conditions and possible lifestyles and dietary habits that impact health or make it difficult for patients to follow treatment plans.<br>▪ Create a core curriculum on cultural competence in healthcare to improve the safety and quality for onboarding new board members and staff.<br>▪ Improve the ability of clinicians to communicate effectively with their patients directly or via interpreters through training in the following:<br>• Communication skills (including how to effectively negotiate a treatment plan which the patient will be able and willing to follow).<br>• Cultural awareness (understanding and acceptance of beliefs and lifestyles different from their own). |

*(continues)*

**Table 4.19** The National CLAS Standards and Patient Safety *(continued)*

| CLAS Standard | Actions/Interventions |
|---|---|
| **Communication and Language Assistance** | |
| 5. Offer language assistance to individuals who have LEP and/or other communication needs, at no cost to them, to facilitate timely access to all healthcare and services. | ▪ Ensure readily available interpreters in the emergency department for LEP patients to avoid delays in care resulting in adverse consequences in the absence of any language assistance service.<br>▪ Use Ask Me 3 from IHI for information and resources to educate patients and providers about health literacy and improving patient–provider communication. |
| 6. Inform all individuals of the availability of language assistance services clearly and in their preferred language, verbally and in writing. | ▪ Put signage in public areas describing the organization's language assistance services and how to access interpretation services.<br>▪ Provide information about language assistance services in admission packets for ambulatory, emergency, and acute care. |
| 7. Ensure the competence of individuals providing language assistance, recognizing that the use of untrained individuals and/or minors as interpreters should be avoided. | ▪ Conduct interpreter certification through oral and written proficiency tests of their knowledge of conversational and medical language in both English and the language of interpretation. Untrained interpreters may lack knowledge of medical terminology and confidentiality. Untrained interpreters are more likely to commit errors in interpretation that can lead to adverse clinical consequences.<br>▪ The presence of interpreters may inhibit discussions of sensitive issues, such as domestic violence, substance use, psychiatric illness, and sexual activity. |
| 8. Provide easy-to-understand print and multimedia materials and signage in the languages commonly used by the populations in the service area. | ▪ Create an indexed resource library of educational materials in threshold and/or preferred languages of patient populations served. Integrate it with the electronic health record if technology permits.<br>▪ Use digital health products such as customized medication instruction programs that provide easy-to-understand, ethnically appropriate medical information on prescribed medications and access to videos that demonstrate how to take medications prescribed.<br>▪ Develop a shared vocabulary. |
| **Engagement, Continuous Improvement, and Accountability** | |
| 9. Establish culturally and linguistically appropriate goals, policies, and management accountability, and infuse them throughout the organization's planning and operations. | ▪ Designate a high-ranking administrator with decision-making power as director of diversity.<br>▪ Form a diversity council or committee to oversee the implementation of the cultural competency program.<br>▪ Include cultural competency as a clearly stated focus in quality plans with measures and goals to evaluate success and progress. |
| 10. Conduct ongoing assessments of the organization's CLAS-related activities and integrate CLAS-related measures into measurement and continuous quality improvement activities. | ▪ Conduct an annual organizational cultural competency assessment using an established tool.<br>▪ Self-audit for cultural and linguistic competency prior to embarking upon a cultural competency initiative. Include items related to safety such as incident reporting and use of interpreters.<br>▪ Develop a disparities dashboard. |
| 11. Collect and maintain accurate and reliable demographic data to monitor and evaluate the impact of CLAS on health equity and outcomes and to inform service delivery. | ▪ Create standardized screening, admission, and intake forms that reflect CLAS-driven demographic data.<br>▪ Collect data on race and ethnicity, country of origin, and language.<br>▪ Stratify data by race/ethnicity, payer proxy, sex at birth, and gender.<br>▪ Gather and compare outcomes statistics for specific populations served with those of the general or majority population for those who do not complete treatment or greater number of repeat clinical presentations of the same complaints. |

**Table 4.19**  **The National CLAS Standards and Patient Safety**                    *(continued)*

| CLAS Standard | Actions/Interventions |
|---|---|
| 12. Conduct regular assessments of community health assets and needs and use the results to plan and implement services that respond to the cultural and linguistic diversity of populations in the service area. | ■ Use U.S. Census data to create organizational snapshot of communities and populations served.<br>■ Use HHS Office of Minority Health "Minority Population Profiles" (2021) for key articles, reports and resources that touch upon diseases, social determinants of health, racial justice, and other important topics.<br>■ Equip the medical center and satellite health centers with interpretation equipment and training for staff.<br>■ Create and distribute community health indicators highlighting population health and disparities. |
| 13. Partner with the community to design, implement, and evaluate policies, practices, and services to ensure cultural and linguistic appropriateness. | ■ Develop local partnerships; partnerships with other organizations; and developing collaborations.<br>■ Maintain a critical mass of influential investigators interested in disparities.<br>■ Focus on conditions prevalent in the community, such as diabetes and cardiovascular disease.<br>■ Develop and implement community-based programs in an ethnically and culturally diverse community.<br>■ Develop partnerships between data analysts and clinical champions to address organizational safety concerns. |
| 14. Create conflict and grievance resolution processes that are culturally and linguistically appropriate to identify, prevent, and resolve conflicts or complaints. | ■ Embed cultural and linguistic elements for complaints and grievances on the complaint form (e.g., race/ethnicity and language spoken/preferred language). This permits analysis of complaints by demographic characteristics of complainants that may be contributing to disparities.<br>■ Create a patient and family relations program with representation from patients and family. |
| 15. Communicate the organization's progress in implementing and sustaining CLAS to all stakeholders, constituents, and the general public. | ■ Develop the business case to address disparities in the healthcare organization or system of care.<br>■ Conduct interactive grand rounds for clinical staff and faculty to develop skills for culturally competent care delivery.<br>■ Report equity measures related to relevant safety activities on the organization's website. |

Data from Alliance for Board Diversity. Missing pieces report: the 2021 Board Diversity Census of women and minorities on Fortune 500 boards. Deloitte Center for Board Effectiveness. Published 2021. Accessed December 8, 2021. https://corpgov.law.harvard.edu/2021/06/25/the-board-diversity-census-of-women-and-minorities-on-fortune-500-boards/; Betancourt JR, Green AR, King RR, et al. *Improving Quality and Achieving Equity: A Guide for Hospital Leaders.* Boston, MA: The Disparities Solutions Center at Massachusetts General Hospital; 2008. Accessed December 8, 2021. http://www.rwjf.org/en/library/research /2008/01/improving-quality-and-achieving-equity.html; California Health Care Foundation. Digitizing the safety net: high tech opportunities for the underserved. Published 2016. Accessed December 8, 2021. http://www.chcf.org/publications/2016/02/digitizing-safety-net; Institute for Healthcare Improvement. Ask me 3: Good questions for your good health. Accessed December 8, 2021. http://www.ihi.org/resources/Pages/Tools/Ask-Me-3-Good -Questions-for-Your-Good-Health.aspx; The Joint Commission. *Advancing Effective Communication, Cultural Competence, and Patient- and Family-Centered Care for the Lesbian, Gay, Bisexual, and Transgender (LGBT) Community: A Field Guide.* Oak Brook, IL: The Joint Commission; October 2011. Accessed December 8, 2021. https://www.jointcommission.org/-/media/tjc/documents/resources/patient-safety-topics/health-equity/lgbtfieldguide_web_linked_verpdf.pdf? db=web&hash=FD725DC02CFE6E4F21A35EBD839BBE97&hash=FD725DC02CFE6E4F21A35EBD839BBE97; Salimbene S. CLAS A-Z: a practical guide for implementing the national standards for culturally and linguistically appropriate services (CLAS) in health care. Published 2001. Accessed December 8, 2021. https://minorityhealth.hhs.gov/assets/pdf/checked/CLAS_a2z.pdf; and U.S. Department of Health & Human Services, Office of Minority Health. Minority health profiles. Published 2021. Accessed December 8, 2021. https://www.minorityhealth.hhs.gov/omh/browse.aspx?lvl=2&lvlID=26

meaningful during the delivery of healthcare services. Healthcare quality professionals can inspire others to provide "care that is respectful of, and responsive to, individual patient preferences, needs and values, and ensuring that patient values guide all clinical decisions" through systematic quality and safety efforts.[1(p40)]

**Box 4.7** shows key points to transforming patient safety.

---

### Box 4.7 Key Points: Transforming Patient Safety in the 21st Century

- Provide leadership in the creation and maintenance of a safety culture throughout the organization.
- Assess needs, develop, and deploy an enterprise-wide safety plan.
- Spread safety concepts using principles such as human factors engineering, high reliability, just culture, and systems thinking.
- Eliminate errors and reduce harm to deliver on the promise of the delivery of care, treatment, and services in a safe environment free of errors and harm.

---

## Summary

Healthcare quality professionals accelerate progress in improving and responding to new challenges for patient safety, including using analytic approaches in patient safety, measurement, and performance improvement. This is accomplished by using evidence-based practices and encouraging the development of learning organizations that integrate continuous learning and the principles of improvement science in day-to-day practice. Attention is given to planning, development, implementation, and evaluation, as well as to continuous improvement. In summary, the following tenets are imperative for an effective patient safety program in any healthcare organization:

- Healthcare leaders set the vision, mission, purpose, intention, and direction and provide the resources necessary to adopt evidence-based patient safety practices.
- Error prevention and harm reduction are the shared responsibility of the board of directors, executive leaders, medical leaders, healthcare personnel, and the patient and family. At every intersection, there is an opportunity to take different actions to mitigate risks and reduce harm.
- Organizations create and maintain a fair and just culture by being mindful, taking actions to reduce preventable errors and mitigate risks, and emphasizing learning to support the workforce in eliminating or preventing future errors.
- Safety program development, implementation, and evaluation considerations include
  - engaging and empowering patients and their support systems;
  - identifying needs and priorities at the organization, department, unit, team, and individual levels;
  - determining how technology can support the program;
  - integrating efforts with risk and infection prevention and control;
  - monitoring and analyzing close calls, near misses, and errors;
  - supporting ethical practices in patient safety using fair and just culture principles; and
  - identifying strategies for adoption, spread, and evaluation of evidence-based safety interventions and innovations.

Patient safety gets better through learning and doing using advanced technology, teamwork, and communication approaches proven to mitigate errors, reduce harm, and save lives. Healthcare quality professionals can inspire, collaborate, and lead on these efforts. They possess the unique experience and expertise to advance safety practices in their organizations and the community at large. This can be accomplished by bringing knowledge, promising practices, improvement tools, and safety innovations to the healthcare setting.

## References

1. Committee on Quality of Health Care in America and Institute of Medicine. *Crossing the Quality Chasm: A New Health System for the 21st Century*. Washington, DC: National Academies Press. 2001.
2. Hughes RG. Tools and strategies for quality improvement and patient safety (Chapter 44). In: Hughes RG, ed. *Patient Safety and Quality: An Evidence-Based Handbook for Nurses*. Rockville, MD: Agency for Healthcare Research and Quality (US); 2008: 3-1-3-39. Accessed December 11, 2021. https://www.ncbi.nlm.nih.gov/books/NBK2682/
3. Kohn LT, Corrigan J, Donaldson MS. *To Err Is Human: Building a Safer Health System*. Washington, DC: National Academies Press; 1999.
4. Aspden P, Corrigan J, Wolcott J, Erickson SM, eds. *Patient Safety: Achieving a New Standard for Care*. Washington, DC: National Academies Press; 2004.
5. Clancy CM, Farquhar MB, Sharp BA. Patient safety in nursing practice. *J Nurs Care Qual*. 2005;20(3):193-197.
6. Agency for Healthcare Research and Quality Patient Safety Network. Glossary. Accessed December 17, 2021. https://psnet.ahrq.gov/glossary-0

7. Emanuel L, Berwick D, Conway J, et al. What exactly is patient safety? In: Henriksen K, Battles JB, Keyes MA, Grady ML, eds. *Advances in Patient Safety: New Directions and Alternative Approaches.* Rockville, MD: Agency for Healthcare Research and Quality; 2008:1-18.

8. Angood P, Colchamiro E, Lyzenga A, Marinelarena M. *Meeting of the National Quality Forum Patient Safety Team.* Washington, DC. Unpublished; August 2009.

9. World Health Organization. Patient safety. Accessed December 11, 2021. https://www.who.int/teams/integrated-health-services/patient-safety/about

10. Marx D. Patient safety and the "Just Culture": A primer for health care executives. Published April 17, 2001. Accessed December 13, 2021. http://www.chpso.org/sites/main/files/file-attachments/marx_primer.pdf

11. Pham JC, Thierry G, Pronovost PJ. What to do with healthcare incident reporting systems. *J Public Health Res.* 2013;2:e27. doi:10.4081/jphr.2013.e27

12. Institute for Safe Medication Practices. Building patient safety skills: common pitfalls when conducting a root cause analysis. *ISMP Medication Safety Alert!* 2011;9(3):1-4.

13. Becher EC, Chassin MR. Improving the quality of health care: Who will lead? *Health Aff.* 2001;20(5):164-179. doi:10.1377/hlthaff.20.5.164

14. Substance Abuse and Mental Health Services Administration. *Key Substance Use and Mental Health Indicators in the United States: Results from the 2020 National Survey on Drug Use and Health.* HHS publication PEP21-07-01-003; NSDUH Series H-56. Rockville MD: Center for Behavioral Health Statistics and Quality, Substance Abuse and Mental Health Services Administration; 2021. Accessed December 13, 2021. https://www.samhsa.gov/data/

15. Berwick DM, Hackbarth AD. Eliminating waste in US health care. *JAMA.* 2012;307(14):1513-1516. doi:10.1001/jama.2012.362

16. Shrank WH, Rogstad TL, Parekh N. Waste in the US health care system: estimated costs and potential for savings. *JAMA.* 2019;322(15):1501-1509. doi:10.1001/jama.2019.13978

17. Dietz DW, Padula WV, Zheng H, Pronovost PJ. Costs of defects in surgical care: a call to eliminate defects in value. *NEJM Catalyst.* Published November 23, 2021. Accessed December 16, 2021. https://catalyst.nejm.org/doi/full/10.1056/CAT.21.0305

18. Association for the Advancement of Medical Instrumentation. *ANSI/AAMI HE75, 2009 R (2013): Human Factors Engineering—Design of Medical Devices.* Arlington VA: AAMI; 2013.

19. Agency for Healthcare Research and Quality. PSNet: Human factors engineering. Published 2019. Accessed January 30, 2022. https://psnet.ahrq.gov/primer/human-factors-engineering

20. Deming WE. *Out of the Crisis.* Cambridge MA: MIT Press; 2000.

21. Institute for Healthcare Improvement. 4 ways to provide safer care every time. Published May 4, 2017. Accessed December 13, 2021. http://www.ihi.org/communities/blogs/4-ways-to-provide-safer-care-every-time

22. Gillespie BM, Gillespie J, Booman, RJ, Granqvist K, Stranne J, Erichsen-Andersson A. The impact of robotic-assisted surgery on team performance: a systematic mixed studies review. *Human Factors.* 2021;63(8):1352-1379.

23. Institute for Healthcare Improvement. Workload, stress, and patient safety: how human factors can help. Published February 5, 2020. Accessed December 13, 2021. http://www.ihi.org/communities/blogs/-workload-stress-and-patient-safety-how-human-factors-can-help

24. The Advisory Board. *Managing Disruptive Behavior: Creating a Healthy Workplace Culture.* Washington, DC: Author; 2010.

25. Hittle BM, Wong IS, Caruso CC. Managing fatigue during times of crisis: guidance for nurses, managers, and other healthcare workers. *NIOSH Science Blog.* Posted April 2, 2020. Accessed December 13, 2021. https://blogs.cdc.gov/niosh-science-blog/2020/04/02/fatigue-crisis-hcw/

26. Institute for Healthcare Improvement. IHI Open School: Patient Safety 102: Human factors and safety. Published 2016. Accessed December 13, 2021. http://www.ihi.org/education/ihiopenschool/Courses/Documents/SummaryDocuments/PS%20102%20SummaryFINAL.pdf

27. Agency for Healthcare Research and Quality. PSNet: Checklists. Published September 7, 2019. Accessed December 8, 2021. https://psnet.ahrq.gov/primer/checklists

28. Gordon S, Mendenhall P, O'Connor BB. *Beyond the Checklist: What Else Health Care Can Learn from Aviation Teamwork and Safety.* Ithaca, NY: Cornell University ILR; 2013.

29. Reason J. Human error: models and management. *BMJ.* 2000;320:768-770.

30. Agency for Healthcare Research and Quality (AHRQ). Patient safety primer: Voluntary patient safety event reporting (incident reporting). Published September 7, 2019. Accessed December 13, 2021. https://psnet.ahrq.gov/primer/reporting-patient-safety-events

31. McKeon LM, Oswaks JD, Cunningham PD. Safeguarding patients: complexity science, high reliability organizations, and implications for team training in healthcare. *Clin Nurse Spec.* 2006;20(6):298-304.

32. Hines S, Luna K, Lofthus J, Marquardt M, Stemokas D. *Becoming a High Reliability Organization: Operational Advice for Hospital Leaders.* Rockville MD: Agency for Healthcare Research and Quality; 2008. AHRQ publication 08-0022.

33. Weick KE, Sutcliffe KM. *Managing the Unexpected—Assuring High Performance in an Age of Complexity.* San Francisco, CA: Jossey-Bass; 2001.

34. Weick KE, Sutcliffe K. *Managing the Unexpected: Resilient Performance in the Age of Uncertainty.* 2nd ed. San Francisco, CA: John Wiley & Sons, Inc.; 2007.

35. Chassin MR, Loeb JM. High-reliability health care: getting there from here. *Milbank Q.* 2013;91(3):459-490.

36. Marx D. Patient safety and the "Just Culture": a primer for health care executives. Published April 17, 2001. Accessed January 14, 2022. https://www.chpso.org/sites/main/files/file-attachments/marx_primer.pdf

37. Outcome Engenuity. The model for engineering better outcomes; 2017. Accessed December 13, 2021. https://www.outcome-eng.com/the-model-for-high-reliability-organizations/

38. Hagg HW, Workman-Germann J, Flanagan ME, Doebbeling BN. Implementation of systems redesign: approaches to spread and sustain adoption. In: Henriksen K, Battles JB, Keyes MA, Grad ML, eds., *Culture and Redesign.* Rockville, MD: Agency for Healthcare Research and Quality (US); 2008. *Advances in Patient Safety: New Directions and Alternative Approaches;* Vol. 2.

39. Advisory Board. *The Journey to Zero: Innovative Strategies for Minimizing Hospital-Acquired Infections.* Washington, DC: Author; 2008.

40. Joint Commission Center on Transforming Healthcare. Get to zero HAIs! Hand Hygiene Targeted Solutions Tool implementation guide for health care organizations. Accessed

December 13, 2021. https://www.centerfortransforminghealthcare.org/-/media/cth/documents/what-we-offer/hh_tst_implementation_guide.pdf

41. Shojania KG, Duncan BW, McDonald KM, Wachter RM. *Making health care safer: A clinical analysis of patient safety practices*. Evidence report/technology assessment no. 43. Revised July 20, 2001. Accessed December 12, 2021. https://archive.ahrq.gov/clinic/ptsafety/pdf/ptsafety.pdf

42. Moody's Global Credit Research. *Clinical Quality Initiatives Have Positive Long-Term Impact on Not-For-Profit Hospital Bond Ratings*. New York, NY: Moody's Investor Services; 2008.

43. Moody's Investors Services. Healthcare Quarterly. Posted April 17, 2017. Accessed April 9, 2022. https://www.moodys.com

44. Grossbart S. Engaging health system boards of trustees in quality and safety: six must-know guidelines. Published June 5, 2019. Accessed December 12, 2021. https://www.healthcatalyst.com/insights/healthcare-boards-quality-safety-pivotal-role/

45. American Society for Health Care Risk Management. Enterprise risk management for health care boards: leveraging the value. Published 2021. Accessed December 13, 2021. https://www.ashrm.org/system/files/media/file/2020/11/ERM_A%20Primer%20for%20Health%20Care%20Boards_2020_final.pdf

46. Daley Ullem E, Gandhi TK, Mate K, Whittington J, Renton M, Huebner J. *Framework for Effective Board Governance of Health System Quality*. IHI white paper. Boston, MA: Institute for Healthcare Improvement; 2018. Accessed December 12, 2021. http://www.ihi.org/resources/Pages/IHIWhitePapers/Framework-Effective-Board-Governance-Health-System-Quality.aspx

47. Millar R, Mannion R, Freeman T, Davies HTO. Hospital board oversight of quality and patient safety: a narrative review and synthesis of recent empirical research. *Milbank Q*. 2013;91(4):738-770.

48. National Quality Forum. Patient safety 2016: final report; 2017. Accessed December 13, 2021. http://www.qualityforum.org/Publications/2017/03/Patient_Safety_Final_Report.aspx

49. Kabcenell A, Nolan TW, Martin LA, Gill Y. *The Pursuing Perfection Initiative: Lessons on Transforming Health Care*. IHI Innovation Series white paper. Cambridge MA: Institute for Healthcare Improvement; 2010.

50. May EL. The power of zero: steps toward high reliability healthcare. *Healthcare Executive*. 2013;28(3):16-22.

51. National Patient Safety Foundation Lucien Leape Institute. Transforming healthcare: a compendium of reports from the NPSF's Lucien Leape Institute. Published 2016. Accessed December 11, 2021. http://www.ihi.org/resources/Pages/Publications/Transforming-Health-Care-Compendium-NPSF-Lucian-Leape-Institute-Reports.aspx

52. Dunham RB, Pierce JL. *Management*. Glenview, IL: Scott Foresman and Company; 1989.

53. Botwinick L, Bisognano M, Haraden C. *Leadership Guide to Patient Safety*. IHI Innovation Series white paper. Cambridge, MA: Institute for Healthcare Improvement; 2006. Accessed December 12, 2021. http://www.ihi.org/resources/Pages/IHIWhitePapers/LeadershipGuidetoPatientSafetyWhitePaper.aspx#:~:text=%20Leadership%20Guide%20to%20Patient%20Safety%20%201,and%20Patients%2FFamilies%20Impacted%20by%20Medical%20Errors%20More%20

54. The Joint Commission. 11 tenets of a safety culture. Published 2017. Accessed April 10, 2022. https://fdocuments.in/download/infographic-11-tenets-of-a-safety-culture-joint-commission-tenets-of-a-safety

55. Reason J. Achieving a safety culture: theory and practice. *BMJ*. 1998;12(3):293-306.

56. Reason J. Human error: models and management. *BMJ*. 2000;320:768-770.

57. Quality Interagency Coordination Task Force. Doing what counts for patient safety: federal actions to reduce medical errors and their impact. Published February 2000. Accessed December 12, 2021. https://archive.ahrq.gov/quic/report/errors6.pdf

58. Agency for Healthcare Research and Quality Patient Safety Network. Adverse events, near misses and errors. Published September 7, 2019. Accessed December 12, 2021. https://psnet.ahrq.gov/primer/adverse-events-near-misses-and-errors

59. The Joint Commission. Sentinel event definition, policy revised. Published 2021. Accessed December 12, 2021. https://www.jointcommission.org/resources/news-and-multimedia/newsletters/newsletters/joint-commission-online/july-21-2021/sentinel-event-definition-policy-revised/

60. Institute for Safe Medication Practices. *Patient Safety: Achieve a New Standard for Care*. Washington, DC: National Academies Press; 2004.

61. Barnard D, Dumkee M, Bains B, Gallivan B. Implementing a good catch program in an integrated health system. *Healthc Qual*. 2006;9: Spec no. 22-27.

62. Kaplan HS, Fastman B. Organization of reporting data for sense making and system improvement. *Qual Safe Health Care*. 2003;12 (Suppl 2: ii68-ii72).

63. Marks CM, Kasda E, Paine L, Wu AW. "That was a close call": endorsing a broad definition of near misses in health care. *Jt Comm J Qual Patient Saf*. 2013;39(10):475-479.

64. Institute of Medicine. *Patient Safety: Achieving a New Standard of Care*. Washington, DC: National Academies Press; 2004.

65. American College of Healthcare Executives, Institute for Healthcare Improvement/National Patient Safety Foundation. *Leading a Culture of Safety: A Blueprint for Success*. Boston, MA: ACHE and IHI; 2017.

66. Paradiso L, Sweeney N. Just culture: it's more than policy. *Nurs Manage*. 2019;50(6):38-45. doi:10.1097/01.NUMA.0000558482.07815.ae

67. Agency for Healthcare Research and Quality. PSNet: Culture of safety. Published September 7, 2019. Accessed December 8, 2021. https://psnet.ahrq.gov/primer/culture-safety

68. Institute for Safe Medication Practices. The differences between human error, at-risk behavior, and reckless behavior are key to a just culture. Published June 17, 2019. Accessed December 13, 2021. https://www.ismp.org/resources/differences-between-human-error-risk-behavior-and-reckless-behavior-are-key-just-culture

69. Rogers EM. *Diffusion of Innovations*. 5th ed. New York: Free Press; 2003.

70. National Quality Forum. *Safe Practices for Better Healthcare—2010 Update: A Consensus Report. Abridged version*. Washington, DC: Author; 2010.

71. Conway J, Federico F, Stewart K, Campbell M. *Respectful Management of Serious Clinical Adverse Events*. 2nd ed. IHI Innovation Series white paper. Cambridge, MA: Institute for Healthcare Improvement; 2011.

72. Pennsylvania Patient Safety Authority. Promote a culture of safety with good catch reports. *Pa Patient Saf Advis*. 2017;14(3).

Accessed December 14, 2021. http://patientsafety.pa.gov/ADVISORIES/Pages/201709_goodcatch.aspx

73. The Joint Commission. Developing a reporting culture: learning from close calls and hazardous conditions. *Sentinel Event Alert*. 2018;60. Accessed December 14, 2021. https://www.jointcommission.org/-/media/tjc/documents/resources/patient-safety-topics/sentinel-event/sea_60_reporting_culture_final.pdf?db=web&hash=5AB072026CAAF4711FCDC343701B0159

74. Agency for Healthcare Research and Quality. Patient safety resources by setting. Published 2018. Accessed December 14, 2021. https://www.ahrq.gov/patient-safety/settings/index.html

75. Centers for Medicare & Medicaid Services. Better care, smarter spending, healthier people: improving our health care delivery system. Published September 29, 2015. Accessed December 10, 2021. https://www.cms.gov/newsroom/fact-sheets/better-care-smarter-spending-healthier-people-improving-our-health-care-delivery-system-0#:~:text=Better%20Care%2C%20Smarter%20Spending%2C%20Healthier%20People%3A%20Improving%20Our,engaged%20consumer%20at%20the%20center%20of%20their%20care

76. Pelletier LR, Stichler JF. Action brief: patient engagement and activation: a health care reform imperative and improvement opportunity for nursing. *Nurs Outlook*. 2013;61(1):51-54. doi:10.1016/j.outlook.2012.11.003

77. Farley DO, Morton SE, Damberg CL, et al. *Assessment of the AHRQ Patient Safety Initiatives: Moving from Research to Practice*. Evaluation report II (2003-2004). Santa Monica, CA: RAND Corporation; 2007.

78. University of California, Los Angeles. UCLA Health System performance improvement & patient safety plan; FY 2020. Published 2020. Accessed December 14, 2021. https://quality.mednet.ucla.edu/files/view/files/quality_initiatives/Performance_Improvement_Plan_FY20.pdf

79. NEJM Catalyst. What is risk management in healthcare? *NEJM Catalyst Innovations in Care Delivery*. April 25, 2018. Accessed December 13, 2021. https://catalyst.nejm.org/doi/full/10.1056/CAT.18.0197

80. Hagg-Rickert S, Gaffey A, eds., American Society for Health Care Risk Management. *Enterprise Risk Management: Implementing ERM*. Chicago, IL: ASHRM; 2020. Accessed December 13, 2021. https://www.ashrm.org/system/files/media/file/2020/12/ERM-Implementing-ERM-for-Suceess-White-Paper_FINAL.pdf

81. Agency for Healthcare Research and Quality (AHRQ). Patient safety primer: voluntary patient safety event reporting (incident reporting). Published September 7, 2019. Accessed December 13, 2021. https://psnet.ahrq.gov/primer/reporting-patient-safety-events

82. Griffin FA, Resar RK. *IHI Global Trigger Tool for Measuring Adverse Events*. 2nd ed. IHI Innovation Series white paper. Cambridge MA: Institute for Healthcare Improvement; 2009.

83. U.S. Department of Health & Human Services, Office of Inspector General. Hospital incident reporting systems do not capture most patient harm. Published January 2012. Accessed December 13, 2021. https://oig.hhs.gov/oei/reports/oei-06-09-00091.pdf

84. Banakhar MA, Tambosi AI, Asiri SA, Yosra BB, Essa YA. Barriers of reporting errors among nurses in a tertiary hospital. *Int J Nurs Clin Pract*. 2017;4:245.

85. Agency for Healthcare Research and Quality. SOPS hospital survey 2.0: 2021 user database report. Published March 2021. Accessed December 6, 2021. https://www.ahrq.gov/sites/default/files/wysiwyg/sops/surveys/hospital/2021-HSOPS2-Database-Report-Part-I-508.pdf

86. National Academy of Sciences. *The Owner's Role in Project Risk Management*. Washington, DC: Author; 2005.

87. MetricSteam. Proactive Risk Assessment—The Key to Business Excellence. 2016. Accessed January 14, 2022. https://www.metricstream.com/insights/proactive-risk-management-approach.htm

88. Oregon Patient Safety Commission. Root cause analysis toolkit. Published 2021. Accessed December 14, 2021. https://oregonpatientsafety.org/tools-and-best-practices/root-cause-analysis-toolkit?rq=Root%20cause%20analysis%20toolkit

89. Institute for Healthcare Improvement, National Patient Safety Foundation. RCA² Improving root cause analyses and actions to prevent harm (version 2). Published 2016. Accessed December 14, 2021. http://www.ihi.org/resources/Pages/Tools/RCA2-Improving-Root-Cause-Analyses-and-Actions-to-Prevent-Harm.aspx

90. Institute for Healthcare Improvement. 5 whys: finding a root cause of a problem. Published 2019. Accessed December 14, 2021. http://www.ihi.org/resources/Pages/Tools/5-Whys-Finding-the-Root-Cause.aspx

91. Jones LK, O'Connor SJ. The use of red rules in patient safety culture. *Univ J Manage*. 2016;4(3):130-139. doi:10.13189/ujm.2016.040306

92. Institute for Safe Medication Practices. Some red rules shouldn't rule in hospitals. Published April 24, 2008. Accessed December 14, 2021. https://www.ismp.org/resources/some-red-rules-shouldnt-rule-hospitals#:~:text=%20Some%20Red%20Rules%20Shouldn%27t%20Rule%20in%20Hospitals,of%20seatbelts%20while%20riding%20in%20an...%20More%20

93. Thomassen O, Storesund A, Softeland E, Brattebo G. The effects of safety checklists in medicine: a systematic review. *Acta Anaesthesiol Scand*. 2013;58(1):5-18. doi:10.1111/aas.12207

94. World Health Organization. Checklists save lives. Published July 2008. Accessed December 14, 2021. https://apps.who.int/iris/bitstream/handle/10665/270232/PMC2647491.pdf?sequence=1&isAllowed=y

95. World Health Organization. Surgical safety checklist. Revised 2009. Accessed December 14, 2021. https://apps.who.int/iris/bitstream/handle/10665/44186/9789241598590_eng_Checklist.pdf;sequence=2

96. National Patient Safety Foundation. Checklist for getting the right diagnosis. Published 2014. Accessed December 14, 2021. https://cdn.ymaws.com/www.npsf.org/resource/collection/930A0426-5BAC-4827-AF94-1CE1624CBE67/Checklist-for-Getting-the-Right-Diagnosis.pdf

97. National Academies Press. Improving diagnosis in healthcare: Resources to facilitate communication between patients and clinicians. Published September 22, 2015. Accessed December 14, 2021. https://www.nap.edu/resource/21794/interactive/

98. Centers for Disease Control and Prevention. Antibiotic prescribing and use: hospital: antibiotic stewardship program assessment tool. Published 2019. Accessed December 14, 2021. https://www.cdc.gov/antibiotic-use/healthcare/pdfs/assessment-tool-P.pdf

99. Centers for Disease Control and Prevention. Antibiotic prescribing and use: outpatient: clinician checklist for outpatient antibiotic use. Published 2021. Accessed December 14, 2021. https://www.cdc.gov/antibiotic-use/community/pdfs/16_268900-A_CoreElementsOutpatient_check_1_508.pdf

100. Pronovost P, Needham D, Berenholtz S, et al. An intervention to decrease catheter-related bloodstream infections in the ICU. *N Engl J Med.* 2006;355:2725-2732. doi:10.1056/NEJMoa061115

101. Gawande A. The checklist. *Ann Med.* 2007. Accessed December 14, 2021. http://www.newyorker.com/magazine/2007/12/10/the-checklist

102. Gawande A. *The Checklist Manifesto: How to Get Things Right.* New York, NY: Metropolitan Books; 2009.

103. Treadwell JR, Lucas S, Tsou AY. Surgical checklists: a systematic review of impacts and implementation. *BMJ Qual Saf.* 2014;3:299-318.

104. Aspden P, Wolcott J, Bootman JL, Cronenwett LR. *Preventing Medication Errors.* Washington, DC: National Academies Press; 2006.

105. The Advisory Board. 5 ways to improve medication adherence—health care's $289 billion problem. Published April 19, 2017. Accessed December 15, 2021. https://www.advisory.com/daily-briefing/2017/04/19/medication-adherence

106. Faraq A, Tullai-McGuinness S, Anthony MK, Burant C. Do leadership style, unit climate, and safety climate contribute to safe medication practices? *J Nurs Adm.* 2017;47(1):8-15.

107. The Joint Commission, Joint Commission International, World Health Organization. Patient safety solutions preamble. *Jt Comm J Qual Pt Safety.* 2007;33(7):427-429.

108. The Joint Commission. Safe use of health information technology. *Sentinel Event Alert.* 2015;54. Accessed April 9, 2022. https://www.jointcommission.org/resources/patient-safety-topics/sentinel-event/sentinel-event-alert-newsletters/sentinel-event-alert-54-safe-use-of-health-information/#.YlIIpJHMKUk

109. Partnership for Health IT Patient Safety. Safe practice recommendations for developing, implementing, and integrating a health IT safety program. ECRI Institute. Published 2018. Accessed January 10, 2022. https://www.ecri.org/hit/safe-practices

110. Institute of Medicine, Committee on Patient Safety and Health Information Technology. *Health IT and Patient Safety: Building Safer Systems for Better Care.* Washington, DC: National Academies Press; 2012.

111. Parente ST, McCullough JS. Health information technology and patient safety: evidence from panel data. *Health Aff.* 2009;28(2):357-360. doi:10.1377/hlthaff.28.2.357

112. Sowan AK, Reed CC. A complex phenomenon in complex adaptive health care systems—alarm fatigue. *JAMA Pediatr.* 2017;171(6):515-516. Published online April 10, 2017. Accessed December 14, 2021. http://jamanetwork.com/journals/jamapediatrics/fullarticle/2614070

113. Woo M, Bacon O. Alarm fatigue. In: Hall KK, Shoemaker-Hunt S, Hoffman L, et al., eds. *Making Healthcare Safer III: A Critical Analysis of Existing and Emerging Patient Safety Practices [Internet].* Rockville, MD: Agency for Healthcare Research and Quality; March 13, 2020; 13-1-13-12. Accessed April 9, 2022. https://www.ncbi.nlm.nih.gov/books/NBK555526/pdf/Bookshelf_NBK555526.pdf

114. Graber ML, Johnston D, Bailey R. *Report of the Evidence on Health IT Safety and Interventions.* Research Triangle Park, NC: RTI International; 2016.

115. Agency for Healthcare Research and Quality. PSNet: Artificial intelligence and diagnostic errors. Published January 31, 2020. Accessed December 14, 2021. https://psnet.ahrq.gov/perspective/artificial-intelligence-and-diagnostic-errors#_ednref1

116. Cohen JK. Building unbiased AI. *Modern Healthcare.* 2021;51(25):18-27.

117. Nationwide Health Information Network (NHIN). Exchange Architecture Overview (Draft 0.9). Published April 21, 2010. Accessed December 14, 2021. https://www.healthit.gov/sites/default/files/nhin-architecture-overview-draft-20100421-1.pdf

118. U.S. Department of Health & Human Services, Office of the National Coordinator. Get the facts about the Nationwide Health Information Network, Direct Project, and CONNECT software. Published 2010. Accessed December 14, 2021. https://www.healthit.gov/sites/default/files/pdf/fact-sheets/get-the-facts-about-nationwide-hit-direct-project-and-connect.pdf

119. Chesapeake Regional Information System for Our Patients. Welcome to CRISP. Published 2020. Accessed December 14, 2021. https://www.crisphealth.org/about-crisp/

120. Delaware Health Information Network. About DHIN. Published 2021. Accessed December 14, 2021. https://dhin.org/about/

121. ECRI Institute for Health IT Patient Safety. Eight safe practice recommendations. Published 2017. Accessed December 6, 2021. https://www.ecri.org/Resources/HIT/Patient%20ID/Recommendations_Patient_ID_Handout.pdf

122. Halpern MT, Roussel AE, Treiman K, Nerz PA, Hatlie MJ, Sheridan S. *Designing Consumer Reporting Systems for Patient Safety Events.* Final report (prepared by RTI International and Consumers Advancing Patient Safety under Contract No. 290-06-00001-5). Rockville, MD: Agency for Healthcare Research and Quality; April 2011. AHRQ publication 11-0060-EF.

123. Health Policy Brief. Public reporting on quality and costs. *Health Aff.* March 8, 2012. Accessed December 10, 2021. http://healthaffairs.org/healthpolicybriefs/brief_pdfs/healthpolicybrief_65.pdf

124. Hanlon C, Sheedy K, Kniffin T, Rosenthal J. *2014 Guide to State Adverse Event Reporting Systems.* Washington, DC: National Academy for State Health Policy; 2015. Accessed December 10, 2021. https://www.nashp.org/wp-content/uploads/2015/02/2014_Guide_to_State_Adverse_Event_Reporting_Systems.pdf

125. U.S. Food & Drug Administration. CFSAN Adverse Event Reporting System (CAERS). Accessed April 10, 2022. https://www.fda.gov/food/compliance-enforcement-food/cfsan-adverse-event-reporting-system-caers

126. U.S. Department of Health & Human Services. Vaccine Adverse Event Reporting System. Accessed April 10, 2022. https://vaers.hhs.gov/

127. The Advisory Board Company. *The Journey to Zero: Innovative Strategies for Minimizing Hospital-Acquired Infections.* Washington, DC: Author; 2008.

128. Centers for Disease Control and Prevention. National Healthcare Safety Network. Published 2021. Accessed December 10, 2021. https://www.cdc.gov/nhsn/

129. Kohn LT, Corrigan J, Donaldson MS. *To Err Is Human: Building a Safer Health System.* Washington, DC: National Academy Press; 1999.

130. Medicare.gov. Find & compare nursing homes, hospitals & other providers near you. Published 2021. Accessed December 16, 2021. https://www.medicare.gov/care-compare/?providerType=Hospital&redirect=true

131. National Committee for Quality Assurance. HEDIS measures. Published 2021. Accessed December 10, 2021. https://www.ncqa.org/hedis/measures/

132. The Joint Commission. ORYX performance measurement reporting. Accessed April 10, 2022. https://www.jointcommission.org/measurement/reporting/accreditation-oryx/

133. The Joint Commission. National patient safety goals. Published 2021. Accessed December 14, 2021. https://www.jointcommission.org/standards_information/npsgs.aspx

134. The Leapfrog Group. The Leapfrog Group mission and vision. Accessed December 10, 2021. http://www.leapfroggroup.org/about/mission-and-vision

135. The Leapfrog Group. Mission and vision. Accessed December 14, 2021. http://www.leapfroggroup.org/

136. National Quality Forum. What we do. Published 2021. Accessed December 14, 2021. https://www.qualityforum.org/what_we_do.aspx

137. National Quality Forum. Field guide to NQF resources. Published 2021. Accessed December 14, 2021. https://www.qualityforum.org/Field_Guide/Field_Guide.aspx

138. Muller M, Jurgens MM, Redaelli M, Klingberg K, Hautz WE, Stock S. Impact of the communication and patient hand-off tool SBAR on patient safety: a systematic review. *BMJ Open.* 2018;8:e022202. doi:10.1136/bmjopen-2018-022202

139. Institute for Healthcare Improvement. SBAR tool: Situation-Background-Assessment-Recommendation. Accessed April 9, 2022. http://www.ihi.org/resources/Pages/Tools/SBARToolkit.aspx

140. Singer SJ, Meterko M, Baker L, Gaba G, Falwell A, Rosen A. Workforce perceptions of hospital safety culture: development and validation of the Patient Safety Climate in Healthcare Organizations survey. *Health Serv Res.* 2007;42(5):1999-2021.

141. Sexton JB, Helmreich RL, Neilands TB, et al. The safety attitudes questionnaire: psychometric properties, benchmarking data, and emerging research. *BMC Health Serv Res.* 2006;6(1):44. doi:10.1186/1472-6963-6-44

142. Thomas EJ, Sexton JB, Helmreich RL. Discrepant attitudes about teamwork among critical care nurses and physicians. *Crit Care Med.* 2003;31(3):956-959. doi:10.1097/01.CCM.0000056183.89175.76

143. University of Texas Health Science Center, McGovern Medical School. Center for Healthcare Quality and Safety: Generating knowledge to improve patient care: Survey. Accessed December 15, 2021. https://med.uth.edu/chqs/survey/

144. Singer SJ, Meterko M, Baker L, Gaba G, Falwell A, Rosen A. Workforce perceptions of hospital safety culture: development and validation of the Patient Safety Climate in Healthcare Organizations survey. *Health Serv Res.* 2007;42(5):1999-2021.

145. Singer SJ, Meterko M, Baker L, Gaba D, Falwell A, Rosen A. Patient safety climate in healthcare organizations (PSCHO). Measurement instrument database for the social sciences. Published 2012. Accessed December 15, 2021. http://www.midss.org/sites/default/files/pscho_survey_2006.pdf

146. Benzer JK, Meterko M, Singer SJ. The patient safety climate in healthcare organizations (PSCHO) survey: short-form development. *J Eval Clin Pract.* 2017;23(4):853-859. doi:10.1111/jep.12731. Epub April 20, 2017.

147. Agency for Healthcare Research and Quality. *Hospital Survey on Patient Safety Culture: 2008 Comparative Database Report.* Rockville MD: Author; 2008. AHRQ publication 08-0039.

148. Famolaro T, Hare R, Yount ND, Fan L, Liu H, Sorra J. Surveys on Patient Safety Culture (SOPS) Hospital Survey 2.0: 2021 user database report (prepared by Westat, Rockville, MD, under contract no. HHSP233201500026I/HHSP23337004T). Rockville, MD: Agency for Healthcare Research and Quality; March 2021. AHRQ publication no. 21-0017. Accessed December 6, 2021. https://www.ahrq.gov/sites/default/files/wysiwyg/sops/surveys/hospital/2021-HSOPS2-Database-Report-Part-I-508.pdf

149. Medical Group Management Association. MGMA survey participation. Published 2021. Accessed December 14, 2021. https://www.mgma.com/participate

150. MGMA. MGMA DataDive and survey participant benefits. Published 2021. Accessed December 15, 2021. https://www.mgma.com/data/landing-pages/mgma-datadive-and-survey-participation-benefits

151. Joint Commission Center for Transforming Healthcare. Cultivate your safety culture with TRIO. Published 2021. Accessed December 14, 2021. https://www.centerfortransforminghealthcare.org/products-and-services/trio/

152. Institute of Medicine. *Best Care at Lower Cost: The Path to Continuously Learning Health Care in America.* Washington, DC: National Academies of Sciences, Engineering and Medicine; 2012.

153. Senge PM. *The Fifth Discipline: The Art and Practice of the Learning Organization* 2nd ed. New York, NY: Doubleday; 2006.

154. Edwards MT. An organizational learning framework for patient safety. *Am J Med Qual.* 2016;32(2):148-155.

155. Institute for Safe Medication Practices. Using information from external errors to signal a "clear and present danger." *Patient Saf Qual Healthcare.* 2017;14(2):32-34.

156. Frankel A, Haraden C, Federico F, Lenoci-Edwards J. *A Framework for Safe, Reliable, and Effective Care.* White paper. Cambridge, MA: Institute for Healthcare Improvement and Safe & Reliable Healthcare; 2017:6-7.

157. Agency for Healthcare Research and Quality Patient Safety Network. Training and education overview. Accessed December 15, 2021. https://psnet.ahrq.gov/training-education

158. Agency for Healthcare Research and Quality. About TeamSTEPPS. Published 2019. Accessed December 15, 2021. https://www.ahrq.gov/teamstepps/about-teamstepps/index.html

159. Agency for Healthcare Research and Quality. Pocket Guide: TeamSTEPPS team strategies & tools to enhance performance and patient safety. Published 2013. Accessed December 15, 2021. https://www.ahrq.gov/sites/default/files/wysiwyg/professionals/education/curriculum-tools/teamstepps/instructor/essentials/pocketguide.pdf

160. ECRI. Partnership for Health IT Patient Safety. Published 2021. Accessed December 15, 2021. https://www.ecri.org/solutions/hit-partnership

161. ECRI. Medical Device Safety Reports. Published 2021. Accessed April 9, 2022. https://www.fda.gov/medical-devices/science-and-research-medical-devices/medical-device-material-safety-summaries-ecri-reports

162. Institute for Healthcare Improvement. IHI Open School online courses: certificates and continuing education. Published 2021. Accessed December 15, 2021. http://www.ihi.org/education/IHIOpenSchool/Courses/Pages/OpenSchoolCertificates.aspx

163. Institute for Healthcare Improvement. Patient safety. Published 2021. Accessed December 8, 2021. http://www.ihi.org/Topics/PatientSafety/Pages/Overview.aspx

164. Institute for Safe Medication Practices. Learn about us: The Institute for Safe Medication Practices. Accessed December 15, 2021. https://www.ismp.org/about

165. Institute for Safe Medication Practices. ISMP Medication Safety Alert! Published 2021. Accessed December 15, 2021. https://www.ismp.org/newsletters

166. The Joint Commission. Patient safety systems. Published 2021. Accessed April 9, 2022. https://www.jointcommission.org/-/media/tjc/documents/standards/ps-chapters/camcah_04a_ps_all_current.pdf

167. The Joint Commission. The Oro 2.0 Resource Library. Published 2021. Accessed December 15, 2021. https://www.centerfortransforminghealthcare.org/products-and-services/oro-2/our-resource-library/

168. National Association for Healthcare Quality. NAHQ's Healthcare Quality Competency Framework: reduce variability in healthcare quality competencies. Published 2021. Accessed December 15, 2021. https://nahq.org/nahq-intelligence/competency-framework/

169. Occupational Safety and Health Administration. Worker safety in hospitals. Accessed April 9, 2022. https://www.osha.gov/hospitals

170. Patient-Centered Outcomes Research Institute. About PCORI. Published 2021. Accessed December 11, 2021. https://www.pcori.org/about/about-pcori

171. Patient-Centered Outcomes Research Institute. Proposed national priorities for health. Published 2021. Accessed December 11, 2021. https://www.pcori.org/sites/default/files/PCORI-Proposed-National-Priorities-for-Health-English-June-2021.pdf

172. World Health Organization. *Patient Safety Curriculum Guide: Multi-professional Edition*. Geneva Switzerland: Author; 2011. Accessed December 15, 2021. https://www.who.int/publications/i/item/9789241501958

173. Agency for Healthcare Research and Quality. *Advancing Patient Safety: A Decade of Evidence, Design and Implementation*. AHRQ publication no. 09(10)-0084; 2009. Accessed December 6, 2021. https://www.ahrq.gov/sites/default/files/publications/files/advancing-patient-safety.pdf.

174. National Quality Forum. *Serious Reportable Events in Healthcare—2011 Update: A Consensus Report*. Washington, DC: Author; 2011.

175. National Priorities Partnership. *Input to the Secretary of Health and Human Services on Priorities for the National Quality Strategy*. Washington, DC: National Quality Forum; 2011.

176. Centers for Medicare & Medicaid Services. CMS quality strategy 2016. Published December 1, 2021. Accessed December 6, 2021. https://www.cms.gov/Medicare/Quality-Initiatives-Patient-Assessment-Instruments/Value-Based-Programs/CMS-Quality-Strategy

177. U.S. Department of Health & Human Services. Report to Congress: national strategy for quality improvement in health care. Published 2020. Accessed December 10, 2021. https://www.ahrq.gov/workingforquality/reports/index.html

178. National Priorities Partnership. *Executive Summary: National Priorities and Goals: Aligning Our Efforts to Transform America's Healthcare*. Washington, DC: National Quality Forum; 2008.

179. Agency for Healthcare Research and Quality. *Strategies to Improve Patient Safety: Final Report to Congress Required by the Patient Safety and Quality Improvement Act of 2005*. Rockville, MD: Agency for Healthcare Research and Quality; 2021. AHRQ publication 22-0009. Accessed December 17, 2021. https://pso.ahrq.gov/sites/default/files/wysiwyg/strategies-improve-patient-safety-final.pdf

180. Agency for Healthcare Research and Quality. *Strategies to Improve Patient Safety: Final Report to Congress Required by the Patient Safety and Quality Improvement Act of 2005*. Rockville, MD: December 2021. AHRQ publication 22-0009. https://pso.ahrq.gov/sites/default/files/wysiwyg/strategies-improve-patient-safety-final.pdf

181. Agency for Healthcare Research and Quality. Patient Safety and Quality Improvement Act of 2005. Accessed December 10, 2021. https://www.gpo.gov/fdsys/pkg/PLAW-109publ41/pdf/PLAW-109publ41.pdf

182. Agency for Healthcare Research and Quality, Office for Civil Rights, & U.S. Department of Health & Human Services. Patient safety and quality improvement; final rule. *Fed Regist.* 2008;73(226):70732-70814.

183. Cartwright-Smith L, Rosenbaum S, Sochacki C. The Patient Safety and Quality Improvement Act regulations: implications for health information access and exchange. *Legal Notes.* 2011;2(2):1-7.

184. Agency for Healthcare Research and Quality. Patient safety organization (PSO) frequently asked questions. Published 2021. Accessed December 10, 2021. https://www.pso.ahrq.gov/faq

185. Connecticut Center for Patient Safety. Annual report. Published 2020. Accessed December 10, 2021. http://www.ctcps.org/pdf/2020%20Annual%20Report.pdf

186. Oregon Patient Safety Commission. Advancing patient safety in Oregon. Director. Accessed December 10, 2021. http://oregonpatientsafety.org/

187. Centers for Medicare & Medicaid Services. About the CMS Innovation Center. Published 2021. Accessed April 9, 2022. https://innovation.cms.gov/about

188. Centers for Medicare & Medicaid Services. Partnership for patients. Published 2021. December 10, 2021. https://innovation.cms.gov/innovation-models/partnership-for-patients

189. Berwick DM, Nolan, TW, Whittington J. The Triple Aim: care, health, and cost. *Health Aff.* 2008;27(3):759-769.

190. Sikka R, Morath JM, Leape L. The quadruple aim: care, health, cost, and meaning in work. *BMJ Qual Saf.* 2015;24(10):608-610. doi:10.1136/bhjqs-2015-004160. Accessed December 10, 2021. http://qualitysafety.bmj.com/content/qhc/24/10/608.full.pdf

191. Bodenheimer T, Sinsky C. From triple to quadruple aim: care of the patient requires care of the provider. *Ann Family Med.* 2014;12(6):573-576.

192. Itchhaporia D. The quadruple aim. Published April 26, 2018. Accessed December 10, 2021. https://www.acc.org/membership/sections-and-councils/cardiovascular-management-section/section-updates/2018/04/26/12/07/the-quadruple-aim

193. American Hospital Association, AHA Physician Alliance: Minnesota Hospital Association. Published 2018. Accessed December 17, 2021. https://www.aha.org/system/files/2018-11/plf-case-study-mha.pdf

194. Centers for Medicare & Medicaid Services. Better care, smarter spending, healthier people: improving our health care delivery system. Published September 29, 2015. Accessed December 10, 2021. https://www.cms.gov/newsroom/fact-sheets/better-care-smarter-spending-healthier-people-improving-our-health-care-delivery-system-0#:~:text=Better%20Care%2C%20Smarter%20

Spending%2C%20Healthier%20People%3A%20Improving%20Our,engaged%20consumer%20at%20the%20center%20of%20their%20care

195. Josie King Foundation. About. Published 2016. Accessed December 12, 2021. www.josieking.org/about

196. Patient Safety Movement. Annual report 2020: Zero because one is too many. Published 2021. Accessed December 12, 2021. https://patientsafetymovement.org/wp-content/uploads/2021/10/Annual-Report.pdf

197. Agency for Healthcare Research and Quality. The SHARE approach—achieving patient-centered care with shared decision making: a brief for administrators and practitioners. Published 2020. Retrieved December 12, 2021. http://www.ahrq.gov/professionals/education/curriculum-tools/shareddecisionmaking/tools/tool-9/index.html

198. Hibbard JH, Greene J. What the evidence shows about patient activation: better health outcomes and care experiences; fewer data on costs. *Health Aff*. 2013;32(20):207-214. doi:10.1377/hlthaff.2012.1061

199. The Joint Commission. Speak up campaigns. Published 2021. Accessed December 12, 2021. https://www.jointcommission.org/resources/for-consumers/speak-up-campaigns/

200. OpenNotes. What is OpenNotes? Accessed December 12, 2021. http://www.opennotes.org/about/

201. OpenNotes. The research continues. Accessed December 12, 2021. https://www.opennotes.org/research/

202. OpenNotes. *OurNotes* for health professionals: creating notes with patients. Accessed December 12, 2021. https://www.opennotes.org/ournotes-professionals/

203. Frampton SB, Guastello S, Hoy L, Naylor M, Sheridan S, Johnston-Fleece M. *Harnessing Evidence and Experience to Change Culture: A Guiding Framework for Patient and Family Engaged Care*. Discussion paper. Washington, DC: National Academy of Medicine; 2017. Accessed December 12, 2021. https://nam.edu/wp-content/uploads/2017/01/Harnessing-Evidence-and-Experience-to-Change-Culture-A-Guiding-Framework-for-Patient-and-Family-Engaged-Care.pdf

204. Institute of Medicine. What healthcare consumers need to know about racial and ethnic disparities in healthcare. Published March 2002. Accessed December 12, 2021. https://www.nap.edu/resource/10260/disparities_patient.pdf

205. Centers for Disease Control and Prevention. COVID-19 racial and ethnic disparities; 2020. Accessed December 12, 2021. https://www.cdc.gov/coronavirus/2019-ncov/community/health-equity/racial-ethnic-disparities/index.html#:~:text=People%20from%20racial%20and%20

ethnic%20minority%20groups%20are,result%20in%20distrust%20of%20government%20and%20healthcare%20systems

206. The Joint Commission. Addressing health care disparities by improving quality and safety. *Sentinel Event Alert*. 2021;64:1-7.

207. Cross TL, Bazron BJ, Dennis KW, Isaacs MR. *Towards a Culturally Competent System of Care*. National Institute of Mental Health, Child and Adolescent Services Program (CASSP). Washington, DC: Technical Assistance Center, Georgetown University Child Development Center; 1989.

208. The Joint Commission. Overcoming the challenges of providing care to LEP patients. *Quick Saf*. 2021;13:1-4. Accessed December 12, 2021. https://www.jointcommission.org/-/media/tjc/newsletters/quick-safety-issue-13-lep-update-10-5-21.pdf

209. Hsueh L, Huang J, Millman AK, et al. Disparities in use of video telemedicine among patients with limited English proficiency during the COVID-19 pandemic. *JAMA Netw Open*. 2021;4(11):e2133129. doi:10.1001/jamanetworkopen.2021.33129

210. Divi C, Koss RG, Schmaltz SP, Loeb JM. Language proficiency and adverse events in US hospitals: a pilot study. *Int J Qual Health Care*. 2007;19:60-67.

211. Rosse F, De Bruijne M, Suurmond J, Essink-Bot M, Wagner C. Language barriers and patient safety risk in hospital care: a mixed methods study. *Int J Nurs Stud*, 2016:54:45-53. doi:10.1016/j.ijnurstu.2015.03.012

212. The Joint Commission. Most commonly reviewed sentinel event types. Updated February 1, 2021. Accessed December 12, 2021. https://www.jointcommission.org/-/media/tjc/documents/resources/patient-safety-topics/sentinel-event/most-frequently-reviewed-event-types-2020.pdf

213. World Health Organization. Social determinants of health. Accessed December 12, 2021. https://www.who.int/health-topics/social-determinants-of-health#tab=tab_1

214. U.S. Department of Health & Human Services, Office of Minority Health, Think Cultural Health. National CLAS standards. Accessed December 12, 2021. https://thinkculturalhealth.hhs.gov/CLAS/

215. Saha S, Beach MK, Cooper LA. Patient centeredness, cultural competence and healthcare quality. *J Natl Med Assoc*. 2008;100(11):1275-1285.

216. U.S. Department of Health & Human Services, Office of Minority Health, Think Cultural Health. National CLAS standards. Accessed December 12, 2021. https://thinkculturalhealth.hhs.gov/CLAS/

## Suggested Readings

Afriyie-Boateng M, Loftus C, Wiesenfeld L, Hunter M, Lawson A. Proactive psychiatry intervention using a nurse-led behavioral response model for hospitalized patients with behavioral disturbances. *J Healthc Qual*. 2019;41(5):267-273. doi:10.1097/JHQ.0000000000000208

Agency for Healthcare Research and Quality, Patient Safety Network (PSNet). Primers. Accessed December 11, 2021. https://psnet.ahrq.gov/primers-0

Alan J, Card JW, Clarkson PJ. Successful risk assessment may not always lead to successful risk control: a systematic literature review of risk control after root cause analysis. *J Healthc Risk Manag*. 2012;31(3):6-12. doi:10.1002/jhrm.20090

Brock JB, Cretella DA, Parham JJ. An antimicrobial stewardship intervention improves adherence to standard of care for *Staphylococcus aureus* bloodstream infection. *J Healthc Qual*. 2019;41(6):e83-e89. doi:10.1097/JHQ.0000000000000191

Card AJ, Ward JR, Clarkson PJ. Beyond FMEA: the structured what-if technique (SWIFT). *J Healthc Risk Manag*. 2012;31(4):23. doi:10.1002/jhrm.20101

Chiswell E, Hampton D, Okoli CTC. Effect of patient and provider education on antibiotic overuse for respiratory tract infections. *J Healthc Qual*. 2019;41(3):e13-e20. doi:10.1097/JHQ.0000000000000144

Dimentberg R, Caplan IF, Winter E, et al. Prediction of adverse outcomes within 90 days of surgery in a heterogeneous orthopedic surgery population. *J Healthc Qual.* 2021;43(4):e53-e63. doi:10.1097/JHQ.0000000000000280

Elias RM, Kashiwagi D, Lau C, Hansel SL. An imaging stewardship initiative to reduce low-value positron emission tomography-computed tomography use in hospitalized patients. *J Healthc Qual.* 2020;42(6):e83-e91. doi:10.1097/JHQ.0000000000000255

Frankel A, Haraden C, Federico F, Lenoci-Edwards J. *A Framework for Safe, Reliable, and Effective Care.* White paper. Cambridge MA: Institute for Healthcare Improvement and Safe & Reliable Healthcare; 2017.

Gleason KM, Brake H, Agramonte V, Perfetti C. *Medications at Transitions and Clinical Handoffs (MATCH) Toolkit for Medication Reconciliation* (prepared by the Island Peer Review Organization, Inc., under Contract No. HHSA2902009000 13C; AHRQ publication 11(12)-0059). Rockville MD: Agency for Healthcare Research and Quality; 2011.

Hessels AJ, Murray MT, Cohen B, Larson EL. Perception of patient safety culture in pediatric long-term care settings. *J Healthc Qual.* 2018;40(6):384-391. doi:10.1097/JHQ.00000000000 00134

Hurtado MP, Swift EK, Corrigan JM, eds. *Envisioning the National Health Care Quality Report.* Washington, DC: National Academies Press; 2001. Accessed April 9, 2022. www.nap.edu/catalog.php?record_id=10073

Institute of Medicine, Committee on Enhancing Federal Healthcare Quality Programs. Corrigan JM, Eden J, Smith BM, eds. *Leadership by Example: Coordinating Government Roles in Improving Health Care Quality.* Washington, DC: National Academies Press; 2003. Accessed December 11, 2021. www.nap.edu/catalog.php?record_id=10537

International Network of Health Promoting Hospitals and Health Services. *2020 Standards for Health Promoting Hospitals and Health Services.* Hamburg, Germany: International HPH Network; 2020.

Kandagatla P, Su WK, Adrianto I, Jordan J, Haeusler J, Rubinfeld I. The effects of harm events on 30-day readmission in surgical patients. *J Healthc Qual.* 2021;43(2):101-109. doi:10.1097/JHQ.0000000000000261

Kim S, Appelbaum NP, Baker N, et al. Patient safety over power hierarchy: a scoping review of healthcare professionals' speaking-up skills training. *J Healthc Qual.* 2020;42(5):249-263. doi:10.1097/JHQ.0000000000000257

Kneeland MD, Ivory CH, Bloomingburg P, Choma NN. Exploring the perceived value of a personalized informatics tool to anticipate and mitigate patient risk. *J Healthc Qual.* 2018:40(3):155-162. doi:10.1097/JHQ.0000000000000100

Lau CY, Seymann G, Imershein S, et al. UC care check—a postoperative neurosurgery operating room checklist: an interrupted time series study. *J Healthc Qual.* 2020;42(4):224-235. doi:10.1097/JHQ.0000000000000246

Leape L. Full disclosure and apology—an idea whose time has come. *Physician Executive.* 2006;32(2):16-18.

Maurer M, Dardess P, Carman KL, Frazier K, Smeeding L. Guide to patient and family engagement: environmental scan report. Published May 2012. Accessed December 11, 2021. https://www.ahrq.gov/sites/default/files/wysiwyg/research/findings/final-reports/ptfamilyscan/ptfamilyscan.pdf

Montgomery AP, Azuero A, Baernholdt M, et al. Nurse burnout predicts self-reported medication administration errors in acute care hospitals. *J Healthc Qual.* 2021;43(1):13-23. doi:10.1097/JHQ.0000000000000274

Morgan CK, Amspoker AB, Howard C, et al. Continuous cloud-based early warning score surveillance to improve the safety of acutely ill hospitalized patients. *J Healthc Qual.* 2021;43(1):59-66. doi:10.1097/JHQ.0000000000000272

National Steering Committee for Patient Safety. *Safer Together: A National Action Plan to Advance Patient Safety.* Boston, MA: Institute for Healthcare Improvement. Published 2020. Accessed April 9, 2022. http://www.ihi.org/Engage/Initiatives/National-Steering-Committee-Patient-Safety/Pages/National-Action-Plan-to-Advance-Patient-Safety.aspx

Nolan K, Zullo AR, Bosco E, Marchese C, Berard-Collins C. Controlled substance diversion in health systems: a failure modes and effects analysis for prevention. *Am J Health Syst Pharm.* 2019;76(15):1158-1164. doi:10.1093/ajhp/zxz116

Pelletier LR. Quality and safety. In: Huber DL, Lindell Joseph M, eds. *Leadership and Nursing Care Management.* 7th ed. St. Louis, MO: Elsevier; 2022:348-384.

Petrovich B, Sweet M, Gillian S, Copenhaver J. Assessing the impact of a pharmacist-managed discharge medication reconciliation pilot at a community hospital system. *J Healthc Qual.* 2021;43(2):e26-e32. doi:10.1097/JHQ.0000000000000282

Reason J. *Human Error.* Cambridge, UK: Cambridge University Press; 1990.

Reason J. Human error: models and management. *BMJ.* 2000;320:768-770. doi:10.1136/bmj.320.7237.768

Shang J, Russell D, Dowding D, et al. Predictive risk model for infection-related hospitalization among home healthcare patients. *J Healthc Qual.* 2020;42(3):136-147. doi:10.1097/JHQ.0000000000000214

Shekelle PG, Sarker U, Shojania K, et al. *Patient Safety in Ambulatory Settings.* Technical brief 27. AHRQ publication 16(17)-EHC033-EF. Rockville, MD: Agency for Healthcare Research and Quality. Published 2016. Accessed April 9, 2022. https://www.ncbi.nlm.nih.gov/books/NBK396055/

Stargell LF, Heatherly SL. Managing what is measured: a rural hospital's experience in reducing patient harm. *J Healthc Qual.* 2018;40(3):172-176. doi:10.1097/JHQ.0000000000000139

Stinehart KR, Spitzer CR, Evans KA, Buehler J, Attar T, Besecker B. Going silent: redesigning the activation process for in-hospital cardiopulmonary arrests. *J Healthc Qual.* 2021;43(4):232-239. doi:0.1097/JHQ.0000000000000303

Weick KE, Sutcliffe KM. *Managing the Unexpected: Resilient Performance in an Age of Uncertainty.* 2nd ed. (MP3-CD ed.). Audible Studios on Brilliance Audio; 2007.

Xie Y, Gunasekeran DV, Balaskas K, et al. Health economic and safety considerations for artificial intelligence applications in diabetic retinopathy screening. *Transl Vis Sci Technol.* 2020;9(2):22. doi:10.1167/tvst.9.2.22. eCollection 2020 Apr. PMID: 32818083.

Zallman L, Finnegan KE, Todaro M, et al. Association between provider engagement, staff engagement, and culture of safety. *J Healthc Qual.* 2020;42(4):236-247. doi:10.1097/JHQ.0000000000000220

# Online Resources

## Agency for Healthcare Research and Quality (AHRQ)

www.ahrq.gov

- **Advances in Patient Safety**
  https://www.ahrq.gov/patient-safety/resources/advances/index.html
- **Advancing Patient Safety: A Decade of Evidence, Design and Implementation**
  https://www.ahrq.gov/sites/default/files/publications/files/advancing-patient-safety.pdf
- **CAHPS Ambulatory Care Improvement Guide**
  https://www.ahrq.gov/cahps/quality-improvement/improvement-guide/improvement-guide.html
- **Education and Training for Health Professionals**
  https://www.ahrq.gov/patient-safety/education/index.html
- **Guidelines and Measures**
  https://www.ahrq.gov/gam/index.html
- **Improving Patient Safety in Nursing Homes**
  https://www.ahrq.gov/sites/default/files/wysiwyg/professionals/quality-patient-safety/patientsafetyculture/nursing-home/resources/nhimpptsaf.pdf
- **Oral, Linguistic, and Culturally Competent Services: Guides for Managed Care Plans**
  https://www.ahrq.gov/ncepcr/tools/cultural-competence/index.html
- **Patient Safety Measure Tools and Resources**
  https://www.ahrq.gov/patient-safety/resources/measures/index.html
- **Patient Safety and Quality: An Evidence-Based Handbook for Nurses**
  https://archive.ahrq.gov/professionals/clinicians-providers/resources/nursing/resources/nurseshdbk/
- **Quality and Patient Safety Resources**
  https://www.ahrq.gov/patient-safety/resources/index.html
- **TeamSTEPPS**
  http://teamstepps.ahrq.gov
- **WebM&M (Morbidity & Mortality Rounds on the web)**
  https://www.ahrq.gov/cpi/about/otherwebsites/webmm.ahrq.gov/index.html

## American Board of Internal Medicine Foundation—Choosing Wisely

www.choosingwisely.org

## American Hospital Association

https://www.aha.org/

- **Center for Health Innovation: Health Research & Education Trust**
  https://www.aha.org/center/hret
- **Hospitals Against Violence**
  http://www.aha.org/advocacy-issues/violence/index.shtml
- **Hospitals in Pursuit of Excellence**
  www.hpoe.org
  - **A Leadership Resource for Patient and Family Engagement Strategies**
    http://www.hpoe.org/resources/hpoehretaha-guides/1407
  - **Patient and Family Resource Compendium**
    http://www.hpoe.org/resources/hpoehretaha-guides/2735
  - **Institute for Diversity and Health Equity: AHA Disparities Toolkit**
    https://ifdhe.aha.org/hretdisparities/toolkit

## American Society for Health Care Risk Management

http://www.ashrm.org/

## American Society of Health-System Pharmacists: Patient Safety Resource Center

https://www.ashp.org/pharmacy-practice/resource-centers/patient-safety

## Canadian Patient Safety Institute

http://www.patientsafetyinstitute.ca/en/pages/default.aspx

## Centers for Disease Control and Prevention

- **Guidelines for the Prevention of Intravascular Catheter-Related Infections**
  http://www.cdc.gov/mmwr/preview/mmwrhtml/rr5110a1.htm
- **Medication Safety Program**
  www.cdc.gov/medicationsafety
- **National Healthcare Safety Network**
  https://www.cdc.gov/nhsn/

- **NHSN Patient Safety Component Manual**
  https://www.cdc.gov/nhsn/pdfs/pscmanual/
  pcsmanual_current.pdf
- **Ten Things You Can Do to Be a Safe Patient**
  http://www.cdc.gov/HAI/patientSafety/patient-
  safety.html

## Centers for Medicare & Medicaid Services

- **Partnership for Patients**
  https://innovation.cms.gov/innovation-models/
  partnership-for-patients
- **A Practical Guide to Implementing the National CLAS Standards: For Racial, Ethnic and Linguistic Minorities, People with Disabilities and Sexual and Gender Minorities**
  https://www.cms.gov/About-CMS/Agency-
  Information/OMH/Downloads/CLAS-Tool-
  kit-12-7-16.pdf

## The Cochrane Collaboration

http://www.cochrane.org

## Cynosure Health

http://www.cynosurehealth.org/

## ECRI Institute

http://www.ecri.org

## Food & Drug Administration

https://www.fda.gov/

- **Medical Devices**
  https://www.fda.gov/MedicalDevices/Safety/
- **Drugs**
  https://www.fda.gov/Drugs/default.htm
- **MedWatch**
  https://www.fda.gov/safety/medwatch-fda-
  safety-information-and-adverse-event-reporting
  -program

## GW Cancer Center: Prepared Patient

https://preparedpatient.org/

## The Health Foundation

- **The Measurement and Monitoring of Safety**
  http://www.health.org.uk/publication/measurement-
  and-monitoring-safety

## Institute for Healthcare Improvement

http://www.ihi.org/

- **Free from Harm**
  http://www.ihi.org/resources/Pages/Publications/
  Free-from-Harm-Accelerating-Patient-Safety-
  Improvement.aspx
- **High-Alert Medication Safety**
  http://www.ihi.org/topics/highalertmedication
  safety/pages/default.aspx
- **Medication Administration**
  http://www.ihi.org/resources/Pages/Changes/
  ImproveCoreProcessesforAdministeringMedica
  tions.aspx
- **National Patient Safety Foundation**
  http://www.ihi.org/Topics/PatientSafety/Pages/
  default.aspx
- **Open School**
  http://www.ihi.org/education/ihiopenschool/
  Pages/default.aspx?msclkid=038248b85bfd1ff3a
  10a2902c1815963
- **Safety Briefings**
  http://www.ihi.org/Engage/Memberships/
  Passport/Documents/SafetyBriefings.pdf

## Institute for Safe Medication Practices

www.ismp.org

## The Joint Commission

www.jointcommision.org

- **Behaviors That Undermine a Culture of Safety**
  https://www.jointcommission.org/resources/
  patient-safety-topics/sentinel-event/sentinel-
  event-alert-newsletters/sentinel-event-alert-issue-
  40-behaviors-that-undermine-a-culture-of-safety/
- **Developing a Reporting Culture: Learning from Close Calls and Hazardous Conditions**
  https://www.jointcommission.org/-/media/tjc/docu
  ments/resources/patient-safety-topics/sentinel-event/
  sea_60_reporting_culture_final.pdf?db=web&hash
  =5AB072026CAAF4711FCDC343701B0159
- **The Essential Role of Leadership in Developing a Safety Culture**
  https://www.jointcommission.org/assets/1/18/
  SEA_57_Safety_Culture_Leadership_0317.pdf
- **Joint Commission Center for Transforming Healthcare**
  https://www.centerfortransforminghealth
  care.org/high-reliability-in-health-care/
- **The Joint Commission International—International Center for Patient Safety**
  www.jointcommissioninternational.org

- **Patient Safety Systems**
  https://www.jointcommission.org/standards/patient-safety-systems-ps-chapter/
- **Sentinel Event**
  www.jointcommission.org/sentinel_event.aspx

*Josie King Foundation*

www.josieking.org

*The Just Culture Company*

https://justculture.com/

*The Leapfrog Group*

www.leapfroggroup.org

*National Academies Press*

www.nap.edu

- **Improving diagnosis in healthcare**
  https://www.nap.edu/resource/21794/interactive/

*National Academy of Medicine (formerly Institute of Medicine)*

https://www.nationalacademies.org/hmd/health-and-medicine-division

*National Association for Healthcare Quality*

www.nahq.org

- **HQ Competency Framework**
  https://nahq.org/nahq-intelligence/competency-framework/
- **HQ Principles**
  https://nahq.org/products/hq-principles/

*National Coordinating Council for Medication Error Reporting and Prevention*

www.nccmerp.org

*National Network of Libraries of Medicine*

https://nnlm.gov/

*Occupational Safety & Health Administration—U.S. Department of Labor*

- **Healthcare**
  https://www.osha.gov/SLTC/healthcarefacilities/index.html

- **Sustainability in the Workplace**
  https://www.osha.gov/sustainability/

*Partnership for Patients, Leadership*

https://innovation.cms.gov/innovation-models/partnership-for-patients

*Patient and Family Engagement in Healthcare*

- **A Roadmap for Patient + Family Engagement in Healthcare**
  http://patientfamilyengagement.org/

*The Patient Safety Group*

https://www.patientsafetygroup.org/

*PubMed*

https://pubmed.ncbi.nlm.nih.gov/

*Quality and Safety Education for Nurses (Case Western Reserve University)*

www.qsen.org

*Safe & Reliable Healthcare*

https://www.safeandreliablecare.com/

*University of Texas Safety Climate Survey*

https://med.uth.edu/chqs/survey/

*U.S. Department of Health & Human Services, Office of Minority Health*

- **Think Cultural Health**
  https://www.thinkculturalhealth.hhs.gov/about

*VA National Center for Patient Safety (NCPS)*

http://www.patientsafety.va.gov/

*World Health Organization*

www.who.int

- **Infection Prevention and Control**
  https://www.who.int/health-topics/infection-prevention-and-control#tab=tab_1
- **Patient Safety**
  https://www.who.int/teams/integrated-health-services/patient-safety

# Performance and Process Improvement

Susan V. White

## SECTION CONTENTS

# Introduction

Through understanding performance and process improvement principles, models, and tools, healthcare quality professionals can apply evidence-based techniques and practices to ensure quality and safety in their healthcare organizations. This section provides an overview of the historical development of performance and process improvement as well as the key principles and practices for performance improvement in healthcare quality and safety. The tenets of quality and safety must first be established through strategic planning to better align the activities with the organization's mission, vision, values, goals, and objectives. Important to an organization's success is establishing priorities for quality and performance improvement activities, translating strategic goals into quality outcomes, and aligning organizational culture and structure to support quality and safety.

A formal quality and performance improvement program with a defined scope and infrastructure is required to identify, prioritize, and evaluate projects and performance toward desired goals. Fundamentals of a quality and performance improvement program are described in this section, including tools and methods for use by healthcare quality professionals to sustain improvement solutions. A summary is provided about innovation as a key to improvement and creating a future-oriented, adaptable, agile organization. An overview of teams and their roles and responsibilities is given as an essential component of working collaboratively on improvement projects (e.g., team effectiveness, process champions, and process owners). Sharing successes, evaluating external award opportunities, and acquiring requisite knowledge and skills to continuously improve are also discussed.

# Evolution of Performance Improvement

There are important individuals in the quality and performance improvement movement who were influential in shaping current performance management and improvement methods. Early pioneers viewed process as a sequence of activities and communications that fulfilled a service need for a client or customer and improving a process to yield quality outcomes. These early pioneers are briefly presented with their major contributions to the development of quality management and improvement.

## Shewhart

In the 1920s, Shewhart, a statistician at Bell Telephone Laboratories, developed the Shewhart cycle, best known as plan-do-check-act (PDCA). This four-step process is designed to continuously improve quality (**Figure 5.1**). The PDCA steps include the following:

**Plan.** Question the capacity or capability of a process. Pose theories on how to improve the process and predict measurable outcomes.

**Do.** Make changes on an experimental, pilot basis.

**Check.** Measure outcomes compared to predicted outcomes.

**Act.** Implement the changes on a broad scale.[1]

Later, Deming adapted the PDCA cycle as the plan-do-study-act (PDSA) cycle; therefore, it also is referred to as the Deming cycle, or the Deming wheel. Both PDCA and PDSA are used as improvement frameworks. Shewhart is also credited with his work on statistical process control charts (see the *Health Data Analytics* section).

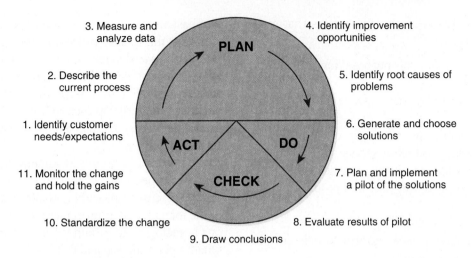

3. Measure and analyze data

4. Identify improvement opportunities

**PLAN**

2. Describe the current process

5. Identify root causes of problems

1. Identify customer needs/expectations

**ACT**

**DO**

6. Generate and choose solutions

11. Monitor the change and hold the gains

**CHECK**

7. Plan and implement a pilot of the solutions

10. Standardize the change

8. Evaluate results of pilot

9. Draw conclusions

**Figure 5.1** The Traditional Plan-Do-Check-Act Cycle

## Ohno

As an industrial engineer known as Ono Taiichi in Japan and as Taiichi Ohno in the West developed methods to improve efficiency and minimize waste in manufacturing by identifying steps to eliminate these types of waste:

1. Waste of overproduction
2. Waste of time on hand (waiting)
3. Waste in transportation
4. Waste of processing itself
5. Waste of stock on hand (inventory)
6. Waste of movement
7. Waste of making defective products

Kanban is one of Ohno's methods that became an integral part of the Toyota Production System to control inventory costs and space without the risk of running short on materials, and it is foundational to Lean manufacturing. Kanban was built upon supermarket practices

> where a customer can get (1) what is needed, (2) at the time needed, (3) in the amount needed. Sometimes, of course, a customer may buy more than he or she needs. In principle, however, the supermarket is a place where we buy according to need. Supermarket operators, therefore, must make certain that customers can buy what they need at any time.[2]

Other quality concepts brought forward through his work are just-in-time (right time, right place) ordering and autonomation (automation with a human touch), which are the two pillars supporting the elimination of waste. Ohno believed in the power of individual skill and teamwork and felt that reducing waste and ensuring the competitive position of

a business required a "revolution in consciousness" where defects and waste must be understood to avoid business losses.

## Deming

Deming is probably the most famous of the industrial quality gurus. A statistician with doctorates in mathematics and physics, he became the philosopher of quality and the learning organization. The story of post–World War II America's rejection of Deming's quality exhortations—and of his subsequent dealings with a receptive Japan—is now legend.[3] In the 1950s, Deming visited the Western Electric Hawthorne Plant in Chicago while the Harvard University study regarding motivation of workers was in progress. The *Hawthorne effect* (change in behavior due to awareness of being observed) was coined from this work. Following this experience, he proposed replacing traditional management techniques with a statistically controlled management process to determine when—and when not—to intervene in a process. Statistical process control techniques allow management to determine a range of random variation that always occurs in a process. Statistical process control describes two types of causes of variation: common cause and special cause. Common-cause problems are rooted in basic processes and systems. Special-cause problems stem from isolated occurrences that are outside the system. Statistical process control is discussed in the *Health Data Analytics* section, which further explains control limits, common cause variation, and special cause variation.

Deming said that 85% of the problems detected are process- or system-related, whereas 15% are traceable to individuals; this is known as the "85/15 theory."[1] Deming's management philosophy is based on the 14 points for businesses that seek to be competitive:

1. Create a constancy of purpose toward quality improvement.
2. Adopt a philosophy that expects good products and services.
3. Cease dependence on mass inspection and build quality into the product or service.
4. Do not award business solely on price tag.
5. Constantly improve the system of production and service.
6. Institute on-the-job training.
7. Institute leadership with an arm to help people and machines do better jobs.
8. Drive out fear.
9. Break down barriers between departments.
10. Eliminate slogans, exhortations, and targets.
11. Eliminate number quotas and management by objective and substitute leadership.
12. Remove barriers to pride of workmanship.
13. Institute education and self-improvement.
14. Take action to accomplish the transformation.[1,3]

## Juran

Juran's background was in engineering and law. He followed Deming to Japan after World War II, emphasizing the key role of top organizational leadership and the quality process in the organization.[4] In *Juran on Leadership for Quality*, Juran states that quality is "product performance that results in customer satisfaction; freedom from product deficiencies which avoid customer dissatisfaction."[5(pp16,31)] This concept is known as fitness for use and is explained in Juran's Trilogy (**Figure 5.2**).

The cost accounting for quality means there is a break-even point of less than 100%. Beyond a certain point, the cost of providing quality exceeds the value of the incremental improvement in quality. Juran's Trilogy is analogous to certain familiar financial processes. Quality planning is equal to budgeting, quality control (sometimes called measurement) is comparable to cost control, and quality and performance improvement relate to cost reduction and margin improvement.[6]

## Crosby

In the 1970s and 1980s, Crosby developed an important concept known as *the cost of [poor] quality*. His work documented that high quality (what he terms *conformance to expectations*) is less costly than the waste and rework that characterizes poor-quality processes. Crosby demonstrated conclusively that investment in quality can offer

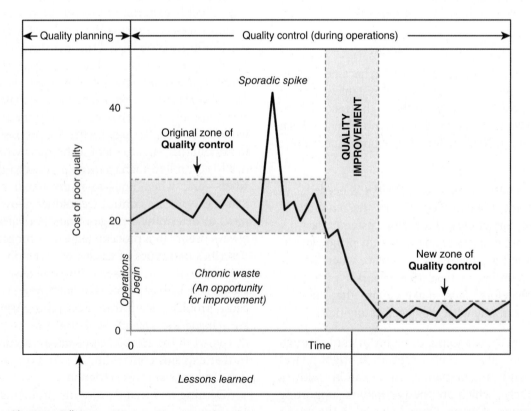

**Figure 5.2** The Juran Trilogy

Reproduced from DeFeo JA. *The Juran Trilogy: Quality Planning*. Published 2019. Accessed January 8, 2022. https://www.juran.com/blog/the-juran-trilogy-quality-planning/

an enormous financial return. Five stages of management maturity are identified in *Quality Is Free*.[7] Crosby's underlying philosophy is "Do it right the first time." The stages are

1. uncertainty,
2. awakening,
3. enlightenment,
4. wisdom, and
5. certainty.[8]

Crosby also identified 14 steps to improve quality and move a company toward certainty, including:

Step 1. Management is committed to quality improvement.

Step 2. A quality improvement team is formed to oversee actions.

Step 3. Quality measurement is undertaken appropriate to the activities undergoing improvement.

Step 4. Quality cost is evaluated, using estimates as necessary.

Step 5. Quality awareness is promoted through various methods and supervisor involvement.

Step 6. Corrective actions are generated in response to steps 3 and 4.

Step 7. Zero-defects planning is tailored to the company and its products.

Step 8. Supervisory training is undertaken at all management levels.

Step 9. A zero-defects day is held to celebrate a new performance standard.

Step 10. Goals are set for individuals and groups.

Step 11. Error cause(s) is removed by management after notification.

Step 12. Goals are met and recognized.

Step 13. The quality council's experiences, problems, and ideas are shared.

Step 14. The process is repeated (the pursuit of quality is never ending).

## Ishikawa

Ishikawa was one of Deming's early Japanese hosts and inventor of the cause-and-effect, or fishbone, diagram. He is credited with using the term *total quality control* to imply not just the operational but also the total organizational commitment (marketing, finance, research) needed to fully actualize all components of the modern quality-committed organization. The preferred American term is *total quality management*.[9]

Key points to the evolution of healthcare quality are listed in **Box 5.1**.

---

**Box 5.1 Key Points: Evolution of Performance Improvement**

- Key leaders in healthcare quality laid the foundation for current frameworks that stand the test of time.
- Values and philosophy derive from long-standing quality leaders.
- Learning comes from theory and experience.

---

# Healthcare Quality Movement into the 21st Century

The U.S. healthcare quality movement began in the 19th century and continues into the 21st century. Highlights are described in the timeline herein and **Figure 5.3**.

## The First Era: Nightingale, Codman, and the American College of Surgeons

In 1863, Nightingale noted that patients seemed to fare better in some London hospitals than in others. She was the first to call for systematic inquiry into the nature of care processes that could be related to outcome variability. Although there is little evidence that Nightingale's quality vision came to fruition during her lifetime, Boston surgeon Codman's early 20th-century efforts had a more direct impact. Codman, who also observed variability in patient outcomes among several hospitals, called for a systematic evaluation process with a view toward improving care.[10] Although these efforts met considerable resistance at the time, Codman's ideas were embodied in the founding of the American College of Surgeons in 1913. Codman's body of work set about the task of establishing quality standards and focus on outcomes. In 1917, the College established a five-part minimum standard, and the Hospital Standardization Program was born.[11] This was the early beginning for hospital accreditation based on standards. The Program was based on Codman's end-result system of standardization in which hospitals would track every patient treated for long enough to determine if the treatment was effective. When treatment was found to be ineffective, the hospital would attempt to determine how similar cases could be treated with success in the future.

| | |
|---|---|
| 1863 | Nightingale calls for a systematic review of patient care. |
| 1910 | Codman proposes an end-result system of hospital standardization and Flexner publishes report calling for American medical schools to enact standards for teaching and research of the medical profession. |
| 1918 | The American College of Surgeons develops minimum standards for hospitals and conducts its first survey. |
| 1950 | Donabedian formulates a theoretical framework for patient care evaluation (structure, process, outcomes). |
| 1951 | The Joint Commission on Accreditation of Hospitals is founded by Codman, introducing quality assurance standards for hospitals. |
| 1960 | Japan focuses on becoming a world quality leader; adopts the Deming management philosophy. |
| 1970 | Juran and Crosby build on Shewhart and Deming's work; plan-do-check-act/plan-do-study-act cycles emerge. |
| 1980 | Berwick, Batalden, and James apply quality improvement methods to healthcare. |
| 1996 | The Health Insurance Portability and Accountability Act of 1996 is enacted. |
| 1999 | Institute of Medicine (IOM) releases the report, *To Err Is Human: Building a Safer Health System*. |
| 2000 | Six Sigma, Lean Enterprise, rapid cycle improvements, safety, and pay for performance begin to have an impact on healthcare quality. |
| 2001 | The Committee on the Quality of Health Care in America released *Crossing the Quality Chasm: A New Health System for the 21st Century* for fundamental change to close the quality gap in the American healthcare system. |
| 2002 | Medicare begins a series of quality measurement and reporting initiatives starting with nursing homes, followed by home healthcare, and eventually hospitals and physicians. |
| 2009 | The American Recovery and Reinvestment Act is signed into law; it includes the Health Information Technology for Economic and Clinical Health Act. |
| 2010 | The Patient Protection and Affordable Care Act is signed into law. |
| 2011 | U.S. Department of Health & Human Services releases the *National Quality Strategy* and presents three aims to guide efforts to improve quality—better care, healthy people/healthy communities, and affordable care. |
| 2011 | IOM publishes *The Future of Nursing: Leading Change, Advancing Health.* |
| 2013 | IOM releases its report, *Best Care at Lower Costs: The Path to Continuously Learning Health Care in America*, looking at economic and quality barriers that hinder progress toward improving health, continuous improvement, and quality care. |
| 2015 | National Academy of Medicine (NAM) releases *Improving Diagnosis in Healthcare*. The Society to Improve Diagnosis in Medicine is established. |
| 2016 | Accreditation and regulatory agencies focus on sepsis and mortality. |
| 2020 | Policy and research emerge on COVID-19 and the worldwide pandemic, including vaccines, personal protective equipment, treatment, and impact on patients and staff (disparities, well-being, and resilience). |
| 2020 | Healthcare organizations expand focus on mental health and well-being of patients and staff including burnout, psychological safety, and whole health. |
| 2020 | National attention grows on diversity, equity, and inclusion in healthcare. |
| 2021 | NAM's *The Future of Nursing 2020–2030: Charting a Path to Achieve Health Equity* is published. |
| 2021 | The voice of patients in performance measurement expands by increasing the number and use of Patient Reported Outcome Measures (PROMs) and Patient Reported Outcome Performance Measures (PRO-PMs). |
| 2022 | CMS National Quality Strategy takes a person-centered approach to quality and safety and seeks to improve the overall care journey across the continuum of care, from home or community-based settings to hospitals and post-acute care. |

**Figure 5.3** Quality Movement Timeline

## The Second Era: Legal Decisions, Donabedian, and The Joint Commission's Monitoring and Evaluation Process

Definitions and requirements for quality in healthcare evolved over the past decades. In the early 1950s, quality care review was conducted exclusively by individual physicians using an unstructured and subjective process that relied on the practitioner's knowledge and experiences. Between 1950 and 1960, the responsibility for quality of care expanded beyond the physician to include both the hospital and the board of directors. Two significant legal decisions marked this transition period:

- *Bing v. Thunig* (1957). In this case, the New York Court of Appeals ruled that the doctrine of charitable immunity no longer applied to hospitals; hospitals are liable for patient injuries sustained through negligence of employees.
- *Darling v. Charleston Community Memorial Hospital* (1965). In this important corporate negligence case, the court ruled that the hospital had a legal responsibility to protect a patient from harm by others by overseeing the quality of patient care.

Accreditation standards evolved slowly throughout the 1950s and early 1960s. At the academic level, the University of Michigan's Donabedian examined existing research, formulating a theoretical framework for patient care evaluation.[9] He is best recognized for the "structure, process, outcomes" model of quality evaluation. This model suggests the importance of relating healthcare structures (qualifications of practitioners and facilities and technology available to them) and processes (activities involved in prevention, diagnosis, and treatment) to outcomes (how patients fare because of their care).

In the past, The Joint Commission accreditation standards reflected the structure and process elements of this model. Surveyors, who reviewed the structures and processes, assessed hospital plans and technology, qualifications of clinicians and administrators, and organizational structures against the annually updated requirements contained in the *Comprehensive Accreditation Manual for Hospitals*. Specialized standards for behavioral health and other services were also developed. Surveyors inferred process from documentation and discussion. They reviewed minutes and interviewed clinical and administrative leaders to ascertain whether designated individuals were following procedures and compliant with quality evaluation processes.

As a matter of policy and practical considerations, accreditation standards did not address patient outcomes directly. First, there were problems with the way quality was measured. Second, no professional consensus existed on systematic measures of patient outcomes. Finally, uniform and comparable clinical databases and registries were nonexistent. The problems of measuring and interpreting patient outcomes precluded their practical use in accreditation. Consequently, the accreditation process was necessarily built on an implicit assumption that if proper structures and processes were in place, good outcomes were likely to follow. As measurement systems matured, the evaluation of patient outcomes became a strong focus for accreditation processes as well as the organizational review of various aspects of care, treatment, and services. See the *Regulatory and Accreditation* section for further details on accreditation.

## The Third Era: Berwick, Batalden, and Deming, Juran, and "Japan, Inc."

The names of Berwick, Batalden, and James are eminent in the field of healthcare quality. Like many of their colleagues, these physicians were dissatisfied with traditional healthcare quality assurance practices. These pioneering physicians, however, went beyond a mere critique of existing quality assurance. Both Berwick and Batalden researched the industrial methods publicized by the Japanese experience. Arising from this research, Berwick's article describing healthcare quality assurance as based upon the theory of the bad apples became a classic.[12] Among his many contributions, Batalden translated Deming's 14 points into a healthcare context.[13] In 1987, these two physicians played key roles in linking with the Juran Institute and a variety of industrial quality consultants to create the National Demonstration Project on Quality Improvement in Healthcare. This multiyear project and its original 21 forward-looking healthcare organizations conclusively demonstrated the applicability of performance improvement processes to healthcare.[14]

James, of the Intermountain Health System, was also a pioneer in applying quality improvement processes directly to patients and clinical outcomes. The success of James and his team measured not only improved results in a single hospital but also across the entire multihospital system.[15,16]

In 1991, Berwick established the Institute for Healthcare Improvement (IHI), a not-for-profit organization that began driving improvements in healthcare. It accomplished this by supporting national projects focused on the six aims—safety, effectiveness, patient-centeredness, timeliness, efficiency, and equity.[17] Collaboratives are one approach involving many organizations trying to affect the same issue and using rapid cycle improvement efforts to implement change. A major benefit of this approach is that the collaborating organizations share their experiences and improvements spread quickly. Projects initiated include improvements in patient safety, chronic care, critical care, falls, and end-of-life care. Berwick was appointed administrator of the Centers for Medicare & Medicaid Services (CMS) in 2010 and served for 18 months in President Obama's administration. While in office, Berwick inculcated the Triple Aim into health policy: improving the patient care experience, improving population health, and reducing health costs. Dr. Berwick was also responsible for initiating major changes under the new health reform legislation known as the Affordable Care Act.[18]

With more experience, the list of visionary leaders, both clinical and managerial, continues to grow as evidenced by recent literature and presentations in public forums. Healthcare organizations are taking the learnings from these leaders as well as newer methodologies and are advancing the science and experience of healthcare quality to serve as role models for others. For example, Virginia Mason led Lean initiatives by modeling the Toyota methods and Catalysis (formerly ThedaCare Center for Healthcare Value) is sharing its Lean journey.

## The Fourth Era: Patient Is Front and Center with Growth of Advocacy, Engagement, and Activation

Healthcare reform stresses an imperative to engage families in their own care. Enhancing patient-centered care that results in empowerment, engagement, and activation is everyone's job. Patients and their families need to understand their role and responsibilities related to quality and safety. Patient-centered communication is shown to improve clinical outcomes.[19,20] More patient-centric technology tools and applications are available and have been found to be most useful in managing chronic disease.

Patient advocacy includes addressing the rights and responsibilities of patients and involving them in shared decision making, obtaining informed consent for treatment, and disclosing unanticipated outcomes. An advocate or ombudsman is often available to manage inquiries, requests, complaints, and grievances, with a process to document and track reported issues to resolution. An ethical framework is often applied with ethics consultation to respond to issues that may create conflict with the rights of the patient and the organization or others.

A patient's bill of rights was first adopted by the American Hospital Association in 1973 and revised in 1992. Additionally, the President's Advisory Commission on Consumer Protection and Quality in Health Care Industry addressed consumer rights as the managed care industry was booming, and there were many questions about services patients could expect to receive.[21] The American Hospital Association published under the Patient Care Partnership, replacing the rights with a plain-language brochure.[22] The protection of patient rights may include a variety of concerns, such as

- abuse, neglect, and exploitation;
- financial responsibility;
- caregiving;
- decision-making ability and use of surrogates or durable power of attorney;
- advance directives or living wills;
- choices about healthcare and treatment;
- care regardless of ability to pay, gender, race, religion, sexual orientation, or any other factor;
- treatment without fear of retaliation; and
- visitation and support.

While the American Hospital Association publication is hospital focused, there are broader patient rights across settings from the 1998 Patients' Bill of Rights Act. Additionally, certain healthcare settings have additional requirements for rights and responsibilities (e.g., patient consent based on 42 CFR Part 2 - Confidentiality of Substance Use Disorder Patient Records). Organizations encode these rights and responsibilities into policies and procedures for the particular healthcare setting and populations served.

*Engagement* is defined as "actions an individual must make to obtain the greatest benefit from the healthcare services available to them."[23(p2)] Engaged patients produce better health outcomes.[24-26] In this context, patient engagement involves an active process of synthesizing health information, recommendations of healthcare professionals, and personal beliefs, values, and preferences to manage one's illness. Advocacy, engagement, and activation all offer opportunities for improved healthcare quality and safety in the current environment.

**Box 5.2** lists the key points of healthcare quality in the 21st century.

# Performance Improvement Approaches

There are a variety of performance improvement (PI) approaches, and they each have value and usefulness depending on the type of problem, scope, and solution needed. The process for determining which performance improvement model or models to use in an organization requires an analysis of the organization and its history of success with current and previous models, level of maturity, and resources. How will the model be communicated across the organization? Are all staff members expected to know how to use it? Which model or models are a good fit with the culture and the current strategies that are working?

Healthcare quality professionals may be asked to provide a review and analysis of the PI methodology currently in use and compare it with alternative options. As more sophisticated tools and methods become available, healthcare quality professionals must keep pace and contribute to the final selection(s) of what approaches and tools to use in which situations. Today, quality, safety, and performance improvement projects call for perspectives beyond unit-based or team activities regardless of healthcare setting. The use of epidemiologic principles in healthcare quality grows as healthcare reform focuses on improving the health of the population, advancing quality of care for the individual, and containing costs—the Triple Aim—and, more recently, workforce engagement and workforce safety. This requires looking at the distribution and determinants of health status and disease states.

Various methods can be used to conduct quality, safety, and performance improvement projects and epidemiologic studies: surveillance, descriptive studies, analytic studies, and systematic review. Outcomes of interest can include injury, disability, and health-related quality of life. Project results can contribute to changing clinical practices and policies at the point of care, developing/validating evidence-based practice, implementing population-based interventions, and preventive medicine targeting health conditions (e.g., cancer, cardiovascular disease, obesity, and diabetes).

## Quality Assurance

Audits led to a preoccupation with meeting audit number requirements. Thus, in 1980, the Joint Commission on Accreditation of Hospitals, now known as The Joint Commission, developed the first quality assurance standards requiring a problem-focused approach to measuring quality. This approach required organizations to identify and monitor problem areas. The combined strengths of criteria-based audits and the epidemiologic approach used in infection control in the 1980s resulted in a new focus on systematic monitoring and evaluation in 1985. From this, a 10-step process for quality and performance improvement evolved in 1986, requiring organizations to evaluate important aspects of care and then use the results to identify opportunities for improvement. Early work focused on this 10-step model and has since evolved into more mainstream tools with Lean and Six Sigma.[27]

## Retrospective Audits

A shift from physician review to medical audits occurred in 1955. Medical audits included a systematic procedure using objective, valid criteria with an orientation on outcomes. In 1966, there was a major change whereby the Joint Commission on Accreditation of Hospitals (as it was called then) focused on optimal, not minimal, standards of care. In 1975, it published the quality of professional services standards, requiring hospitals to demonstrate optimal care using valid and reliable measures.

Although *optimal* was never defined, this new focus led to one-time audits of care, known as performance evaluation program audits. During that period, monitoring quality was focused on the acute care setting. Later, as care in the outpatient and homecare setting grew, additional monitoring and performance measures were established. Specialty organizations and accreditations also grew to meet this need. However, some office and outpatient settings were not accredited and had less oversight by regulatory agencies. Quality monitoring was slower to mature in these settings. Additionally, the major costs in healthcare occurred in the hospital setting. Audits continue to be a useful tool to collect data for analysis and compliance, but more real-time data allow for timely quality care and assessment of that care.

## Reengineering and System Redesign

In the 1990s, reengineering was one of the major initiatives in hospitals with efforts focused on workforce redesign. There was typically a focus on restructuring or redesigning systems and departments into more efficient processes. For example, hospitals experimented with creating new positions that combined work from different areas. A focus on cross-functional capabilities led to the dissolution of departmental silos. A patient service associate or technical associate would deliver meals, clean patient rooms, stock supplies, and provide patient transportation. Many hospitals thought that reengineering would increase profit margins and create financial stability. The problem was that reengineering often became associated with mergers, acquisitions, downsizing, and layoffs. When this happened, employee morale declined, and productivity suffered. Because of these negative connotations, reengineering fell out of vogue and was replaced by other improvement models and initiatives. The newer approach is to consider adopting the Lean Enterprise method to increase financial stability by eliminating waste.

The key components and tools of Lean Enterprise include identifying value (value stream mapping and voice of the customer), eliminating waste, establishing smooth flow, enabling pull (instead of push) systems, and pursuing perfection. The Six Sigma method includes a five-step process: define, measure, analyze, improve, and control (DMAIC). See **Table 5.1** and **Figure 5.4** for key questions/steps in the improvement process and common tools used. Lean Enterprise and Six Sigma are complementary tools. Lean focuses on dramatically improving flow in the value stream and eliminating waste to improve efficiency and speed.[28] Six Sigma focuses on eliminating defects and reducing variation in processes to improve effectiveness.[29] Both are extremely effective in and of themselves, but together they offer a powerful approach to improvement.

## Rapid Cycle Improvement

IHI developed the collaborative approach, termed the *Breakthrough Series*, to bring about rapid cycle

**Table 5.1** The DMAIC Methodology

| Phase | Key Questions | Common Tools |
|---|---|---|
| **D**efine | <ul><li>What is the problem?</li><li>Why are we working on this project?</li><li>Who is going to be working on this project?</li><li>What resources do we need to complete this project? What is the scope?</li><li>By when must the project be completed?</li><li>Who is the customer?</li><li>Who are key stakeholders?</li><li>What key metrics are important?</li><li>What does the current process look like?</li></ul> | Project Charter<br>SIPOC (supplier-input-process-output-customer)<br>Voice of the Customer<br>Run Chart<br>Process/Flow Map |
| **M**easure | <ul><li>How can we measure the process or performance?</li><li>What data sources are available, and what is the data collection method?</li><li>What is our current or baseline performance of the process? What data display (graphs) is useful?</li><li>What does our customer define as a defect?</li><li>How can we stratify data or measure defects?</li><li>What benefits do we hope to achieve through solving this problem?</li></ul> | Control Charts<br>Pareto<br>Histogram<br>Other Analysis |
| **A**nalyze | <ul><li>Why is there a gap between current performance and customer expectations?</li><li>What are the root causes of variability in our processes and have they been verified?</li><li>What root causes are the highest priority to focus efforts?</li><li>Where is waste in the process and what type of waste?</li></ul> | Process Map<br>Value Stream Map<br>Risk Analysis<br>Cause and Effect Diagram (Fishbone/Ishikawa Diagram) |

*(continues)*

**Table 5.1** The DMAIC Methodology                                                      *(continued)*

| Phase | Key Questions | Common Tools |
|---|---|---|
| Improve | ▪ What are potential solutions to the root causes?<br>▪ What solutions have been verified and are the highest priority?<br>▪ How will we track implementation?<br>▪ Are there any anticipated barriers to improvement?<br>▪ How can we best translate the details into standard work expectations?<br>▪ What will the redesigned process look like, and how will it be tested, measured, and validated?<br>▪ Does the redesigned process reduce waste or variation? | Brainstorming<br>Risk Analysis<br>Standard Work<br>Mistake Proofing<br>Visual Workplace Tools |
| Control | ▪ How will the improved process be sustained?<br>▪ Who will be responsible for maintaining/monitoring the improvements and measures?<br>▪ How will we communicate the new process expectations?<br>▪ How will we eliminate deviations from standard work and prevent backsliding?<br>▪ How will we share best practices and lessons learned?<br>▪ What were the benefits realized from the project? | Control Plan<br>Control Charts<br>Dashboard<br>Standard Operating Procedures and Policy Revision<br>Checklist/Audits |

**Define** — Tollgate — **Measure** — Tollgate — **Analyze** — Tollgate — **Improve** — Tollgate — **Control** — Tollgate

| Define | Measure | Analyze | Improve | Control |
|---|---|---|---|---|
| Step 1: Define problem and scope | Step 5: Refine operational definitions | Step 9: Identify VA/NVA steps | Step 13: Generate prioritized solutions | Step 17: Create control plan |
| Step 2: Determine project objectives | Step 6: Develop data collection plan | Step 10: Identify potential causes (X's) and wastes | Step 14: Develop pilot plan and execute | Step 18: Publish revised process documentation |
| Step 3: Create project charter in database | Step 7: Collect baseline data | Step 11: Validate and prioritize X's | Step 15: Validate and implement solutions | Step 19: Finalize handoff to owner and follow-up plan |
| Step 4: Create visualization of process | Step 8: Update database | Step 12: Update database | Step 16: Update database | Step 20: Close project in database |

*Actions: Define* — *Actions: Measure* — *Actions: Analyze* — *Actions: Improve* — *Actions: Control*

**Deliverables** (Define)
1. Problem statement
2. Goal statement
3. Stakeholder analysis
4. High level process map
5. Primary and secondary metrics
6. Project scope
7. Project champion and process owner
8. Project timeline

**Potential tools**
• Project charter template
• Stakeholder power/ interest grid
• SIPOC
• Affinity diagrams
• Swimlane diagram

**Deliverables** (Measure)
1. Measurement system analysis
2. Baseline data summary
3. Financial and operational benefits estimate

**Potential tools**
• Data collection plan template
• Pareto charts
• Minitab graphical summary
• Control charts
• Graphical analysis tools (boxplots, etc.)

**Deliverables** (Analyze)
1. Detailed current state process map
2. Analyzed data (graphical, statistical, and/or process)
3. Risk analysis
4. Prioritized and validated root causes (X's)

**Potential tools**
• Mapping (value stream, swimlane) w/VA analysis
• Cause and effect analysis (diagram or matrix)
• Pareto charts
• Hypothesis tests (ANOVA, 1 and 2 sample t, etc.)
• 8 wastes (DOWNTIME)
• Graphical analysis tools
• 5 whys analysis

**Deliverables** (Improve)
1. Prioritized solutions
2. Future state map
3. Action plan for pilot
4. Pilot results and improvement validation
5. Full implementation plan

**Potential tools**
• Brainstorming
• Cause and effect analysis (diagram or matrix)
• Decision matrix
• 5 cycle PDSA
• Standard work
• Mistake proofing
• Visual workplace tools
• Pull systems
• Action plan templates

**Deliverables** (Control)
1. Control plan
2. Future state process documentation
3. Update risk assessment
4. Final financial and operational benefits
5. Executive summary and final report

**Potential tools**
• Control plan template
• Final standard work and policies
• Risk assessment
• Executive summary template
• Metrics dashboard
• Action plan templates

**Figure 5.4** DMAIC with Steps and Tools

Reproduced from Canode C. *Veterans Integrated Service Network (VISN 8) Lean Six Sigma Belt Training*. U.S. Department of Veterans Affairs.

improvements. Fundamental to the collaborative approach is the acceptance of a model and the establishment of an infrastructure through which collaborating organizations can identify and prioritize aims for improvement and gain access to methods, tools, and materials to conduct sophisticated, evidence-based activities that they could not successfully conduct on their own. The key elements of success are enlisting a broad range of stakeholders and partners, using evidence-based practice to improve quality of care, and developing toolkits that contain essential information and resources to manage change.

At the core of the collaborative approach is the PDCA cycle that builds on incremental improvements. The real benefits to organizations that participate in the Breakthrough Series are that they can learn from other organizations' successes and failures. Another key principle in the IHI approach is the concept of spread where successful small-scale improvement efforts with an individual organization are disseminated or spread later to the industry (i.e., other hospitals) and eventually to the entire national healthcare system. The spread is fostered through learning sessions in which organizations share their experiences.

The IHI approach also can be adapted to a single organization (the work begins with a few units or teams and then is spread to other units and, eventually, to the entire organization). **Figure 5.5** illustrates how the multiple improvement cycles in a collaborative occur.[27] Another method for rapid improvement is the rapid process improvement workshop or rapid improvement event in which the DMAIC process is condensed into a focused weeklong event including preevent and postevent work (some organizations use the term *workout*). Reasons to do a rapid process improvement workshop/rapid improvement event are the importance of the project to the organization

or action is needed in a short amount of time. These events are resource intense with planning, meetings, staffing, and other supplies. They can also be highly effective in developing actions and solutions for immediate implementation.

## Six Sigma

Six Sigma is a business management strategy, originally developed by Motorola. This rigorous methodology, used in different industry sectors, uses data and statistical analyses to measure and improve performance through the reduction of variation. Quality is improved by eliminating errors in production and service-related processes. Six Sigma is based on the concept of the normal distribution or curve and the belief that there is a point, six standard deviations from the mean, where there should be almost zero defects. Therefore, error rates do not exceed 3.4 defects per million opportunities. Six Sigma can be characterized as obtaining the right measures (or metrics) of quality, using rigorous statistical methods, and possessing a customer-focused and data-driven philosophy.

In 1998 Chassin concluded, "We can learn a good deal from industries that are working toward the Six Sigma goal. Let's try it in healthcare and see how close we can get."[30(p587)] Over the past years, this approach was adopted by many hospitals and health systems. With cost, quality, and regulatory pressures continuing to increase within the healthcare industry, Six Sigma gained more attention from hospitals and health systems seeking a better approach to achieving long-term results. This approach to improving quality can be used to address many of the challenges facing healthcare, including resource utilization, patient safety, appropriate use of technology, and increasing market share. Six Sigma efforts typically include a methodology that

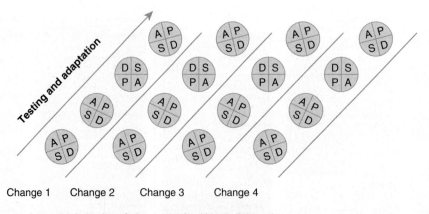

**Figure 5.5** Process for Testing Multiple Cycles of Change as Used in a Collaborative

Reproduced from Testing and Adaptation. Institute for Healthcare Improvement. Available on www.IHI.org. Derived from Langley GL, Moen R, Nolan KM, Nolan TW, Norman CL, Provost LP. *The Improvement Guide: A Practical Approach to Enhancing Organizational Performance.* 2nd ed. San Francisco, CA: Jossey-Bass Publishers; 2009.

addresses variation and goes by the acronym *DMAIC* (define, measure, analyze, improve, and control). See Table 5.1 and Figure 5.4 for key questions and tools for the healthcare quality professional to consider during each step in the DMAIC process.

A Six Sigma project can address process redesign, a problem that needs to be solved, a change that needs to be instituted, or a process that needs to be monitored. Six Sigma projects are managed by Black Belts, who oversee the project. Black Belts are members of the organization who are extensively trained in Six Sigma methods. Black Belts also must be experienced in statistical analysis and able to teach others. Projects normally are conducted by Green Belts. Green Belts are organization members who are knowledgeable about Six Sigma methods but received less training than Black Belts. For major projects, an organization also assigns a senior manager or executive to function as a sponsor or champion. Six Sigma shows success in reducing emergency room wait times, lost charges for billing in financial services, delinquent medical records, diagnostic result turnaround times, account receivable days, patients' length of stay, and medication errors.[31] Some articles found in the *Journal for Healthcare Quality* discussing examples of these projects include "Improving Operating Room Efficiency: First Case On-Time Start Project" (**Figure 5.6** and **Figure 5.7**).[32]

## Lean Enterprise

The Japanese automotive industry initiated the concept of Lean manufacturing, whereby significant importance is given to reducing waste and focusing on those activities that add value for the customer. Interest in applying similar principles in service industry environments, including healthcare, continues to grow. Lean Enterprise includes five basic principles:

1. Specify value from the end customer's perspective.
2. Identify all steps in the value stream for each service, eliminating the non–value-added steps.
3. Make the value-adding steps flow without interruption to the customer.
4. Implement a pull system based on customer demand.
5. As value is specified, value streams are identified, non–value-added steps are removed, and flow and pull are introduced, go back to the first step and continue until a state of perfection is achieved.[33]

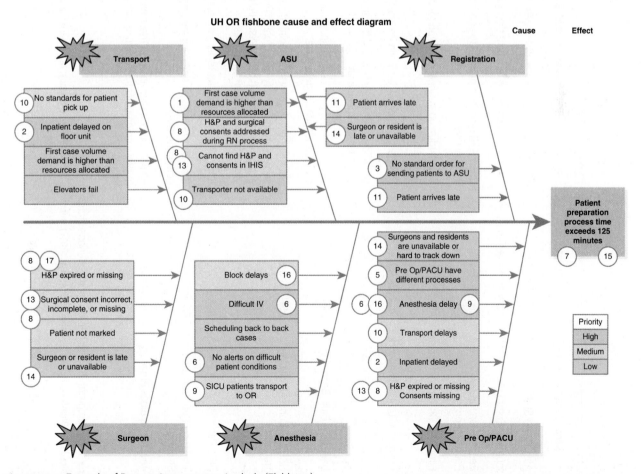

**Figure 5.6** Example of Process Improvement Analysis (Fishbone)

Reproduced from Phieffer L, Hefner JL, Rahmanian A, et al. Improving operating room efficiency: First case on-time start project. *J Healthc Qual*. 2017;39(5):e70–e78.

| # | Area of Improvement | Location | Solution/Next Step | Feasability | Benefit | Total Score | Implemented | Date |
|---|---|---|---|---|---|---|---|---|
| 1 | ASU/Preop Staffing | ASU/PreOP | Share/pool staff between ASU and Pre-op | 5 | 5 | 25 | Yes | 9/10/2012 |
| 2 | Inpatient Communication | Inpatient Floor/Front Desk | Place follow up call to inpatient floor DOS & Check List | 5 | 5 | 25 | Yes | 8/1/2012 |
| 3 | Registration Patient Prioritization | Registration | Change Registration process to prioritize patients by surgery time | 5 | 5 | 25 | Yes | 8/15/2012 |
| 4 | First Case On Time Definition | All Areas | Standardize operational definition for scorecard and daily report | 4 | 5 | 20 | Yes | 6/13/2012 |
| 5 | Pre-op/PACU Standard Work | PreOp/PACU | Standardize process between Pre-op/PACU | 4 | 5 | 20 | No | NA |
| 6 | Anesthesia - OPAC Alerts | OPAC - Anesthesia | OPAC identifies patients with difficult anesthesia conditions to anesthesia | 4 | 5 | 20 | Yes | 3/23/2012 |
| 7 | Daily First Case Reporting | All Areas | Report out first case performance daily to improve communication - current state | 3 | 5 | 15 | Yes | 4/18/2012 |
| 8 | H&P and Consent Missing Tracking | ASU/PreOp | Submit monthly report to appointed surgeons and service chairs; identify to IT (John O'Brien) for support; assign new projects (Leslie Weist) focus on standardize processes on surgeon clinic sites | 3 | 5 | 15 | Yes | 3/23/2012 |
| 9 | SICU Patients | SICU | Improve SICU flow/Create flex process for SICU | 3 | 5 | 15 | Yes | 9/5/2012 |
| 10 | Transport Communication/Strategy | Transport | Standardize Transport process and improve communication | 3 | 5 | 15 | No | NA |
| 16 | Anesthesia Block Process | Anesthesia | Identify block cases and plan these cases as priority; improve communication within anesthesia and block teams | 3 | 5 | 15 | No | 3/23/2012 |

**Figure 5.7** Example of Process Improvement Solutions Matrix

Reproduced from Phieffer L, Hefner JL, Rahmanian A, et al. (2017). Improving operating room efficiency: first case on-time start project. *J Healthc Qual.* 2017;39(5):e70–e78.

**Table 5.2** Types of Waste in Lean Production Systems

| Type of Waste | Waste Description | Lean Strategy to Eliminate Waste |
|---|---|---|
| **T**ransportation | Moving material or information | One-piece flow, avoid batching |
| **I**nventory (overproduction) | Having more material than you need | Standard work, 6S tool |
| **M**otion | Moving people to access or process material or information | Quick changeover, work cell, standard work |
| **W**aiting | People waiting for material or information, or material or information waiting to be processed | Quick changeover, one-piece flow, avoid batching |
| **O**verproduction | Creating too much material or information | Standard work, one-piece flow, avoid batching |
| **O**verprocessing | Processing more than necessary to achieve the desired output | Mistake-proofing, standard work |
| **D**efects (necessitating rework) | Errors or mistakes necessitating rework to correct the problem | Mistake-proofing, standard work |
| **U**nderutilizing resources | Not utilizing or underutilizing the talent (scope) of employees or use of resources, staff not involved in improvement projects | Process mapping and Value Stream mapping to identify key resources needed |

*Note*: Type of waste may be abbreviated as TIMWOODU or DOWNTIME.

A key focus in a Lean Enterprise is to eliminate waste in eight key areas: defects, overproduction, waiting, nonutilized talent/resources, transportation, inventory, motion, and extra processing.[34] An explanation of wastes found in healthcare (with examples in each category and the common strategy to address the waste) is given in **Table 5.2**. One of the major distinctions of the Lean approach versus traditional quality improvement is its emphasis on investigating new ways of getting things done and making the changes in a brief period. The basic idea is to identify new procedures that are designed to be more effective than existing systems, resulting in eliminating waste. Quality improvement typically used the incremental change model, but Lean Enterprise is more concerned with speed and total redesign. A key element of success is the commitment and involvement of frontline workers and staff in the change process. The typical project includes cross-functional teams with training in Lean principles and tools.

Organizations usually implement Lean methods before considering Six Sigma, because waste should be eliminated prior to fine-tuning the system to deliver excellence. The newer approach is a combination of both Lean and Six Sigma, as there is value in reducing waste, speeding up the process, and reducing variation. Naik and colleagues applied Lean principles to their emergency department, which improved overall length of stay, time of arrival to triage completion, time of arrival to being seen by a provider, and increased provider productivity. Significant improvements in workflow were realized.[35]

Of note, the Lean philosophy encompasses the concept of *True North*. True North is a key concept in Lean process improvement that emerged from Toyota and connotes the compass needle for Lean transformation. True North works like a compass, providing a guide to take an organization from the current condition to where it wants to be. It might be viewed as a purpose of the organization and the foundation of a strategic plan. Later in this section, other approaches are explained that determine the organization's direction, pillars, dashboard metrics, or key success factors. In Lean management, continuous improvement is also known as *Kaizen*. Continuous improvement seeks to improve every process in the organization by focusing on enhancing activities that generate the most value for the customer while removing as many waste activities as possible. There are Lean terms with which to become familiar. Healthcare quality professionals should at least have a basic understanding of the key terms. The three types of waste in Lean are Muda (the eight wastes), Mura (the waste of unevenness), and Muri (the waste of overburden). Other key terms are *Kaizen* (continuous improvement), *Kanban* (a workflow management method for defining, managing, and improving services that deliver knowledge work), and *Gemba* (the real place).[36,37]

The use of Lean and Six Sigma constitutes what The Joint Commissions refers to as *robust process improvement,* which supports organizations to be highly reliable.[38] While Lean methodology has specific terminology addressing continuous improvement, the general trend in organizations is to create continuous learning and improvement, especially by engaging frontline staff. Improvement occurs in the daily operations by people doing the work who understand the process—including the barriers and bottlenecks. While large cross-functional teams can address complex system and process issues, there is immense value in the daily focus on continuous improvement, patient safety, and innovation.

**Box 5.3** lists the key points in performance improvement structure, processes, and models.

### Box 5.3  Key Points: PI Structure, Processes, and Models

- Quality and performance improvement must be integrated into the overall organizational strategy and goals.
- Lean/Six Sigma, PDSA, and other models have value. No single model perfectly fits all situations.
- Learning from other industries on improvement models and tools is important for continued development.
- Dashboards are useful to visually monitor trends and patterns and to identify when to act.
- Performance improvement should be part of routine operations and discussions.
- Go to the *Gemba* to understand how processes actually work.

## Strategic Management Systems

Although there are a variety of quality performance evaluation programs, including the Baldrige Performance Excellence Framework and the European Foundation for Quality Management, a significant percentage of government agencies and Fortune 1000 companies use the balanced scorecard (BSC) as an approach to performance management. BSCs are completely compatible with other quality performance programs but go beyond such programs by embedding quality and performance improvement in the strategic framework of the organization.[39]

This framework to implement and manage strategy was developed by Norton and Kaplan in the early 1990s. This approach is

> . . . consistent with the initiatives under way in many companies: cross-functional integration, customer–supplier partnerships,

global scale, continuous improvement, and team rather than individual accountability. By combining the financial, customer, internal process and innovation, and organizational learning perspectives, the balanced scorecard helps managers understand, at least implicitly, many interrelationships. This understanding can help managers transcend traditional notions about functional barriers and ultimately lead to improved decision making and problem solving. The balanced scorecard keeps companies looking—and moving—forward instead of backward.[40(p79)]

The basic idea is that performance measures provide a comprehensive view of organizational performance, not overly dependent on choice indicators. Unlike other performance models, the BSC helps organizations better link long-term strategy with short-term activities.[41]

The BSC approach views the organization from four different perspectives or categories:

1. Financial (How do we look to providers of financial resources?)
2. Customer (How do our customers see us?)
3. Internal business processes (At what must we excel?)
4. Learning and growth (Can we continue to improve and create value for customers?)

Answers to these questions influence the nature of the strategic goals and objectives that are set and what performance measures are used. The critical aspect of performance indicators is that they must reflect the organization's strategic goals and objectives.

There are likely to be strategic objectives corresponding to each of the four perspectives. Each of these objectives has at least one measure with vetted measurement properties (e.g., reliability, validity, qualitative data, quantitative data) and can be collected through a variety of means (e.g., surveys, focus groups, patient chart reviews). The Health Resources & Services Administration suggests that development and use of different types of measures (i.e., structure, process, outcomes) in each of the categories is an important approach.[42]

The foundation for an organization's strategic success begins with its people, who must be willing to learn and grow. To meet the changing needs of customers, they must, for example, learn new technology and acquire new skills to take on new responsibilities. The strategic goal "Develop a state-of-the-art program for breast cancer detection and treatment" could consider measures such as:

- *Structure.* The quantity of imaging equipment
- *Process.* The number of patients diagnosed with imaging technology
- *Outcome.* The higher percentage of early diagnoses, due to use of imaging technology

It is necessary to monitor and improve key processes so that employees can convert learning and growth into products and services or quality outcomes. "Be recognized as one of the top healthcare providers in the community" could be another strategic goal. Measures might include the following:

- *Structure.* The resources available for care delivery (e.g., nurse–patient ratio or number of primary care providers)
- *Process.* Care (how patients are diagnosed and treated or access to an appointment)
- *Outcomes.* The results of care (e.g., satisfaction, length and quality of life, turnover rates or completed preventive cancer screening)

Just as different organizational levels and units develop goals and objectives based on corporate strategy, different levels and units also can use the BSC. Note that for the same strategic goal (e.g., be recognized as one of the top healthcare providers in the community) there are several measures of performance across different perspectives. Organizations use dashboards with specific metrics and do not refer to the term *BSC* (e.g., utilization management, experience of care). Emerging models now include a tiered approach with real-time data at the work unit level, management level, and senior leader level with both horizontal and vertical communication. These tiered huddles include visual daily management that may address operational, patient safety, and quality improvement topics.[43,44]

# Performance Management and Organizational Strategy

This section describes various aspects of the organization's strategy for performance management. *Performance management* is defined as "the use of performance management information to effect positive change in organizational culture, systems, and processes by helping to set agreed-upon performance goals, allocating and prioritizing resources, informing managers to either confirm or change current policy or program direction to meet those goals, and sharing results of performance

in pursuing those goals."[41(p1)] The goal of a performance management system is to make certain that the vision of the organization is being met by defining and measuring outcomes reflected in that vision.

The development of meaningful governance in quality and safety requires assessment of the governing body's knowledge of performance improvement. This is a key role of healthcare quality professionals responsible for organizing and coordinating quality management and performance improvement activities for the organization and its medical staff. Healthcare quality professionals can promote the commitment to quality of the governing body and organizational leadership by providing useful information in a format easily understood by individuals who may lack familiarity with healthcare terminology and procedures (see the *Quality Review and Accountability* section for reporting principles and examples). There are leadership frameworks with similarities. As is true with the system framework, often it is less important to choose a specific framework than simply having one to guide behavior.

*Leadership* is the ability to influence an individual or group toward achievement of goals.[45] Leadership and management are not identical. *Leadership* is determining the correct direction or path, whereas *management* is doing the correct things to stay on that path. Kotter notes that management is about coping with complexity through planning and budgeting; setting goals; organizing, staffing, and creating a structure to foster goal attainment; setting up mechanisms for monitoring; and controlling results.[46] In contrast, leaders are responsible for coping with change by developing a vision for change and aligning the subsystems of the organization. Both strong leadership and management are necessary for high performance. Some people are great leaders but poor managers and vice versa; in some cases, a person may be successful in both roles. Key points on leadership and performance improvement are listed in **Box 5.4**.

---

### Box 5.4 Key Points: Leadership and Performance Improvement

- Leadership vision, strategic goals/direction, and support are essential to quality.
- Quality leaders establish and communicate strategically aligned improvement goals.
- Leaders empower managers and frontline staff to engage in performance improvement initiatives.
- Quality improvement planning is systems based and integrates processes with business and operational needs.

The organization's governing body bears ultimate responsibility for setting policy, financial and strategic direction, as well as for the quality of care and services provided by all its practitioners. Together with the organization's management and medical staff leaders, the governing body sets priorities for quality improvement activities. The American Hospital Association outlined principles of accountability for hospitals and healthcare organizations, with specific directives for governing boards and leadership.[47] These government and leadership directives are shown in **Table 5.3**.

The American Hospital Association and American Medical Association published a joint statement called *Integrated Leadership for Hospitals and Health Systems: Principles for Success*,[48] which addresses integrated leadership and includes six principles summarized here:

1. Physicians and hospital leaders who share similar values and expectations; aligned incentives; goals aligned across the board with appropriate means of measuring them; responsibility for financial, cost and quality targets; accountable service line teams; shared strategic planning; and a focus on engaging patients as partners
2. A structure incorporating all disciplines and supporting collaborative decision making between doctors and hospital executives, with physicians maintaining their clinical autonomy
3. Integrated hospital and clinical leadership at all levels of the health system; and inclusion of nursing and other caregivers participating in all key management decisions
4. Collaborative, participatory partnership built on trust, with interdependence and a thrust toward achieving the Triple Aim being "crucial to alignment and engagement"[48(p3)]
5. Transparency of both clinical and business information, across the entire enterprise, by all parties
6. An information technology system that allows clinicians to capture and report quality and performance data of all participants, with leadership holding its workforce accountable for those measurements

Other settings address rights specific to special populations such as those in behavioral health (mental health and substance use) and long-term care, as well as consumer rights. For practical purposes, day-to-day leadership is the responsibility of the chief executive officer and senior management (sometimes called the *C-Suite*), elected or appointed members of the medical staff (e.g., chairs), and administrative and clinical staff (e.g., practitioners, quality improvement staff).

---

**Table 5.3** The American Hospital Association's Principles of Accountability for Hospitals and Healthcare Organizations: Governance/Leadership

**Mission and Vision.** The organization's governing body and leadership should articulate clearly defined mission and vision statements. With these statements as a foundation, the organization's leadership should develop an action plan with specific goals, time frames for accomplishment, and linked measures of performance for a regular assessment of achievement, with oversight by the governing body. As part of this development process, the organization's governing body and leadership should seek input from relevant stakeholders concerning their needs and interests relative to the organization. The plan and the results should be widely communicated to all individuals who are employed by or affiliated with the organization.

**Executive Management Oversight.** The organization's governing body is responsible for the oversight of the organization's leadership performance and should periodically evaluate that performance relative to the organization's achievement of its stated strategic goals. As part of the process of evaluating the organization's leadership, the governing body should periodically and systematically assess its own performance relative to defined goals and measures of performance.

**Quality Oversight.** The organization's governing body and leadership, in conjunction with the clinical staff, are responsible for developing and implementing, in a comprehensive manner, systems and procedures for safeguarding and enhancing the quality of patient care and services. The governing body and leadership, in conjunction with the clinical staff, are also responsible for actively monitoring and immediately acting upon, where appropriate, the results derived from those systems and procedures such that patient and staff safety is ensured or improvements in patient care occur.

**Financial Stability.** The organization's governing body is responsible for ensuring the financial well-being of the organization and, in conjunction with the organization's leadership, for overseeing the appropriate and most optimal allocation of financial and physical resources for the improvement of patient care. The organization's mission and duty to improve patient care and community health must not be obstructed by (and must take precedence over) the financial interests of individuals or groups employed by or affiliated with the organization.

Reproduced from American Hospital Association. *Accountability—The Pathway to Restoring Public Trust and Confidence for Hospitals and Other Health Care Organizations.* Chicago, IL: American Hospital Association; 1999:8, with permission.

Innovation goes hand in hand with improvement. Improvement optimizes existing processes, while innovation creates new products and services. Improvement is often incremental and continuous while innovation is usually short term and often dramatic in its effect. Improvement is based on structured steps while innovation is based on flexibility in steps often with great speed. Improvement creates change that is usually gradual, constant, and sustained, while innovation is abrupt and volatile. Improvement requires time, effort, and experienced staff; innovation requires financial investment in new products but does not require sustainment in the same way. Finally, improvement is process focused to create strong outcomes; innovation is immediate results focused.

**Box 5.5** lists key points of performance management and organizational strategy.

---

### Box 5.5 Key Points: Performance Management and Organizational Strategy

- Systems and processes, not individuals, should be the focus of improvement efforts.
- There are multiple improvement tools and models. Choose the best fit for the improvement need (problem solving, analysis, root cause, or solution).
- Follow the steps in the performance improvement models for a consistent and standardized approach.
- Baseline data are needed to demonstrate improvement.

---

See the *Quality Leadership and Integration* section for more information on models, frameworks, culture, and impact on performance and process improvement.

## Setting Priorities and Decision Support

Every organization should have an organization-wide plan for performance improvement. The plan defines examples of key activities and quality control methods for each service. There are regulations at the federal, state, and local level and accreditation standards that govern quality monitoring, evaluation, and reporting. This is especially true for diagnostic services such as pathology and laboratory services, radiology, nuclear medicine, and pharmacy. Content experts in these services lead the identification of regulations or other requirements and the specific quality control processes and measures that must be maintained. The requirements may include provisions for employee exposure monitoring, including issuance of individual radiology

badges (dosimeters) or devices. Quality management personnel are often involved in the direct monitoring within services or the aggregation of data or reports from different services in the organization.

Regulations such as those set forth by CMS have increased along with insurance requirements on every healthcare setting so that each setting needs to develop a plan specific to its needs. The unit or service level is considered a microsystem, and it is at this level that change happens and improvements occur. The plan includes the following:

- Identifying populations served
- Describing services provided
- PI priorities at the service level, aligned with the organization's goals and strategic plan
- Identifying any requirements related to PI, quality control, and quality monitoring (e.g., accreditation standards, regulations, and device monitoring)
- Selecting valid and reliable metrics for the service
- Developing a monitoring plan (e.g., sample, frequency, and reporting)
- Planning for evaluating performance and comparison data and benchmarking
- Methods for improving performance

A standard format can make the development of plans or quality monitoring across multiple services and sites more efficient and effective for tracking, trending, and reporting. Discussion about the various aspects to consider in the planning process follows.

## Planning and Setting Priorities

The road to quality begins with strategic planning to guide the organization in focusing on the most important aspects or priorities. Priorities for performance and process improvement activities are based on standard approaches. The first approach is aligning the priorities with the organization's strategic priorities to maximize resources for improvement. The second is a criteria-based approach considering risk, volume, problem proneness, patient safety, cost, customer satisfaction, and other criteria established specifically by the organization. The pillars identified by Studer—quality, people, finance, service, growth, and community—are also often used as the categories of improvement priorities.[49] Safety and innovation have recently been added to the pillars of excellence model.

A framework for leadership of improvement is the first step in turning the strategic plan into an operational plan for improvement. In this framework leaders apply the mission, vision, values, and strategic plan to set direction. This framework is built on a foundational leadership team to support improvement capability and three components that contribute to a leadership system of change:

1. The will to prepare for change
2. Ideas to generate new ways of performing
3. Execution of change

Models depicting the framework and how the framework operates in an integrated system are shown in **Figure 5.8** and **Figure 5.9**.

Prioritizing evaluates key processes against key business drivers to identify the most important processes to improve and measure in evaluating performance. Applying priorities determines the initiation of an improvement action, based on the analysis of data collection. The goals and drivers of the system are depicted in **Figure 5.10**.

Leaders identify a priority list of processes or services for improvement.[50] Healthcare quality professionals facilitate development of priorities by

- establishing criteria for priority assessment (e.g., volume, risk, problem proneness);
- using data on past performance to assess gaps (internal performance);
- using external drivers for consideration (new regulations, standards, technology);
- providing information to leaders with a basis for recommendations;
- using tools to create a matrix for priorities for decision making;
- involving key stakeholders for input; and

- identifying internal and external requirements that influence priorities.

In addition, healthcare quality professionals and their teams use the described criteria to prioritize performance and process improvement activities based on the quantitative and qualitative data available to them. By using past performance, aligned with the criteria and strategic initiatives, the team can determine the priorities for action and establish a plan approved by the clinical leaders to ensure success of the activities, especially in applying resources for the effort required for the team. The use of a priority matrix or impact grid can be applied in evaluating priorities in a structured manner.

The initiatives tackled first are often those having the most opportunity for improvement. Usually, the initiatives selected focus on core clinical processes, high-risk processes, high-risk patients and populations, high-risk medications, or high-risk actions or interventions. The level of risk is based on the potential consequences of injury or harm to patients (severity).

Another aspect in assessing level of risk is the frequency with which the process or procedure is performed. For example, responding to a case of malignant hyperthermia would hold considerable risk for the patient, and if the staff does not manage this scenario often, they may not respond as a highly effective team and the outcome could be death. Therefore, it may be a priority to perform drills to ensure that staff is competent. Managing high-risk patients and processes significantly affect morbidity and mortality. Examples of high-risk processes include:

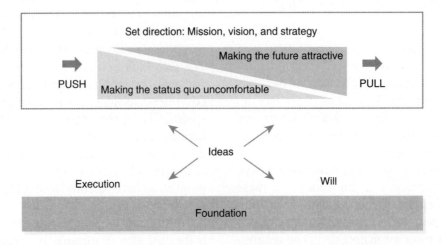

**Figure 5.8** Framework for Leading Improvement

Adapted from Reinertsen JL, Bisognano M, Pugh MD. *Seven Leadership Leverage Points for Organization-Level Improvement in Health Care.* 2nd ed. Cambridge, MA: Institute for Healthcare Improvement; 2008. Available on www.ihi.org

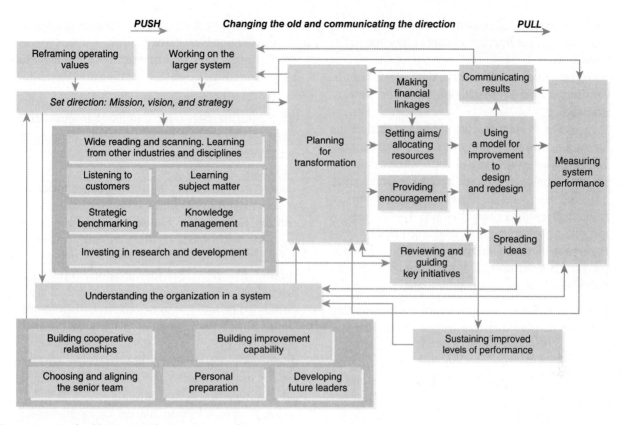

**Figure 5.9** Leadership Framework as an Integrated System

Reproduced from Massoud MR, Nielsen GA, Nolan K, Nolan T, Schall MW, Sevin C. *A Framework for Spread: From Local Improvements to System-Wide Change.* IHI Innovation Series white paper. Cambridge, MA: Institute for Healthcare Improvement; 2006. Available on www.IHI.org

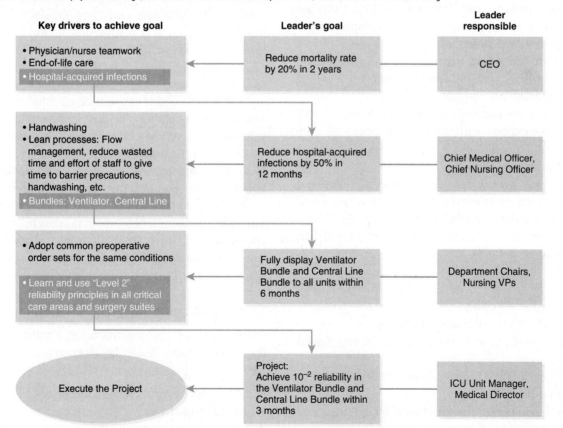

**Figure 5.10** Cascading Series of Goals and Drivers for Improvement

Reprinted from Reinertsen JL, Bisognano M, Pugh MD. *Seven Leadership Leverage Points for Organization-Level Improvement in Health Care.* 2nd ed. Cambridge, MA: Institute for Healthcare Improvement; 2008. Available on www.ihi.org

- *Core processes.* Admission, transfer, discharge, transitions, coordination of care, other handoffs/handovers
- *High-risk processes.* Medication delivery or administration, surgery, resuscitation, infection prevention and control
- *High-risk patients.* Patients with reduced renal function, immunocompromised patients, neonates, patients in critical care units, suicidal patients, dementia patients at risk for wandering
- *High-risk medications.* Heparin (and oral anticoagulants), insulin, chemotherapy, opiates, neuromuscular blocking agents, psychotropics
- *High-risk actions and interventions.* Blood and blood product transfusions, use of restraints, extracorporeal circulation, moderate sedation[51]

See the *Patient Safety* section for more information about high-risk areas such as infection prevention and control.

After priorities are established, specific initiatives or activities are undertaken. Key steps to implementing PI activities to ensure success of the PI priorities follow:

1. Ensure leadership support and commitment for the PI initiative.
2. Assess priority and feasibility of the initiative based on risk, resources, leadership support, and organizational strategies.
3. Identify the aim of the initiative and include the topic, process, or problem to be improved within a manageable scope (rationale).
4. Convene an interprofessional team of content and process experts with all key disciplines as participants (involve all the right stakeholders with a champion for change).
5. Use tools and techniques to analyze processes, best practices, research, and consensus-based evidence for the desired change.
6. Develop the change to be implemented and add timelines (tollgates or milestones) and accountability for the project.
7. Identify the measures to demonstrate that the change resulted in improvement; set performance goals.
8. Educate staff on the desired change.
9. Implement and test the change via the redesigned processes.
10. Collect, analyze, and evaluate data on the redesigned process.
11. Make additional changes based on findings and disseminate to all areas.
12. Report and display results to reward staff for improvements.
13. Continue to monitor performance to ensure that the change is sustained.
14. Compare performance internally and externally.
15. Celebrate successes internally and externally.[51,52]

When choosing between improvement activities, use a prioritization matrix to assist in evaluating the items against specific criteria. After leaders determine the improvement priorities for process improvement, they make decisions about the need to organize a team. A prioritization matrix organizes tasks, issues, or actions and prioritizes them based on agreed-upon criteria (**Figure 5.11**). The tool is helpful in identifying criteria for specific priorities and applying a rating scale to help make decisions for the selection of specific activities. This matrix applies options under discussion to the priority considerations of the organization. The tool combines the tree diagram and the *L*-shaped matrix diagram, displaying the best possible effect. The prioritization matrix is often used before more complex matrices are needed. This matrix applies options under discussion to the priority considerations of the organization.

A project selection matrix ranks and compares potential project areas for implementation. Ranking criteria may include organizational and strategic goals, potential financial impact to the organization, effect on patient and employee satisfaction, likelihood of success, and completion within a specified time frame (**Figure 5.12**).

An impact effort matrix (risk/frequency chart, ease impact matrix, or *Possible, Implement, Challenge, and Kill* [PICK] chart) can also be used to compare the ease of implementation and cost to implement specific solutions. It is very useful to identify root causes of an event from a fishbone or other analysis to determine most important cause(s) and assist with decisions on where to focus attention first. The matrix identifies the quadrant of where to focus efforts in priority order. This is an excellent tool to use in process improvement efforts, after a fishbone analysis and during a root cause analysis (**Figure 5.13**). The logical next step after determining priorities is to develop an action plan.

## Projects and Action Plans

Once priorities are identified, an action plan puts them into motion. A standard format includes

- who (accountability),
- what (specific actions or steps to be followed),
- when (time frame),
- status (progress made and ongoing monitoring), and
- completion (closure or closing the loop).

| | High Risk | High Volume | Problem Prone | Cost | Customer Satisfaction | Regulatory | Total |
|---|---|---|---|---|---|---|---|
| Infection rates | 3 | 2 | 2 | 3 | 1 | 3 | 14 |
| Surgical complications | 2 | 1 | 2 | 3 | 1 | 3 | 12 |
| Emergency department time to treatment | 1 | 3 | 1 | 1 | 3 | 0 | 9 |
| Falls with injuries | 2 | 1 | 1 | 2 | 2 | 2 | 10 |
| Medication safety | 3 | 3 | 3 | 2 | 1 | 2 | 14 |

### How to construct
1. Create an *L*-shaped matrix.
2. Prioritize and assign weights to the list of criteria that will be used in the prioritization.
3. Prioritize the list of options based on each criterion.
4. Prioritize and select the items across all the criteria.

### When to use
- When problems are identified and options must be narrowed down, when options have strong interrelationships, and when all options need to be done but prioritization or sequencing is required

**Figure 5.11** Prioritization Matrix: Clinical Improvement Priorities

| | Low Cost | High Strategic Priority | Meets Accreditation Standards | MD Concern | Staff Concern | Totals |
|---|---|---|---|---|---|---|
| Repair roof | 3 | 4 | 2 | 3 | 4 | 16 |
| Purchase new X-ray machine | 5 | 2 | 0 | 1 | 5 | 13 |
| Develop skilled nursing unit | 4 | 1 | 0 | 2 | 2 | 9 |
| Develop better communications with home health | 2 | 3 | 1 | 4 | 3 | 13 |
| Develop staff newsletter | 1 | 5 | 3 | 5 | 1 | 15 |

### How to construct
1. Create an *L*-shaped matrix.
2. Prioritize and assign weights to the list of criteria that will be used in the prioritization.
3. Prioritize the list of options based on each criterion.
4. Prioritize and select the item(s) across all the criteria.

### When to use
- When issues are identified and options must be narrowed down
- When options have strong interrelationships
- When options all need to be done, but prioritization or sequencing is needed

**Figure 5.12** Prioritization Matrix: Project Selection Decision Example

Projects vary, ranging from improving a defined process to complete redesign or even designing a new process or system. Although the scope varies, the key format remains constant. The level of detail, number of steps, and length of time to complete will vary greatly. **Figure 5.14** shows the framework for execution of plans for a performance improvement project.[53]

## Planning and Evaluation

Healthcare quality professionals often guide the planning and evaluation for projects and activities. The first step is to understand data and tools to construct an overall plan—specifically the data collection plan. This includes the following steps:

Risk/Frequency chart (root causes)

| | | Low | High |
|---|---|---|---|
| **Risk** | **High** | Focus here 2nd<br>1. Root cause<br>2. Root cause | Focus here 1st<br>1. Root cause<br>2. Root cause |
| | **Low** | Focus here 4th<br>1. Root cause<br>2. Root cause | Focus here 3rd<br>1. Root cause<br>2. Root cause |
| | | **Low** | **High** |
| | | **Frequency** | |

Note: Used to determine which root cause or action to address

**Figure 5.13** Risk/Frequency Chart

*Note*: Used to determine which root cause or action to address.
Reproduced from Canode C. *Veterans Integrated Service Network (VISN 8) Lean Six Sigma Belt Training*. U.S. Department of Veterans Affairs.

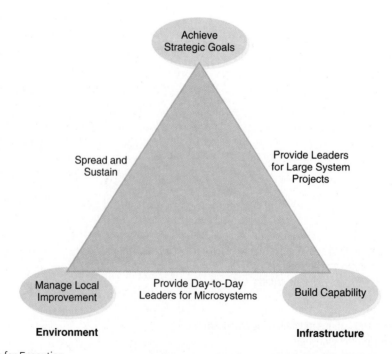

**Figure 5.14** Framework for Execution

Adapted from Reinertsen JL, Bisognano M, Pugh MD. *Seven Leadership Leverage Points for Organization-Level Improvement in Health Care*. 2nd ed. Cambridge, MA: Institute for Healthcare Improvement; 2008. Available on www.ihi.org

- Determine who, what, when, where, how, and why.
- Structure the design.
- Choose and develop a sampling method.
- Determine and conduct training.
- Delegate responsibilities.
- Facilitate coordination.
- Forecast budget.
- Conduct pilots or tests of change.

A clear understanding of data and tools to assist in problem identification and solutions is needed to facilitate planning and evaluating improvement projects. An overview of data and data management is provided with some of the more common tools used in these processes later in the section.

## Evidence-Based Practice Guidelines

*Evidence-based medicine* is the "conscientious, explicit, and judicious use of current best evidence in making decisions about the care of individual patients."[54(p71)] Because multiple disciplines participate in healthcare delivery, however, the term *evidence-based practice* (EBP) is more appropriate than evidence-based medicine from a healthcare quality perspective. Clinicians not only base their care on the experimental evidence but also consider experiential evidence, physiologic principles, patient and professional values, and system features in their decision making. This allows individualized application and dissemination of aggregate research evidence.[55]

EBP promotes patient safety (and quality) through the provision of effective and efficient healthcare, resulting in less variation in care and fewer unnecessary or nontherapeutic interventions.[56] EBP and outcomes measurement are iterative; one facilitates the other.[57] They complement the principles of continuous quality improvement. Outcome evaluation at the individual and aggregate level is an essential step in evaluating the impact.

Evidence-based quality management is based on two types of research: clinical research and health services research. Clinical research evaluates the impact of interventions on patient outcomes. Outcome measures may include clinical outcomes, functional outcomes, and patient satisfaction. This type of research assists healthcare quality professionals in determining clinical evidence-based best practices. Health services research evaluates the health system at the micro and macro levels. Results from this type of research guide healthcare quality professionals in improving work processes and systems of care.

In recent years, the process of putting research into practice quickly to improve outcomes has come to be known as implementation science or translational research.[58]

To facilitate research-based practice—that is, to promote research use—healthcare quality professionals must collaborate with organizational leaders to promote a culture of excellence. Healthcare providers must be motivated to provide the best possible care and to use the best system processes based on the evidence in the research literature or on data obtained in their own organizations. A key strategy is to keep all discussions based on improving the patient's experience and outcomes and keep personality conflicts out of the conversation, based on previously established ground rules. Research use is a key aspect of the continuous quality improvement process and critical to obtaining healthcare quality.

The rating of evidence for EBP is often based on the U.S. Preventive Services Task Force (USPSTF) levels of evidence and grading system.[59,60] Evidence for practice can be classified by certain levels or strength of the evidence. USPSTF also defined levels of certainty about net benefit (**Table 5.4**). USPSTF levels of evidence are often used to rate the evidence so that practitioners can make wise decisions about care and treatment options with some degree of certainty about outcomes. Strong evidence is transformed into practice and then measured in standardized formats. For example, there is convincing evidence that blood pressure control decreases morbidity and mortality. Evidence-based practices are often applied in measures such as CMS, The Joint Commission, and the National Quality Forum. Organizations make this practice operational by using clinical pathways, standard order sets, plans of care, and ongoing measurement processes.

Common sources for EBP guidelines and national measures include the following:

- Agency for Healthcare Research and Quality (e.g., the National Clinical Guideline)[61]
- Cochrane (e.g., clinical evidence comparisons)
- The Leapfrog Group (e.g., hospital-based measures)
- National Quality Forum (e.g., never events, nurse sensitive measures, ambulatory sensitive measures, long-term care measures, and hospital measures)
- Specialty professional associations and societies (e.g., the American Cardiology Association)

USPSTF updated the definitions of the grades it assigns to recommendations and now includes

**Table 5.4** Levels of Certainty About Net Benefit

| Level of Certainty* | Description |
| --- | --- |
| High | The available evidence usually includes consistent results from well-designed, well-conducted studies in representative primary care populations. These studies assess the effects of the preventive service on health outcomes. This conclusion is therefore unlikely to be strongly affected by the results of future studies. |
| Moderate | The available evidence is sufficient to determine the effects of the preventive service on health outcomes, but confidence in the estimate is constrained by such factors as:<br>▪ The number, size, or quality of individual studies.<br>▪ Inconsistency of findings across individual studies.<br>▪ Limited generalizability of findings to routine primary care practice.<br>▪ Lack of coherence in the chain of evidence.<br>As more information becomes available, the magnitude or direction of the observed effect could change, and this change may be large enough to alter the conclusion. |
| Low | The available evidence is insufficient to assess effects on health outcomes. Evidence is insufficient because of:<br>▪ The limited number or size of studies.<br>▪ Important flaws in study design or methods.<br>▪ Inconsistency of findings across individual studies.<br>▪ Gaps in the chain of evidence.<br>▪ Findings not generalizable to routine primary care practice.<br>▪ Lack of information on important health outcomes.<br>More information may allow estimation of effects on health outcomes. |

* The U.S. Preventive Services Task Force (USPSTF) defines certainty as "likelihood that the USPSTF assessment of the net benefit of a preventive service is correct." The net benefit is defined as benefit minus harm of the preventive service as implemented in a general primary care population. The USPSTF assigns a certainty level based on the nature of the overall evidence available to assess the net benefit of a preventive service.
Reproduced from U.S. Preventive Services Task Force. Update on methods: estimating certainty and magnitude of net benefit. Published April 2019. Accessed January 10, 2022. https://uspreventiveservicestaskforce.org/uspstf/about-uspstf/methods-and-processes/update-methods-estimating-certainty-and-magnitude-net-benefit

suggestions for practice associated with each grade (**Table 5.5**). These definitions apply to USPSTF recommendations voted on after July 2012. USPSTF is a group of independent experts in prevention and evidence-based medicine that makes evidence-based recommendations about clinical preventive services.

## Pathways, Guidelines, and Standardization

Clinical guidelines are consensus statements developed to assist in clinical management decisions, and clinical pathways are tools to manage quality outcomes and cost of care based on clinical guidelines and current evidence. Clinical pathways are document-based tools providing a link between the best available evidence and clinical practice. Clinical pathways, also known as care pathways, critical pathways, integrated care pathways, or care maps, are one tool used to manage the quality in healthcare concerning the standardization of care processes. A variety of terms are used for this tool. For simplicity, the term *clinical pathway* is used here.

Clinical pathways support EBP and clinical guidelines in a time-oriented plan. The use of pathways or guidelines reduces variation of clinical practice to optimize patient outcomes. The concept was introduced by Zander and Bower at the New England Medical Center in Boston. They were early nursing pioneers in applying process management thinking and techniques to improve patient care.[62] Clinical pathways operationalize evidence into daily practice for patient care. Clinical pathways are intended to create an integrated comprehensive approach or plan to the patient's care rather than individual professions functioning independently. Interdisciplinary communication, collaboration, and teamwork are enhanced by working from one pathway, and continuity and care coordination are achieved for the patient. Care coordination across multiple providers and healthcare settings is a frequent opportunity for improvement due to handoffs/handovers/care transitions.

The clinical pathway shapes expectations or outcomes of care as the patient progresses, based on what is the best practice for most patients most of the time. The pathway is written and deployed in a manner to

**Table 5.5** USPSTF Grade Definitions (After July 2012)

| Grade | Definition | Suggestions for Practice |
|---|---|---|
| A | The USPSTF recommends the service. There is high certainty that the net benefit is substantial. | Offer or provide this service. |
| B | The USPSTF recommends the service. There is high certainty that the net benefit is moderate or there is moderate certainty that the net benefit is moderate to substantial. | Offer or provide this service. |
| C | The USPSTF recommends selectively offering or providing this service to individual patients based on professional judgment and patient preferences. There is at least moderate certainty that the net benefit is small. | Offer or provide this service for selected patients depending on individual circumstances. |
| D | The USPSTF recommends against the service. There is moderate or high certainty that the service has no net benefit or that the harms outweigh the benefits. | Discourage the use of this service. |
| I Statement | The USPSTF concludes that the current evidence is insufficient to assess the balance of benefits and harms of the service. Evidence is lacking, of poor quality, or conflicting, and the balance of benefits and harms cannot be determined. | Read the clinical considerations section of USPSTF Recommendation Statement. If the service is offered, patients should understand the uncertainty about the balance of benefits and harms. |

ensure that actions or interventions are completed at designated points with the expected outcome. They are designed to support clinical management, clinical and nonclinical resource management, audit management, and fiscal management. Often, the improved clinical outcomes are intended to support cost-effective use of resources such as length of stay, diagnostic tests, and pharmaceutical management. Because there are differences in the responses for the same condition or treatment, individual variances must be captured, documented, and addressed. This continuous monitoring and data evaluation component is essential to pathway improvement through continual revision of pathways. It is expected that over time, variation decreases through standardization, costs decrease, and the value of care improves.

Although standardization is important to pathways, they are not intended to be overly prescriptive and should still allow personalized care. However, one critique of pathways is that not all variation in patient care is negative, and standardized care or "cookbook medicine" would be a detriment to patient care and clinician autonomy. Individual patient factors may contribute to variation that cannot be controlled by the system. Pathways tend to address processes in the ideal or uncomplicated patient and may not address problems in most patients. It is

important to identify which patients are appropriate for the pathway. In general, pathways are more applicable to patients with uncomplicated illnesses undergoing procedures or surgery. Complex cases with multiple comorbidities may be more difficult to fit into a standard pathway. These pathways have been incorporated into decision support systems in electronic health records (see more in the *Health Data Analytics* section).

The standardized approach is designed to empower patients such that each patient knows the plan and their expected outcome at each phase of recovery (e.g., on postoperative day one, the hip replacement patient is expected to ambulate a defined number of steps or feet and void without a urinary catheter). Standardization also helps reduce clinical risk by ensuring that for specific conditions there are no lapses in care to be provided, and if outcomes are not met there is an immediate assessment of the reason for the variation. When differences or unwanted variances do occur, they are noted, and accommodations are made in the plan of care to ensure safety and effectiveness. Common areas addressed by clinical pathways include orthopedic surgery such as hips, knees, and shoulders. Surgical care is more conducive to clinical pathways than medical conditions, where more differences in the patient's condition occur.

Clinical pathways facilitate the development of standardized physician order sets, interventions for the patient, and documentation of the patient's condition. They are often used in the following situations:

- Prevalent pathology in the care setting (e.g., pain)
- Pathology with a significant risk for patients (e.g., venous thromboembolism)
- Pathology with an excessive cost for the hospital (e.g., total joint replacement)
- Predictable clinical course (e.g., total knee or hip replacement)
- Pathology that is well defined and permits homogeneous care (e.g., laminectomy, transurethral prostate resection)
- Existence of recommendations of good practices or expert opinion (e.g., diabetes, heart failure)
- Possibility of obtaining professional agreement (e.g., coronary angioplasty)
- Multidisciplinary implementation (e.g., joint replacement)
- Relatively mature guidelines (e.g., stroke)[63]

Although it is based on current evidence or clinical guidelines, the clinical pathway details processes of care for the specific condition and, in noting any variances, highlights inefficiencies. Twenty-seven studies involving 11,398 participants were included in a meta-analysis of clinical pathway effectiveness.[64] Twenty studies compared stand-alone clinical pathways to usual care. These studies indicated a reduction in in-hospital complications and improved documentation. There was no evidence of differences in readmission to hospital or in-hospital mortality. Length of stay was the most commonly employed outcome measure, with most studies reporting significant reductions. A decrease in hospital costs or charges was also observed. Seven studies compared clinical pathways as part of a multifaceted intervention with usual care. No evidence of differences was found between intervention and control groups. There are both strengths and limitations of the pathway process that an organization must consider in its development and use of the tool. The development of a clinical pathway includes the following steps:

1. *Select the topic.* The topic concentrates on high-volume, high-cost diagnoses and procedures; higher mortality; longer length of stay; or greater number of outcome variations. Surgical procedures are more suitable for pathways because of the predictable course of events that occur during the hospitalization.
2. *Select a team.* Create a multidisciplinary team including representatives from all groups that would be affected by the pathway. Without physician support of the pathway, it is unlikely to be successful or achieve any of the stated goals.
3. *Evaluate and map current process.* Examine care for the condition or procedure to identify current variation and create an idealized process.
4. *Evaluate the current evidence.* In the absence of best practices, comparison with other organizations, or benchmarking, is the best method to use. Look to the literature to inform work.
5. *Determine the clinical pathway.* Use a form to support this work. This may be a hardcopy checklist placed in the patient's medical record or at bedside or an electronic tool capable of tracking variances.
6. *Educate all users.* Learn how to use the tool and implement it. It is critical to define roles within the pathway for it to be successful.
7. *Document and analyze.* When variances do not meet the expectation of the pathway, identify factors that contribute to the variance. Select interventions to improve those factors are the key features of process improvement.

Often, a case manager or other utilization management staff member collects data on use of the pathway and variances. These data must then be analyzed, and processes must be improved to achieve cost savings, quality, and safety.

A *clinical practice guideline* is defined by the IOM as a "statement that includes recommendations that intend to optimize patient care. Guidelines are informed by a systematic review of evidence and an assessment of the benefits and harms of alternative care options."[65(pp25-26)] A medical guideline (also called a clinical guideline, clinical protocol, or clinical practice guideline) is a document with the aim of guiding decisions and criteria regarding diagnosis, management, and treatment in specific areas of healthcare. Following a guideline is never mandatory.

The National Guideline Clearinghouse was a publicly available database of evidence-based clinical practice guidelines and related documents. As of June 18, 2018, it is no longer federally funded, but the National Guideline Clearinghouse guidelines are archived. The new Alliance for the Implementation of Clinical Practice Guidelines will soon update guidelines as a resource.[66]

Another tool to apply evidence into practice to improve healthcare quality is the concept of bundles.[67] IHI developed the concept of the bundle in 2001, and it is now commonly used for selected conditions. The original initiative was a joint development of IHI and the Voluntary Hospital Association, focused on improving critical care and increasing reliability of processes and thereby improving outcomes.

A *bundle* is defined as "a small set of evidence-based interventions for a defined patient segment/population and care setting that, when implemented together, result in significantly better outcomes than when implemented individually."[67(pp1-2)] There are guidelines to the bundle design that include the following:

- The bundle has three to five interventions (elements), with strong clinician agreement.
- Each bundle element is relatively independent.
- The bundle is used with a defined patient population in one location.
- The multidisciplinary care team develops the bundle.
- Bundle elements are descriptive rather than prescriptive, which allows for local customization and use of clinical judgment.[67(p5)]

The first two bundles included ventilator-associated events and central-line–associated bloodstream infections. Through ongoing testing and application of the bundles in clinical practice, modifications were made to the original elements, and new bundles such as the sepsis bundle and perinatal care bundle developed. "The use of bundles of care interventions as an approach to improving the reliability of care received by patients and preventing certain serious clinical outcomes has been demonstrated successfully for nearly ten years, with a growing body of published results."[67(pp2-5)]

When assessing processes of bundle use and outcomes, an all-or-none measurement is used to ensure reliability in providing care that offers the best evidence to prevent adverse events and improve outcomes. Often healthcare quality professionals are directly involved in data collection or reporting of bundle compliance as well as the outcomes of care such as ventilator-associated events or central-line–associated bloodstream infections—key measures of harm to patients.

Newer modalities such as telehealth and videoconferencing visits are increasing in use, but the evidence base is slowly growing so frequent review of the literature is needed to determine the level of evidence and effectiveness and what quality monitoring tools might look like.

# Performance Monitoring and Evaluation

Performance monitoring is an important role for the healthcare quality professional. Areas for monitoring and evaluation are identified in accreditation standards, regulatory requirements, and organizational demands. These areas are high risk or problem prone. When quality or safety issues are identified, they may be subject to review or audit. General criteria to be considered for a review or audit include the following:

- Was the intervention used? Was it performed using specific criteria? Was it performed safely?
- Was there any adverse effect or outcome to the patient?
- Was staff competent to perform the intervention?
- Was it effective (this may include cost-effectiveness)?
- Was there a better alternative to the intervention?

In the discussions that follow, areas most monitored that demonstrate specific monitoring and evaluation processes are presented: medication use; blood, blood products and biologics use; restraints; operative and invasive procedures; cardiopulmonary resuscitation; morbidity and mortality; medical records; diagnostic monitoring; suicide prevention; and pain management.

## Medication Use

Safe medication practices, including medication use evaluation, pharmacy and therapeutics, adverse drug reactions, and adverse drug events, are reviewed in healthcare organizations. The types of medications and the setting in which they are used indicate which medications are high risk, high alert, frequently used, and most vulnerable to underuse, overuse, and misuse. Thousands of drugs are currently on the market. Many are hazardous to use but show beneficial effects for patients. Organizations can identify the drugs they provide in a standard formulary and identify methods to obtain nonformulary items. Then the use of nonformulary medications is monitored, usually by pharmacy staff, to determine cost-effective, safe medications for administration and ways to integrate new medications into use.

The purpose of medication use monitoring is to improve the efficiency and effectiveness of medication use and the appropriate use of medication. Because of the frequent use of medications in healthcare, ongoing monitoring is needed. Priorities for monitoring are based on the numbers of patients affected (volume), the degree of risk associated with the drug's use (risk), the degree to which the medication is known to be problem prone, and other criteria developed by the medical staff. For example:

- High-risk medications include antibiotics, opioids, insulin, anticoagulants/direct oral anticoagulants, chemotherapy, and benzodiazepines.

- High-risk populations may include infants and children, frail older adults, immunocompromised patients, critically ill patients, those with multiple chronic conditions, patients with spinal cord injury and disorders, and transplant recipients.

The usual steps in measuring improvement include the following:

1. Prescribing appropriate medication
2. Preparing and dispensing medications
3. Administering medications
4. Improving adherence
5. Eliminating disparities
6. Monitoring the effects of medications on patients
7. Medication reconciliation

Trends and patterns of usage can be presented in several different ways, which may include a description of use in the steps just listed. Trends can be described in terms of specific medication types, such as antibiotic usage, and compared with antibiograms for specific organisms. Patterns can be presented relative to overuse, underuse, and misuse. **Table 5.6** uses the basic monitoring criteria to illustrate medication monitoring of a specific case that can be used to

aggregate the data into trends. If a pattern or trend is identified, then a deeper review of the data is needed to determine what caused or contributed to the trend, how significant the trend is, and what action should be taken to prevent further impact or harm. A trend or pattern should be an alert that something has changed, and the performance is changing—this could be favorable or unfavorable. A trend or pattern is not necessarily statistically significant but may be empirically significant.

In recent years, antibiotics have been found to be overused and overprescribed. Various professional and government organizations have developed strategies to reduce the inappropriate use of antibiotics. A partnership of the National Quality Forum, National Quality Partners, and the Antibiotic Stewardship Action Team published a *National Quality Partners Playbook: Antibiotic Stewardship in Acute Care*.[68] It was written to support the call by the Centers for Disease Control and Prevention in 2014 to meet the urgent need of changing antibiotic use in hospitals.[68(p5)] The core elements of an antibiotic stewardship program include:

1. *Leadership commitment.* Dedicate necessary human, financial, and information technology resources.

## Table 5.6 Medication Use Monitoring

| General Criteria | Specific Criteria |
|---|---|
| Was the intervention used? | What class or type of medication is being monitored (e.g., antibiotic, opioid, insulin, anticoagulant, psychotropic)?<br>Were there barriers to use of the intervention (e.g., adherence, social determinants of health)? |
| Was it performed properly according to specific criteria? | Was the medication administered in accordance with policy, criteria, or current evidence (e.g., was the proper antibiotic preoperatively administered and within one hour)? |
| Was it performed safely? | Was the medication administered safely (e.g., should the medication be administered by an infusion device to control the rate, should it be administered in a central versus peripheral site, was it diluted properly)? |
| Was there any adverse effect or outcome to the patient? | Were there any adverse effects to patients (e.g., medication reactions or complications, allergies, errors, interactions with other medications or foods)? |
| Was staff competent to perform the intervention? | Was the staff who administered the medication competent in the procedure (e.g., does the route of administration require special knowledge and skill, does the type of medication require a certain setting for observation, is there a specific staff competency)? |
| Was it effective? | Did the medication achieve the desired result or an untoward result? |
| Was there a better alternative to the intervention? | Were there clearly documented indications for use of the medication?<br>If the medication is high risk, high alert, or nonformulary, was there documentation on usage? |

2. *Accountability.* Appoint a single leader responsible for program outcomes who is accountable to an executive-level or patient quality-focused hospital committee.
3. *Drug expertise.* Appoint a single pharmacist leader responsible for working to improve antibiotic use.
4. *Action.* Implement at least one recommended action.
5. *Tracking.* Monitor process measures, impact on patients, antibiotic use, and resistance.
6. *Reporting.* Report information regularly to doctors, nurses, and relevant staff.
7. *Education.* Educate clinicians about disease state management, resistance, and optimal prescribing.[68(p5)]

While antibiotic stewardship has been more focused on the acute care setting, there is a definite role in the outpatient setting with most care occurring outside of the hospital.

# Blood, Blood Products, and Biologics Use

The administration of blood, blood products, and other biologics is a high-risk aspect of care. Staff must consider the risk and the therapeutic benefit, including the risk of blood-borne pathogens, transfusion reactions, and transfusion errors. It is also a high-cost item. The key elements to be monitored include ordering, distribution (availability and timeliness of administration), handling and dispensing, administration, and monitoring of the effects on patients. Individual cases are reviewed (**Table 5.7**), and then an evaluation of product usage practices for providers and the organization can be performed. An evaluation might include a determination of whether blood/blood product is administered when not indicated, not administered when indicated, or administered incorrectly. Specific standards from the College of American Pathologists

**Table 5.7**  Blood, Blood Product, and Biologic Usage Monitoring

| General Criteria | Specific Criteria |
| --- | --- |
| Was the intervention used? | Was blood or blood components administered? Were there barriers to use of the intervention (e.g., adherence, social determinants of health)? |
| Was it performed properly according to specific criteria? | Was the order for the blood products clear and documented in the medical record? Was blood administration performed using defined policy including vital signs before, during, and after administration? Were proper tubing, filters, and administration devices used? |
| Was it performed safely? | Was the patient monitored during the administration? Was the rate of administration in accordance with policy, orders, and the patient's condition? |
| Was there any adverse effect or outcome to the patient? | Were there any adverse reactions to the administration (immediate or delayed)? If there was a reaction, was the response in accordance with policy? |
| Was staff competent to perform the intervention? | Were the staff who administered the blood products competent in the procedure (is there a specific competency)? |
| Was it effective? | Was the most appropriate blood product administered for the patient's condition? |
| Was there a better alternative to the intervention? | Was there a review of lab results, vital signs, and other results before the order to determine whether the particular blood product was indicated (e.g., iron, watchful waiting)? Was there a review of any special considerations before administration, such as religious beliefs? |
| Was there proper consent and education done? | Was informed consent provided prior to administration? If not, were there special exceptions such as trauma or other emergency conditions? Was the patient educated on the process including discharge instructions in the event of delayed reaction? |

and the American Association of Blood Banks may be useful for evaluating transfusion services. Blood products and biologics are administered in the outpatient setting and require strict monitoring of practices and patient outcomes.

## Seclusion and Restraint

Restraint use is another high-risk procedure that may be used with certain populations. It is no longer allowed in the long-term care setting but may be used in acute hospitals in medical–surgical units, inpatient behavioral health departments, and emergency departments for highly unpredictable patients and situations. National and state organizations are calling for the eradication of restraint use in behavioral health settings altogether because of high-profile adverse events related to their use and due to the organizations' adoption of trauma-informed principles and practices. The Joint Commission's Hospital-Based Inpatient Psychiatric Services (HBIPS) measures for seclusion and restraint ensure these are used only when clinically justified or when warranted by patient behavior that threatens the physical safety of the patient, staff, or others. These core measures include HBIPS-2 Hours of physical restraint use and HBIPS-3 Hours of seclusion use.

CMS established specific rules related to restraint usage, and these were adopted by The Joint Commission, which has deemed status with CMS. The monitoring of this process includes each episode of restraint application (**Table 5.8**). Similar monitoring can be used for seclusion. When restraints are used, a checklist is employed to ensure that all required components are met, and each episode can be easily monitored according to criteria. An aggregate utilization summary allows the organization to determine any trends. Such trends may reveal patterns associated with

- time of day or day of week in which restraint use may be higher, such as nights or weekends;
- units in which restraint use may be higher, such as geropsychiatric units or units with higher numbers of patients with tubes and other devices; and
- providers whose ordering practices reveal higher restraint use.

## Operative and Invasive Procedures

Operative, invasive, and noninvasive procedures are important diagnostic and therapeutic interventions occurring in all settings. They often pose risks to patients and must be monitored systematically (**Table 5.9**). Aspects for monitoring may include

- selection of the appropriate procedures;
- patient preparation for procedures;
- consent for procedures;

**Table 5.8** Seclusion and Restraint Use Monitoring

| General Criteria | Specific Criteria |
| --- | --- |
| Was the intervention used? | Were restraints applied to the patient (what type of restraint and what limb or body part was restrained)? <br> What was the reason for the restraint, and was it documented? |
| Was it performed properly according to specific criteria? | Were restraints applied properly in accordance with policy, CMS regulations, and The Joint Commission standards? <br> Was there compliance with requirements for orders, timeliness, trial releases, alternatives, initial face-to-face assessment, and ongoing monitoring? |
| Was it performed safely? | Were restraints applied safely so that the patient was not at risk for injury or harm? |
| Was there any adverse effect or outcome to the patient? | Were there any adverse effects (e.g., physical, emotional) to the patient related to the application of restraints? |
| Was staff competent to perform the intervention? | Were the staff who applied the restraints competent in the procedure (is there a specific competency)? |
| Was it effective? | Did the use of the restraints achieve the desired result? |
| Was there a better alternative to the intervention? | Were other alternatives tried before restraints were applied (and documented)? <br> Was seclusion used with restraints? |

**Table 5.9** Operative and Invasive Procedure Monitoring

| General Criteria | Specific Criteria |
|---|---|
| Was the intervention used? | What was the surgical or invasive procedure performed? <br> Were there barriers to use of the intervention (e.g., adherence, social determinants of health)? |
| Was it performed properly according to specific criteria? | Were there documented indications for the procedure? <br> Was the patient properly informed of risks, benefits, and alternatives and did the patient provide consent? |
| Was it properly consented? | Was oral or written consent required? <br> Was consent documented per policy? |
| Was it performed safely? | Was the procedure performed using policy, guidelines, or other criteria? <br> Was a time-out performed prior to the procedure (if required)? |
| Was there any adverse effect or outcome to the patient? | Was there any adverse effect on the patient before, during, or after the procedure? <br> Was any action taken to prevent, mitigate, or respond to an adverse event (e.g., preprocedure positioning to prevent injury, postprocedure X-ray if a retained object was suspected)? |
| Was staff competent to perform the intervention? | Were staff performing the procedure competent? <br> Were providers privileged to perform the procedure? |
| Was it effective? | What was the result or outcome for the patient? |
| Was there a better alternative to the intervention? | Was the procedure elective, urgent, or emergent? <br> Were all viable options considered and discussed with the patient? <br> Was patient education completed? Documented? <br> Were specialists consulted if needed? <br> Was the procedure performed in the right setting (e.g., inpatient or outpatient, or in a specialty hospital, or a hospital that performs a high volume of procedures vs. a hospital that infrequently performs a procedure, especially one of considerable risk and complexity)? |

- performance of the procedure and patient monitoring;
- postprocedure care;
- preprocedure and postprocedure patient education;
- preprocedure and postprocedure diagnostic discrepancies;
- moderate sedation monitoring; and
- complications or adverse events related to the procedure.

Procedures always carry the risk of complications even when performed properly. Risk is greater with procedures performed when not indicated, not performed when indicated, and performed poorly or incorrectly. Outcomes are influenced by clinical performance of all preprocedure processes; clinical performance of the procedure; and

patient monitoring before, during, and after the procedure.

Common errors in the operating room reported as sentinel events to The Joint Commission include

- wrong patient, wrong site, or wrong procedure;
- unintended retention of foreign objects; and
- operative/postoperative complications.[69]

Kim and colleagues[70] also identified quality issues in surgery as

- a breakdown in communication within and among the surgical team, care providers, patients, and their families;
- a delay in diagnosis or failure to diagnose; and
- a delay in treatment or failure to treat.

National databases allow comparisons of organizational data with risk-adjusted surgical cases for observed-to-expected ratios of morbidity and mortality. This allows the organization to use an external comparison or benchmark to assess its rate of complications as a trigger or threshold for action (e.g., the National Surgical Quality Improvement Program; the Chevron Supplier Quality Improvement Process, and the Society of Thoracic Surgeons National Database).

## Cardiopulmonary Resuscitation

Monitoring cardiopulmonary resuscitation (CPR) and outcomes is important to include in any quality improvement program (**Table 5.10**). Cardiopulmonary resuscitation is defined as the application of chest compressions, defibrillation, and artificial respirations or rescue breathing. One consideration in CPR monitoring is whether the patient exhibited any signs or symptoms that could have been identified for early intervention before a full arrest occurred. If CPR must be performed, there are specific guidelines on chest compressions, airway maintenance and breathing, defibrillation, and medications. Advanced care and treatment depend on the setting and the patient's underlying condition.

A national registry for data on CPR events collects detailed information on exact interventions, times, and results (including electrocardiograms). The use of a registry allows comparison of data on process and outcome measures. Associated with cardiopulmonary resuscitation are the use of advanced care planning, preferences for CPR initiation, and other prolonging or removal actions for life-sustaining treatment. The whole continuum can be monitored in some fashion to include the following:

- Presence of advance directive (at home, hospital, long-term care, other setting)
- Knowledge of CPR status prior to need
- Identification of deteriorating status for action to prevent full arrest
- Timely initiation of CPR if indicated
- Proper use of procedures (e.g., airway, compressions, medications, defibrillation, documentation, personal protective equipment, formal algorithms)
- Any issues during CPR (e.g., airway, compressions, equipment, teamwork, medications, defibrillation, and documentation)
- Corrective action as needed
- Family support

## Morbidity and Mortality

Review of morbidity and mortality is often based on specific criteria. For mortality, a review of expected or unexpected mortality (observed vs. expected) is performed by condition, within specific time frames (e.g., immediately in the operating room, in the hospital setting, or within 30 days after discharge), and based on inclusion and exclusion criteria. For example, patients are usually excluded from review if they are expected to die based on a terminal condition with a do not resuscitate/do not intubate/allow natural death order, who are in hospice, or who have an end-stage condition. Other mortalities are then reviewed as outcomes that can provide information about the quality of care provided. Similarly, complications are also

**Table 5.10** Cardiopulmonary Resuscitation (CPR) Monitoring

| General Criteria | Specific Criteria |
|---|---|
| Was the intervention used? | Was CPR performed (defined by defibrillation and chest compressions or similar definition)? |
| Was it performed properly according to specific criteria? | Was CPR performed correctly and promptly in accordance with basic life support or advanced cardiac life support guidelines including timeliness? |
| Was it performed safely? | Was CPR performed safely (e.g., consider the location of the victim, defibrillation, and other safety factors)? |
| Was there any adverse effect or outcome to the patient? | What was the outcome (immediate, defined intervals, at discharge)? |
| Was staff competent to perform the intervention? | Were staff trained and certified in the proper level of response? Was certification current? |
| Was it effective? | Were compressions and rescue breathing effective in sustaining perfusion? Was CPR initiated timely? |
| Was there a better alternative to the intervention? | Were there early warning signs for rapid response team (RRT) to intervene before full arrest? RRT may be monitored separately for outcomes. |
| Outcomes | Immediate survival Survival at discharge |

reviewed, and the criteria for cases and conditions to be reviewed are established by the medical staff. Individual cases are then identified and reviewed, and aggregated reports are trended to identify opportunities for improvement. Comparisons of trends can be made internally over time or externally compared with national databases.

Morbidity and mortality data are often risk adjusted to compare similar patients (usually with similar conditions, procedures, or diagnosis-related groups). National databases allow comparison of morbidity and mortality using a risk-adjusted model. Typical occurrence screening examples for mortality include

- death within 24 hours of admission to a hospital;
- death within 72 hours of transfer out of a special care unit;
- lack of documentation of deterioration during the 48 hours preceding death;
- failure of a physician to respond to a notification of change in a patient's condition during the 48 hours preceding death;
- lack of documentation indicating death was expected (consider suicide, oxygen/fire, and other high risks);
- lack of concordance between premortem and postmortem diagnoses;
- clinically significant incident or occurrence within 72 hours of death;
- clinically significant complication of surgical procedure within 72 hours of death;
- clinically significant complication of invasive procedure within 72 hours of death;
- death during surgery;
- unplanned organ removal during operative procedure within two months preceding death;
- surgical procedure to repair a perforation, laceration, or other injury of an organ during an invasive procedure within two months preceding death;
- repeat of any surgical procedure within two months preceding death;
- myocardial infarction within 24 hours of a surgical or invasive procedure;
- death within 48 hours of an elective surgical procedure; and
- lack of concordance between preoperative and postoperative diagnoses.

Whether or not the death was preventable is another important consideration.

## Medical Records

Health information comes in many types such as e-prescribing, personal health record, and dental

records. Health information as a medical record is held in a paper-based chart, within an electronic health record, or a combination of both. The monitoring of the medical record usually includes elements such as:

- *Required documentation content.* The requirements vary by setting, procedure, and even profession. For example, the requirements for a treatment plan/individualized plan of care are different for an acute care hospital and a long-term care facility. The requirements for surgery with general anesthesia are different from those for an outpatient procedure with moderate sedation. Each facility must first identify the required content for the record and then develop a process to monitor essential elements. Checklists, databases, or other tools make this process more efficient. This step often reflects the presence or absence of the required content.
- *Timeliness of documentation.* The next requirement is the time requirement of specific documentation. Most common elements monitored for timeliness include history and physical exam, preoperative and postoperative notes, and discharge summaries. This step reflects whether the documentation met or did not meet the required timeline.
- *Appropriateness of documentation (clinical pertinence).* The monitoring of clinical pertinence requires an assessment of the documentation in terms of the patient's condition, diagnostic results, intervention procedures, vital signs, and other information. This review may determine that documentation was appropriate or not appropriate to the standard of care, key elements of the assessment, treatment plan, interventions, and medication management.

## Diagnostic Monitoring

In 2015, the National Academies of Sciences, Engineering, and Medicine published *Improving Diagnoses in Healthcare*, which acknowledged that diagnosis has been an underappreciated component of quality and safety.[71] Increasingly, tests of all kinds are done to diagnose a patient's condition. If tests are not completed, reported, or communicated, or if the provider does not make the correct diagnosis, then the patient might not receive the proper treatment, timely treatment, or any treatment. The generally accepted definition of *diagnostic error* is the failure to establish an accurate and timely explanation of the patient's health problem(s) or to communicate that explanation to the patient.[71(pxiii)] While diagnostic testing occurs in any setting, it may be more likely to result in problems in the outpatient setting due to the large numbers of outpatient tests (e.g., laboratory, radiology). Examples of criteria that can be used for monitoring include

- identification of high risk or critical tests;
- patient has the test (e.g., preventive cancer screenings);
- timeliness of receiving results from the diagnostic service (e.g., turnaround time);
- timeliness of reporting results to the patient (e.g., normal versus abnormal results);
- timeliness of referral to specialty care if needed; and
- independent validation of test interpretation (e.g., with imaging studies and pathology reports).

Diagnostic errors related to actual diagnosis of medical conditions occur but are difficult to monitor, and problems are usually identified by a reviewer after an error. The processes for clinical review are often with risk management or peer review.

## Suicide Screening and Prevention

Suicide screening and prevention is a heightened area of concern, therefore, the need for quality monitoring has increased. Suicide screening occurs in most healthcare settings, including primary care, emergency care, acute care, long-term care, home care, and behavioral health specialty care. Initial screening is done using an evidence-based tool. Screening helps identify risk levels for further evaluation by a provider or mental health specialist. The monitoring often includes a review of documentation for timely screening and timely evaluation as well as referral based on the level of risk. A particularly important component with suicide or self-harm prevention is the identification and removal of ligature points within any environment of care.

## Pain Management

Pain management has been a focus primarily in the acute care hospital setting due to standards related to the types of medications, the route, and the effectiveness. However, pain management, both acute and chronic, has continued to grow across all settings and includes a variety of medications, routes, and techniques, as well as integrative approaches. An awareness of the modalities used in the work setting will guide the type of monitoring, which may include

- documentation of pain type, location, characteristics, and aggravating and relieving factors;

- appropriate prescribing of medications (especially for controlled substances);
- dispensing processes;
- documentation of administration;
- the patient's response to pain treatment; and
- the timeliness of documentation of response.

Organizations may have a committee that addresses pain management due to the highly regulated environment for controlled substances and the risk for abuse or addiction.

Key points for performance monitoring and evaluation are listed in **Box 5.6**.

---

**Box 5.6  Key Points: Performance Monitoring and Evaluation**

- Monitor required regulatory and accreditation indicators applicable to the organization (e.g., hospital, skilled nursing facility, health plan).
- Apply criteria to determine priority measures such as risk, volume, problem prone, safety, and cost.
- Establish a data collection plan for measures including definition, technical specifications, analysis approach, actions/intervention, and goals for improvement.

---

# Performance Improvement Tools

Described next are methods and tools for decision making and process improvement. Detailed descriptions and examples of these tools follow. More information on data analysis and statistical process control are described in the *Health Data Analytics* section.

## A3 Tool

The *A3* tool is considered a Kanban (workflow management) tool for process and problem solving based on the PDCA method (**Figure 5.15**). This summary of improvement steps on a single form fosters continuous improvement by following structured steps.[72,73] This tool and exercise are typically covered in Six Sigma White and Yellow Belt training.

## Activity Network Diagram

This tool is also known as an *arrow diagram* or called the program evaluation and review technique or a

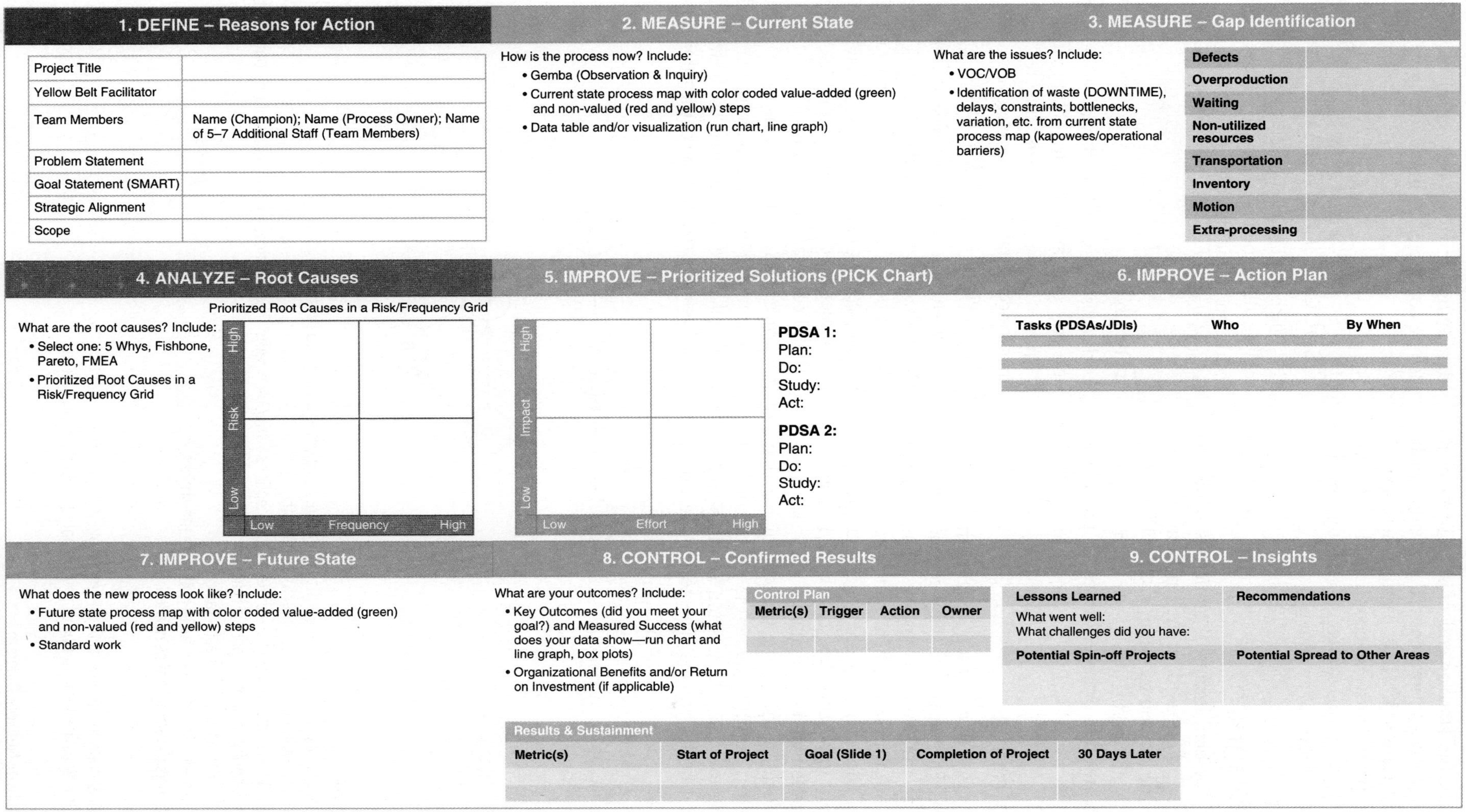

## 1. DEFINE – Reasons for Action

| Project Title | |
| --- | --- |
| Yellow Belt Facilitator | |
| Team Members | Name (Champion); Name (Process Owner); Name of 5–7 Additional Staff (Team Members) |
| Problem Statement | |
| Goal Statement (SMART) | |
| Strategic Alignment | |
| Scope | |

## 2. MEASURE – Current State

How is the process now? Include:
- Gemba (Observation & Inquiry)
- Current state process map with color coded value-added (green) and non-valued (red and yellow) steps
- Data table and/or visualization (run chart, line graph)

## 3. MEASURE – Gap Identification

What are the issues? Include:
- VOC/VOB
- Identification of waste (DOWNTIME), delays, constraints, bottlenecks, variation, etc. from current state process map (kapowees/operational barriers)

- **Defects**
- **Overproduction**
- **Waiting**
- **Non-utilized resources**
- **Transportation**
- **Inventory**
- **Motion**
- **Extra-processing**

## 4. ANALYZE – Root Causes

What are the root causes? Include:
- Select one: 5 Whys, Fishbone, Pareto, FMEA
- Prioritized Root Causes in a Risk/Frequency Grid

Prioritized Root Causes in a Risk/Frequency Grid

(Risk: High / Low, Frequency: Low / High grid)

## 5. IMPROVE – Prioritized Solutions (PICK Chart)

(Impact: High / Low, Effort: Low / High grid)

**PDSA 1:**
Plan:
Do:
Study:
Act:

**PDSA 2:**
Plan:
Do:
Study:
Act:

## 6. IMPROVE – Action Plan

| Tasks (PDSAs/JDIs) | Who | By When |
| --- | --- | --- |
| | | |
| | | |
| | | |

## 7. IMPROVE – Future State

What does the new process look like? Include:
- Future state process map with color coded value-added (green) and non-valued (red and yellow) steps
- Standard work

## 8. CONTROL – Confirmed Results

What are your outcomes? Include:
- Key Outcomes (did you meet your goal?) and Measured Success (what does your data show—run chart and line graph, box plots)
- Organizational Benefits and/or Return on Investment (if applicable)

**Control Plan**

| Metric(s) | Trigger | Action | Owner |
| --- | --- | --- | --- |

**Results & Sustainment**

| Metric(s) | Start of Project | Goal (Slide 1) | Completion of Project | 30 Days Later |
| --- | --- | --- | --- | --- |

## 9. CONTROL – Insights

**Lessons Learned**
What went well:
What challenges did you have:

**Potential Spin-off Projects**

**Recommendations**

**Potential Spread to Other Areas**

**Figure 5.15** A3 Tool

Reproduced from Canode C. *Veterans Integrated Service Network (VISN 8) Lean Six Sigma Belt Training.* U.S. Department of Veterans Affairs.

critical path method chart. In the arrow diagram, arrows connect the start or end of an activity in a sequence. These nodes represent the start and finish of activities (**Figure 5.16**). It is useful when several simultaneous paths must be coordinated and best case/worst case scenarios are considered that might impact the completion of an activity.

## Affinity Diagram

The *affinity diagram* organizes numerous ideas or issues into groupings based on their natural relationships within the groupings (**Figure 5.17**). These diagrams typically are used to analyze or chart a process and to structure and organize issues to provide a new perspective.

## Brainstorming

*Brainstorming* is a free-flowing generation of ideas (**Figure 5.18**). This approach can generate excitement, equalize involvement, and result in original solutions to the problem. There is no censoring or discussion of ideas as they are generated, but the team can build upon the ideas of others. It is especially important that no judgments are made concerning the idea's worth to the process, or whether the idea is even feasible (money is no object in a brainstorming exercise). Discussion of ideas comes at a later point in the process. This technique works well to generate ideas related to cause and effect or identifying paths toward a goal. This activity can also be conducted as brainwriting.

## Cause-and-Effect, Ishikawa, or Fishbone Diagram

The *Ishikawa diagram* is used to display, explore, and analyze all the potential causes related to a problem or condition and to discover the root causes of variation (**Figure 5.19**).

## Checklist

A *checklist* is a standard way to ensure completion of critical tasks for a process or activity (**Figure 5.20**). The checklist ensures accuracy, timeliness, accountability, completeness, and efficiency. Ways to organize a checklist include:

- *Ordered list.* A list of tasks needed to be accomplished in a particular order. The checklist is numbered, starting at the first task or step and proceeding to the last task or step, in increasing numerical order. The ordered list ensures correct and complete processing.
- *Itemized list.* A list of items to be addressed, with meaningful information alongside; used as a guide or reference. An itemized list provides a complete accounting or reporting of the information present.

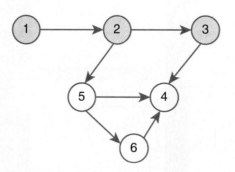

**How to construct**
1. List all the necessary tasks, one per card, to complete a project from start to finish.
2. Use the cards to sequence the activities for each path.
3. Identify the places in the paths where there are connections with other paths. These places identify parts of one path that cannot be initiated until a point in another path is reached.
4. Determine the time duration for each task.
5. Calculate the shortest possible time to complete the project.
6. Review and revise the diagram as needed.

**When to use**
- When a task is complex or crucial to an organization.
- When simultaneous implementation of several paths must be coordinated.

**Figure 5.16** Activity Network Diagram

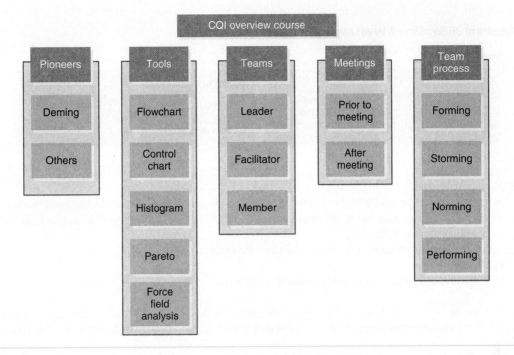

**How to construct**

1. Define the issue.
2. Brainstorm and record ideas on cards.
3. Randomly display the cards on a board.
4. Have the group silently sort the issues into groups.
5. Create header cards for groupings.
6. Draw a diagram based on the groupings (it will look like an organizational chart).

**When to use**

- To analyze or chart a process
- To structure and organize issues to provide a new perspective

**Figure 5.17** Affinity Diagram

- *Sublist.* A sublist is a branch or subset of an ordered list. Sublists can exist for almost any of the other types of checklists.
- *Prioritized list.* Any of the aforementioned lists placed into an order based on a priority scheme. It helps use time effectively, focus energy where it's most needed, and address the important items or tasks first.
- *General list.* Any of the previous lists with a space for a check mark, initials, or additional information. As tasks or items are completed, the line is checked or initialed.[74]

## Deployment Chart or Planning Grid

A *deployment chart,* also called a *planning grid,* is used to project schedules for complex tasks and their associated subtasks (**Figure 5.21**). It usually is used with a task for which the time for completion is known. The tool also is used to determine who has responsibility for the parts of a plan or project. The grid helps the group organize key steps in the project to reach milestones and the desired goal. Shaded boxes may be used to indicate the people who primarily are responsible, with ovals indicating an assistant or adviser.

## Delphi Method

The *Delphi method* is a combination of the brainstorming, multivoting, and nominal group techniques. This technique is used when group members are not in one location and often is conducted by email when a meeting is not feasible. After each step in the process, the data are sent to one person, who compiles the data and sends out the next round for participants to complete.

## Failure Mode and Effects Analysis

A *failure mode and effects analysis (FMEA)* is a preventive approach to identify failures and opportunities for

---

**Topic: Why Patients in OB/Gyn Clinic A Have Long Wait Times for Appointments**

Post-its

| | | | |
|---|---|---|---|
| Dr. A likes to spend extra time with patients. | Doctors are called to labor and delivery with no backup clinic coverage. | Physician assistant A and nurse practitioner B are double booked on a regular basis. | Don't use open-access scheduling practices. |

---

**How to construct**

1. Define the brainstorming topic.
2. Bring together the best group to address the topic (e.g., practice manager, physicians, physician assistants, nurse practitioners, nursing staff)
3. Inform participants of the ground rules that (a) "all ideas are good ideas" and (b) "all comments/evaluation should be held in abeyance until the brainstorming is complete."
4. Brainstorm in silence. Give everyone a few minutes to think about the topic.
   a. Write down their ideas.
   b. Use sticky notes to encourage participation and ensure an equal voice.
5. Gather ideas.
   a. *Flip chart.* Have the team members call out their ideas. This can be free-flowing, or a structure can be used, such as going around the table with each person verbalizing one idea each time around. As the ideas are generated, one person should write the ideas on a flip chart.
   b. *Sticky notes.* Place the sticky notes on a flat surface (e.g., on butcher paper on a table or on a wall).
6. Organize and summarize ideas.

**When to use**

- Use when a list of possible ideas is needed.
- This technique works well to generate ideas for such tools as the cause-and-effect diagram and the tree diagram.

**Figure 5.18** Brainstorming

---

error and can be used for processes as well as equipment. The traditional techniques for an FMEA originated in manufacturing and other industries and were adapted to healthcare. The Veterans Affairs National Center for Patient Safety created the Healthcare FMEA (HFMEA). There are six main steps to the HFMEA, as displayed in **Figure 5.22**.[75]

## Flowchart, Process Flowchart, or Process Map

The *flowchart* or *process flowchart* or *process map* is a graphical display of a process as it is known to its authors, owners, or teams (**Figure 5.23**). The flowchart outlines the sequence and relationship of the steps of the process. Through management of data and information, the team comes to a collective understanding and knowledge concerning the process. Information is discussed about the structure (who carries out the specific step in the identified process), the activity that is occurring, and the outcome or the results. Flowchart examples are available on websites.[76] An example

of a healthcare process flowchart/map is depicted in **Figure 5.24**.

## Force Field Analysis

*Force field analysis* is a method to systematically identify the various forces that facilitate or increase the likelihood of success, and the opposite factors that decrease or restrain the likelihood of success or improvement in the process. This tool serves as a root cause analysis with listing the pros and cons of an action as shown in **Figure 5.25**.

## Human-Centered Design

*Human-centered design* is a problem solving, design-based discipline to move ideas and innovations from concept to prototype to implementation (**Figure 5.26**). This can be used to

- problem solve a process through a human-centered approach;
- identify stakeholders who are responsible for processes or tasks; and
- demonstrate current processes (current state; problems) and the future state (solution).

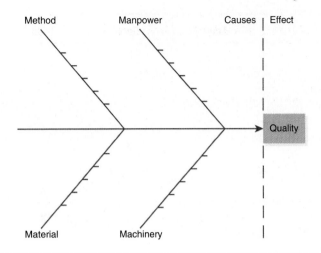

**How to construct**
1. Determine the effect or the label for the diagram, and put it on the far-right side of the diagram.
2. Draw a horizontal line to the left of the effect.
3. Determine the categories (the four Ms or the six Ps).
   a. Four Ms: Machine (technology), Method (process), Material (includes Raw Material, Information), and Manpower
   b. Six Ps: Policy, Process, People, Plant, Program, and Product
4. Draw a diagonal line for half of the categories above the line and half below the line.
5. Brainstorm the list for each of the categories.
6. Organize each of the causes on each bone.
7. Draw branch bones to show the relationships.

**When to use**
- To identify and organize potential causes of problems
- To identify factors that will lead to success
- As part of a root cause analysis

**Figure 5.19** Cause-and-Effect, Ishikawa, or Fishbone Diagram

| Task | Completed |
|------|-----------|
| Process 1 | |
| Task 1, a | |
| Task 1, b | |

**How to construct**
1. Identify critical elements or tasks to be completed for a process.
2. Make a list of all elements with a space to indicate completion of the task before moving to the next task or process.

**When to use**
- When reliance on memory is not sufficient
- When tasks for a process or activity are critical and omission may cause harm
- When the process is complicated and the tasks are many

**Figure 5.20** Checklist

The design process must include the people (stakeholders) who will use the product or service. The process includes steps to frame (empathize, define), discover (ideate), design (prototype), and deliver (test, implement).

## Interrelationship Diagram

The *interrelationship diagram* requires multidirectional thinking when there is not a straight-line cause-and-effect relationship (**Figure 5.27**). This

| | Amy | Gary | Todd | Alia | Jaxson |
|---|---|---|---|---|---|
| Chart Review at Hospital | X | | | | |
| Chart Review at MD Ambulatory Care | | | | X | |
| Interview Drs #123 and #456 | | | | | X |
| Interview Office Nurses #123 and #456 | | X | | | |
| Compile Data | | | X | | |
| Create Graphics | | | X | | |
| | | | | | |
| | | | | | |
| | | | | | |

**How to construct**
1. Specify the desired outcome.
2. Identify the last step necessary (e.g., a report to a committee with the team's recommendations).
3. Identify the starting point.
4. Brainstorm a list of the necessary steps between the starting and final steps.
5. Refine the list by combining like steps and defining the sequence steps.
6. Design a grid with important items (e.g., who is responsible, due date, budget/cost) listed across the top.
7. Arrange the list of tasks or steps in sequence down the left column.
8. Fill in the appropriate columns, including tentative dates.
9. Revise the planning grid, as necessary.

**When to use**
- Use as a planning tool to identify steps to be taken, timelines, and responsibility for those steps.
- Use for project and management teams to determine what needs to be done, in what sequence, who is responsible for what, and how that relates to others.

**Figure 5.21** Deployment Chart or Planning Grid

**How to construct**

There are six main steps to HFMEA:

1. Define a topic and process to be studied.
2. Convene an interdisciplinary team with content and process experts.
3. Develop a flow diagram of the process with consecutive numbering of each step and lettering of all subprocesses.
4. List all possible failure modes of each subprocess, including the severity and probability of the failure mode, and then number these failure modes (brainstorming may be helpful to identify failure modes).
5. After analyzing the failure modes, determine the action for each failure mode to eliminate, control, or accept.
6. Identify the corresponding outcome measure to test the redesigned process.

**Figure 5.22** Healthcare Failure Mode and Effects Analysis (HFMEA)

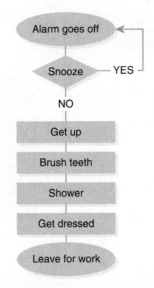

**How to construct**

1. Define the process that will be represented in the flowchart.
2. Determine all individuals, departments, and groups involved in the process.
3. Brainstorm the steps in the process.
4. Construct the flowchart graphically using rows or columns corresponding to the associated work units.
5. Arrange the steps sequentially.
6. Draw arrows between the steps to show the process flow.
7. Review the flowchart and validate its accuracy with other individuals who are involved in the process.

**When to use**

- To show steps in a process
- To find one or multiple sources of a problem or identify potential areas for improvement
- To examine the handoffs that occur in a process
- To identify personnel, groups, or entire departments that are responsible for processes or tasks
- To demonstrate current processes (current state)

**Figure 5.23** Flowchart or Process Flowchart

Data from Agency for Healthcare Research and Quality. Workflow assessment for health IT: Flowchart. Accessed May 31, 2022. https://digital.ahrq.gov/health-it-tools-and-resources/evaluation-resources/workflow-assessment-health-it-toolkit/all-workflow-tools/flowchart

tool organizes complex problems, issues, or ideas by sorting and displaying their interrelations. It is useful to address both operational and organizational issues.

## Matrix Diagram

A *matrix diagram* can show the relationship between two items as well as the strength of the relationship (**Figure 5.28**). This tool displays the connection between each idea or issue in one group to one or more groups. Many matrix diagram formats are available, but the *L*-shaped matrix is the most common. Other common formats include the *T*-shaped, *Y*-shaped, *X*-shaped, and *C*-shaped matrices.

## Multivoting

*Multivoting* is an easy, quick method for determining the most popular or important items from a list (**Figure 5.29**). The method uses a series of votes to cut the list in half each time, thus reducing the number of items to be considered.

## Nominal Group Technique

The nominal group technique is a group decision-making process for generating many ideas by each group member working alone and then bringing all the group ideas together. The *nominal group technique* is used when group members are new to each other or when they have different

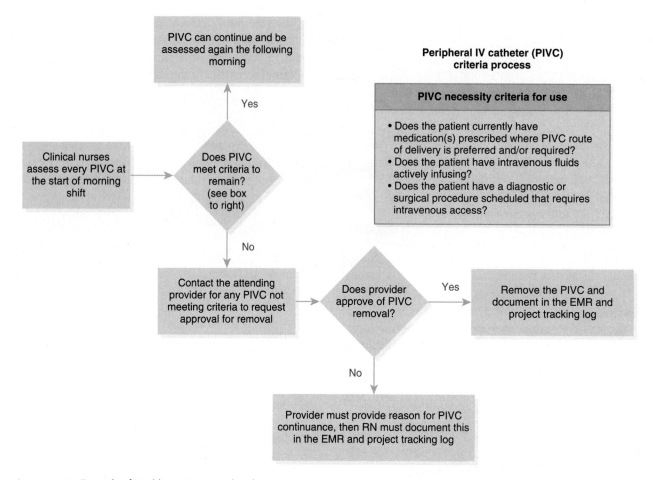

**Figure 5.24** Example of Healthcare Process Flowchart

Reproduced from Loudermilk RA, Steffen LE, McGarvey JS. Strategically applying new criteria for use improves management of peripheral intravenous catheters. *J Healthc Qual.* 2018;40(5):274–282.

CQI education program

| Strengths | Barriers |
|---|---|
| Management supports program ⟶ | ← Lack of time |
| Physicians support program ⟶ | ← Lack of commitment of all participants |
| Have committed time and other resources to complete program ⟶ | ← Viewed as not important |

**How to construct**

1. Identify the issue.
2. Create two columns on a piece of paper. Label one "strengths" and one "barriers."
3. Brainstorm and list potential strengths and barriers on the chart.
4. Determine actions to be taken to increase the strengths and to decrease or eliminate the barriers.

**When to use**

Identify the strengths and barriers for the success of the project

**Figure 5.25** Force Field Analysis

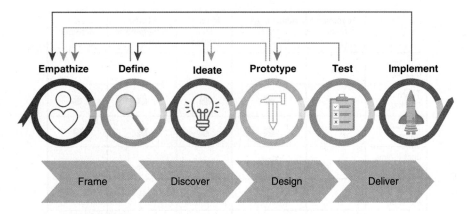

**Figure 5.26** Human-Centered Design Model
Reproduced from Bielicki K. Human centered design. Department of Veterans Affairs (VA) Innovation Network.

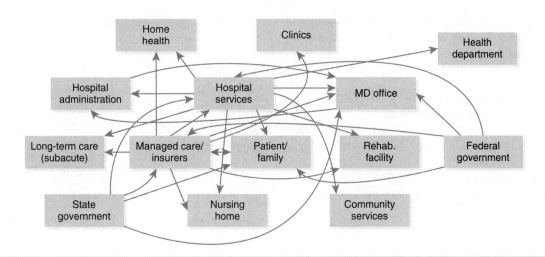

## How to construct

1. Determine the issue/problem.
2. Generate ideas through brainstorming and other methods regarding the steps in the processes or issues.
3. Write the steps on cards and arrange them in similar groups (as with the affinity diagram) in cause-and-effect sequence. This technique is most effective when dealing with 15 to 50 items that may be interrelated. Discussion is appropriate throughout this process to ensure that no steps are missed.
4. Allow at least 1/2 inch of space between the cards so that relationship arrows can be drawn.
5. Fill in the relationship arrows that indicate what leads to what.
   a. This is done one card at a time until all cards have been discussed and relationship arrows drawn.
   b. Each card should be examined in terms of what happens when this card (process step) occurs; two-way arrows should be avoided.
6. Review and revise the diagram, transfer the information to a sheet of paper, and distribute it to team members for their review and revision before the next meeting.
7. Identify cards with the most arrows leading to them and cards with the most arrows leading away from them.
   a. Cards with incoming arrows represent a secondary issue or bottleneck in a process.
   b. Cards with outgoing arrows indicate a basic cause/issue that, if solved or overcome, will affect many other items.
   c. Cards with the most arrows are key factors in the process and should be addressed first.

## When to use

- When the correct sequencing of events is critical
- When the issue/problem is complex and contains interrelationships among and between ideas/steps

**Figure 5.27** Interrelationship Diagram

| | Governing body | Administrative team | Medical staff leaders | Middle management | Staff member |
|---|---|---|---|---|---|
| Overview course | ▲ | ▲ | ▲ | ▲ | ▲ |
| Team training | | ■ | ■ | ■ | ● |
| Facilitator training | | ■ | ■ | ■ | ● |
| Just-in-time training | | ● | ▲ | ▲ | ▲ |
| Systems thinking | ▲ | ▲ | ▲ | ● | |
| Principle centered leadership | ▲ | ▲ | ▲ | ● | |

**How to construct**

1. Select the appropriate matrix format (e.g., *L*-shaped: two sets of items; *T*-shaped: three sets of items showing both indirect and direct relationships). Place the appropriate items on each axis of the matrix.
2. Determine the relationship symbols to be used (for example, the following symbols may be selected: ▲ = very important; ■ = moderately important, as appropriate; ● = as needed.
3. Create the matrix and indicate the relationships.

**When to use**

- When defined tasks are to be assigned to employees
- When comparing tasks to a set of criteria
- When evaluating products or services against certain criteria
- When determining the relationship between patient satisfaction and certain factors

**Figure 5.28** Matrix Diagram

**How to construct**

1. Generate a list of items and number them.
2. If the group agrees, combine items that seem similar.
3. If necessary, renumber all items.
4. Each member lists on a sheet of paper the items they consider the most important (the number of items chosen should be at least one-third of the total number of items on the list).
5. Tally the votes beside each item on the list.
6. Eliminate items with the lowest scores.
7. Repeat the above process until the list is narrowed down to an appropriate number for the group to focus on or the item with the top priority is identified.

**When to use**

Use after a brainstorming session to identify the key items on which the group will focus.

**Figure 5.29** Multivoting

opinions and goals (**Figure 5.30**). This approach is more structured than brainstorming and multivoting.

## Pareto Chart

The *Pareto chart* contains bars in descending order with a line graph representing the cumulative total by percentage (**Figure 5.31**). The chart is related to the Pareto principle that finds 80% of the problems or effects come from 20% of the causes. Therefore, by tackling 20% of the most frequent causes, an 80% improvement can be achieved. It represents the most common sources of defects, problems, or categories for improvement to help narrow the focus.

**How to construct**

1. Define the task as you would for brainstorming.
2. Describe the purpose of this technique and the process to the group.
3. Write the question to be answered for all to see. Be sure to clarify the question as needed for the group.
4. Generate ideas to address the identified question by having the group write down their ideas in silence.
5. List all the items as you would in brainstorming. Only be sure to use a structured approach so that all ideas are listed (again, there is to be no discussion of the items at this time).
6. Clarify and discuss the ideas one at a time.
7. Give each member 4–8 cards or pieces of paper.
8. Members write one selection from the list on each card and assign a point value to each item. The highest value should be assigned to the most important item (i.e., if there are four cards, the most important card is numbered 4, next important 3, etc.).
9. The cards are collected and the votes are tallied; mark each item on the list with the value on the cards for that item.
10. The item with the largest number becomes the group's selection/priority.

**When to use**

- Use when team members are new to each other.
- Use when dealing with a controversial topic.

**Figure 5.30** Nominal Group Technique

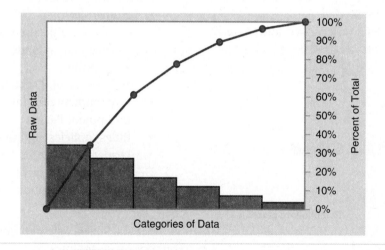

**How to construct**

1. Define your problem of focus. From your data set of categories, areas or factors identify the actual number of elements per category.
2. Most software programs have a wizard to create a Pareto Chart. Use the wizard. Without software you can manually calculate the percent each category contributes as a percent. One column of data will list the categories and the second column will include the corresponding actual number of elements in that category.
3. Either using software or manually create the categories on the horizontal X-axis and the raw data on the left vertical Y-axis. The categories should be sorted in descending order.
4. Calculate the total number of elements and the percent that each category makes up of the total number.
5. Add the cumulative percentage of each category until 100% is achieved on the right vertical Y-axis.

**When to use**

- Used to narrow the scope of a project by identifying areas contributing the most categories or areas to a process, especially for root causes.
- Displays the relative importance of these problems or categories in a simple visual format.
- The tallest bar can be broken down into another Pareto Chart as part of the drill down process.
- Use a pre- and post-chart display after a project is completed to show the change in categories or problems.

**Figure 5.31** Pareto Chart

## Plan-Do-Study-Act

The basic plan-do-study-act (PDSA) model is depicted in **Figure 5.32**. Specific strategies that can be used to test and link tests of change using PDSA cycles and the IHI model[77] include the following:

- Plan for multiple cycles of improvement in advance to support rapid cycle movement.
- Scale the scope and size of tests so that small tests can be done rapidly (e.g., with a few patients, with one provider, in a single day).
- Choose people who want to work on the improvement change process.
- Capitalize on existing resources, best practice, and research. Don't reinvent the wheel.
- Select opportunities for change that are readily achievable (low-hanging fruit or easy, visible wins) first. Make the test feasible and practical.
- Don't delay a project because technology is not available; for small projects, paper and pen or other simple methods may be sufficient.
- Collect useful, meaningful measures and review results of every change cycle to determine any modifications that are needed.
- Test the change under a variety of conditions (e.g., different shifts and on weekends).

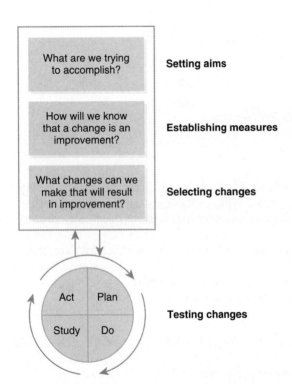

**Figure 5.32** Process Improvement Model (Plan-Do-Study-Act)

Reproduced from Langley GL, Moen R, Nolan KM, Nolan TW, Norman CL, Provost LP. *The Improvement Guide: A Practical Approach to Enhancing Organizational Performance.* 2nd ed. San Francisco, CA: Jossey-Bass Publishers; 2009.

- Be prepared to stop or abandon the process if no improvement is observed.

## Root Cause Analysis

When variation is inherent in the process and a reduction of the variation is desired, the root cause of the variation must be identified to eliminate tampering with the effective components of the process. The Joint Commission requires a root cause analysis in response to sentinel events (unexpected serious adverse events).

1. Identify potential causes of the variation. An interdisciplinary team familiar with the process can use brainstorming, flowcharts, cause-and-effect diagrams, or other process to determine these potential causes.
2. Verify the potential causes by collecting data about the process. After the data are collected and analyzed using the tools discussed in this module, the actual causes of the variation (or at least the most probable causes) can be identified. The following areas are addressed in the analysis:
   - Human factors
     - Communications and information management systems
     - Training
     - Fatigue and scheduling
   - Environmental factors
   - Equipment factors
   - Rules, policies, and procedures
   - Leadership systems and culture[51]
3. Develop and implement an action plan designed to eliminate or minimize the root causes of the variation.

   See the *Patient Safety* section for more information on root cause analyses.

## 6S

Another performance improvement tool is 6S, a Lean tool that is modeled after the 5S process improvement system designed to reduce waste and optimize productivity. 6S has the added pillar of safety (**Figure 5.33**). It is used in the workplace to (1) create and maintain organization and orderliness, (2) use visual cues to achieve more consistent operational results, and (3) reduce defects and make accidents less likely.

## Spaghetti Diagram

A *spaghetti diagram*, also called a layout diagram, is a graphic representation of the flow of traffic or movement (**Figure 5.34**).

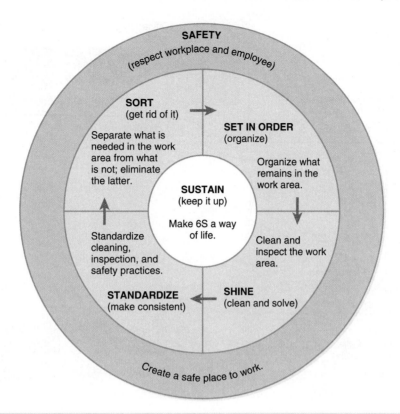

**How to construct**

1.  Sort (Get rid of it): Separate what is needed in the work area from what is not; eliminate the latter.
2.  Set in order (Organize): Organize what remains in the work area.
3.  Shine (Clean and solve): Clean and inspect the work area.
4.  Safety (Respect workplace and employee): Create a safe place to work.
5.  Standardize (Make consistent): Standardize cleaning, inspection, and safety practices.
6.  Sustain (Keep it up): Make 6S a way of life.

**When to use**

- To establish orderly flow, eliminate waste, and organize the workplace
- To standardize the work setting

**Figure 5.33** 6S

Reproduced from U.S. Environmental Protection Agency. Lean & Environment Toolkit: Chapter 5. Accessed January 9, 2022. https://www.epa.gov/lean/lean-environment-toolkit-chapter-5#definition

## Supplier-Input-Process-Output-Customer

A supplier-input-process-output-customer is a tool in process management to identify key drivers of a process (**Figure 5.35**). The healthcare quality professional may hear of a variety of models for process steps pertaining to understanding of data, types of data, and tools (e.g., PDSA; PDCA; assess, plan, implement, evaluate), but the models include similar components. No specific improvement model is endorsed in this section so that the healthcare quality professional can use tools depending on the improvement question and the organizational context. Regardless of the improvement model, the improvement process seeks to accomplish the following:

- Ensure the project is a priority for the organization and is aligned with the strategic plan.
- Ensure leadership support and commitment.
- Assess the priority and feasibility of initiatives based on risks, resources, leadership support, and organizational strategies.
- Clarify the aim, stated in specific measurable terms.
- Present baseline data analysis that illustrates the problem. Use tools and techniques to analyze.
- Demonstrate that the aim is based on the organization's own data and identifies the specific problem to be solved, the program to be enhanced, or the process or system to be redesigned.

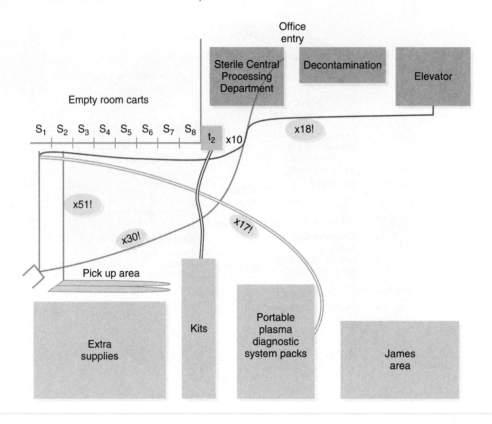

### How to construct
1. Get a layout or blueprint of the area.
2. Pick the subject to follow for the flow.
3. Record every movement until completed.

### When to use
- To demonstrate flow or movement in a process
- To identify excess or wasted travel or movement

**Figure 5.34** Spaghetti Diagram (or Layout Diagram)

| S | I | P | O | C |
|---|---|---|---|---|
| Supplier name | Process input | Process step 1 | Process output | Customer name |
| Supplier name | Process input | Process step 2 | Process output | Customer name |
| Supplier name | Process input | Process step 3 | Process output | Customer name |

### How to construct
1. Identify each element of the SIPOC and list across the top of a page.
2. Under each heading of SIPOC list the suppliers, their inputs, the process, the customers, and the outputs.

### When to use
To identify internal and external customer needs in a process and to use with other Lean tools for process improvement

**Figure 5.35** Supplier Input Process Output Customer

- Select an interprofessional team with content and process experts and all key disciplines as members.
- Map the as-is or current state process and collect data on key aspects of the process.
- Continue to use data and tools to identify bottlenecks, constraints, delays, and other barriers.
- Define measures and collect data. Indicate how a change results in improvement.
- Describe the change to be made.
- Implement the change (small tests of change or pilot tests).
- Study the effects of the change and decide whether to adopt, adapt, or abandon the specific change.
- Map the new to-be or future state process.
- Spread the change throughout the organization in a defined implementation plan (include a communication plan and an education plan).
- Sustain the improvement by monitoring.

Another approach called customer-output-process-input-supplier is also used. It is an outward–in approach to begin with the customer's viewpoint. Both the supplier-input-process-output-customer and customer-output-process-input-supplier approaches are used in Six Sigma, and both complement DMAIC.

## Three-Box Solution

The *three-box solution* is a strategy for leading innovation associated with human-centered design (**Figure 5.36**). The three boxes include the present, the past, and the future.[78]

## Tree Diagram

This tool maps out the full range of paths and tasks in the process that must be accomplished to achieve a goal. A *tree diagram* resembles an organizational chart (**Figure 5.37**). The tree diagram can be presented as an organizational chart or placed on its side.

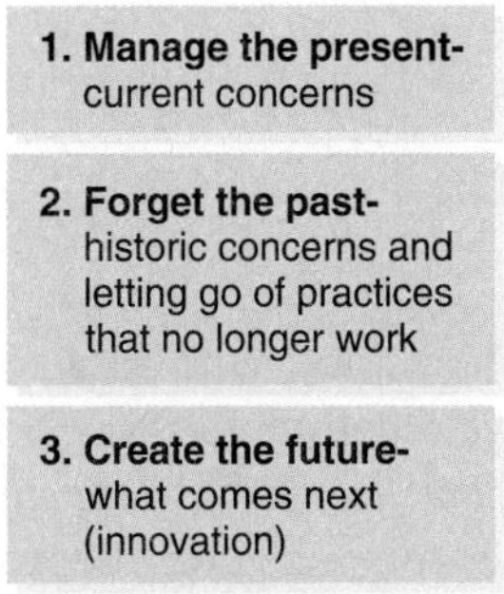

**1. Manage the present-**
current concerns

**2. Forget the past-**
historic concerns and
letting go of practices
that no longer work

**3. Create the future-**
what comes next
(innovation)

**Figure 5.36** Three-Box Solution

Data from Govindarajan V. *The Three Box Solution*. Recorded Books Publisher; 2017.

## Value Stream Mapping

*Value stream mapping* is a map of the process in which only value-added steps for the customer are retained and waste is removed. This Lean tool analyzes a process from a systems perspective and creates a visual depiction of the sequential steps in a process from beginning to end. A value stream map example from an emergency department project follows (**Figure 5.38**).

## Voice of the Customer

*Voice of the customer* is a tool conducted at the start of any new product, process, or service design initiative to understand better the customer's wants and needs (**Figure 5.39**). The voice of the customer can serve as key input for new product definition, quality function deployment, or the setting of detailed design specifications. Four aspects of the voice of the customer are customer needs, a hierarchical structure, priorities, and customer perceptions of performance.[79] The product is a list of needs, wants, and desires of the customer of a process output (e.g., specifications, requirements).

Key points for performance improvement tools are listed in **Box 5.7**.

# Leading Organization Change and Excellence

Change management is a critical component to ensure personal concerns, resistance, and other barriers are identified and addressed for an improvement project or even a simple change to a process. Using change management models and tools will support effective implementation and sustainability. Organizations use teams to work on one or more targeted improvement opportunities. Teams may report up to an established quality operational structure or to a group of individuals with responsibility for the area where the improvement opportunity exists. The composition and size of each team depend on the specific aim of the team. Including the right stakeholders on the team is critical to success.

IHI identified three categories of team membership with impact on team success: (1) clinical leadership representation to bring the authority necessary to test and implement the recommended change and to help overcome issues; (2) technical expertise to ensure relevant understanding of related technical content areas; and (3) day-to-day leadership to include front-line leadership and physician representation to serve as a driving force during the project and the champion

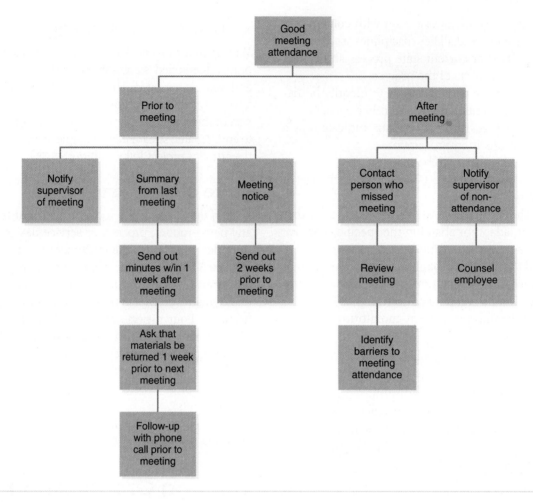

**How to construct**
1. Identify the overall goal that can be broken down into the steps necessary to achieve it.
2. Position the paper you are working on vertically because the diagram usually is long rather than wide; work from left to right.
3. Select the appropriate tree branches (categories/groups) to investigate (an affinity diagram often is helpful to identify the first level of detail, which always is the broadest level); create headers for each of these branches.
4. For each header, ask: What needs to happen to achieve the header and goal statement? Write ideas on cards and place them to the right of the appropriate first-level idea. This level should have a direct cause-and-effect relationship with the previous level.
5. When complete, ask the following questions to each level of detail: Will these lead to the results? Do we really need to do this task to reach the results?

**When to use**
- When it is crucial that a step/task not be overlooked
- When a specific task has become the focus, but it is a complicated task to complete
- When there have been numerous roadblocks to implementation

**Figure 5.37** Tree Diagram

for change during implementation of improvements.[80] In addition, each team selects a project sponsor or champion with executive authority who serves as liaison to other areas of the organization as well as to other members of senior management. The project sponsor checks in periodically on the team's progress and helps remove barriers to progress.

What is a team? A *team* is "a group of people who are interdependent with respect to information, resources, and skills and who seek to combine their efforts to achieve a common goal."[81(p2)] An important structural element for healthcare quality is creating a team-based organization. Because patient care involves multiple professional disciplines, the linchpin for improvement is an employee base with regular communication and contact that allows them to coordinate and problem solve to continuously improve quality of care. The organization must develop an

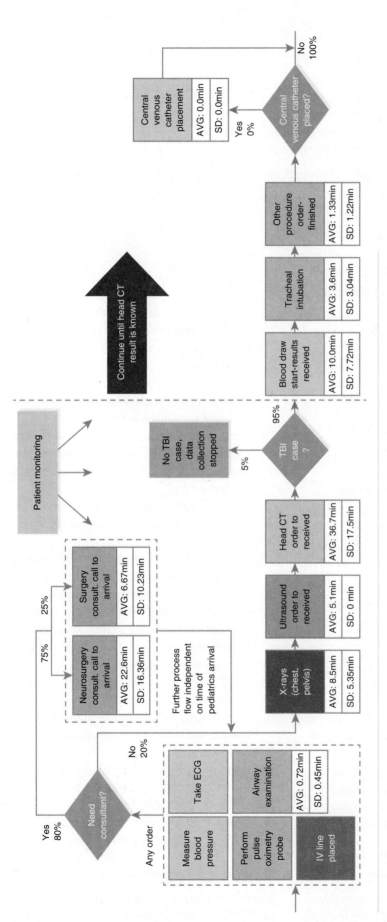

**Figure 5.38** Value Stream Mapping: Emergency Department Processes

**How to construct**

1. Identify the current process (mark steps that are of no value to the customer or required by a regulatory body).
2. Identify the ideal process state.
3. Close the gap between the two states.

**When to use**

To improve flow of the process, reduce waste, and implement Lean functioning

Reproduced from Ajdari A, Boyle L, Kannan N, et al. Examining emergency department treatment processes in severe pediatric traumatic brain injury. *J Healthc Qual.* 2017;39(6):334–344. doi:10.1097/ JHQ.0000000000000052

- What do you like about the current process?
- What do you think needs improvement?
- What would you recommend for improving the current process?
- What could threaten the success of the project?

**How to construct**
1. Identify customers of a process output.
2. Develop a list of questions to ask customers about the process and their needs.
3. Refine the list to use with the process review and improvement.

**When to use**
To improve a process

**Figure 5.39** Voice of the Customer

---

**Box 5.7  Key Points: Performance Improvement Tools**

- Evidence-based tools are used for decision making and process improvement.
- The healthcare quality professional uses tools based on the improvement question and the situational context.
- Regardless of the improvement model, the improvement process seeks to
  - ensure the project is a priority for the organization and is aligned to the strategic plan;
  - clarify the aim, stated in specific measurable terms;
  - select an interprofessional team composed of content and process experts and key disciplines;
  - describe the change to be made and explain what it will look like; and
  - spread the change and sustain the improvements by monitoring (sustain the gains).

---

infrastructure within which the cycle of improvement can operate. One feature of this infrastructure is teams. Teamwork in healthcare is

> a dynamic process involving two or more health professionals with complementary backgrounds and skills, sharing common health goals, and exercising concerted physical and mental effort in assessing, planning, or evaluating patient care. This is accomplished through interdependent collaboration, open communication, and shared decision-making. This in turn generates value-added patient, organizational and staff outcomes.[82(p238)]

Nancarrow and colleagues identified 10 competencies of effective interprofessional teams:

1. Identify a leader who establishes a clear direction and vision for the team, while listening and providing support and supervision to the team members.
2. Incorporate a set of values that clearly provide direction for the team's service provision; these values should be visible and consistently portrayed.
3. Demonstrate a team culture and interdisciplinary atmosphere of trust where contributions are valued and consensus is fostered.
4. Ensure appropriate processes and infrastructures are in place to uphold the vision of the service (for example, referral criteria, communications infrastructure).
5. Provide quality, patient-focused services with documented outcomes; utilize feedback to improve the quality of care.
6. Utilize communication strategies that promote intrateam communication, collaborative decision making, and effective team processes.
7. Provide sufficient team staffing to integrate an appropriate mix of skills, competencies, and personalities to meet the needs of patients and enhance smooth functioning.
8. Facilitate recruitment of staff who demonstrate interdisciplinary competencies including team functioning, collaborative leadership, communication, and sufficient professional knowledge and experience.
9. Promote role interdependence while respecting individual roles and autonomy.
10. Facilitate personal development through appropriate training, rewards, recognition, and opportunities for career development.[83(pp5-11)]

## Types of Teams

There are many types of teams; they can be classified along five major dimensions: purpose or mission, time, degree of autonomy, authority structure, and physical presence.[84] Teams are of great importance—there are many types of formal and informal teams (**Figure 5.40**).

- *Temporary project*. Teams working on a temporary project have a special focus on improvement, problem solving, or product development. There are often both core and resource members. Core members participate throughout the project and have complementary skills needed for the desired work output. Resource members may be critical only for specific phases of the project and may move in and out of the team. Other ongoing or functional work teams are usually permanent or may be long-standing.
- *Natural work*. Teams doing natural work involve the people in each work setting who share responsibility for a process, workflow, or type of work. Members are those who work together each day to complete the task. These teams can be cross-functional, as with an operating room team, or intact, such as a team of nurses in a unit. Autonomy varies, but there typically is a leader. These teams can be temporary (e.g., brought together to solve a single problem) or permanent (e.g., continuous improvement teams).

- *Self-directed*. A self-directed work team is a type of natural work team that shares management responsibilities, such as scheduling work, managing budgets, evaluating performance, and hiring new team members.
- *Process management*. The process management team focuses on sharing responsibility for monitoring and controlling a work process, such as new product development. Members may rotate on and off the team based on their contributions (subject matter expertise).
- *Virtual teams*. These teams typically use technology-supported communications rather than face-to-face interactions to accomplish their tasks. They may cross boundaries, such as time zones, geography, and organizational units. Virtual teams can be either project teams or ongoing teams.

## Steering Committees

Steering committees (often known as a quality council) are permanent quality improvement teams consisting of cross-functional members, and in patient-centered care environments, they include patients and family members. These committees are self-managed teams that provide direction and focus by identifying and prioritizing improvement opportunities in

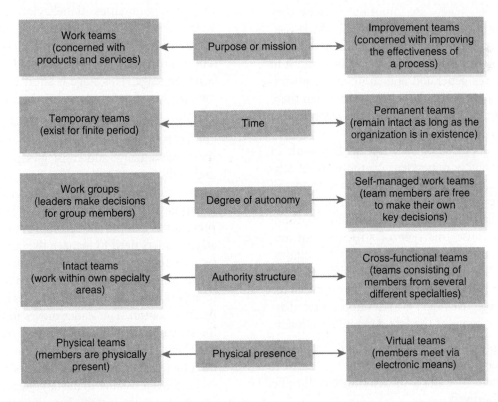

**Figure 5.40** Classification of Teams

the organization. The role of the steering committee or quality council is to sustain, facilitate, and expand the performance and process improvement initiatives based on the strategic plan. It comprises top leaders in the organization, including medical staff. The main responsibilities of the quality council include

- lending legitimacy to the quality efforts;
- maintaining organization focus on the identified goals and priorities;
- fostering teamwork for improvement;
- providing necessary resources (e.g., human, financial, educational); and
- formulating organizational policies regarding quality and safety priorities, participation, annual self-assessments, and reward and recognition systems.

## When to Use Teams

Three aspects of the required task are examined before deciding whether to use a team: task complexity, task interdependence, and task objectives.[85] Tasks are complex when they involve large amounts of information, they are performed under conditions of high uncertainty, they contain many subtasks that require people with specialized skills and knowledge, and there are no standardized procedures for completing the tasks. Teams are important because they bring larger numbers of specialized individuals (i.e., subject matter experts) to carry the burden and offer greater diverse inputs that are more likely to result in more alternatives generated and more creative solutions. Creativity is particularly important when there are no standardized procedures and the environment is uncertain.

Task interdependence means that the work of one person is highly dependent on the work of others. Patient care typically involves a multitude of disciplines that must coordinate their work, and this requires intense communication. Teams therefore are appropriate because this type of structure can foster communication between the various disciplines. Finally, teams are appropriate to use when the task objectives are clear and time bound. One approach for making task objectives clear is to develop a team charter. The charter contains the following information:

- A description of the process, why it needs improvement, and who is affected
- Development of criteria to demonstrate that the process improved
- A timeline for meetings
- Resources available

- The structure of leadership (e.g., self-managed, leader-directed)
- Expected communication of progress and results[86]

## How Teams Develop or Grow

Teams develop, mature, and change over time. Tuckman described four stages of development in one popular model with somewhat predictable stages.[87] This classic framework continues to be used to this day.

*Stage 1: Forming.* During the first stage, the members try to get to know each other, agree on the goal or vision, and delegate tasks. They cautiously explore boundaries to determine acceptable group behavior. Discussions focus on how to accomplish the tasks and the information and resources needed, and the team accomplishes little at this stage. This is a period of testing to find out what kind of behavior is appropriate. Members tend to defer to the leader or dominant member for guidance. In this stage, team leaders need to be directive and provide role clarification. Members get to know each other, agree on goals, and delegate tasks; members may feel anxiety, excitement, and uncertainty, and they may test boundaries of behavior. The team leader needs to be directive, with high-task relationships, and provide role clarification. The team depends on the leader during this learning stage. This stage is short if the tasks are clearly defined and easily achievable.

*Stage 2: Storming.* This second stage is where conflict typically arises. Members try to express their individuality and resist group pressures and influence. There often are emotional responses to group demands, especially if the group is under pressure to achieve results. To prevent the group from becoming stuck at this stage, leaders need to manage the conflict, not by suppressing it but by using it to energize the team. Conflict and tension often arise, and members assert their individual roles and compete for control. The leader moves to a coaching style of leadership. At this stage, reality sets in. There is the realization that the task may be difficult, they notice their lack of progress, and there is resistance to the task. Resources are applied to the task rather than education about the problem. People are willing to suggest tasks, and the leader then delegates the tasks.

People do not take responsibility for problems, yet the team is building cohesion. This is likely the most difficult stage. Arguing, defensiveness, disunity, and tension are often evident.

*Stage 3. Norming.* In this stage, members develop close ties and a strong identity with the team. There is a shift from *I* to *we* and a willingness to accept the views of others. Team members develop feelings of mutual respect, harmony, and trust. Group standards and members' roles emerge. Leaders need to challenge the team members to continue to grow and guard against too much conformity to group norms. The team develops close ties and a strong identity; members develop harmony by avoiding conflict. Tentative constructive criticism is allowed. A supporting leadership style evolves. Concern moves from silos to the interprofessional group. Members volunteer evidence-based solutions instead of just providing vague suggestions. There is an emerging leadership or ownership of functional roles by the members. There is acceptance of team rules, norms, and roles and finally optimism that things work out. More harmony, cohesion, and discussion of team dynamics occur.

*Stage 4. Performing.* In the fourth stage, the team works harmoniously toward a common goal and is very productive. The team develops a functional but flexible structure, and roles are interrelated. Interpersonal conflicts are resolved, and the group is highly task oriented. In this stage, the leader needs to develop mechanisms for sharing leadership responsibilities. The team works harmoniously and gains insight into the team's process. Improvement of the team's process and team identification begins to predominate. The team is task oriented and accomplishes its work. Goal orientation is now optimized, and task competency is high. High morale, support, and appreciation come from team members. Roles diminish, and participation by all is encouraged. The team may begin to take on additional responsibilities and is functioning at an optimal level.

Not all teams progress through these four stages, and if they do, they move back and forth through the stages as new issues are identified. Nevertheless, the stages point to important developmental issues having implications for team leaders, facilitators, and coaches. Lack of effectiveness often results from leadership and facilitation problems and a lack of clear goals and expectations. Teamwork components of cohesiveness, communication, role clarity, and goal clarity from *The Team Handbook* are integrated into these specific roles found in stages in **Table 5.11**.[88]

## Characteristics of Effective Teams

It is widely known that teams often fail to produce the results for which they were brought together. What makes a team successful? Abundant research and practice demonstrate the following important predictors of team success:

- Competent members with technical, problem-solving, interpersonal, and organizational skills
- Commitment to clear, common goals
- Standards of excellence
- Contributions from every member
- Collaborative environment (culture to support teamwork)
- Leadership support
- Nonhierarchical structure
- External support and recognition[89-93]

Characteristics of effective and ineffective teams are further described in **Table 5.12**. Four key traits can predict a team's success: (1) cohesiveness, (2) communication, (3) clear roles, and (4) clear goals.[88]

Cohesiveness is the social glue that binds the team members together as a unit. Cohesiveness can be increased by the establishment of ground rules, or norms, addressing how meetings are run, how team members interact, and what kind of behavior is acceptable. Each member is expected to respect these rules, which usually prevents misunderstandings and disagreements. Balanced participation is encouraged to strengthen the team's cohesion. Because every team member has a stake in the achievements, everyone participates in discussions and decisions, shares the commitment to the project's success, and contributes their talents. The use of brainstorming or a nominal group technique to obtain input from all team members during discussions is one method to encourage members to bond. When a team is cohesive, members are attracted to the team; find membership in the team to be a personally meaningful experience; enjoy the company of the other team members; support, nurture, and care for each other; feel free to share ideas and suggest ways to improve team function; feel they are using their

**Table 5.11** Team Roles

| | |
|---|---|
| Sponsor | Sponsors are the formal leaders and prime movers of the project. They align resources and monitor progress. Sponsors hold others accountable to get on with change. The sponsor inspires the team members to say, "I believe in this project." Project tasks may require sponsors at multiple levels to obtain adequate resources and buy-in from the entire project team. |
| Champion | Champions are the respected opinion leaders who provide credibility to the project and are integral to the social structure. The champions are respected clinicians or staff with influence through clinical reputation or leadership qualities. Their experience provides credibility for the project team and task. They support the change and work for its implementation by speaking favorably about it and sharing their first-hand knowledge or experience. |
| Leader | Leaders guide the team to achieve successful outcomes and attain the established aims or goals. They provide direction and support. The team leader knows meeting procedures and has effective communication and people skills. |
| Timekeeper | Monitors meeting agendas, ensures the team is aware of the time allotted for each agenda item, and reminds the team when they go over the allotted time. |
| Process Owner | The process owner is the leader among frontline staff directly involved in the process. This is the team member who is responsible and accountable for sustaining improvements during and after implementation. Ideally, the process owner should be someone with authority over frontline staff directly involved in the process evaluation. |
| Facilitator | Although facilitators (change agents or coaches) have no formal authority over other team members, they are instrumental in implementing the change through planning, helping, and facilitating. The facilitator is not vested in the project but is skilled in problem solving and adult learning and has excellent communication and people skills. As change agents, they are the technical experts on the team; they influence progress by gathering measurable data and information. They listen to the concerns of other team members and help remove barriers. They support the sponsors by advancing the team's work to goal achievement. They promote effective group dynamics and are concerned with how decisions are made. They may also serve as coaches or consultants. They keep the team on track. They provide expertise on using tools. Coaches focus on helping the team to learn rather than teaching them. The facilitator needs to have a clear perception of the facts and information and the ability to determine what is relevant. That ability includes an understanding of systems, dynamics, relationships between system components, and psychology. The facilitator, change agent, or coach needs to understand when and how emotions or desires distort one's perception. |
| Member | Actual representative on the team. Although project team composition varies, in most cases the project team includes the frontline staff (e.g., nurses, physicians, clerks, ancillary services staff) and area supervisors directly affected by the project task. To identify these personnel, consider all relevant stakeholders to the process. The ideal team size is 8–12 people. Unless necessary, team size should not exceed 15 people. They can collect data and information related to the process of focus. For the stakeholders not represented, develop a communication mechanism (team minutes, session report). Designate one or more people to disseminate this information regularly. Chosen team members must be able to commit to attend team meetings and meet their responsibilities. |
| Scribe | This role may be assigned to one person or rotated between members. The role includes documenting minutes of meetings and other recordkeeping activities. |

unique skills for the benefit of the team; have a strong *we* feeling; and routinely develop creative solutions to problems.

Communication is the next key component to successful teams. Communication involves a full range of topics, including decision making and problem solving. Effective communication becomes easier once the team develops a certain level of cohesiveness. Communication is key because further team development and effective functioning cannot occur without team communication. When a team is communicating effectively, team members

- freely say what they feel and think;
- are always direct, truthful, respectful, and positive;

**Table 5.12** **Team Characteristics**

| Effective Teams | Ineffective Teams |
|---|---|
| ▪ Mutual agreement and identification with respect to the team goal<br>▪ Have open communication between members<br>▪ Have mutual trust and support<br>▪ Management of human differences<br>▪ Selective use of the team<br>▪ Appropriate member skills<br>▪ Leadership<br>▪ Values and goals of the members interpreted as needs and values of the team<br>▪ Team believes it can accomplish the impossible<br>▪ Understand the value of constructive team cohesiveness and how to use it<br>▪ Mutual influence between members and the leader<br>▪ Exhibit clear goals, purposes, discussions, and decisions<br>▪ Agree on the goal<br>▪ Have formally defined roles<br>▪ Revise plan as needed<br>▪ Use tool to map the process and project steps<br>▪ Effectively use talents of members<br>▪ Balance participation of all members<br>▪ Discuss issues openly<br>▪ Clarify ideas or issues<br>▪ Use consensus-based decision making<br>▪ Use data for problem solving<br>▪ Apply resources and training throughout the project | ▪ Do not distinguish between facts, opinions, and feelings<br>▪ Do not separate idea generation from idea evaluation<br>▪ Prematurely close discussion before all alternatives identified<br>▪ Dominated by aggressive members<br>▪ Fail to assign specific responsibilities<br>▪ Do not review minutes, tasks, or due dates<br>▪ Work on problems that are outside the scope of the team<br>▪ Exhibit uncertainty about the team's direction<br>▪ Launch many improvement projects without clear objectives<br>▪ Fail to apply discussion skills<br>▪ Hide a secret agenda<br>▪ Rely on one person to manage discussion without sharing responsibility<br>▪ Discuss the project outside the meeting rather than bringing issues to the team<br>▪ Repeat points of discussion<br>▪ Concede to opinions rather than fact-based data<br>▪ Use majority rule rather than consensus in disagreements<br>▪ Use decision by default, with silence assumed as consent<br>▪ Avoid certain topics<br>▪ Do not acknowledge ground rules<br>▪ Have recurring differences on acceptable behavior<br>▪ Have conflicting expectations<br>▪ Do not deal with clues or shifts in the team mood<br>▪ Have members who make remarks that discount someone's behavior or contribution |

- openly discuss all decisions before they are made;
- handle conflict in a calm, caring, and healing manner;
- openly explore options to solve problems when they arise; and
- do not gossip about each other, have unknown alliances, or hidden agendas.

Effective, clear communication depends on how well information is passed between team members. Ideally, team members speak clearly, directly, and succinctly. They ask questions in an inviting way. Members listen actively and avoid interrupting when others are speaking. The team encourages all members to use the skills and practices that make discussions and meetings more effective. Team members initiate discussions, seek information and opinions, suggest procedures, elaborate on ideas, complete assignments on time, and summarize.

Team leaders and facilitators function as gatekeepers during communication by managing member participation, keeping discussion focused, and resolving differences creatively. Considering the stage of team development, such as storming, leaders and facilitators may need to ease tension and work through difficulties. Communication also includes well-defined decision-making procedures.

The role of champion can benefit engagement in a quality or safety effort. The ideal champion is perceived as credible and able to influence others to adopt or implement a new process as part of the patient safety or quality effort. Physician champions are especially effective in improving physician engagement in quality and safety efforts. Champions are also critical for successful teams in healthcare settings. They can contribute to the success of projects, innovations, and other organizational change initiatives.

A team is always aware of the different ways it reaches consensus. The team discusses how decisions are made, explores important issues by polling, tests for agreement, and uses data as the basis for decisions. Occasionally, the team may want to designate a member to observe team interactions and give feedback on how decisions are made so the group can talk about any changes it needs to make. Team members are also sensitive to nonverbal communication. This includes seeing, hearing, and feeling the team dynamics.

Role clarity is the next area to facilitate team success. The roles are common among teams, but they may differ slightly depending on the type of team that is convened. The role of team member supersedes individual professional roles. Although professional roles brought to the team give the team its potential strength, it is also important for team development that individuals feel equally valued. In addition, team members know who is doing what and what other team members expect of them. When a team achieves role clarity, members feel that accomplishments of the team are placed above those of individuals and understand the roles and responsibilities of all other team members, and there is a clear understanding of what other team members expect of them. A team facilitator is clearly identified. Facilitation requires skills that are both art and science. A skilled facilitator guides group process in an unbiased manner ensuring that the meeting agenda is carried out and decisions are responsibly reached with independent contributions from all team members.

The final component of team development to become a fully functioning and high-performing team is clearly defining team goals and the means used to reach these goals. When a team achieves goal clarity, team members agree on what the real work of the team is, clearly understand the goals, agree on how to reach the goals, and agree on clear criteria for evaluating the outcomes of the team. Teams operate most efficiently when they tap everyone's talents and when all members understand their duties and know who is responsible for what issues and tasks. Goal clarity begins with a charter.

Successful teams are one of the most important aspects of effective organizational functioning and quality, safety, and performance improvement. Two special team types have patient safety as their focus but include essential elements of teams that increase their ability to address patient safety and error reduction. The first is Team Strategies and Tools to Enhance Performance and Patient Safety (TeamSTEPPS), a teamwork system designed for healthcare professionals (**Figure 5.41**). This is an evidence-based teamwork system designed to improve communication and teamwork skills. Team members learn four primary teamwork skills: leadership, communication, situation monitoring, and mutual support. Three types of team outcomes are desired: performance, knowledge, and attitudes. The TeamSTEPPS tools, barriers, and outcomes are listed in **Figure 5.42** as a summary of the training materials to support positive team behaviors.

The TeamSTEPPS model is based on lessons learned, change models, the literature of quality and patient safety, and culture change. Phase 1 assesses an organization's readiness for undertaking the initiative.

Phase 2 includes planning, training, and implementation; options in this phase include tools and strategies. Phase 3 sustains and spreads improvements in teamwork performance, clinical processes, and outcomes.[94,95]

The second special type of team is crew resource management. A specific crew resource management training program based on airline safety was developed for healthcare. Although the team is focused on patient safety, the effectiveness of team functioning is a first critical component.[96] Additional elements include a focus on the patient safety mindset and high-reliability functioning. The team learns skills in decision making under stressful situations through continued practice, simulation, and use of checklists to embed teamwork behaviors into daily work and provide opportunities to practice the desired behaviors.

For those organizations employing Six Sigma or Lean methods, a *workout* is a fast-track change acceleration process developed originally at General Electric. The workout is conducted by a group of team members in a brief time (hours or days).[97]

## Evaluating Team Performance

Evaluating team performance is important to the overall effectiveness of an organization's operations and improvement strategy. Three key actions determine the success of any team:

1. Developing shared goals and methods to accomplish outcomes
2. Developing methods and skills to communicate and make decisions across systems and organizations
3. Engaging leadership that balances getting input and making decisions, so work moves ahead

Team performance also requires formal evaluation. In general, evaluation of a team includes three criteria:

1. *Productivity or results.* This is the extent to which the goals were met. Did the team accomplish what it set out to do and within the defined time frame?
2. *Satisfaction of team members.* It is important that team members can work together in the future. To the extent that members are satisfied with the team, they are more likely to work well together in the future.
3. *Individual growth.* This is the extent to which individual members developed professionally by serving as team members.

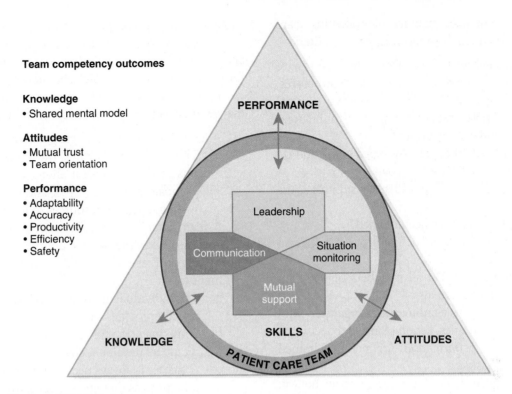

**Figure 5.41** The TeamSTEPPS Model

Reproduced from Agency for Healthcare Research and Quality. *Pocket Guide: TeamSTEPPS 2.0: Team Stratergies & Tools to Enhance Performance and Patient Safety*. Published 2013. Accessed December 7, 2021. https://www.ahrq.gov/sites/default/files/wysiwyg/professionals/education/curriculum-tools/teamstepps/instructor/essentials/pocketguide.pdf

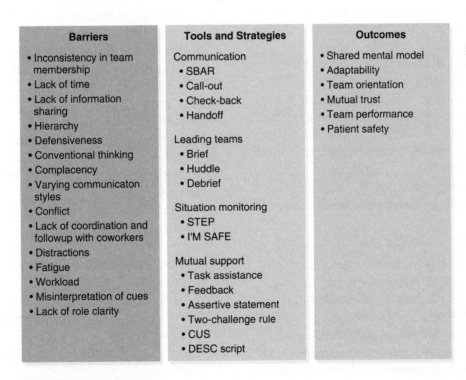

**Figure 5.42** The TeamSTEPPS Tools, Barriers, Outcomes

Reproduced from Agency for Healthcare Research and Quality, U.S. Department of Health & Human Services. *Pocket Guide: TeamSTEPPS 2.0: Team Stratergies & Tools to Enhance Performance and Patient Safety*. Rockville, MD: AHRQ; 2012. Accessed January 10, 2022. https://www.ahrq.gov/teamstepps/instructor/essentials/index.html

A more formalized manner of evaluating team performance includes the following process criteria:

- *Organizational alignment.* Does the team have statements of mission, vision, values, structures, roles, and goals? Does the team have a charter? Are the purpose and goals important to the organization's strategic priorities?
- *Goal clarity.* Are there clearly stated goals, and do actions exist to achieve the goals?
- *Leadership.* Is there clear leadership support of the team?
- *Roles.* Have team roles been defined?
- *Norms.* Does the team define ground rules and abide by them?
- *Team participation.* Do all members of the team participate and share tasks?
- *Team meetings.* Are team meetings organized with agendas, time frames, action plans, and decisions?
- *Competency to perform tasks.* Are members trained to work on tasks?
- *Communication.* Is communication open, honest, and constructive?
- *Atmosphere.* Is the atmosphere warm, accepting, and supportive for all team members?
- *Decision making.* Does the team achieve consensus on decisions and look at multiple alternatives before reaching a decision?
- *Problem solving.* Is the team able to validate problem identification before moving to a solution by using sound data and tools?
- *Conflicts.* Does the team have a process for constructively managing interpersonal conflict?
- *Performance management.* Does the team manage its performance, or must management intervene?
- *Work tools and training.* Has the team been trained on tools and data management to function effectively?
- *Boundary management.* Has the team developed relationships with other teams, stakeholders, and customers?

Healthcare quality professionals play a vital role in leading or facilitating performance improvement projects. Different types of improvement projects may be chartered. They vary in breadth, scope, and duration. There are also different names that may be assigned to projects, but they all can be categorized under the umbrella of quality and safety. For example, there may be rapid process improvement teams, Green Belt project teams, Black Belt project teams, Lean projects, Six Sigma projects, and redesign projects. They are similar in their basic approach. The types of tools and level of statistical analysis may vary by type of team.

Depending on the complexity of the project, a simple action plan may be sufficient, or the use of a Gantt chart or program evaluation review technique chart for project management might be more helpful.

A basic approach and actual steps in a performance improvement project include the following:

1. Align priorities and strategic goals and objectives.
   a. This first step ensures the leaders support this project because it aligns with the strategic goals and PI priorities, and the leaders are willing to devote resources to it.
2. A team charter is usually written at this point and describes the scope, boundaries, expected results, and resources used by a process improvement team.
   a. The individual or group who formed the team usually provides the charter.
   b. Sometimes the process owner or the team members develop a charter.
   c. A charter is always needed for a team working on a process that crosses departmental lines.
   d. A charter may not be necessary for a team that is improving a process found solely within a work center or office space.
3. Basic team functions are identified, including
   a. members of the team,
   b. roles within the team,
   c. meeting schedule,
   d. project timeline,
   e. resources available and needed to complete the improvement project, and
   f. expected communication of progress and results.
4. A clearly defined aim must be identified for the team to work toward a common goal.
5. Analysis of baseline performance and problem identification is needed to determine the level of improvement.
6. A map of the process (current and ideal) is developed.
7. A description of the process explains why it needs improvement and who is affected.
8. Criteria must be developed to demonstrate that the process is improved.
9. A measurement of success is established; this includes the numerator and denominator for a percentage, rate, or other weighted measure.
10. Changes to be tested and implemented must be determined.
    a. Tests of change supported by data collection, analysis, and reporting.
    b. Control or methods to sustain the change.
11. Results or outcomes of the project are noted.

12. The project and results are reported to leaders, the organization, or others.
13. Evaluation tools for the team process are selected.

**Box 5.8** lists the key points of leading change and organizational excellence through teamwork.

---

**Box 5.8  Key Points: Leading Change and Organizational Excellence Through Teamwork**

- Teamwork is a dynamic process involving two or more health professionals with complementary backgrounds and skills, common goals, and concerted physical and mental effort in assessing, planning, or evaluating patient care.
- Four stages of team development include forming, storming, norming, and performing.
- High-functioning teams improve clinical and financial outcomes.

---

# Aligning Rewards to Support Quality

Reward systems are critical to the success of quality, safety, and performance improvement initiatives. In fact, "The most damaging alignment problem to which many total quality failures have been attributed is the lack of alignment between expectations that arise from total quality change processes and reward systems."[98(p362)] Rewards are important because they can motivate people. Motivating people to provide excellent customer service is a top priority for most organizations. Therefore, before discussing rewards, it is important to understand motivation.

## Basics of Motivation

*Work motivation* is "the psychological forces that determine the direction of a person's behavior in an organization, a person's level of effort, and a person's level of persistence."[99(p181)] There are many theories of motivation, and each has different but complementary implications for actions that can be taken to motivate employees. Therefore, a basic understanding of all the major theories is important. One way to view all theories is through the motivation equation.[100] Each theory stresses different parts of the equation (**Figure 5.43**).

### Need Theories

Need theories center on what employees are motivated to obtain from work (outcomes). These theories include Maslow's hierarchy of needs, McClelland's need theory, and Hertzberg's two-factor theory.

Maslow's need theory was first published in 1943. Maslow, a psychologist, believed that human needs could be arranged in a hierarchy from the most basic to higher order needs, as follows:

- Physiological or survival needs (basic survival needs such as food and water)
- Safety or security needs (protection from harm or physical deprivation)
- Belongingness or social needs (the need for interaction with others, companionship, belonging, and friendship)

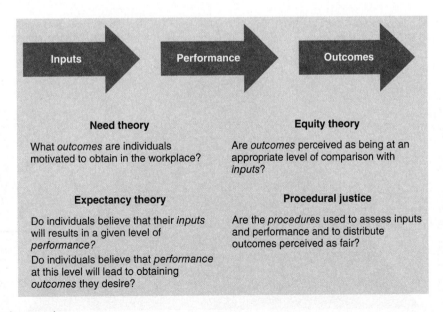

**Figure 5.43** Motivation Equation

Reproduced from George JM, Jones GR. *Understanding and Managing Organizational Behavior.* Upper Saddle River, NJ: Prentice Hall; 2002.

- Esteem or status needs (needs for recognition and appreciation)
- Self-actualization needs (the need for self-fulfillment or to reach one's highest potential)[100]

Maslow believed that basic needs had to be met before higher order needs. For example, in a workplace, basic survival needs are met (e.g., working in a safe environment) before employees focus on esteem needs. In addition, Maslow maintained that only unsatisfied needs served to motivate people; people want what they do not have.

McClelland proposed a concept like Maslow's, narrowing the number of needs to three types: achievement, power, and affiliation.[101]

Finally, Herzberg's two-factor theory classified the elements of motivation into two categories: motivators and hygiene factors.[102] Motivators are the elements of a job that increase job satisfaction, including challenging work, achievement, recognition, growth, and advancement. Hygiene factors, on the other hand, do not contribute to motivation, but their absence leads to dissatisfaction. Hygiene factors include company policy and administrative issues such as supervision, working conditions, interpersonal relations, safety, salaries, morale, and productivity. Herzberg expanded on Maslow's theory, making a distinction between factors that motivate and factors that maintain motivation.

At least two managerial implications for motivation are clear from need theories:

1. There are diverse needs, and these differ between employees.

2. If employees are not motivated, managers seek to determine the needs of employees and which are satisfied or dissatisfied.

The relationship between Maslow's hierarchy of needs and employee engagement is shown in **Figure 5.44**.

## Expectancy Theory

Expectancy theory is concerned with how people decide which behaviors to engage in and the effort they give to that behavior. This theory focuses on the person's perception of effort-to-performance and performance-to-outcome links. A person asks, "If I work hard (effort), will I be able to perform?" Motivation is improved by strengthening that link. Managers want to be certain that employees believe that if they work hard, they will achieve high performance. Thus, providing training and education so that they have the appropriate skills to perform the work would improve motivation. In accordance with this theory, managers do the following:

- Be certain employees possess the necessary skills to perform well.
- Coach employees to believe that if they work hard, they will be successful.
- Know what outcomes employees perceive as important (as detailed by needs theory).
- Establish clear policies about what levels of performance are rewarded (result in outcomes) and which levels are not.

Individuals also ask themselves, "If I perform at a high level, will there be an outcome, and is it

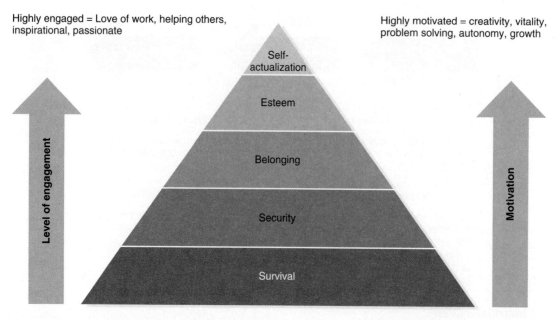

**Figure 5.44** Maslow's Hierarchy of Needs Applied to Employee Engagement

something I care about?" To strengthen this performance-outcome link, managers want employees to believe that if they perform at a high level, there is an outcome that they desire. Managers can strengthen this link by having valid performance appraisal systems that capture quality and safety performance and by having systems in place to reward such performance. For example, when an employee reports an adverse event, there should be an immediate outcome that is positive in the eyes of that employee.

## Equity Theory

Equity theory centers on the input and outcomes part of the motivation equation. The overall idea is that employees are motivated when there is fairness in the workplace. This theory contends that employees determine fairness by looking at the ratio of their inputs (work effort) to their outcomes (e.g., rewards, benefits). For example, Employee A may be motivated if they receive a financial bonus that they perceive to be equitable given their effort on the PI project. According to this theory, however, employees also compare the ratio of their inputs to outcomes with others' inputs and outcomes. Therefore, if Employee B in the same department is awarded a larger financial bonus for the same amount of effort, Employee A's motivation would drop. Ways for managers to motivate employees include the following:

- Acknowledge different performance levels with various levels of rewards.
- Employ just culture principles and practices.
- Periodically check employees' perceptions about their own input and outcomes as well as those of others (through annual employee engagement surveys).
- Know what outcomes are desirable and tie those to performance in a timely manner.

## Procedural Justice

*Procedural justice* is a theory of motivation that focuses on fairness with respect to processes or procedures used to allocate outcomes. Research demonstrates that people are more likely to see outcome allocations as fair when the following conditions exist:

- Input from employees is sought and considered when decisions are made.
- There is an opportunity for performance errors to be corrected.
- Rules and policies for allocation of outcomes are applied consistently.
- Decisions are made in an unbiased manner.

## What Employees Say

There is research support for these various motivation theories. In the past 25 years, the Gallup Organization undertook two extremely large studies. The first asked, "What do the most talented employees need from their workplace?" For this part of the research, Gallup interviewed more than one million people who were employed across a broad range of companies, industries, and countries. This study's most powerful conclusion is that the retention and performance of an employee is determined "by his relationship with his immediate supervisor."[103] So, what makes a good supervisor? Gallup's data indicate that there are 12 factors critical to the retention and performance of employees:

1. Do I know what is expected of me at work?
2. Do I have the materials and equipment I need to do my work correctly?
3. Do I have the opportunity at work to do what I do best every day?
4. In the last seven days, did I receive recognition or praise for doing good work?
5. Does my supervisor, or someone at work, seem to care about me as a person?
6. Is there someone at work who encourages my development?
7. Do my opinions seem to count at work?
8. Does the mission or purpose of my work organization make me feel my job is important?
9. Are my coworkers committed to doing high-quality work?
10. Do I have a best friend at work?
11. In the last 6 months, has someone at work talked to me about my progress?
12. This past year, have I had opportunities at work to learn and grow?

More recently, Harter and Adkins discussed the fact that employees want more from their managers. They found that

1. managers account for up to 70% of variance in engagement;
2. consistent communication is connected to higher engagement; and
3. managers must help employees develop their strengths.[104]

These factors clearly are consistent with the theories of motivation discussed previously.

## Setting Up a Reward System

Given the role rewards play in employee motivation, setting up an effective reward system is important. Seven steps are fundamental to a reward system:

1. Determine priorities and values; rewarded behaviors are prioritized.
2. Identify the criteria or milestones.
3. Establish a budget for recognition.
4. Determine who is accountable for managing the recognition.
5. Develop specific procedures and features of the rewards and recognition.
6. Obtain feedback from employees on desired rewards and recognition.
7. Modify the program based on feedback.[105]

The most crucial step is to reward the desired behavior.[106]

## Sharing Successes of Teams, Projects, and Initiatives

Sharing organization success stories internally and externally is important. As described earlier, it motivates employees and serves as both reward and recognition to them. The value is demonstrated to the employees in increasing knowledge transfer, learning from experience, sharing best practices, and stimulating innovation within the organization. Value is next demonstrated to the customer in showcasing successful processes and outcomes to the people served. Communicating successes also demonstrates accountability and transparency to the community and public served. There may be other stakeholders for whom communicating success is also important.

Externally, sharing of lessons learned with other organizations, professional groups, online communities, and the public might be performed in different ways. Common audiences are professional conferences, committees, and professional organizations. The report format often includes an abstract, title, objectives, outline, content (may include data analysis, implementation, and process maps), results, and references. Additionally, sometimes the A3 format is used (seven or nine blocks) to address an improvement process (Figure 5.15). This format is usually standardized from Lean or Six Sigma projects. This usually includes the background; current condition; goal; analysis; proposal/recommendation/countermeasure; plan; and follow-up.[73]

The form in which communication takes place can also include face-to-face presentations, webinars, posters and storyboards, publications, and social networking tools. Publications may be local newsletters, peer-reviewed journals, or online forums including blogs. It is necessary to follow specific submission guidelines for a poster, abstract, or article. The publishing organization defines poster measurements, labeling design, and key elements for text and graphics. Abstract criteria focus on topics of interest, maximum and minimum word limits, and categories to include. Journal articles must conform to author guidelines and use a specific writing style. In preparing for any of these external communication methods, it is essential to have samples of the work product reviewed to increase the chances of acceptance and to ensure no protected health information is used.

## Recognition and Quality Awards

Quality professionals are often instrumental in completing applications for external quality awards as well as addressing internal quality awards. One framework used to understand performance improvement in complex systems is the Baldrige National Health Care Criteria for Performance Excellence Framework. The Baldrige Award was created in 1987, named for former U.S. Secretary of Commerce Malcolm Baldrige in tribute to his managerial ability (for more information, see the *Quality Leadership and Integration* section). The award is given to organizations demonstrating a commitment to quality excellence. This model displays the principles of performance improvement and shows the relationships between the structural, process, and outcome factors. Other quality and recognition awards are shown in **Table 5.13**.

There are other external awards not necessarily called quality awards but acknowledge high-performing organizations that demonstrate evidence of that performance per defined criteria. Usually through a rigorous evaluation process, the organization is selected for the award, prize, or designation.

Steps in evaluating readiness to apply for external quality awards include the following:

1. Demonstrate ownership and commitment to the cultural transformation for performance excellence.
2. Make the pursuit of quality an organizational commitment for the sake of intrinsic improvement, not just to win an award.
3. Create the organization cultural transformation by upholding the standards in daily practice.
4. Identify the specific quality reward or recognition program and requirements.
5. Review the standards and criteria.
6. Determine eligibility.

**Table 5.13 Common Quality and Recognition Awards**

| Name | Sponsor | Eligible Organizations | Key Focus |
|---|---|---|---|
| Beacon Award for Excellence | American Association of Critical-Care Nurses | Any unit where the patient receives principal nursing care after admission can apply | Sets the standard for excellence in patient care environments by collecting and utilizing evidence-based information to improve patient outcomes, and patient and staff satisfaction |
| John M. Eisenberg Patient Safety and Quality Award | National Quality Forum and The Joint Commission | Eisenberg award recognizes major achievements by individuals and organizations to improve patient safety and healthcare quality. | Best examples of individual, local, and national efforts to improve patient safety and healthcare quality |
| Deming Prize | Union of Japanese Scientists and Engineers | Any organization under certain conditions, be it public or private, large or small, domestic or overseas, or part of or entire organization | Recognizing businesses worldwide for excellence in applying the principles of Total Quality Management |
| Nicholas E. Davies Award of Excellence | Healthcare Information and Management Systems Society | Hospitals and specialty hospitals, integrated care delivery networks, academic medical centers<br>Independent ambulatory practices<br>Community health organizations<br>Enterprise clinics<br>State or local public health organizations | Showcases healthcare organizations that demonstrate globally innovative, thoughtful applications of information and technology to drive and redefine evidence-based best practices so that others can learn, adapt, and improve population health and patient outcomes |
| Healthcare Quality Recognition Awards | National Association for Healthcare Quality | Individual professional recognition, state recognition | Healthcare quality and safety |
| Malcolm Baldrige National Quality Award | National Institute of Standards and Technology | U.S. organizations in the business, healthcare, education, and nonprofit sectors for performance excellence | Performance excellence focusing on performance in five key areas: product and process outcomes; customer outcomes; workforce outcomes; leadership and governance outcomes; and financial and market outcomes |
| Leapfrog Top Hospital | The Leapfrog Group | Hospitals | Better systems in place to prevent medication errors, higher quality on maternity care and high-risk procedures, and lower readmission rates |

*(continues)*

**Table 5.13** Common Quality and Recognition Awards *(continued)*

| Name | Sponsor | Eligible Organizations | Key Focus |
|---|---|---|---|
| Magnet Recognition Program Pathway to Excellence | American Nurses Credentialing Center | All entities (hospitals, long-term care, rehab center, hospice, surgicenters, ambulatory clinics, etc.) and all settings (MedSurg, OB, NICO, ICU, CCU, Step-Down, Rehab, Pediatrics, Psych, ER, Dialysis, Home Care, Long-Term Care, etc.) | Organizations worldwide where nursing leaders successfully align their nursing strategic goals to improve the organization's patient outcomes |
| NCAL Awards Program ▪ The Jan Thayer Pioneer Award ▪ National Quality Award Program | American Health Care Association/National Center for Assisted Living (AHCA/NCAL) | National quality awards for long-term care and assisted living facilities | Commitment, achievement excellence |
| Shingo Prize for Operational Excellence | Utah State University | Any industry Any part of world | Frequency, duration, intensity, and scope of the desired principle-based behavior. Degree to which leaders focus on principles and culture, and managers focus on aligning systems to drive ideal behaviors at all levels |
| Bernard J. Tyson National Award for Excellence in Pursuit of Healthcare Equity | The Joint Commission and Kaiser Permanente | Tyson award recognizes all types of organizations that directly deliver healthcare. | Initiatives that achieve a measurable, sustained reduction in one or more healthcare disparities. |
| U.S. News Best Hospitals | U.S. News & World Report | Hospitals | Scores based on data that include survival, patient safety, nurse staffing, and other factors |

**Table 5.14** Framework for Performing a Gap Analysis

| Standard | Importance High, Medium, Low | For High-Importance Areas | | | |
| --- | --- | --- | --- | --- | --- |
| | | Stretch (Strength) or Improvement Goal | What Action Is Planned? | By When? | Who Is Responsible? |
| **Standard** | | | | | |
| Strength or Evidence | | | | | |
| 1. | | | | | |
| 2. | | | | | |
| Opportunity for Improvement | | | | | |
| 1. | | | | | |
| 2. | | | | | |
| | | | | | |
| **Standard** | | | | | |
| Strength or Evidence | | | | | |
| 1. | | | | | |
| 2. | | | | | |
| Opportunity for Improvement | | | | | |
| 1. | | | | | |
| 2. | | | | | |

Reproduced with permission of the Baldrige Performance Excellence Program. *2021–2022 Framework: Leadership and Management Practices for High Performance.* Gaithersburg, MD: U.S. Department of Commerce, National Institute of Standards and Technology; 2021.

7. Develop a team approach to self-assessment (facilitator or coordinator and subject matter experts).
8. Perform a self-assessment or gap analysis of current performance compared with the standards or criteria (**Table 5.14**).
9. Identify strengths or evidence of compliance for each criterion.
10. Identify opportunities for improvement based on the criteria.
11. Prioritize findings from the self-assessment or gap analysis.
12. Plan a course of action to meet the standards; perform benchmarking (see the *Health Data Analytics* section for more information on benchmarking).

13. Develop an action plan based on the priority for each criterion.
14. Perform ongoing feedback and update evidence of compliance.
15. Determine who coordinates the application submission process.
16. Complete an application.
17. Submit the application.
18. Plan for a site visit and documentation of evidence.
19. Sustain the process.
20. Integrate into daily operations.
21. Celebrate successes.
22. Plan for redesignation if applicable.

# Recognition of Internal Customers

An important structural element in the quality, safety, and performance improvement program is recognizing internal customers. Every process has both internal and external customers. Most people readily understand the concept of being a supplier of goods to an external customer. However, the idea of internal customers is equally important.

An employee can be a customer when they receive material, information, or services from others in the organization. Conversely, an employee also can be a supplier when they provide material, information, or services to others in the organization or to external customers. For example, when a nurse sends a specimen to the laboratory, the nurse is the supplier, and the laboratory is the customer. When the laboratory sends a report back to the nurse, the laboratory is the supplier, and the nurse is the customer. Just as there are suppliers to internal customers, those internal customers can, in turn, be suppliers to external customers. This approach can help to

- remind departments without direct contact with external customers that they are still a critical link to customer satisfaction,

- improve relationships,
- make the work process flow smoothly, and
- avert potential bottlenecks.

**Table 5.15** provides an example of an approach one organization followed to ensure the recognition of internal customers. Notice that the customer service standard pledge reflects the values necessary to make quality a reality (e.g., teamwork, information sharing).

In most healthcare organizations and as in Table 5.15, service excellence is as important as clinical excellence. For example, Sharp HealthCare, a Malcolm Baldrige award recipient, implemented initiatives that formed the foundation of service excellence—what it referred to as the Sharp Experience.[107] These include

1. *AIDET.* Acknowledge, introduce, duration, explanation, thank you
2. *Behavior standards.*
   - Attitude is everything—Create a lasting impression.
   - Thank somebody—Reward and recognition.
   - Make words work—Talk, listen, and learn.
   - All for one—And one for all; teamwork.
   - Make it better—Service recovery.

**Table 5.15** Customer Service Standards and Pledge

| Respect Me and My Job | We Are All Professionals | Work and Communicate with Me | Smile—It's Contagious |
|---|---|---|---|
| *Our need:* Respect. *Our response:* I understand the need to be respectful, and I will<br>■ acknowledge you,<br>■ be sensitive to your point of view,<br>■ thank you for a job well done,<br>■ value your time and priorities,<br>■ discuss my concerns with you in private,<br>■ value your job and its contribution to the organization,<br>■ treat you as I would like to be treated, and<br>■ speak to you in a pleasant tone in person or on the phone. | *Our need:* Professionalism. *Our response:* I understand the need to represent the hospital in a professional manner, and I will<br>■ take responsibility for my actions,<br>■ protect confidential information about patients and fellow employees,<br>■ look professional in dress, grooming, and manner,<br>■ coach others when necessary, and<br>■ follow through on my promise to you. | *Our need:* Teamwork. *Our response:* I understand the need for teamwork, and I will<br>■ pitch in and offer to help you whenever possible,<br>■ ask for your input before making a decision that may affect you,<br>■ talk to you directly instead of talking to others secretly if I have a concern,<br>■ listen to you, offer positive advice, and not interrupt until you are finished,<br>■ recognize that everyone has a valid opinion, and<br>■ seek out information and share what I have learned. | *Our need:* Positive attitude. *Our response:* I understand the need for a positive work environment, and I will<br>■ be sensitive to the effects my actions have on others,<br>■ replace criticism with positive ideas,<br>■ try to see things through the other person's eyes,<br>■ attempt to leave any personal problems at home,<br>■ coach my coworkers in portraying a positive attitude, and<br>■ project a caring and concerned attitude. |

Reproduced from Baird K. *Customer Service in Health Care: A Grassroots Approach to Creating a Culture of Service Excellence.* New York, NY: Wiley; 2000. Copyright 2000 by Jossey-Bass with permission of John Wiley & Sons, Inc.

- Think safe, be safe—Safety at work.
- Look sharp, be sharp—Appearance speaks.
- Keep in touch—Ease waiting times.
- It's a private matter—Confidentiality.
- To email or not to email—Email manners.
- *Vive la différence!*—Diversity.
- Get smart—Increasing skills and competence.

3. *Must haves.*
   - Greet people with a smile and "Hello," using their name when possible.
   - Take people where they are going, rather than pointing or giving directions.
   - Use key words at key times: "Is there anything else I can do for you? I have the time."
     - Foster an attitude of gratitude. Send thank-you notes to deserving employees.
     - Round with reason to better connect with staff, patients, family, and other customers.

4. *On stage/off stage.* This framework allows employees to stage patient and guest experiences, based on the premise that every action, object, and detail can either add to an experience or detract from it. Even small acts can be of immense importance to patients and their families.

5. *Storytelling.* The development and sharing of stories can be a potent means of promoting values and beliefs in an organization. StoryCorps, a non-profit organization, helps organizations "remind one another of our shared humanity, strengthen and build the connections between people, teach the value of listening, and weave into the fabric of our culture the understanding that every life matters."[108(p2)]

The measurement of customer perception, satisfaction, and loyalty is important for healthcare organizations to determine how their customers like the services provided. There are vendors who survey these customers and provide data back to the organization for tracking, trending, and benchmarking performance.

CMS identified customer perception as a key component of measuring hospital performance and developed the Hospital Consumer Assessment of Healthcare Providers and Systems (HCAHPS) survey as a standardized method to compare performance and link payment to performance. HCAHPS is the first national, standardized, publicly reported survey of patients' perspectives of hospital care. Before the advent of HCAHPS, there was no national standard for collecting and publicly reporting information about patient experience of care that allowed comparisons across hospitals locally, regionally, and nationally.

The survey is designed to produce data about patients' perceptions of care that allow objective comparisons of hospitals on topics that are important to consumers. Public reporting of the survey results increases accountability by increasing transparency in the quality of care. CMS and the HCAHPS project team take steps to ensure the survey is credible, useful, and practical.

In 2002, CMS partnered with AHRQ to develop and evaluate the HCAHPS survey. In May 2005, the HCAHPS survey was endorsed by the National Quality Forum, and approval for the national implementation for public reporting occurred in March 2008. The survey, methods, and results are in the public domain. The Deficit Reduction Act of 2005 created an additional incentive for acute care hospitals to participate in HCAHPS. As of July 2007, hospitals must collect and submit HCAHPS data to receive their full inpatient prospective payment system annual payment update. Inpatient prospective payment system hospitals that fail to publicly report the HCAHPS survey may receive an annual payment update that is reduced. The Patient Protection and Affordable Care Act of 2010 (P.L. 111-148) includes HCAHPS among the measures to be used to calculate value-based incentive payments in the Hospital Value-Based Purchasing program, with discharges since October 2012. HCAHPS results are published on the Care Compare website.[109] The survey consists of both inpatient and outpatient items depending on the population assessed. Instruments for long-term care and home care are available, but there are no comparative data collected or published for this measure for this population. See the *Quality Review and Accountability* section for more information about activities that support compliance with voluntary, mandatory, and contractual reporting requirements for data acquisition, analysis, reporting, and improvement.

**Box 5.9** lists key points in recognition and quality awards.

---

### Box 5.9  Key Points: Recognition and Quality Awards

- Healthcare quality professionals are instrumental in assessing and applying for external quality awards as well as establishing internal awards.
- State and national quality awards acknowledge organizations that demonstrate excellence in quality, process, and results.
- Most awards are outcomes focused and criteria-based.

# Education and Training in a Learning Organization

This section addresses competencies as the base for organizational learning. Because the most common cause of failure in any performance or process improvement effort is uninvolved or indifferent top and middle management, it is essential that all leaders be educated and onboard from the start. Training begins at the top and cascades down through the learning organization. Senior and middle management are part of the teaching team; this demonstrates to frontline employees that they are committed to quality and safety.

Senge's concept of the learning organization can be applied to healthcare. The definition of a *learning organization* is one "where people continually expand their capacity to create the results they truly desire, where new and expansive patterns of thinking are nurtured, where collective aspiration is set free, and where people are continually learning to see the whole together."[110(p3)] A *learning healthcare system* "is designed to generate and apply the best evidence for the collaborative healthcare choices of each patient and provider; to drive the process of discovery as a natural outgrowth of patient care; and to ensure innovation, quality, safety, and value in health care."[111(pix)] The most pressing needs for change identified by IOM roundtable are those related to adaptation to the pace of change; the stronger synchrony of efforts; a culture of shared responsibility; a new clinical research paradigm; clinical decision support systems; universal electronic health records; and tools for database linkage, mining, and use, among others.[111(p5)]

In a learning organization, learning needs to be embedded in the way the organization operates. When learning is embedded, it means that learning is a regular part of work and results in solving problems at their source (root cause). Building and sharing knowledge is deployed throughout the organization and is driven by opportunities to effect significant, meaningful change and to innovate. Sources for learning include staff and physicians' ideas; research findings; patient and other customer input; best-practice sharing; and benchmarking.

Organizational learning has multiple benefits. It can result in increased value to patients through new and improved healthcare services as well as the development of new healthcare business opportunities. Organizational learning can lead to the development of evidence-based approaches and new healthcare delivery models. Patient safety can be enhanced through reduced errors, defects, waste, and related costs. Finally, organizational learning can lead to greater agility in managing change and disruption in the current healthcare environment.[112] Gallup defined *agility* as "employees' capacity to gather and disseminate information about changes in the environment, and respond to that information quickly and expediently."[113(p3)] Gallup found that cooperation is key to an agile workplace and proposed seven shifts to an agile culture (**Figure 5.45**).

## Staff Knowledge and Competency

To evaluate needs and ensure general staff knowledge and competency, the healthcare quality professional needs first to evaluate their own knowledge and competency for the area of education and training being offered. NAHQ offers the Healthcare Quality Competency Framework as a structure to support healthcare quality professionals in assessing and expanding their professional knowledge and abilities for specific job requirements and capabilities.[114] Healthcare quality professionals are encouraged to review the Framework, which organizes healthcare quality work into eight domains, composed of 29 competency statements and

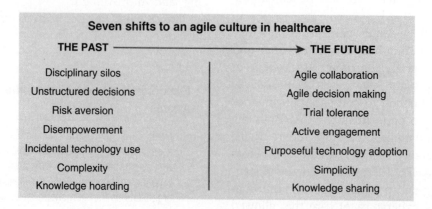

**Figure 5.45** Seven Shifts to an Agile Culture in Healthcare
Courtesy of GALLUP.

486 skill statements. These skills are required to achieve quality objectives and are stratified by levels of progression (i.e., foundational to proficient to advanced).[114]

## Quality, Safety, and Performance Improvement

Providing training on quality, safety, and performance improvement is often a collaborative effort between healthcare quality professionals who are subject matter experts and educators who are experts on teaching and learning modalities. Education to achieve varying levels of understanding of principles related to quality, safety, and performance improvement has been incorporated into the basic training programs for many different health professions. Healthcare quality professionals should collaborate with organizational leaders to gain an understanding of which health professions have students in their organizations and work with key leaders to align, to the extent possible, quality training projects with organizational quality priorities.

Health professions have professional associations or societies that offer education and training in healthcare quality and safety. The healthcare quality professional may be called upon to assist leaders and clinicians in assessing the value of available educational offerings. There are multiple approaches to education using adult learning principles and accelerated learning methods, including the following:

- Engage multiple senses to enhance experiential learning (auditory, visual, kinesthetic).
- Use concepts and principles, then add application into practice.
- Integrate self-directed learning with follow-up that includes simulation, role playing, and critical reflection.
- Utilize interactive tools in virtual learning (annotation, hand raising, chat, polling, breakout rooms) to activate the brain and keep the learner engaged to facilitate learning and retention.
- Allow students to teach each other key concepts; acting as a teacher promotes a stronger focus on learning and encourages learners to be reflective in their practice.
- Embrace the pause; use a 7-second rule to allow students to formulate questions and engage.
- Cluster learning material into key categories and teach in segments, building on easier concepts and then adding more difficult ones.

The use of simulation and case studies to apply concepts or tools is another effective way to enhance training. Most types of hands-on experience and practice will make the learning fun and more relevant and increase muscle memory for the task.

Training on quality, safety, and performance improvement must address the current employee base, physicians, new employees, and students/trainees. Although core concepts and tools can be taught and reemphasized to embed the improvement philosophy into the culture, there will be degradation in memory unless the information is clearly integrated into daily work and used often. For this reason, just-in-time training is often used for teams or projects.

By building a learning organization, leaders foster an environment conducive to learning about quality, safety, and performance improvement. This opens boundaries across departments, disciplines, and professions and stimulates the exchange of ideas. The way to foster this development is to create learning forums, which may take many forms to achieve innovation and learning. The learning organization will excel in a culture of performance excellence and improvement because the cultural foundation will support ongoing learning, change, and improvement. Organizations can also collaborate with other healthcare facilities through state initiatives (i.e., California Health Collaborative), or national programs (i.e., Quality and Safety Education for Nurses Teaching and Practice Strategies; IHI Collaboratives).

AHRQ provides free continuing education events in the areas of comparative effectiveness, quality and patient safety, and prevention/care management.[115] IHI offers Open School online courses in quality, safety, and performance improvement[116] and online courses with coaching. Quality and Safety Education for Nursing (QSEN) prepares nurses using learning modules for new and experienced nursing faculty on various quality and safety issues.[117]

## Training Effectiveness

Kirkpatrick's foundational principles for evaluating effectiveness of training, first published in 1959, continue to be relevant and used by healthcare quality professionals today. The focus was a return on expectations as the ultimate indicator of value, and value must be created before it can be measured. The framework for evaluation can be envisioned as a compelling chain of evidence that demonstrates the bottom-line value to the organization.

### Framework for Evaluating the Results of Training

As an expert in the field of training, Kirkpatrick perceived three reasons for evaluating training programs, namely,

1. to determine how to improve future training,
2. to determine whether the current training continues, and
3. to justify the existence of the training department.[118]

To the extent trainers can demonstrate important outcomes from training, they will be important to the quality and safety culture and the organization itself. Kirkpatrick suggests there are four important levels of training evaluation: reaction, learning, behavior, and results.[119] This model is often used to describe various levels of measuring training effectiveness.

**1. Reaction** This is the extent to which the participants are satisfied (favorability, engagement, relevance) with training. Because negative attitudes toward the program can interfere with learning, this is an important measurement. Reactions are often measured at the end of the training program or soon after the program ends through use of a questionnaire about what participants thought and felt about the training. For example, here are two ways of measuring reactions:

1. Customer (learner) satisfaction, or their opinion (What did they like? What did they learn? Was anything missing?), using a Likert rating scale for feedback.
2. Good facilitator, interesting or useful subject, adequate facilities (or virtual environment managed well), opinion of conduciveness to learning, scheduling, additional comments.

**2. Learning** When participants change attitudes, improve knowledge, or increase skill because of the program, learning occurred. Unless one of these parameters changes, it is unlikely that behavior will change. Learning is best measured both before and after training and, where possible, includes a control group for comparison. The type of measure used will depend on what is being evaluated. For example, increased skill may need to be evaluated by a thought leader, specialist, or subject matter expert, whereas a change in attitude can be measured using a before-and-after questionnaire. For example, learning can be measured by a change in attitude, skills, or knowledge and using valid and reliable pretests and posttests, test performance, engagement in interactive tools (chat, polling, etc.), and demonstrations/simulation or role play in virtual breakout rooms.

**3. Behavior** This level refers to behavioral change (application) because of training. It focuses on the transfer of knowledge, skills, or attitudes from the classroom to the job. Although positive reactions may produce a desire to change behavior and learning may give participants the skills to know how and what to change, it does not necessarily follow that behavior will change. In addition to positive reactions and

learning, employees must work in a climate supportive of change, and they must see rewards associated with changing their behaviors. These do not have to be tangible rewards; intangible rewards such as a feeling of achievement are important motivators for change. The climate depends heavily on the support of the leader, manager, or supervisor, further supporting the importance of all levels of management being involved in quality, safety, and performance improvement education and training.

Ideally, behaviors are measured both before and after training, allowing ample time for behavioral change to occur. Pretraining and posttraining information can be collected by questionnaires, informal polling, and interviews, and from those who can observe participants' behaviors (e.g., immediate supervisor, customers, and peers). Relevant examples of behavioral changes relating to quality and safety may include the extent to which

- department heads deploy quality, safety, and performance improvement concepts, methods, and tools;
- more and more staff receive formal training in performance improvement models;
- the number of performance improvement, evidence-based initiatives, and safety projects increase;
- staff report variances in processes and near misses;
- safety culture metrics improve;
- senior leaders communicate the organization's values (measured by employee engagement surveys and focus groups); and
- leadership practices reflect employee involvement, engagement, and participation.

**4. Results** This is the last—and probably the most important—level of program evaluation described by Kirkpatrick. Indicators used to measure targeted outcomes are tied to the driving force behind conducting training in the first place. For example, did quality of care improve, and was this a function of quality, safety, and performance improvement training? Did adverse event reporting (including near misses) increase? Were overall errors reduced through organization-wide quality and safety training? As with evaluation of behavioral changes, result evaluation is conducted before and after training, uses a control group, allows ample time for results to be achieved, monitors results over time, and compares the cost of the training program with the benefit. A direct link between training and results may be difficult to prove because other factors might influence an outcome. However, evidence that supports the link should be gathered. Examples of results may include

- final overall change for the business because of the training program;
- improved quality, improved production, or decreased costs;
- increased job satisfaction and engagement;
- reduced problems or accidents; and
- increased number of programs and/or market share to meet merging population needs.

## Return on Investment

Return on investment evaluation addresses how the bottom line changed because of training. The return on investment asks the question, "Were the benefits greater than the cost?"[120] Phillips suggests a fifth level of evaluation in which the fourth level of the standard model is compared with the overall costs of training.[120,121] Phillips describes methods for isolating the effects of the program or process, methods of converting data to monetary values, cost categories, intangible benefits, and communication targets. For quality, safety, and performance improvement, questions to consider include:

- Are staff using the tools and methods (e.g., more improvement projects being initiated)?
- Are outcomes improving, and if so, is value being demonstrated beyond the cost of the training?

**Box 5.10** lists the key points of education and training in learning organizations.

---

**Box 5.10  Key Points: Education and Training in Learning Organizations**

- A learning healthcare system uses the best evidence for patient and provider collaboration; drives discovery as a natural outgrowth of patient care; and ensures innovation, quality, safety, and value.
- Adult learning principles and accelerated learning methods inform educational approaches.
- Kirkpatrick's foundational principles for evaluating effectiveness of training are relevant and used by healthcare quality professionals today.

---

Everyone in the organization is responsible for quality and safety. Therefore, educating staff at all levels of the organization is critical to the success of quality and PI. The NAHQ Healthcare Competency Framework includes performance and process improvement as a domain. Three key competencies include implement standard performance and process improvement methods; apply project management methods; and use change management principles and tools.[122] Specific skills and proficiency levels are further identified

to support organizational learning for the healthcare quality professional.

The method of education or training must be tailored to the audience and use tools and methods to match the audience needs and learning styles. Governing body or board members must also be included in understanding and their accountability for quality of care in the organization. Board training is often included for new members. A comprehensive program for all levels of employees, management, board, and physicians is designed to meet the needs of these distinct groups. For example, governing board training includes

- a review of oversight responsibility for the organization's quality and safety performance;
- quality, safety, and PI committee or review functions;
- use of quality performance as a criterion in rating executive performance; and
- trends and public reporting of the organization's data and its image in the community.

## Determining Education and Training Needs

There are ways to determine the educational needs of the healthcare workforce. Methods to obtain information include

- evaluating knowledge and skills contained in the job description,
- asking participants,
- asking participants' supervisors,
- asking others who are knowledgeable about the job (e.g., customers, peers, experts in quality, safety, and PI),
- testing participants on their skills and knowledge, and
- analyzing the participant's past performance appraisals.[105,118,119]

## Elements of Performance Improvement Curriculum

The curriculum includes the following elements:

- An explanation of the need for organizational improvement, including individual and collective benefits of performance and process improvement
- Development and use of common quality language or taxonomy
- A discussion of the organization's quality and safety goals
- A definition of the program structure
- Articulation of the organization's philosophy and a model for improvement

- A description of the improvement process
- A description and clarification of responsibilities
- Tools and techniques to participate in teams and to manage work processes
- A description of how change may affect the individual's job and work relationships
- Metrics for the organization
- A reporting structure for leaders and staff

Tailor training to the specific needs of each group (i.e., top management, middle management, frontline staff). **Table 5.16** offers a comparison of topics addressed across major groups in a quality, safety, and performance improvement curriculum. Another approach to considering training is the IHI Improvement Advisor Professional Development Program,[77] which includes the following agenda for training:

- Science of improvement (includes high reliability organizations)
- Model for improvement
- Scoping improvement efforts
- Understanding systems and processes
- Using data for improvement
- Understanding relationships
- Gathering information
- Organizing information

- Developing powerful ideas for change
- Testing changes
- Implementing changes
- Decision making
- Working with people
- Planned experimentation

## Requisite Knowledge and Skills

The key operating assumption of building capacity is that people have various levels of need for knowledge and skills. A teaching plan ensures each group receives the knowledge and skill sets they need, when they need them, and in the appropriate amounts. **Figure 5.46** shows a pyramid model in which experts need an elevated level of specific knowledge on

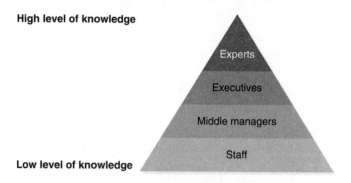

High level of knowledge

Low level of knowledge

Experts

Executives

Middle managers

Staff

**Figure 5.46** Levels of Knowledge

---

**Table 5.16** Substantive Issues for Education and Training

| Top Management Topics | Middle Management Topics | Staff Topics |
|---|---|---|
| ■ Role of board in quality and safety<br>■ Quality and safety as strategic advantages<br>■ Role of leadership in creating and sustaining quality vision<br>■ Integrating quality values and safety culture into day-to-day leadership<br>■ Indicators for measuring, evaluating, and improving quality and organizational performance<br>■ Components of quality, safety and performance excellence and implementation process<br>■ Basic quality and performance improvement tools<br>■ Role as team leaders, champions, and sponsors<br>■ Awareness of accreditation standards | ■ Key concepts of quality and performance management (e.g., customer satisfaction, process management, teamwork, continuous improvement methods)<br>■ Management practices for building teamwork, employee involvement, and recognition for customer service<br>■ Team building and contributions for quality, team leadership skills, conflict resolution<br>■ Communication skills, listening, and giving feedback<br>■ Principles of customer service<br>■ Managing process performance (measurement, quality and performance improvement tools, variation, problem solving, data collection and analysis)<br>■ Measurement of quality outcomes<br>■ Accreditation standards | ■ Organization's mission, vision, and performance improvement plan<br>■ Quality awareness, definition of quality<br>■ Fundamental training in quality and performance improvement, including process improvement tools and techniques<br>■ Concepts of quality management: customer satisfaction, process improvement, teamwork, continuous improvement<br>■ Promoting cooperation between coworkers within and between departments<br>■ Communication skills<br>■ Customer service<br>■ Relevant accreditation standards |

performance improvement, quality management, and tools, whereas most staff need a much lower level of knowledge in this area.

There are common reasons why managers are often reluctant to support training in quality, safety, and PI. These barriers must be overcome for the organization to develop the infrastructure necessary to support healthcare quality and safety. They include

- no results from the training;
- too costly;
- no input on the content, process, or timing;
- no relevance of the content to actual work;
- no involvement in the process;
- no time for staff to participate;
- lack of preparation of programs;
- lack of knowledge about learning and development; and
- no requirements for the training (e.g., no regulations).[123(pp2-4)]

**Box 5.11** lists key points for organizational learning and knowledge.

## Summary

A formal quality, safety, and performance improvement program and infrastructure are required to

> ### Box 5.11  Key Points: Organizational Learning and Knowledge
>
> - A comprehensive training program is designed to meet the needs of different audiences and all levels of employees, management, the board, and medical staff.
> - The training program addresses knowledge barriers using different methods to inform curriculum, such as evaluating skills in the job descriptions.
> - Developing the learning infrastructure necessary for healthcare quality and safety advances the organization's growth and professional development of the workforce.

ensure quality and safety. The tenets of quality and safety must first be developed through strategic planning. Strategic planning is supported by the establishment of priorities for performance and process improvement activities, translating strategic goals into quality outcomes, and aligning culture and structure. Through the understanding of principles and practices reviewed herein and in other *HQ Solutions* sections, the healthcare quality professional can apply evidence-based techniques to ensure quality and safety in their respective organizations—every day.

## References

1. Deming WE. *Out of the Crisis*. Cambridge, MA: MIT Press; 2000.
2. Ono T. *Toyota seisan hoshiki* (translated to *Toyota Production System: Beyond Large-Scale Production*). Tokyo: Diamond, Inc.; 1978.
3. The W. Edwards Deming Institute. Deming the man: Dr. W. Edwards Deming. Published 2022. Accessed January 13, 2022. https://deming.org/deming-the-man/
4. The Juran Institute. About us. Published 2022. Accessed January 13, 2022. https://www.juran.com/about-us
5. Juran JM. *Juran on Leadership for Quality: An Executive Handbook*. New York, NY: The Free Press; 1989.
6. DeFeo JA. The Juran trilogy: quality planning. Published April 15, 2019. Accessed February 5, 2022. https://www.juran.com/blog/the-juran-trilogy-quality-planning/
7. Crosby PB. *Quality Is Free: The Art of Making Quality Certain*. New York, NY: McGraw-Hill; 1979.
8. Hunt VD. *Quality in America: How to Implement a Competitive Quality Program*. Homewood, IL: Business One Irwin; 1992.
9. Donabedian A. *The Definition of Quality and Approaches to its Assessment*. Ann Arbor, MI: Health Administration Press; 1980.
10. Codman EA. *A Study of Hospital Efficiency*. Ann Arbor, MI: University Microfilms; 1916 and 1972.
11. Roberts JS, Redman RR, Coate JG. A history of the Joint Commission on Accreditation of Hospitals. *JAMA*. 1987;258, 936-940. doi:10.1001/jama.1987.03400070074038
12. Berwick DM. Continuous improvement as an ideal in health care. *NEJM*. 1989;320(21):53-56. doi:10.1056/NEJM198901053200110
13. Buchanan ED, Batalden PB. Knowledge for improvement: initiating continual improvement at the Hospital Corporation of America. In: Goldfield N, Nash DB, eds. *Providing Quality Care*. Philadelphia, PA: American College of Physicians; 1995:99-114.
14. Berwick DM, Godfrey AB, Roessner J. *Curing Health Care*. San Francisco, CA: Jossey-Bass Publishers; 1990.
15. James BC. *Quality Management for Health Care Delivery*. Chicago, IL: The Hospital Research and Education Trust; 1990.
16. White SV. Interview with a quality leader: Brent James on reducing harm to patients and improving quality. *J Healthc Qual*. 2007;29(5):35-44. doi:10.1111/j.1945-1474.2007.tb00211.x
17. Institute of Medicine Committee on Quality of Health Care in America. *To Err Is Human: Building a Safer Health System*.

Kohn LT, Corrigan JM, Donaldson MS, eds. Washington, DC: National Academies Press; 2000.

18. Berwick DM, Nolan TW, Whittington J. The triple aim: care, health and cost. *Health Aff.* 2008;27(3):759-769. doi:10.1377/hlthaff.27.3.759

19. Epstein RM, Street RL. *Patient-Centered Communication in Cancer Care: Promoting Healing and Reducing Suffering.* Bethesda, MD: National Cancer Institute; 2007.

20. Pelletier LR, Stichler JE. Patient-centered care and engagement: Nurse leaders' imperative for health reform. *J Nurs Adm.* 2014;44(9):473-480. doi:10.1097/NNA.0000000000000102

21. Agency for Healthcare Research and Quality, President's Advisory Commission on Consumer Protection and Quality in the Health Care Industry. Consumer bill of rights. Published 1998. Accessed December 1, 2021. https://archive.ahrq.gov/hcqual/cborr/

22. U.S. Department of Health & Human Services. Partnership for Patients: a common commitment. Published 2011. Accessed December 1, 2021. https://innovation.cms.gov/innovation-models/partnership-for-patients

23. Center for Advancing Health. *A New Definition of Patient Engagement: What Is Engagement and Why Is It Important?* Washington, DC: Author; 2010.

24. Glascow R. Technology and chronic care. Paper presented at the Congress on Improving Chronic Care: Innovations in Research and Practice; September 8-10, 2002; Seattle, WA.

25. Kaplan S, Greenfield S, Ware JE. Assessing the effects of physician–patient interactions on the outcomes of chronic disease. *Med Care.* 1989;27(3)(suppl):S110-S127. doi:10.1097/00005650-198903001-00010

26. Von Korff M, Gruman J, Schaeffer J, Curry SJ, Wagner EH. Collaborative management of chronic illness. *Ann of Int Med.* 1997;127(12):1097-1102.

27. Institute for Healthcare Improvement. How to improve: science of improvement: testing multiple changes. Published 2017. Accessed December 1, 2021. http://www.ihi.org/resources/Pages/HowtoImprove/ScienceofImprovementTestingMultipleChanges.aspx

28. Institute for Healthcare Improvement. *Going Lean in Healthcare.* Cambridge, MA: IHI; 2005.

29. Pyzdek T, Keller P. *The Six Sigma Handbook: A Complete Guide for Greenbelts, Blackbelts, & Managers at All Levels.* New York, NY: McGraw Hill; 2018.

30. Chassin MR. Is health care ready for six sigma quality. *Milbank Q.* 1998;76(4):565-591. doi:10/1111/1468-9990.00106

31. Ahmed S, Manaf NH, Islam R. Effects of Lean Six Sigma application in healthcare services: a literature review. *Rev Environ Health.* 2013;28(4):189-194. doi: 10.1515/reveh-2013-0015

32. Phieffer L, Hefner JL, Rahmanian A, et al. Improving operating room efficiency: first case on-time start project. *J Healthc Qual.* 2017;39(5):e70-e78.

33. Lean Enterprise Institute. Principles of Lean. Accessed December 1, 2021. www.lean.org/WhatsLean/Principles.cfm

34. MoreSteam. Lean Six Sigma on-line training. Published 2012. Accessed December 1, 2021. www.moresteam.com/lean-six-sigma/green-belt.cfm

35. Naik T, Duroseau Y, Zehtabchi S, et al. A structured approach to transforming a large public hospital emergency department via Lean methodologies. *J Healthc Qual.* 2012;34(2):86-97. doi:10.1111/j.1945-1474.2011.00181.x

36. Graban M, Swartz JE. *Healthcare Kaizen: Engaging Front-Line Staff in Sustainable Continuous Improvement.* Boca Raton, FL: CRC Press; 2012.

37. Arthur J. *Lean Six Sigma for Hospitals: Simple Steps to Fast Affordable and Flawless Healthcare.* New York, NY: McGraw Hill; 2011.

38. Chassin MR. Is health care ready for Six Sigma quality? *The Milbank Quart.* 1998;76(4):565-591. doi:10.1111/1468-0009.00106

39. Kaplan R, Bower M. The balanced scorecard and quality programs. *Balanced Scorecard Report* [Newsletter]. Cambridge, MA: Harvard Business School Publishing; March 15, 2001:3-6.

40. Kaplan RS, Norton DP. The balanced scorecard: measures that drive performance. *Harv Bus Rev.* 1992;70(1):71-79.

41. Kaplan R, Norton D. Using the balanced scorecard as a strategic management system. *HBR.* 1996;74:75-85.

42. U.S. Department of Health & Human Services, Health Resources & Services Administration. Performance measurement and management. 2021. Accessed December 1, 2021. https://www.hrsa.gov/quality/toolbox/508pdfs/performancemanagementandmeasurement.pdf

43. Goldenhar LM, Brady PW, Sutcliffe KM, Muething SE. Huddling for high reliability and situation awareness. *BMJ.* 2013;22:899-906. doi:10.1136/bmjqs-2012-001467

44. U.S. Department of Energy, Office of Management. Balanced scorecard program. Accessed December 1, 2021. http://energy.gov/management/office-management/operational-management/procurement-and-acquisition/balanced-scorecard

45. Robbins SP. *Organizational Behavior.* 8th ed. Upper Saddle River, NJ: Prentice Hall; 2001.

46. Kotter JP. What leaders really do. *HBR.* 1990;68:103-111.

47. American Hospital Association. Accountability: The pathway to restoring public trust and confidence for hospitals and other healthcare organizations. Published 1999. Accessed December 1, 2021. www.aha.org/content/00-10/AHAPrinciplesAccountability.pdf

48. American Hospital Association and American Medical Association. Integrated leadership for hospitals and health systems: principles for success. Published 2015. Accessed December 1, 2021. https://www.ama-assn.org/sites/default/files/media-browser/public/about-ama/ama-aha-integrated-leadership-principles_0.pdf

49. Studer Group. Studer Group. Accessed December 1, 2021. https://az414866.vo.msecnd.net/cmsroot/studergroup/media/studergroup/pages/who-we-are/about-studer-group/studergroup_infographic.pdf

50. Provost L, Miller D, Reinertsen J. *A Framework for Leadership for Improvement.* Cambridge, MA: Institute for Healthcare Improvement; 2006.

51. White SV. Interview with a quality leader: David Brailer on information technology and advancing healthcare quality. *J Healthc Qual.* 2004;26(6):20-25. doi:10.1111/j.1945-1474.2004.tb00531.x

52. Rosati RJ. Creating quality improvement projects. In: Siegler EL, Mirafzali S, Foust JB, eds. *A Guide to Hospitals and Inpatient Care.* New York, NY: Springer; 2003:326-338.

53. Reinertsen JL, Bisognano M, Pugh MD. *Seven Leadership Leverage Points for Organization-Level Improvement in Health Care.* 2nd ed. Cambridge, MA: Institute for Healthcare Improvement; 2011.

54. Sackett D, Rosenberg WMC, Muir-Gray JA, Haynes RB, Richardson WS. Evidence-based medicine: what it is and what it isn't. *BMJ.* 1996;312(13):71-72. doi:10.1136/bmj.312.7023.71

55. Tonelli M. The limits of evidence-based medicine. *Respir Care.* 2001; 46(12):1435-1440. doi:10.1097/00001888-199812000-00011

56. Institute of Medicine, Committee on Quality of Health Care in America. *Crossing the Quality Chasm: A New Health System for the 21st Century.* Washington, DC: National Academies Press; 2001.

57. Deaton C. Outcomes measurement and evidence-based nursing practice. *J Cardiovasc Nurs.* 2001;15(2):83-86.

58. Khoury MJ, Gwinn M, Yoon PW, Dowling N, Moore CA, Bradley L. The continuum of translation research in genomic medicine: how can we accelerate the appropriate integration of human genomic discoveries into health care and disease prevention? *Genet Med.* 2007;9(10):665-674.

59. US Preventive Services Task Force. Grade definitions. Published June 2016. Accessed December 1, 2021. https://www.uspreventiveservicestaskforce.org/Page/Name/grade-definitions

60. US Preventive Services Task Force. Update on methods: Estimating certainty and magnitude of net benefit. Published 2017. Accessed January 10, 2022. https://uspreventiveservicestaskforce.org/uspstf/about-uspstf/methods-and-processes/update-methods-estimating-certainty-and-magnitude-net-benefit

61. Agency for Healthcare Research and Quality. National Guideline Clearinghouse. Accessed January 10, 2022. https://www.ahrq.gov/gam/index.html

62. Zander K, Bower K. *Nursing Case Management, Blueprint for Transformation.* Boston, MA: New England Medical Center Hospitals; 1987.

63. Every NR, Hochman J, Becker R, Kopecky S, Cannon CP, for the Committee on Acute Cardiac Care, Council on Clinical Cardiology, American Heart Association. Critical pathways: a review. *Circulation.* 2000;101:461-465. doi:10.1161/01.CIR.101.4.461

64. Rotter T, Kinsman L, James EL, et al. Clinical pathways: effects on professional practice, patient outcomes, length of stay and hospital costs. Cochrane Database of Systematic Reviews. 2010;March 17(3). CD006632. doi:10.1002/14651858.CD006632

65. Institute of Medicine. *Clinical Practice Guidelines We Can Trust.* Washington, DC: The National Academies Press. Published 2011. Accessed January 10, 2022. https://www.nap.edu/catalog/13058/clinical-practice-guidelines-we-can-trust

66. Alliance for the Implementation of Clinical Practice Guidelines. One-click access and free decision support from guideline developers in the new AiCPG Guideline Clearinghouse. Accessed December 1, 2021. www.aicpg.org

67. Resar R, Griffin FA, Haraden C, Nolan TW. *Using Care Bundles to Improve Health Care Quality.* IHI Innovation Series white paper. Cambridge, MA: Institute for Healthcare Improvement; 2012. http://www.IHI.org

68. National Quality Forum. *National Quality Partners Playbook: Antibiotic Stewardship in Acute Care.* Washington, DC: Author; 2016. Accessed January 10, 2022. https://store.qualityforum.org/collections/antibiotic-stewardship

69. Stempniak M. Patient safety in the OR. *Hospitals & Health Networks.* 2012:86(10):40-47. Accessed February 6, 2022.

70. Kim FJ, da Silva RD, Gustafson D, Nogueira L, Harlin T, Paul DL. Current issues in patient safety in surgery: a review. *Patient Saf Surg.* 2015;9:1-26. Accessed January 10, 2022. doi:10.1186/s13037-015-0067-4

71. National Academies of Sciences, Engineering, and Medicine (NASEM). *Improving Diagnoses in Healthcare.* Washington, DC: NASEM; 2015. Accessed January 10, 2022. https://www.nap.edu/catalog/21794/improving-diagnosis-in-health-care

72. Shook J. *Managing to Learn: Using the A3 Management Process to Solve Problems, Gain Agreement, Mentor and Lead.* Cambridge, MA: Lean Enterprise Institute; 2008.

73. Shook J. *A3 templates from Lean Enterprise Institute.* Cambridge, MA: Lean Enterprise Institute; 2010. Accessed January 10, 2022. http://www.lean.org/common/display/?o=1314

74. World Health Organization. Checklists save lives. Published 2008. Accessed December 14, 2021. https://apps.who.int/iris/bitstream/handle/10665/270232/PMC2647491.pdf?sequence=1&isAllowed=y

75. U.S. Department of Veterans Affairs. National Center for Patient Safety. Healthcare Failure Mode and Effect Analysis (HFMEATM). Published 2001. Accessed December 1, 2021. https://webarchive.library.unt.edu/eot2008/20090118025109/http://www.patientsafety.gov/SafetyTopics.html#HFMEA

76. Agency for Healthcare Research and Quality. Workflow assessment for health IT: Flowchart. Accessed April 24, 2022. https://digital.ahrq.gov/health-it-tools-and-resources/workflow-assessment-health-it-toolkit/all-workflow-tools/flowchart

77. Institute for Healthcare Improvement. Improvement advisor: professional development program. Accessed December 1, 2021. www.ihi.org/offerings/Training/ImprovementAdvisor/Pages/default.aspx

78. Govindarajan V. *The Three Box Solution.* Recorded Books Publisher; 2017.

79. Gaskin SP, Griffin A, Hauser HR, Katz GM, Klein RL. Voice of the customer. Massachusetts Institute of Technology. Accessed January 10, 2022. http://www.mit.edu/~hauser/Papers/Gaskin_Griffin_Hauser_et_al%20VOC%20Encyclopedia%202011.pdf

80. Institute for Healthcare Improvement. Science of improvement: forming the team. Accessed December 12, 2021. http://www.ihi.org/resources/Pages/HowtoImprove/ScienceofImprovementFormingtheTeam.aspx

81. Thompson L. *Making the Team: A Guide for Managers.* Upper Saddle River, NJ: Prentice Hall; 2000.

82. Xyrichis A, Ream E. Teamwork: A concept analysis. *J Adv Nurs.* 2008;61:232-241. doi:10.1111/j.1365-2648.2007.04496.x

83. Nancarrow SA, Booth A, Ariss S, Smith T, Enderby P, Roots A. Ten principles of good interdisciplinary work. *Hum Resour Hlth.* 2013;11:1-19. doi:10.1186/1478-4491-11-19

84. Greenberg J, Baron RA. *Behavior in Organizations.* 8th ed. Upper Saddle River, NJ: Prentice Hall; 2003.

85. Luecke R. *Creating Teams with an Edge: The Complete Skill Set to Build Powerful and Influential Teams.* Harvard Business Essentials Series. Boston, MA: Harvard Business School Press; 2004.

86. Schwarz M, Landis S, Rowe J. A team approach to quality improvement. *Fam Pract Man.* 1999;6:25-31.

87. Tuckman W. Developmental sequence in small groups. *Psych Bulletin.* 1965;63:384-399. doi:10.1037/h0022100

88. Scholtes PR, Joiner BL, Streibel B. *The Team Handbook.* 3rd ed. Madison, WI: Joiner/Oriel; 2003.

89. Campion MA, Medsker GJ, Higgs CA. Relations between work group characteristics and effectiveness: implications for designing effective work groups. *Personnel Psychol.* 1993;46:823-850. doi:10.1111/j.1744-6570.1993.tb01571.x

90. George JM. Leader positive mood and group performance: the case of customer service. *J App Social Psych.* 1995;25:778-794. doi:10.1111/j.1559-1816.1995.tb01775.x

91. Katzenbach JR, Smith DK. *The Wisdom of Teams: Creating the High-Performance Organization*. Boston, MA: Harvard Business School Press; 1994.

92. Saunier AM, Hawk EJ. Realizing the potential of teams through team-based rewards. *Compensation Benefits Rev.* 1994;10:24-33. doi:10.1177/088636879402600404

93. Wageman R. Critical success factors for creating superb self-managing teams. *Organizational Dynamics*. 1997;26:49-61. doi:10.1016/S0090-2616(97)90027-9

94. Agency for Healthcare Research and Quality. About TeamSTEPPS. Accessed December 1, 2021. http://teamstepps.ahrq.gov/about-2cl_3.htm

95. Agency for Healthcare Research and Quality. Essential instructional module and course slides. Accessed December 1, 2021. https://www.ahrq.gov/teamstepps/instructor/essentials/index.html

96. American Combatives, Inc. Airline crew safety training program. Published 2009. Accessed January 10, 2022. www.americancombatives.com/index.php?option=com_content&view=article&id=66&Itemid=79

97. Zuzelo PR. *The Clinical Nurse Specialist Handbook*. 2nd ed. Sudbury, MA: Jones and Bartlett; 2010.

98. Evans JR, Dean JW. *Total Quality: Management, Organization and Strategy*. 3rd ed. Mason, OH: Thomson South-Western; 2003.

99. George JM, Jones GR. *Organizational Behavior*. 3rd ed. Upper Saddle River, NJ: Prentice Hall; 2002.

100. Maslow A. *Motivation and Personality*. New York, NY: Harper and Row; 1954.

101. McClelland DC, Atkinson JW, Clark RA, Lowell EL. *The Achievement Motive*. New York, NY: Irvington; 1976.

102. Herzberg F, Maysner B, Snyderman B. *Works and the Nature of Man*. New York, NY: John Wiley & Sons; 1966.

103. Buckingham M, Coffman C. *First, Break All the Rules: What the World's Greatest Managers Do Differently*. New York, NY: Simon & Schuster; 1999.

104. Harter J, Adkins A. Employees want a lot more from their managers. *Gallup Business J.* 2015. Accessed January 10, 2022. http://www.gallup.com/businessjournal/182321/employees-lot-managers.aspx

105. Gaucher EJ, Coffey RJ. *Total Quality in Healthcare: From Theory to Practice*. San Francisco, CA: Jossey-Bass; 1993.

106. Gunawardena I. Reward management in healthcare. *Br J Healthcare Manage.* 2011;17(11):527-530.

107. Penso J. The Sharp Experience: a journey to healthcare excellence. *Group Pract J.* 2009;59(4):9-18. Accessed April 24, 2022. http://www.sharp.com/about/sharp-experience/

108. StoryCorps. About StoryCorps. Retrieved December 1, 2021. http://storycorps.org/about

109. Centers for Medicare & Medicaid Services. HCAHPS: Patients' perspectives of care survey. Published 2021. Accessed February 6, 2022. https://www.cms.gov/Medicare/Quality-Initiatives-Patient-Assessment-Instruments/HospitalQualityInits/HospitalHCAHPS

110. Senge PM. *Fifth Discipline: The Art and Practice of the Learning Organization*. New York, NY: Doubleday; 1990.

111. Institute of Medicine, Roundtable on Evidence-Based Medicine. *The Learning Healthcare System: Workshop Summary*. Washington DC: National Academies Press; 2007.

112. Deming WE. *Out of the Crisis*. Cambridge MA: MIT Press; 2000.

113. Gallup. The real future of work. Accessed November 29, 2021. https://www.gallup.com/workplace/241295/future-work-agility-download.aspx#ite-241304

114. National Association for Healthcare Quality. NAHQ's healthcare quality competency framework. Accessed November 29, 2021. https://nahq.org/nahq-intelligence/competency-framework/

115. Agency for Healthcare Research and Quality. AHRQ-sponsored continuing education activities. Published 2019. Accessed November 29, 2021. https://www.ahrq.gov/patient-safety/education/continuing-ed/index.html

116. Institute for Healthcare Improvement. IHI Open School. Published 2021. Accessed November 29, 2021. http://www.ihi.org/education/ihiopenschool/overview/Pages/default.aspx

117. Quality and Safety in Nursing. Faculty learning modules. Published 2020. Accessed November 29, 2021. https://qsen.org/faculty-resources/courses/learning-modules/

118. Kirkpatrick DL. *Another Look at Evaluating Training Programs*. Alexandria, VA: American Society for Training & Development; 1998.

119. Kirkpatrick Partners. The Kirkpatrick model. Published 2021. Accessed November 16, 2021. https://www.kirkpatrickpartners.com/the-kirkpatrick-model/

120. Phillips JJ. ROI. *Training Dev.* 1996;50:42-47.

121. Phillips JJ, Phillips PP. *ROI at Work: Best-Practice Case Studies from the Real World*. Alexandria VA: American Society for Training and Development (now the Association for Talent Development); 2005.

122. Schrimmer K, Williams N, Mercado S, Pitts J, Polancich S. Workforce competencies for healthcare quality professionals: leading quality-driven healthcare. *J Healthc Qual.* 2019;41(4):259-265.

123. Phillips JJ, Phillips PP. How to measure the return on your HR investment: using ROI to demonstrate your business impact. *Strategic HR Rev.* 2002;1(4):1-9. Accessed January 10, 2022. https://roiinstitute.net/wp-content/uploads/2017/02/How-to-Measure-the-Return-on-your-HR-Investment.pdf

## Suggested Readings

American Association of Critical Care Nurses. Beacon Award for Excellence. Published 2012. Accessed January 10, 2022. https://www.aacn.org/nursing-excellence/beacon-awards/get-started

American Nurses Credentialing Center. 2023 Magnet application manual. Accessed January 10, 2022. https://www.nursingworld.org/organizational-programs/magnet/

Bailit M, Dyer M. *Beyond Bankable Dollars: Establishing a Business Case for Improving Healthcare*. New York, NY: The Commonwealth Fund; 2004.

Barry R, Murcko AC, Brubaker CE. *The Six Sigma Book for Healthcare*. Chicago, IL: Health Administration Press; 2002.

Bayer ND, Taylor A, Atabek Z, Santolaya JL, Bamat TW, Washington N. Enhancing residents' warmth in greeting caregivers: an inpatient intervention to improve family-centered communication. *J Healthc Qual.* 2021;43(3):183-193. doi:10.1097/JHQ.0000000000000263

Becher EC, Chassin MR. Improving the quality of healthcare: who will lead? *Health Aff.* 2001;20:164-179. doi:10.1377/hlthaff.20.5.164

Beckerleg W, Hasimja-Saraqini D, Kwok ES, Hamdy N, Battram E, Wooller KR. Improving timeliness of internal medicine consults in the emergency department: a quality improvement initiative. *J Healthc Qual.* 2020;42(5):294-302. doi:10.1097/JHQ.0000000000000235

Berwick DM. Continuous improvement as an ideal in health care. *NEJM.* 1989;320:53-56. doi:10.1056/NEJM198901053200110

Berwick DM, Godfrey AB, Roessner J. *Curing Health Care.* San Francisco, CA: Jossey-Bass; 1990.

Berwick DM, Nolan TW, Whittington J. The triple aim: care, health and cost. *Health Aff.* 2008;27(3):759-769. doi:10.1377/hlthaff.27.3.759

Donabedian, A. *Exploration in Quality Assessment and Monitoring.* Ann Arbor, MI: Health Administration Press; 1980.

Fottler MD, Ford RC, Heaton CP. *Achieving Service Excellence: Strategies for Healthcare.* Chicago, IL: Health Administration Press; 2002.

Fried BJ, Johnson JA. *Human Resources in Healthcare: Managing for Success.* Chicago, IL: Health Administration Press; 2001.

Gaucher EJ, Coffey RJ. *Breakthrough Performance: Accelerating the Transformation of Health Care Organizations.* San Francisco, CA: Jossey-Bass; 2000.

Gawande A. *The Checklist Manifesto.* New York, NY: Metropolitan Books; 2009.

Gerard B, Robbins M, Putra J, et al. Applying Lean Six Sigma to improve depression screening and follow-up in oncology clinics. *J Healthc Qual.* 2021;43(3):153-162. doi:10.1097/JHQ.0000000000000294

Griffith JR, White KR. *Thinking Forward: Six Strategies for Highly Successful Organizations.* Chicago, IL: Health Administration Press; 2003.

Helmrich RL, Merritt AC. *Culture at Work in Aviation and Medicine.* Aldershot, England: Ashgate; 1998.

Holleran L, Baker S, Cheng C, et al. Using multisite process mapping to aid care improvement: an examination of inpatient suicide-screening procedures. *J Healthc Qual.* 2019;41(2):110-117. doi:10.1097/JHQ.0000000000000182

Hughes MC, Roedocker A, Ehli J. A quality improvement project to improve sepsis-related outcomes at an integrated healthcare system. *J Healthc Qual.* 2019;41(6):369-375. doi:10.1097/JHQ.0000000000000193

James BC. *Quality Management for Health Care Delivery.* Chicago, IL: The Hospital Research and Education Trust; 1990.

The Joint Commission. Center for Transforming Healthcare. Oro 2.0. Accessed January 28, 2022. www.centerfortransforminghealthcare.org

Juran JM. The QC circle phenomenon. *Industr Contr.* 1967;23:329-336.

Juran JM. Quality and its assurance: an overview. Presented at the Second NATO Symposium on Quality and Its Assurance; 1977; London, England.

Kollipara U, Varghese S, Mutz J, et al. Improving diabetic retinopathy screening among patients with diabetes mellitus using the define, measure, analyze, improve, and control process improvement methodology. *J Healthc Qual.* 2021;43(2):126-135. doi:10.1097/JHQ.0000000000000276

Konda SR, Johnson JR, Kelly EA, Egol KA. Pull the foley: improved quality for middle-aged and geriatric trauma patients without indwelling catheters. *J Healthc Qual.* 2020;42(6):341-351. doi:10.1097/JHQ.0000000000000241

Loudermilk RA, Steffen LE, McGarvey JS. Strategically applying new criteria for use improves management of peripheral intravenous catheters. *J Healthc Qual.* 2018;40(5):274-282.

Marszalek-Gaucher E, Coffey RJ. *Transforming Healthcare Organizations: How to Achieve and Sustain Organizational Excellence.* San Francisco, CA: Jossey-Bass; 1991.

National Academies of Sciences, Engineering, and Medicine. *Improving Diagnosis in Health Care.* Washington, DC: The National Academies Press; 2015. Accessed April 24, 2022. https://www.nationalacademies.org/our-work/diagnostic-error-in-health-care

Novak P, Bloodworth R, Green K, Chen J. Local health department activities to reduce emergency department visits for substance use disorders. *J Healthc Qual.* 2019;41(3):134-145. doi:10.1097/JHQ.0000000000000161

Plsek P, Omnias A. *Juran Institute Quality Improvement Tools: Problem Solving/Glossary.* Wilton, CT: Juran Institute; 1989.

Rever H. IIL blog: Applying the DMAIC steps to process improvement projects. "Define, measure, analyze, improve, control" is the roadmap to improving processes. Posted August 8, 2016. Accessed January 28, 2022. https://blog.iil.com/applying-the-dmaic-steps-to-process-improvement-projects/

Shinwa M, Bossert A, Chen I, et al. "THINK" before you order: multidisciplinary initiative to reduce unnecessary lab testing. *J Healthc Qual.* 2019;41(3):165-171. doi:10.1097/JHQ.0000000000000157

Tham E, Nandra K, Whang SE, Evans NR, Cowan SW. Postoperative telehealth visits reduce emergency department visits and 30-day readmissions in elective thoracic surgery patients. *J Healthc Qual.* 2021;43(4):204-213. doi:10.1097/JHQ.0000000000000299

Tyler JL, Biggs E. *Practical Governance.* Chicago, IL: Health Administration Press; 2001.

Wackerbarth SB, Bishop SS, Aroh AC. Lean in healthcare: time for evolution or revolution? *J Healthc Qual.* 2021;43(1):32-38. doi:10.1097/JHQ.0000000000000253

Walker M, Gay L, Raynaldo G, et al. Impact of a resident-centered interprofessional quality improvement intervention on acute care length of stay. *J Healthc Qual.* 2019;41(4):212-219. doi:10.1097/JHQ.0000000000000156

Warring CD, Pinkney JR, Delvo-Favre ED, et al. Implementation of a routine health literacy assessment at an academic medical center. *J Healthc Qual.* 2018;40(5):247-255. doi:10.1097/JHQ.0000000000000116

Wilson J, Swee M, Mosher H, et al. Using Lean Six Sigma to improve pneumococcal vaccination rates in a Veterans Affairs rheumatology clinic. *J Healthc Qual.* 2020;42(3):166-174. doi:10.1097/JHQ.0000000000000218

Wu S, Brown C, Black S, Garcia M, Harrington DW. Using Lean performance improvement for patient-centered medical home transformation at an academic public hospital. *J Healthc Qual.* 2019;41(6):350-361. doi:10.1097/JHQ.0000000000000197

Yaqoob M, Wang J, Sweeney AT, Wells C, Rego V, Jaber BL. Trends in avoidable hospitalizations for diabetes: experience of a large clinically integrated health care system. *J Healthc Qual.* 2019;41(3):125-133. doi:10.1097/JHQ.0000000000000145

Youl P, Philpot S, Theile DE. Cancer Alliance Queensland outcomes after rectal cancer surgery: a population-based study using quality indicators. *J Healthc Qual.* 2019;41(6):e90-e100. doi:10.1097/JHQ.0000000000000200

Young T, Brailsford S, Connell C, Davies R, Harper P, Klein JH. Using industrial processes to improve patient care. *BMJ.* 2004;328:162-164. doi:10.1136/bmj.328.7432.162

## Online Resources

### Agency for Healthcare Research and Quality (AHRQ)

- **Patients and Consumers**
  www.ahrq.gov/consumer/i ndex.html
- **Quality and Patient Safety Resources**
  www.ahrq.gov/qual/pips/issues.htm
- **Talking Quality: Reporting to Consumers on Health Care Quality**
  www.talkingquality.ahrq.gov/content/about/default.aspx

### ANCC Magnet Recognition Program

https://www.nursingworld.org/organizational-programs/magnet/

### Baldrige Performance Excellence Program

- **State, Local, and Regional Baldrige-Based Award Programs**
  www.nist.gov/baldrige/community/state_local.cfm
- **National Institute of Standards and Technology**
  www.nist.gov/baldrige/

### The Commonwealth Fund

http://www.commonwealthfund.org/

### The Leapfrog Group

- **Hospital Ratings and Reports**
  http://www.leapfroggroup.org/ratings-reports

### National Association for Healthcare Quality

- **Healthcare Quality Competency Framework**
  https://nahq.org/nahq-intelligence/competency-framework/

### Partnership for Patients

https://partnershipforpatients.cms.gov/

### Quality and Recognition Awards

- **AHCA/NCAL National Quality Award Program**
  www.ahcancal.org/quality_improvement/quality_award/pages/default.aspx

- **American Association of Critical-Care Nurses Beacon Award for Excellence**
  https://www.aacn.org/nursing-excellence/beacon-awards
- **National Association for Healthcare Quality—Professional Recognition Awards**
  https://nahq.org/individuals/manage-your-career/professional-recognition/awards/
- **National Quality Forum and Joint Commission John M. Eisenberg Patient Safety and Quality Awards**
  https://www.jointcommission.org/resources/awards/john-m-eisenberg-patient-safety-and-quality-award/
- **Union of Japanese Scientists and Engineers Deming Prize**
  http://www.juse.or.jp/english/
- **Utah State University Shingo Prize for Operational Excellence**
  https://shingo.org/awards/

### Society for Healthcare Epidemiology of America (SHEA)

https://shea-online.org/

### United Kingdom National Health Service

- **Falls Prevention**
  https://www.gov.uk/government/publications/falls-applying-all-our-health/falls-applying-all-our-health

### U.S. Department of Health & Human Services, Health Resources & Services Administration

https://www.hrsa.gov/

### U.S. News & World Report

- **Best Hospitals Rankings and Ratings**
  http://health.usnews.com/best-hospitals

# SECTION 6

# Health Data Analytics

Christy L. Beaudin, Pradeep S.B. Podila, and Deborah J. Bulger

## SECTION CONTENTS

# Introduction

Data analytics is a major component of quality improvement across the continuum of healthcare delivery. Data analytics is the process and practice of analyzing data to answer questions, draw valuable information and insights from the analysis, identify trends and patterns, and make data-informed decisions to improve quality and safety. Organizations invest heavily in building the infrastructure to enhance capabilities to gather, analyze, and report valid and reliable quality, safety, and performance data. This section describes the foundational steps to plan and deploy a data management system to support the quality improvement (QI) program, measure identification, measurement selection, sampling, balanced scorecards, dashboards, incorporating external data sources, identifying appropriate benchmarks, data collection, and data validation. There is discussion on the characteristics of data management systems, tools to display data, the application of statistical analysis, and how to interpret and compare data. How to interpret data is essential to the success of the organization. Finally, the principles presented throughout the section are applicable to reporting and setting goals to improve performance.

# Health and Data Informatics

The need for quality has always existed. However, the means for meeting that need—the processes of managing and improving for quality—have undergone extensive and progressive change.[1] Before the 20th century, managing quality was based on principles that included product inspection by consumers (still employed in today's world), and marketplaces concept, where buyers rely on trained, experienced craftsmanship.[2] When the Industrial Revolution spread to the United States, Americans followed European practices. The Industrial Revolution accelerated the growth of additional strategies, including written specifications for materials, processes, finished goods, and tests; measurement and the associated measuring instruments and testing laboratories; and standardization in different forms.

A new strategy emerged during World War II—statistical quality control. To improve the quality of military goods, the War Production Board sponsored training courses on the statistical techniques developed by the Bell System in the 1920s. W. E. Deming, a widely known proponent of QI during the 1980s, lectured at some of the War Production Board courses.[3] Participants of these courses organized themselves as the American Society for Quality Control. Now known as American Society for Quality, it was strongly oriented toward statistical quality control in its early years.[2]

While drivers for change in using data for decision making and process changes cut across the centuries, most innovations and disruptions occurred in the late 19th century and accelerated in the 21st century. These include the following:

- *1880s and 1890s.* Taylor analyzed workflows to improve economic efficiency, especially labor productivity. This scientific management theory was popular in the U.S. manufacturing industries, social science, and industrial engineering.
- *1940s.* Predictive analytics first started as governments began using the early computers.
- *1960s.* Computers became decision-making support systems. Major drivers for data analytics and information systems were the inception of the Medicare and Medicaid programs.
- *1970s.* Communication between departments in healthcare organizations and the need for discrete departmental systems were drivers. Relational databases were built. These are used by modern data services today. These databases store information in a hierarchical format to be accessed by anyone who knows what they are looking for. Relational databases allowed users to write in structured English query language and retrieve data from databases.
- *1980s.* The amount of data collected continued to grow significantly. Architecture of data warehouses helped transform data coming from operational systems into decision-making support systems. Diagnosis-related groups (DRGs) and reimbursement were launched.
- *1990s.* Data mining—the process of discovering patterns within large data sets—began. Page and Brin designed Google's search engine to search a specific website while processing and analyzing big data in distributed computers.
- *2000s.* Focus on value and outcomes-based reimbursement are major drivers for health data analytics and information systems. The Health Information Technology for Economic and Clinical Health Act (HITECH Act) lays the foundation of electronic health records (EHRs) across the industry. The Obama administration announced in 2012 the Big Data Research and Development Initiative with a $200 million commitment, citing a need to improve the ability to extract valuable insights

from data. The 21st Century Cures Act, signed into law in 2016, places the patient first in health technology. Innovative tools for better healthcare such as artificial intelligence and machine learning emerge as technologies with potential to transform the quality and safety of healthcare delivery.[4]

**Figure 6.1** outlines other milestones in the evolution of data analytics that have paved the way to the new era of analytics and consumerism in healthcare.

# Data Analytics

Data are a valued asset and a *currency* of the modern world. The use of data and information for improvement continues to rapidly evolve. If organizations are going to succeed, they need to compete on analytics.[5] This means exploring big data with emphasis on population health, targeted incentives, and value-based care. The analytics strategy uses all the data captured by the organization's disparate systems (e.g., electronic/paper medical records, human resources, finance, imaging) to support improvements in staffing, customer relationships, financial performance, services provided, product development and managing the supply chain. Davenport proposed that being successful would require an executive commitment to recognizing the importance of analytics capabilities, sophisticated information systems, and employing people with analytical skills.[6]

By 2013, McKinsey & Company reported that the big data revolution was substantially under way in healthcare.[6] Major health systems were using data to deliver better care, provide increased value, and innovate. Today, almost every segment of the healthcare industry invests in big data. The scale of the investment varies depending on how much the organizations can afford to allocate to expand analytic capabilities. Competing on analytics is necessary to survive in the current and future healthcare environment. This becomes particularly evident with the shift to population health and value-based care.

With the proliferation of EHRs and health information exchanges, large data sets are now available to healthcare quality professionals and health services researchers. The National Institutes of Health Big Data to Knowledge initiative acknowledges improvement areas for big data in healthcare, which impedes rapid translation of data into useful information at the service level (e.g., appropriate tools, data accessibility, and sufficient training). The four aims of the Big Data to Knowledge initiative in using big data include:

1. Facilitate broad use of biomedical digital assets by making them findable, accessible, interoperable, and reusable.
2. Conduct research and develop the methods, software, and tools needed to analyze biomedical big data.
3. Enhance training in the development and use of methods and tools necessary for biomedical big data science.
4. Support a data ecosystem that accelerates discovery as part of a digital enterprise.[7]

By utilizing a big data infrastructure, organizations can monitor populations (e.g., people with diabetes and asthma) to determine if patients are getting the right care at the right time in the right place. Further, it is possible to assess outcomes and drill down to specific providers and benchmark their performance.

What is big data? Big data consists of "extensive datasets—primarily in the characteristics of volume, velocity, and/or variability—that require a scalable architecture for efficient storage, manipulation, and analysis."[8(p5)] Based on current literature and practices, big data has 10 characteristics and dimensions.[9]

1. *Volume.* The physical size of the data and number of records are dramatically higher than what is managed in a traditional data system.
2. *Velocity.* Data are received in near or real time or as a continuous stream and should be made available to inform decisions as quickly as possible (predictive, prescriptive analytics).
3. *Variety.* Data include structured records, unstructured text, images (medical imaging), audio, video, and biomedical sensor traces.
4. *Veracity.* The vast amounts of structured and unstructured data come from sources that may be uncertain or imprecise or noisy (low veracity).[10(p1)] High veracity data benefit the organization since it may contain many records to support analysis and interpretation.
5. *Variability.* Data have multiple and multidimensional disparate data types and sources.
6. *Validity.* Data are found to be accurate for their intended use.
7. *Vulnerability.* Security concerns are managed to minimize data breaches.
8. *Volatility.* Costs and complexity of storage and retrieval process are magnified with big data. A sound data governance process is paramount (e.g., how long are the data stored to avoid performance-related issues).
9. *Visualization.* Meaningful visualizations with a billion data points using the traditional graphs are a

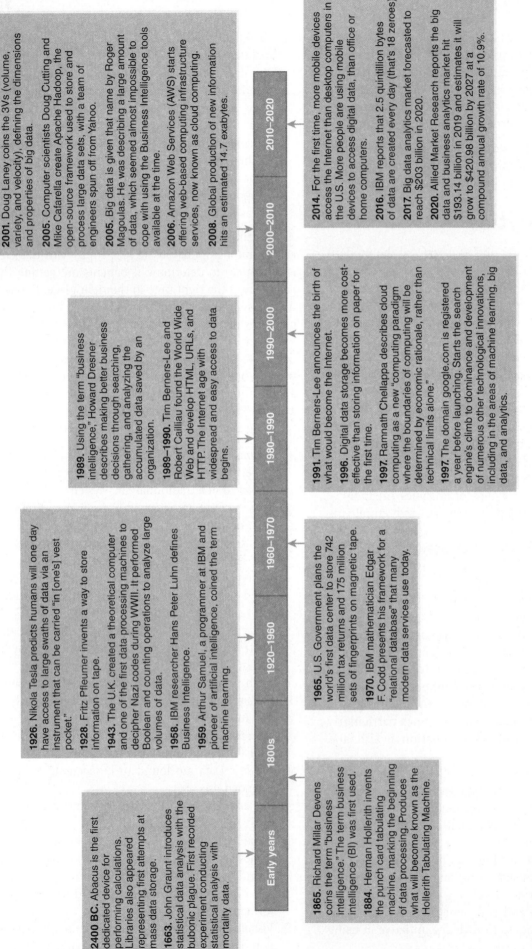

**Figure 6.1** Milestones in Data Analytics

Data from Marr B. A brief history of big data everyone should read. *World Economic Forum.* Published February 25, 2015. https://www.weforum.org/agenda/2015/02/a-brief-history-of-big-data-everyone-should-read/; Phillip A. A history and timeline of big data. Published April 1, 2021. https://www.techtarget.com/whatis/feature/A-history-and-timeline-of-big-data; and Foote KD. A brief history of analytics. Published September 20, 2021. Accessed February 19, 2022. https://www.dataversity.net/brief-history-analytics/

challenge. Find new ways to represent the multi-dimensional data.

10. *Value*. Data add value by helping organizations understand customers better, optimize the processes, and improve overall performance.

Hospitals that manage clinical bundles can use the data to evaluate the care delivered prior to discharge and to assess which postacute providers deliver the best outcomes at the lowest cost. For example, a hospital could look at 30-, 60-, and 90-day readmission rates for heart failure patients with care transitions to skilled nursing facilities, home healthcare, or home with no services. Choosing the organizations to partner with in the future might rely on performance. With a focus on data comes the need to accelerate the adoption and expansion of health information technology (IT).

Technology is widely recognized and was singled out as a key goal by the Health Care Delivery and Information Technology Subcommittee of the President's Information Technology Advisory Committee.[11] Studies suggest that the quality of healthcare can improve with the appropriate use of technology.[12,13] These studies specifically highlight the need to facilitate the transmission of clinical information contained in the medical record between healthcare providers. A second goal is use of health IT to achieve substantial economic and social benefits (such as reducing medical errors, eliminating unproductive healthcare expenditures, and improving quality of care). As of 2017, nearly 9 of 10 (86%) office-based physicians adopted any EHR, and four in five (80%) adopted a certified EHR. Since 2008, office-based physician adoption of any EHRs more than doubled, from 42% to 86%. The Office of the National Coordinator for Health Information Technology and the Centers for

Disease Control and Prevention (CDC) began tracking adoption of certified EHRs by office-based physicians in 2014.[14] Trends are shown in **Figure 6.2**. However, electronic health records systems in the United States lack interoperability and user satisfaction.[15]

A lack of standards hindered the adoption of IT tools in the healthcare industry.[16] The National Committee on Vital and Health Statistics began to standardize formats and data for the electronic exchange of patient health record information in 2002,[17] which progressed to the Healthcare Information and Management Systems Society developing a set of principles to support IT interoperability in the United States.[18] In addition, other organizations and task forces continue to work on international protocols and frameworks for data exchanges between heterogeneous systems in the healthcare industry. The industry Health Level 7, the Systemized Nomenclature of Medicine (SNOMED), and extensible markup language special interest groups were leaders in defining EHR standards. As these standards evolved, more comprehensive EHRs were developed and shared among all the providers in the healthcare system. EHRs pertain to records used and held by healthcare providers but can be referred to as *personal health records* geared more toward consumers.

Federal support increased since the 2004 announcement of the U.S. Department of Health & Human Services' 10-year plan to create a new national health information infrastructure to include an EHR for every American and a new network to link health records nationwide. Health IT and interoperable systems are requisites for healthcare delivery in the 21st century. Health IT potentially includes products such as EHRs, patient engagement tools such as personal health records; secure, private Internet portals; and health information exchanges. An Institute of

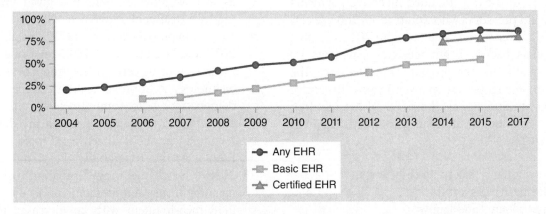

**Figure 6.2** Office-Based Physician Electronic Health Record Adoption

Reproduced from Office of the National Coordinator for Health Information Technology. Office-based physician electronic health record adoption, health IT quick-stat #50. U.S. Department of Health and Human Services. August 6, 2021. Accessed March 17, 2022. https://www.healthit.gov/data/quickstats/office-based-physician-electronic-health-record-adoption

Medicine (now the National Academy of Medicine) report examined the state of the art in system safety and opportunities to build safer systems, concluding that safety is an emergent property of a larger system that considers not just the software but also how it is used by clinicians.[19] Considerations for safe IT systems include:

- The sociotechnical system:
  - Technology (software, hardware)
  - People (clinicians, patients)
  - Processes (workflow)
  - Organization (capacity, IT applications, incentives)
  - External environment (regulations, public opinion)
- Safer implementation and use of health IT are part of a complex, dynamic process with shared responsibility between vendors and healthcare organizations.
- Poor user-interface design, poor workflow, and complex data interfaces threaten patient safety.
- Lack of system interoperability is a barrier to improving clinical decisions and patient safety.
- Constant, ongoing commitment to safety is needed—from acquisition to implementation and maintenance—to achieve safer, more effective care.[19(ppS2-S4)]

The HITECH Act was enacted under Title XIII of the American Recovery and Reinvestment Act of 2009 (Pub L No. 111-5). Under the HITECH Act, the U.S. Department of Health & Human Services authorized spending $25.9 billion to promote and expand the adoption of health IT. The HITECH Act also established meaningful use of interoperable and incentivized EHR adoption in the healthcare system as a critical national goal.

Title IV of the Act included incentive payments for Medicaid providers who would adopt and use certified EHRs over 6 years beginning in 2011. Eligible professionals had to begin receiving payments by 2016 to qualify for the program. For Medicare, the maximum payments were set over 5 years. To receive the EHR stimulus money, the HITECH Act required providers to show meaningful use of certified EHR technology to

- improve quality, safety, and efficiency;
- reduce health disparities;
- engage patients and family;
- improve care coordination and population and public health; and
- maintain privacy and security of patient health information.[20]

Meaningful use compliance results include better clinical outcomes, improved population health outcomes, increased transparency and efficiency, empowered consumers, and more robust research data on health systems. Meaningful use outlines specific objectives that eligible professionals and hospitals must achieve to qualify for the financial incentive programs. The Centers for Medicare & Medicaid Services (CMS) established the Medicare and Medicaid EHR Incentive Programs (now known as the Medicare Promoting Interoperability Program) to encourage eligible providers and organizations to adopt, implement, upgrade, and demonstrate meaningful use of certified electronic health record technology. These objectives are defined as the stages of meaningful use intended to guide organizations in their adoption of standards and requirements.[21]

- *Stage 1: Data capture and sharing (2011–2012).* Stage 1 established requirements for the electronic capture of clinical data, including providing patients with electronic copies of health information. This Stage set the foundation by establishing requirements for the electronic capture of patient data such as demographic information, family medical history, and clinical data, including providing patients with electronic copies of health information.
- *Stage 2: Advance clinical processes (2014).* Stage 2 expanded upon the Stage 1 criteria with a focus on advancing clinical processes and ensuring that the meaningful use of EHRs supported the aims and priorities of the U.S. National Quality Strategy. This Stage encouraged continuous quality improvement at the point of care and the exchange of information in the most structured format possible between providers and patients as well as providers within a given practice to improve treatment adherence.
- *Stage 3: Improved Outcomes (2017).* Established in 2017 and because of the 2015 final rule, Stage 3 focuses on using certified electronic health record technology to improve health outcomes. Further demonstrating its commitment to the interoperability and exchange of healthcare data, CMS renamed the EHR Incentive Programs to the Promoting Interoperability Programs in April 2018. This change moved programs beyond the meaningful use requirements to a new phase of EHR measurement with an increased focus on interoperability and improving patient access to health information. There are Stage 3 objectives and measures for eligible professionals and eligible hospitals, critical access hospitals, and

**Table 6.1** Stage 3 Objectives and Measures for Medicaid EHR (Eligible Professionals)

Eligible Professional
Medicaid EHR Incentive Program
Stage 3 Objectives and Measures
Table of Contents
Updated: August 2017

**Eligible Professional Objectives and Measures**

| | |
|---|---|
| **(1)** | Protect electronic protected health information (ePHI) created or maintained by the CEHRT through the implementation of appropriate technical, administrative, and physical safeguards. |
| **(2)** | Generate and transmit permissible prescriptions electronically (eRx). |
| **(3)** | Implement clinical decision support (CDS) interventions focused on improving performance on high-priority health conditions. |
| **(4)** | Use computerized provider order entry (CPOE) for medication, laboratory, and diagnostic imaging orders directly entered by any licensed healthcare professional, credentialed medical assistant, or a medical staff member credentialed to and performing the equivalent duties of a credentialed medical assistant, who can enter orders into the medical record per state, local, and professional guidelines. |
| **(5)** | Patient Electronic Access - The EP provides patients (or patient-authorized representative) with timely electronic access to their health information and patient-specific education. |
| **(6)** | Coordination of Care - Use CEHRT to engage with patients or their authorized representatives about the patient's care. |
| **(7)** | Health Information Exchange - The EP provides a summary of care record when transitioning or referring their patient to another setting of care, receives or retrieves a summary of care record upon the receipt of a transition or referral or upon the first patient encounter with a new patient, and incorporates summary of care information from other providers into their EHR using the functions of CEHRT. |
| **(8)** | Public Health Reporting - The EP is in active engagement with a public health agency or clinical data registry to submit electronic public health data in a meaningful way using certified EHR technology, except where prohibited, and in accordance with applicable law and practice. |

Note: CEHRT = Certified EHR Technology
Reproduced from Centers for Medicare & Medicaid Services. Eligible professional Medicaid EHR incentive program stage 3 objectives and measures. Updated August 2017. Accessed February 15, 2022. https://www.cms.gov/Regulations-and-Guidance/Legislation/EHRIncentivePrograms/Downloads/TableofContents_EP_Medicaid_Stage3.pdf

dual-eligible hospitals. **Table 6.1** displays the objectives and measures eligible professionals for Medicaid.

The 21st Century Cures Act was signed into law on December 13, 2016. This places the patient first in health technology and puts them in charge of their health records.[22] The intent behind the Cures Act was to

- enable patients to make choices that work for them by increasing transparency into the cost and outcomes of care;
- allow patients to shop for and understand their options in getting medical care;
- provide patients with convenient, easy access and visualizations of health information through smartphone apps; and

- support an app economy that provides innovation and choice to patients, physicians, hospitals, payers, and employers.[23]

With the Cures Act final rule, there are a variety of benefits to participants in the U.S. healthcare system as shown in **Figure 6.3**.

In summary, while the HITECH Act (2009) laid the foundation of EHRs across the industry, the Cures Act (2016) focused on using EHRs to get better healthcare, population health, and public health.

The impact of the federal initiatives that supplied the stimulus funding and the requirements for meaningful use (promoting interoperability) benefit the use of data for quality, safety, and performance improvement efforts. Certified EHRs can potentially be a rich source of standardized and structured information.

| The Difference for Patients | The Difference for Doctors and Hospitals | The Difference for Health IT Developers |
|---|---|---|
| **Providing Access to Their Chart in Novel and Modern Ways** Provides patients with control of their health care and their medical record through smartphones and modern software apps. There will likely be disease- and condition-specific apps that offer patients complementary services (i.e., patient education, progress metrics, and community support). | **Making Responses to Patient Data Requests Easy and Inexpensive** Patients will be able to access their health information from EHRs using an app of their choice in an automated fashion without any additional action on the part of the provider other than the initial effort to enable the technical capabilities. | **Minimizing API Development and Maintenance Costs** Makes significant effort to minimize developer costs. The certified API requirements focus on standardized data sets, notably the U.S. Core Data for Interoperability (USCDI). Most major health IT developers already have the necessary infrastructure (i.e., HL7® FHIR® servers). |
| **Protecting Patient Privacy and Security** Industry standard technical security requirements are included as part of certification. They enable patients to choose which data in their electronic medical record they authorize an app to receive. Health care providers and other stakeholders are permitted to educate patients on privacy and security matters without implicating information blocking. | **Allowing Choice of Software** Allows providers to choose software that helps them provide better care. Providers should be allowed to benefit from a vibrant competitive marketplace where the choice of software services lies with them and not a health IT developer. | **Respecting Intellectual Property** Certified EHR developers are permitted to first negotiate agreeable terms in the open market for the licensing of their intellectual property (IP) that is needed for the access, exchange, and use of EHI. If they are unable to reach agreement, developers can meet their regulatory obligations through specified alternative means. Health IT developers also may restrict certain communications under the Certification Program that include IP so long as the restrictions are no broader than necessary and meets other specified limitations. |
| **Enabling the Ability to Shop for Care and Manage Costs** Expands patient choice in health care through increased transparency about care quality and costs. Mobile apps will be used to deliver information to patients to assist in making decisions. | **Improving Patient Safety** Permits the sharing of patient safety concerns arising from certified EHRs. Protects patients and others by recognizing practices that prevent the sharing and use of health information that may cause harm through the Preventing Harm Exception for information blocking. Supports improved patient matching through the exchange of the USCDI and its patient demographic data elements. | |

**Figure 6.3** Why the Cures Act Matters

Reproduced from The Office of the National Coordinator for Health Information Technology. The ONC Cures Act final rule. U.S. Department of Health & Human Services. 2020. Accessed February 15, 2022. https://www.healthit.gov/sites/default/files/cures/2020-03/TheONCCuresActFinalRule.pdf

Quality, safety, and performance improvement teams can use this information to measure the impact of interventions and assess patient clinical outcomes. See the *Quality Review and Accountability* section for discussion of value-based programs related to measurement and improvement.

For the healthcare quality professional, shepherding the new era requires attentiveness to an evolving data landscape shaped by policy and the change in stakeholder appetite for improved processes and outcomes. This includes developing a consciousness about what's ahead and anticipating change through a systems framework. Data's impact on healthcare strategy and decision making is evident. Healthcare quality professionals should be mindful of the emerging and evolving areas described here.

- *Data lakes.* A data lake is a storage repository with raw data in its native format. Data lakes are the key for storing and sorting big data. They allow multiple points of access and collection while preserving the data in their original raw form. Data lakes can offer solutions and better ways to the following:
  - *Ingest and transform.* Move and convert different kinds and formats of data.

- *Persist and access.* Ensure data are secure, readily discoverable by the user, easily scaled, and accessible as needed.
- *Analyze and use data science.* Uncover insights and trends within data.[24]
- *Predictive analytics.* Used by clinical and nonclinical staff (finance departments, human resources, information technology, and supply chain) to identify new ways to improve the overall operations of the organization. Predictive models can improve efficiencies for operational management of healthcare business operations, accuracy of diagnosis and treatment of health conditions, and increased insights to enhance population health management.[25]
- *Artificial intelligence (AI).* Organizations can utilize both structured and unstructured data sources to develop new AI algorithms to address issues related to data fragmentation and data quality. They can help predict health trajectories, recommend treatments, and automate administrative tasks. Clinical AI tools show promise in the following:
  - Predicting health trajectories of patients, recommending treatments, guiding surgical care, monitoring patients, and supporting population health management (i.e., efforts to improve the health outcomes of a community). AI is at varying stages of maturity and adoption except for population health management tools.
  - Reducing provider burden and increasing efficiency by recording digital notes, optimizing

operational processes, and automating laborious tasks. These tools are also at varying stages of maturity and adoption, ranging from emerging to widespread.[26]

**Figure 6.4** illustrates the use of AI as an administrative tool.

- *Smart operations.* Smart operating systems digitally rewire healthcare operations to orchestrate meaningful outcomes. Smart operations look beyond command and control to orchestrate several programs including hospital at home, discharge management (discharge as a service), care orchestration (enhanced recovery after surgery, heart failure, care transitions, level of care, and palliative care), and staffing orchestration (huddle automation and staffing management).[27]

**Box 6.1** lists key points in historical perspectives and the new era of data analytics.

### Box 6.1  Key Points: Historical Perspectives and New Era of Data Analytics

- Medicare and Medicaid were major drivers for healthcare data analytics and information systems in the 1960s.
- The 10 dimensions of big data are volume, velocity, variety, veracity, variability, validity, vulnerability, volatility, visualization, and value.
- The HITECH Act laid the foundation for EHRs across the industry.
- The 21st Century Cures Act puts patients first in health technology and in charge of their health records.

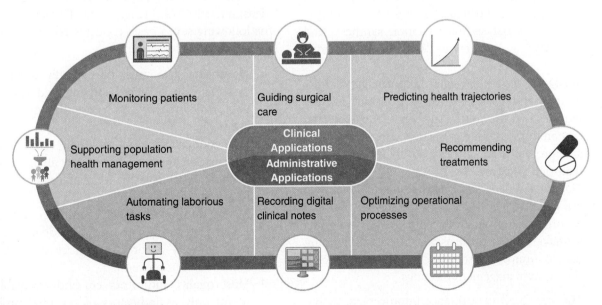

**Figure 6.4** AI as an Administrative Tool

Reproduced from U.S. Government Accountability Office. Artificial intelligence in health care: benefits and challenges of technologies to augment patient care. 2020. Accessed February 15, 2022. https://www.gao.gov/products/gao-21-7sp

# Data for Improvement

Healthcare quality professionals are constantly challenged by sifting through and interpreting the vast amount of data available and then distinguishing what is relevant, meaningful, and important to plan a course of action. Simply, why do certain things happen and how to use data to improve? Nutley and Reynolds described eight activities to encourage and improve the use of health data to strengthen health systems.[28] These include the following:

1. *Assess and improve the data use context*. Organizational and behavioral factors influence whether an organization uses data to inform decision making and whether it promotes a culture of information.
2. *Engage data users and data producers*. Lack of communication is a barrier in those who produce data and those who need data to make decisions.
3. *Improve data quality*. For managers to make sound decisions for improving processes, they need to be confident that the data they are relying on is sound—accurate, complete, and timely.
4. *Improve data availability*. This includes data synthesis, data communication, and access to data. A management information system can facilitate data being available to decision makers.
5. *Identify information needs*. Various stakeholders have various data and information needs, and their audiences may be different. Healthcare quality professionals can help managers prioritize those data that will be useful in monitoring and evaluating a program or service.
6. *Build capacity in the data use core competencies*. Frontline staff and managers need to be competent in data analysis, interpretation, synthesis, and presentation, and how to develop data-informed recommendations.
7. *Strengthen the organization's data demand and use infrastructure*. Data-informed decision making requires that the culture supports the use of data, that an infrastructure exists to ensure data quality, and processes are in place to obtain and report data-rich outcomes.
8. *Monitor, evaluate, and communicate results of data use interventions*. Data must be top of mind in an organization and value placed on using data to make important decisions. Successes in using data to improve must be intentional and explicitly shared in management meetings.

The key to all performance improvement activities is the collection of meaningful data and the communication of useful information. The art of quality, safety, and performance improvement is to communicate the right information the right way at the right time to the right people. There is a distinction between data and information.

- *Data* are the representation of things, facts, concepts, and instructions stored in a defined format and structure on a passive medium (e.g., paper, computer, microfilm). For leadership to be confident that the data they are using to make decisions are sound, there must be an emphasis on data quality. The top four processes for data are application, collection, warehousing, and analysis. The American Health Information Management Association defined 10 characteristics of data quality (**Table 6.2**).
- *Information* is created from meaning attached to data. Data are translated into results and useful statements for decision making. For information to be meaningful, consider data within the context of how obtained and intent for their use.[29,30]

Information contained in data helps leaders to focus on goals and proof points as well as demonstrating value.[31] See **Table 6.3** for how data can help leaders.

A major barrier to success of data analytics is thinking that this complex topic is only understood by statisticians and subject matter experts. As data are more accessible to individuals outside of data domain, it is important for everyone across an organization to have an appreciation of data literacy and the data journey. Data journey steps are shown in **Table 6.4**.

The American Hospital Association's Quality Measurement and Management Project developed the following seven basic concepts related to quality-management information:

1. Healthcare data must be carefully defined and systematically collected and analyzed in their full context before they can be useful in quality management.
2. Tremendous amounts of healthcare data and information are available, but not all of it is useful for quality control, quality management, or quality improvement.
3. Mature information revolves around clearly established patterns of care, not individual cases. Patterns identify a consistent process that can be studied and improved.
4. Most quality indicators currently available are useful only as indicators of potential problems and not as definitive measures of quality.

**Table 6.2** Data Quality Characteristics

| Data Quality Characteristic | Meaning |
| --- | --- |
| Accuracy | Data represent correct and valid values that are attached to the correct patient record. |
| Accessibility | Data items easily obtained with legal access.<br>Strong protections and controls built into the process. |
| Comprehensiveness | All required data items included.<br>Entire scope of data is collected with documented intentional limitations. |
| Consistency | Data are reliable and the same across applications. |
| Currency | Data are up to date. |
| Definition | Clear definitions are provided so current and future data users will know what the data mean.<br>Each data element has clear meaning and acceptable values. |
| Granularity | Attributes and values of data are defined with the correct level of detail. |
| Precision | Data values are just large enough to support the application or process. |
| Relevancy | Data are meaningful to the performance of the process or application for which they are collected. |
| Timeliness | Timeliness is determined by how the data are used and by their context. |

Modified from The American Health Information Management Association (AHIMA). Statement on quality healthcare data and information. 2007. Accessed February 12, 2022. http://bok.ahima.org/doc?oid=101304#.WSXX5WgrKM8

5. Integrating multiple measures provides a clearer picture of quality of care in an organization or system of care.
6. Developing outcomes information without monitoring the process of care, when warranted, is inefficient because it cannot lead directly to improvement in quality.
7. Cost and quality are inseparable issues.[32(p28)]

Bader and Bohr translated the seven concepts to a seven-step strategy for the interpretation and use of quality-of-care information, which are still relevant today and outlined in the following sections.[32]

## Step 1. Planning and Organizing for Data Collection, Interpretation, and Use

Planning for collection and utilization of internally and externally generated data leads to a higher likelihood of success. Anticipating barriers, identifying responsibilities, and laying the groundwork for multidisciplinary and interprofessional collaboration will smoothly guide the process toward improvement. Consider whether the data will be quantitative (e.g., clinical values) or qualitative (e.g., a review of clinical notes). Qualitative data require a rigorous process that delineates exactly where to find and capture data. In addition, a data dictionary that defines all data elements and calculations of indicators can be invaluable to improve the communication of information.

## Step 2. Verifying and Correcting Data

The purpose of verifying data is to identify data limitations and opportunities to improve internal systems that lead to better data quality, provide an opportunity to correct data (e.g., find missing data), and to review data to become familiar with it. For qualitative data, it is necessary to establish inter-rater reliability to ensure that staff who reviewed clinical records consistently captured the same information.

## Step 3. Identifying and Presenting Findings

The first step in this process is to perform preliminary data analysis, often descriptive analyses. When conducting this type of analysis, several questions should be asked.

**Table 6.3** How Data Help Leaders

### Better Care

| Mission and vision | ▪ Assess the extent to how the organization is achieving the mission, vision, and values<br>▪ Develop a vision and evaluate program achievements |
|---|---|
| Clinical quality | ▪ Understand the mechanism for provider appointment and recredentialing while knowing their performance review process is effective<br>▪ Decide on individual credentialing recommendations |
| Performance improvement | ▪ Determine priorities for continuous improvements<br>▪ Monitor aspects of organizational performance and take corrective action<br>▪ Help the governing body evaluate and improve its performance |

### Smarter Spending

| Strategic planning | ▪ Prioritize strategic goals, including programs, to support or discontinue<br>▪ Judge progress toward strategic goals and objectives<br>▪ Identify the need for policy implementation effectiveness |
|---|---|
| Resources | ▪ Understand changes in community needs, financial resources, and technology<br>▪ Weigh long- and short-term financial viability<br>▪ Weigh the impact of budgetary decisions on quality of care/service<br>▪ Secure an organization's resources, efficiency, and effectiveness based on accurate information |

### Healthier People

| Individual health improvement | ▪ Managing one's own health and well-being<br>▪ Making personal choices that reduce risk of harm, injury, illness and/or death<br>▪ Managing long-term conditions particularly for the frail or persons with multiple long-term conditions<br>▪ Navigating the end of life |
|---|---|
| Community health improvement | ▪ Determine goals for improving the health status of the community<br>▪ Evaluate the effectiveness of programs designed to improve health |

### Joy in Work

| Meaning and purpose | ▪ Engaging colleagues in efforts to improve joy in work and address issues identified by the workforce<br>▪ Personal resilience (i.e., the ability to bounce back quickly from setbacks) and stress management<br>▪ Taking care of oneself is part of a larger systems approach to joy in work, not a standalone solution |
|---|---|
| Recognition and accomplishments | ▪ Celebration of individual and team accomplishments<br>▪ Utilize routine and reliable practices to amplify feelings of gratitude |

Data from O'Rourke LM, Bader BS. An illustrative quality and performance report for the governing board. *Qual Lett Healthc Lead*. 1993;5(2):15-28; Perlo J, Balik B, Swensen S, Kabcenell A, Landsman J, Feeley D. *IHI Framework for Improving Joy in Work*. IHI white paper. Cambridge, MA: Institute for Healthcare Improvement; 2017; and Whittington JW, Nolan K, Lewis N, Torres T. Pursuing the Triple Aim: the first 7 years. *Milbank Q*. 2015 Jun;93(2):263-300.

- Who receives the data? For what purpose?
- Are the data likely to be interpreted (or misinterpreted) correctly?
- How do these data compare with other organizations (mortality rates) or with previously trended internal data (healthcare-associated infection rates)?

- What is the trend or pattern over time? Improving, static, or degrading?
- Is there opportunity for improvement?

Translate data into meaningful information using different techniques while presenting information in a clear and concise manner.

**Table 6.4** Steps in the Data Journey

| Data Step | Details | Resources/Tools | Personas |
|---|---|---|---|
| Generation | Gather data from both internal and external sources | Structured data<br>Unstructured data | Organization wide |
| Storage | Store the gathered data | MS SQL server<br>Oracle<br>Excel | Organization wide |
| Processing | Extract the data from sources, transform it into a uniform format, and load it into databases | Data pipeline<br>Data integration<br>Data warehouse | Data engineers |
| Aggregation | Pool the data sources required to answer a question of interest | Data warehouse<br>Data lake | Data engineers<br>Business intelligence (BI) developers |
| Modeling | Create relationships between data and tables | Tables<br>Views | BI analysts<br>BI developers |
| Visualization | Develop visualizations for an easier view of the data | Machine learning<br>Natural language processing | BI analysts |
| Analytics | Extend analytics by creating applications easily accessed by customers | Actionable insights | BI developers |

Data from content published in Murray A. The data journey: from raw data to insights. Published December 16, 2020. Accessed February 6, 2022. https://www.sisense.com/blog/the-data-journey-from-raw-data-to-insights/

## Step 4. Ongoing Study and Recommendations for Change

When further study of the data is warranted, a variety of methods are available. These include variation analysis, review of additional data, retrospective medical reviews, and process analysis. Variation analysis seeks an explanation for statistically significant differences. These differences may reflect clinical factors, patient characteristics, data collection (such as sampling characteristics), or organizational characteristics (such as staffing). Consider collecting and reviewing additional data to completely understand variations. The review can include focused/intensive retrospective review and process analysis as described below.

- *Focused/intensive retrospective review.* This refers to an activity for which processes or outcomes use preestablished criteria or indicators. For example, a hospital may show a steady increase in mortality rates. Additional data related to hospital case mix, diagnostic categories, mortality within a specified time from date of hospital admission, and other hospital characteristics are used to fully interpret the data.
- *Process analysis.* This refers to a method of analyzing data using industrial performance improvement techniques. Process analysis occurs when a group diagrams a healthcare process. The group then measures process variations and looks for ways to improve the process and the administrative or clinical outcome.

## Step 5. Taking Action

*Taking action* implies that people, teams, departments, and committees are empowered to make decisions and implement changes based on information discovered through data analysis. Actions may occur in forms such as education and training of staff, simulation, reporting of findings to outside vendors or the public, changes in organizational or departmental policies and processes, and changes in practice patterns.

## Step 6. Monitoring Performance

Monitoring performance entails monitoring the influence and effectiveness of a quality, safety, or performance improvement action and involves the collection of additional data. Consider the following questions.

- Were proposed changes implemented? To what extent?
- How could adherence to process changes be enhanced?
- What effect are the changes having on patient outcomes? Financial outcomes? Population health outcomes? Are these the desired effects?
- Are process changes modified and then tested further, communicated on a wider scale, tested for a longer period before drawing conclusions, or ended because they are ineffective?

## Step 7. Communicating Results

Three basic barriers to the interpretation of data and use of information are statistical factors, human factors, and organizational factors.

1. Statistical factors include flawed data, missing data, untimely data, poorly displayed data, and data that are difficult to integrate with other organizational data.
2. Human factors include fear of the data; resentment of external data; unrealistic expectations about data (including the myth that all data must be perfect); and lack of training related to planning, organizing, and analyzing data.
3. Organizational factors include data overload; a poor data retrieval system; lack of resources (time, people, money); and poor relationships among administration, physicians, and staff.

Communication is an integral component in each of the previous steps. Striving for healthcare quality is a journey. Performance improvement begins with the communication of where an organization is and where it is going. Effective communication requires providing information to the appropriate staff so they can act. Consider which audiences and methods of communication will be most effective in bringing about change (e.g., peer review committee, medical staff committee, board committee). Depending on the findings, audiences may include frontline clinical staff for patient issues, administration for service delivery failures, or the human resources department for staffing concerns. See the *Performance and Process Improvement* and

*Quality Review and Accountability* sections for additional details on data for improvement.

# Information Systems

Information systems support a variety of activities within healthcare organizations. Effective processes for information gathering and dissemination include considerations such as

- identifying who needs to know the information (this may include various stakeholders such as senior management, board members, customers, physicians, other providers, etc.);
- determining which information stakeholders need to know to make decisions related to improving the quality of care; and
- developing a system that ensures the right people receive the right information at the right time in the right way.[33]

Areas commonly supported include quality, safety, and performance improvement; cost control and productivity; patient registration; utilization management; program planning and evaluation; external reporting; research; and education. Information systems groupings are clinical, diagnostics (e.g., laboratory, imaging), pharmacy, patient experience, administrative, human resources, financial, and decision support.

An organization, such as a primary care clinic, needs to select the best health information system and technology that supports quality, safety, and performance improvement practices to "enable the practice to measure, track, and share health care delivery performance measures and monitor how refinements to clinical workflow process (both internal and external) affect the overall patients experience and care coordination across care settings, while seeking to reduce costs and improve health outcomes."[34(p4)]

An organization can use a checklist to evaluate various system options. While buy or build were common in the 1990s, rarely do organizations currently build their own information management systems. If an organization chooses to buy or build its own, there are considerations when looking at functionality, developing the architecture, and implementing and maintaining the system. When looking to select a system for the organization, there is core information to gather such as

- vendor profile and references;
- market characteristics;
- product specifications;
- an implementation plan with estimated timeline;

- security and technology including hardware requirements and configuration options; and
- cost estimates.

See **Table 6.5** for systems procurement considerations.

Design information systems gather, process, store, integrate, and disseminate information to inform decision making (e.g., clinical decisions, business operations). Systems are classified by characteristics such as

- transactions and decision support,
- software and hardware, and
- users and outputs.

---

**Table 6.5** Information Systems Procurement Checklist

| | |
|---|---|
| ☐ | What are the vendor's market characteristics, such as number of years as a vendor, live sites, size of existing user base, and retention rate? |
| ☐ | Does the system provide for capture, storage, and retrieval of clinical and financial information from a variety of sources (e.g., health information management, medical records/EHRs, admission, discharge, transfer, billing, laboratory, pharmacy, blood bank, operating room schedule, and radiology)? |
| ☐ | What expertise does the organization have in-house to implement and customize the system, database software, analytic tools, and hardware? |
| ☐ | How much money and time must be invested to procure this expertise? |
| ☐ | Does the system interface with the organization's existing information systems? |
| ☐ | Do health information management; IT; or quality, safety, and performance improvement staff have the full industry knowledge required to develop and deploy the information system to support clinical and financial needs of the organization (architecture, nomenclature, and other national standards)? |
| ☐ | Does the system allow for the establishment of triggers or thresholds for important measures of performance and signal an alert when these thresholds are exceeded? |
| ☐ | Can staff provide necessary documentation, training, support, and maintenance for the system on an ongoing basis? If so, will changing priorities interfere with the sustainability of the program? |
| ☐ | Does the system have critical alerts such as abnormal laboratory values, drug interactions, and others to promote patient safety (e.g., identifying serious reportable or never events)? |
| ☐ | How will the organization be able to sustain the system? Are resources available to keep the program up to date in an ever-changing clinical, regulatory, and accreditation environment? |
| ☐ | Does the system have rules-based processing or an algorithm (i.e., the system automatically provides a complete list of cases that meet or fail criteria)? |
| ☐ | Is there flexibility for future data demands of accreditation organizations, regulatory agencies, third-party payers, employers, and other external stakeholders? |
| ☐ | Is the system flexible enough to allow for prospective, concurrent, and retrospective reviews? |
| ☐ | Will there be long-term dedicated resources to enhance such an application for quality, safety, and performance improvement (including various functions such as credentialing, provider profiling)? |
| ☐ | Does the system support accreditation and regulatory reporting requirements? |
| ☐ | Does the system have integrated analytic capabilities like AI and machine learning, data management, and patient- or program-level dashboards? |
| ☐ | Does the system have the capability for data mining reporting or statistical analysis? |
| ☐ | Is the more cost-effective alternative for the organization to develop applications in-house or purchase software dedicated to needs? |
| ☐ | Does the system allow for multiple users to access the same programs at the same time? |
| ☐ | Is it an open operating system (a system that enables users to operate on a variety of different hardware platforms)? |
| ☐ | Does the system have networking capabilities? |
| ☐ | Will the system display data in graphic form (patient dashboards, provider tasks)? |
| ☐ | Is there the capability for drill-down analysis of outcomes? |
| ☐ | Does the system allow access to reports via a secure Intranet website within the organization? |

Several types of information systems are described in the following sections.

## Administrative Support Information System

The administrative support information system supports day-to-day operations in healthcare organizations, including

- financial information systems (payroll, accounts payable, patient accounting, cost accounting, forecasting, budgeting, and asset management);
- human resources information systems (recruitment, employee record, time and attendance, position and performance [talent] management, labor analysis, turnover, and absenteeism); and
- office automation systems (word processing, email, scheduling, facsimile, scanning, and spreadsheets).

## Management Information System

A management information system (MIS) can contain both the manual and the automated methods that provide information for decision making. Other names for an MIS used interchangeably include data-processing structure, medical information system, hospital information system, or decision support system. As commonly used, the term refers to an automated or computerized system. Information plays a key role in decision making in each stage of the management process. Whether a staff member or manager is trying to establish goals; estimate resources; allocate resources; evaluate a quality, safety, or performance process; or monitor a system, access to accurate and timely information is an ongoing requirement of any MIS. The quality of judgments and decisions directly correlates with availability and reliability of data and its synthesis into meaningful, timely information.

Choices for the design or flow of information are so important that they can be a determining factor in the survival of a patient or organization. Although accurate and timely healthcare information provides the rationale for management decisions, this often is not the case. O'Rourke and Bader explain that information often is incomplete, confusing, and not sufficiently relevant to the organization's mission, strategic goals, or customer and stakeholder needs when it is presented in many governing body reports.[35] From a managed care perspective, Rontal outlined the following criteria as being needed for an MIS: appropriate use, place of service, specific procedures, preventive care, cost-effectiveness, patient satisfaction, chronic

illness management, access to care, and patient education.[36] Also needed are outcomes of care for mortality, morbidity, complications, readmissions, quality of life, and disability. Clinical information systems often depend on integration with administrative information systems for data.

## Clinical Information System

Designed to support direct patient care processes, automated clinical information systems or clinical informatics have enormous potential for analyzing and improving the quality of patient care. Barriers to implementation include normal resistance to change, the mindset that patient care is best managed by people, lack of exposure to the application of information science and computers in healthcare educational and training programs, and inadequate resources. In 2008, only 9.4% of nonfederal acute care hospitals had a basic EHR system; in 2014, that percentage rose to 75.5%, due in large part to the passage of the HITECH Act of 2009.[37] Nearly all reported hospitals had a certified EHR—one that met the technological capability, functionality, and security requirements adopted by the U.S. Department of Health & Human Services, Office of the National Coordinator for Health Information Technology.[38(p1)]

Currently, expanded clinical information systems include EHRs and their retrieval systems, computer-assisted medical decision making for history and physicals and antibiotic selection, clinical application programs for health-risk programs, health maintenance organization encounter data, clinical algorithms, predictive modeling, and simulation. To analyze and interpret outcomes data, EHR-based systems allow healthcare providers to identify positive and negative outcomes so as to take appropriate action. Both types of systems serve to focus users on areas of concern regarding outcomes performance. Energy can be focused on analyzing and controlling deviations from the baseline resulting in cost savings.

## Decision Support System

Decision-support data facilitate cross-functional analyses to improve patient care processes and outcomes. Decision support systems address strategic planning functions such as

- strategic planning and marketing,
- resource allocation,
- performance evaluation and monitoring,
- product evaluation and services, and
- medical management (e.g., evidence-based practice, clinical guidelines, and pathways).

When integrating financial and clinical data, there is an opportunity to perform highly sophisticated data analysis involving predictive outcome management. These data help the healthcare quality professional and executive leadership evaluate current operations and the feasibility of the development of new product lines and services. Healthcare quality professionals coordinate outcome and decision-support data by posing pertinent questions such as:

- What kinds of comparative analyses are most important?
- With whom can these comparisons be made?
- What is the certainty that data are comparable?
- What happens when data reveal significant differences in outcomes when compared to benchmarks?

Organizations use decision support systems to develop an outcomes information management plan, which includes evaluating performance outcomes measurement systems. View outcomes in terms of various clinical topics including mortality, complication rates, infection rates, cesarean section rates, fall rates, and other clinical outcomes measurement categories. Categories may or may not reflect the resources (cost, charges, length of stay) associated with a given outcome.

Bright and colleagues assessed healthcare process measures and clinical outcome measures associated with the commercially and locally developed clinical decision support system (CDSS).[39] This study found that a CDSS is effective in improving healthcare process measures across diverse settings. Evidence is limited about the impact on certain outcome measures (i.e., economic, financial) and successful CDSS implementation. More research is needed. Recently Shahmoradi and colleagues reported CDSSes as a promising strategy to prevent medication errors, specifically for improving prescriptions, avoiding adverse events, and optimizing correct drug dosing.[40]

**Box 6.2** outlines key points in information systems.

---

#### Box 6.2  Key Points: Information Systems

- Administrative support information systems (financial/human resources/office automation) support day-to-day operations in healthcare organizations.
- Management information systems contain both the manual and the automated methods that provide information for decision making.
- Clinical information systems are designed to support direct patient processes and have immense potential for analyzing and improving the quality of patient care.

---

## Distributed Health Data Network

Data generated or captured by healthcare systems have many uses. Data not only help the organization where originally generated or collected for conducting day-to-day operations, but they also support health services research and population health efforts. In addition, such data also serve as a great resource for governmental entities (federal or state or local public health agencies) to better understand the needs of the population in those focused regions as well as to populate disease registries to track the progress of conditions such as cancer and other health disease states. In other words, the utility of healthcare data goes beyond assisting the parent organization in generating revenue by adding value from a societal aspect. But the rate at which the data are growing internally (generated for research or surveillance purposes) is many folds greater than the rate at which it could be shared outside of the healthcare entity. This is because of the sensitivity that comes with healthcare data.

Data security is high priority for healthcare organizations, especially in the wake of an increased number of cybersecurity incidents such as malware attacks, phishing attacks, ransomware attacks, and high-profile data breaches. Thefts of laptops and electronic devices with personally identifiable information (PII) or protected health information (PHI) has become a major concern and vulnerability. Governmental agencies and healthcare entities have established security rules to prevent, address, and protect individuals' and entities' sensitive health information records.

In the United States, the Health Insurance Portability and Accountability Act (HIPAA) was signed into law by President Clinton in August 1996.[41] This led to the development of the HIPAA Privacy Rule in 2003 and the HIPAA Security Rule in 2005. The Security Rule and the HITECH Act of 2009 come with a very long list of necessary technical safeguards for organizations storing PII/PHI in addition to data transmission, security authentication protocols, access controls and audit checks, and integrity checks. Despite these efforts, the fallibility of humans (staff members) in handling sensitive information and adhering to best practices can result in security breaches. Healthcare entities safeguard their institutional data and adhere to essential data governance protocols and procedures such as business associate agreements, data use agreements, or data sharing agreements before sharing any sensitive institutional information to external entities.

The U.S. Department of Health & Human Services stressed the importance of increasing access to population-level data sources by integrating data systems to drive health planning and research. Distributed health data networks (DHDNs) support

- health services research;
- evaluation of interventions and comparative effectiveness and patient-centered outcomes research (comparative effectiveness/patient-centered outcomes research [PCOR]); and
- public health surveillance.

DHDNs are gaining momentum due to the increased concerns related to data sharing, privacy, and governance. This is a paradigm shift in health data sharing.[42]

Data within a DHDN are not centralized. Rather, data reside behind the firewalls of the participating organizations or disparate data sources within the network. Participating organizations standardize their in-house or organizational-level data to a single data schema known as a common data model (CDM). The PCORnet is an example of a CDM, which is supported by all networks in the Patient Centered Outcomes Research Institute.[43] It is derived from the mini-sentinel data model, and over 80 institutions have transformed their data into this model. PCORnet focuses on bringing together data and resources to support comparative effectiveness/ patient-centered outcomes research. The PCORnet CDM version 6.0 consists of 19 tables with 355 attributes (data elements or variables) available to support research (**Table 6.6**). Captured data are used by partners within a network to answer important patient outcomes–related questions.

**Table 6.6** PCORnet Common Data Model

| Data Table | Description |
| --- | --- |
| DEMOGRAPHIC | Demographics record of individual patients |
| ENROLLMENT | Insurance enrollment information |
| ENCOUNTER | Healthcare delivery interactions |
| DIAGNOSIS | Diagnosis codes as a result of diagnostic processes and medical coding within healthcare delivery |
| PROCEDURES | Procedure codes such as surgical procedures and lab orders delivered within a healthcare context |
| VITAL | Captures vital signs such as height, weight, systolic, and diastolic blood pressure that directly measure an individual's current state of attributes |
| DISPENSING | Prescriptions filled through a community, mail-order, or hospital pharmacy |
| LAB_RESULT_CM | Stores quantitative and qualitative measurements from blood and other body specimens |
| CONDITION | Represents the patient's medical history and current state |
| PRO_CM | Stores responses to patient-reported outcome measures or questionnaires |
| PRESCRIBING | Provider orders for medication dispensing and/or administration |
| PCORNET_TRIAL | Patients enrolled in PCORnet clinical trials and PCORnet studies |
| DEATH | Reported mortality information for patients |
| DEATH_CAUSE | The individual causes associated with a reported death |
| MED_ADMIN | Records of medications administered to patients by healthcare providers |
| PROVIDER | Data about the providers involved in care processes |
| OBS_CLIN | Standardized qualitative and quantitative clinical observations about a patient |
| OBS_GEN | Table to store everything else |
| HARVEST | Attributes associated with the specific PCORnet DataMart implementation, including data refreshes |

Modified from PCORNet. Common data model (CDM) specification, version 6.0. Published 2020. Accessed February 6, 2022. https://pcornet.org/wp-content/uploads/2022/01/PCORnet-Common-Data-Model-v60-2020_10_221.pdf

DHDNs do have limitations: (1) they are limited to the data generated by the participating institutes collected as a part of their day-to-day business and operations; (2) the local data documentation practices at individual DHDN participating sites may not be resolved using standardized CDMs; and (3) ongoing maintenance of a DHDN requires dedicated resources such as human capital, time, and quality checks to refresh the data at regular intervals.

**Box 6.3** lists the key points of a distributed health data network.

---

**Box 6.3  Key Points: Distributed Health Data Network**

- Data governance protocols and procedures such as business associate agreements, data use agreements, and data sharing agreements should be in place before sharing any sensitive institutional information to external entities.
- DHDNs help improve the sample size by fostering the data sharing in a federal model by giving due importance to privacy and security of sensitive, personal health information.
- DHDNs exist based on the presumption that organizations participating in multi-institutional activities standardize their in-house or organizational-level data to a single data schema known as a common data model.

---

# Design and Management

Quality, safety, and performance improvement and research exist on a continuum of rigor of soft science and hard science. Hard science is the most sophisticated method of acquiring knowledge and involves inductive and deductive reasoning. Hard science might be considered superior based on tradition, authority, and experience (**Table 6.7**). The underlying assumptions are similar for the design, measurement, and interpretation of research studies and continuous quality improvement projects. Research utilization is a key aspect of the QI process and is critical to achieving healthcare quality as defined by the local, state, and federal regulations and standards. Healthcare quality professionals use the level of research rigor that best answers the specific performance improvement question and area of study balancing rigor and practicality. They evaluate research studies and systematic reviews to a practice setting using critical appraisal tools. These tools guide healthcare quality professionals

through the research critique process, allowing effective evaluation and synthesis of research findings for use in performance improvement activities.[44]

When the healthcare quality professional begins the design process for improvement activities, the goodness of project fit (QI process versus research process) is established by examining the question to answer, data collection, analysis plan, and application of findings. **Table 6.8** provides an overview of the processes.

## Data Fundamentals

Organizations are going to make gains and sustain their operations in the future using voluminous data and processing it with advanced methodologies to identify actionable intelligence. This section highlights topics elevating the importance of healthcare data and the importance of data engineering to identify key actionable insights.

## Healthcare Data

Healthcare data sets serve as a key source of information for understanding the disease burden and health disparities that exist within patient populations; they also inform strategies for addressing health inequities. **Table 6.9** provides an overview of the generators and users of healthcare data.[45]

### Common Types of Healthcare Data

Drawing knowledge from mathematics and statistics, healthcare data were often classified into two major categories—quantitative data (e.g., age, admission dates and discharge dates, lab values) and qualitative data (text captured within medical records such as a progress note). With the exponential increase of data captured with the databases, the ability to access such large data sets using high-powered computing resources and the development of standards to document encounter data has led to the usage of slightly different terms or categories to describe the major categories of healthcare data—*structured data* and *unstructured data*.

- Structured data are the information collected and stored in a highly organized and standardized format. Examples of this data type include *quantitative data fields* such as age, admission and discharge dates, and *standard data formats* used for documenting problem lists (SNOMED Clinical Terms [SNOMED CT]), diagnosis codes (International Classification of Diseases ICD-11),

**Table 6.7** Continuous Quality Improvement (Soft Science) and Research (Hard Science)

| Applied | | | | Theoretical |
|---|---|---|---|---|
| Soft | | | | Hard |
| Social sciences | | Biological sciences | | Physical sciences |
| Descriptive | | Inferential | | Predictive |
| Problem-solving | | Fundamental functions | | Hypothesis testing |
| **Observational data** | **Integrative data** | **Survey data** | **Secondary data** | **Output data** |
| Qualitative studies | CQI studies | Program evaluations | Efficacy research | Experimental studies |
| Focus groups | Meta-analysis | Epidemiological investigations | Case-control studies | Randomized clinical trials |
| Retrospective chart reviews | Methodologic reviews | Practice change evaluations | Quasi-experimental research | Longitudinal experimental studies |
| **CQI studies** | **Evaluation research** | **Outcomes research** | **Health services research** | **Clinical research** |

Modified with permission from Wolters Kluwer Health, Inc. Byers JF, Beaudin CL. The relationship between continuous quality improvement and research. *J Healthc Qual.* 2002:24(1):8.

**Table 6.8** Quality Improvement and Research Processes

| QI Process | Research Process |
|---|---|
| Identify the process improvement, survey the literature, and make a flowchart of the process. | Identify information need(s) or ask the question to be investigated. |
| Define the customers and problem. | Define the variable(s) or the elements for which data are required. |
| Formulate a plan. | Formulate a plan of study or hypotheses. |
| Choose one or a combination of basic or quality-management and planning tools. | Choose or design the research design and collection tools/instruments. |
| Collect the data. | Collect the data. |
| Analyze the data and look for root causes. | Analyze the data. |
| Display the data. | Display the data. |
| Report the data and findings. | Report the data and findings. |
| Draw conclusions. | Draw conclusions. |
| Act upon recommendations deduced from the conclusions. | Act upon recommendations deduced from the conclusions. |
| Continue to monitor the process. | Continue to monitor the process. |
| Evaluate and communicate conclusions. | Evaluate and communicate conclusions. |
| Hold the improvement. | Generalize the results. |

procedure codes (Current Procedural Terminology [CPT]), lab values (Logical Observation Identifiers Names and Codes [LOINC]), and drugs (RxNorm, National Drug Code).

- Unstructured data include qualitative data such as clinical notes, progress notes, free text, and images (medical imaging), audio, video, and biomedical sensor traces.

## Patient-Generated Health Data

Digital technologies now allow patients to track health data outside of the clinical setting. This impacts the delivery of healthcare. Healthcare organizations maintain adequate medical/health records to serve as a basis for planning care and for communicating about the patient's conditions and treatments with other

**Table 6.9** Healthcare Data Generators and Users

| Entity | Generator | User | |
|---|---|---|---|
| Patients | Yes | Yes | ▪ Generate data such as heart rate, blood pressure, etc., by using wearable devices.<br>▪ Use data to make informed decisions.<br>▪ Provide PII, which includes demographic data and insurance information at the time of service. |
| Health plans and payers/managed care organizations/employers | Yes | Yes | ▪ Generate data for the healthcare services provided to the enrollees.<br>▪ Use the data to generate bills and pricing models. |
| Healthcare providers | Yes | Yes | ▪ Generate diagnosis, procedure, and lab data to provide a timely health service.<br>▪ Use the data to generate trends over time to understand the burden of disease conditions. |
| Healthcare delivery systems | Yes | Yes | ▪ Generate data for the healthcare services provided.<br>▪ Use the data to create trends over time to understand the burden of disease conditions in their market service area. |
| Suppliers | Yes | Yes | ▪ Generate data for the healthcare services provided.<br>▪ Use the data to understand the trends over time of medications or implants. |
| Public health agencies | Yes | Yes | ▪ Generate the prevalence statistics for disease conditions to inform the key stakeholders and policy makers.<br>▪ Use the data to generate the vital statistics (birth and death data). |

Data from Data Across Sectors for Health. Healthcare 101. Published 2018. Accessed February 6, 2022. http://dashconnect.org/wp-content/uploads/2018/03/Health-Care-Data-101.pdf

healthcare providers. The medical or health record serves other purposes as well. For example, medical records are reviewed by administrative staff performing quality, utilization, and risk management functions and by physicians and other providers engaged in peer review. Outside organizations also use the medical record for matters relating to payment and accreditation. In malpractice cases, the medical record serves as the major source of evidence about the care the patient received. Information contained in medical records is also used for retrospective clinical research. Board approval is needed for PHI collected for research. The term *PII* is used interchangeably with PHI, although PII is a subset of PHI.

Information is often exchanged for the purposes of health treatment and payment. Healthcare organizations effect clear policies for access to medical records, whether records are written, computerized, or otherwise maintained. Policy statements make clear what, other than actual medical records, constitutes a portion of the record. For example, with the advent of and frequent use of photography, videotaping of procedures or fetal heart monitoring

strips, it is important to address (based on state law and legal advice) whether such media are part of the medical record.

Federal and state statutes required organizations to maintain the security, integrity, and confidentiality of the patient's personal data and other information. An organizational plan for health information management (HIM) addresses the critical balance between timely data sharing and data confidentiality. The organization is responsible for safeguarding records against loss, defacement, tampering, and unauthorized use.

Each organization must determine the level of security, integrity, and confidentiality for various categories of information. Access to each category of information must have a functioning mechanism designed to preserve the confidentiality of data and information identified as sensitive or requiring extraordinary means to protect patient privacy. Organizations must follow the standards developed by their accreditation organization (e.g., CARF International, The Joint Commission [TJC], National Committee for Quality Assurance, and URAC). Training programs and reminders must be in place to educate staff about these requirements and consequences of not adhering to institutional policies.

The organization also must identify sanctions for employees who breach confidentiality. Healthcare organizations must keep confidential all PHI pertaining to medical peer review, quality, safety, and performance improvement, and the monitoring and evaluation of patient care. HIPAA defines personal health information. Records with patient and/or provider identifiers are kept confidential. This includes the medical record (in any format, hard copy or electronic) and may also include reports, data abstracts, and supplies. Effective information management security and confidentiality policies and procedures in a healthcare organization contain the following elements:

- HIPAA requirements for release of health information
- Protection of PHI
- Identification of people with access to information
- Delineation of specific information to which people have access
- Requirements for people with access to information to keep that information confidential
- Requirements for removal of medical records (a patient's medical record is the property of the healthcare facility), which are removed from the organization authority and into safekeeping only in accordance with a court order, subpoena, or statute
- Mechanisms for securing information against unauthorized intrusion, corruption, and damage
- Handling the root cause analysis reporting requirements as directed by regulators, accreditation standards, and/or contractual arrangements

**Figure 6.5** lists the elements of PHI in the HIPAA regulations. Examples of information management confidentiality and security methods include the following:

- Organizations can restrict access to records or portions of records with the use of security codes or by restricting certain operations to specific devices or people.
- An organization relying on computerized information has an adequate backup plan for each computer application and extensive security firewall.
- Portions of medical records may be stored separately, for example, if the record contains information regarding certain types of psychiatric and addictions treatment.
- The complete medical record would have to be available as needed for medical care and follow-up, utilization review, or in quality, safety, and performance improvement activities.

- Names
- All geographic subdivisions smaller than a state, including street address, city, county, precinct, zip code, geocodes (in some instances, the first three numbers of a zip code may be collected)
- Birth dates, admission dates, discharge date, date of death, all ages over 89 unless aggregated to 90 or older; only year data may be collected
- Telephone and fax numbers
- Electronic mail addresses, Web universal resource locators (URLs), and Internet protocol (IP) addresses/numbers
- Medical record, health plan beneficiary, and account numbers
- Certificate/license numbers
- Vehicle identification and license plate numbers
- Device identifiers and serial numbers
- Biometric identifiers, including finger and voice prints
- Full-face photographic images and any comparable image
- Any other unique identifying number, characteristic, or code that could be used alone or in combination to identify a person:
  - Patient name
  - Name of individual/organization requesting information
  - Reason for release of information
  - Anticipated use of information released
  - Exact material to be released, including reference to PHI
  - Period during which the release of information is valid
  - Documentation that information is released only to the individual/organization named previously
  - Signature and date of the patient or legal representative (as defined by policy/state law)

**Figure 6.5** HIPAA and Protected Health Information

Data from U.S. Government Publishing Office. U.S. Code of Federal Regulations. 2002. Accessed February 16, 2022. www.gpo.gov/fdsys/pkg/CFR-2002-title45-vol1/xml/CFR-2002-title45-vol1-sec164-514.xml

The legal basis for confidentiality derives from the physician–patient privilege, set forth by statute in almost all states. This is one of several relationships recognized as special by law. The preservation of confidentiality is essential to the maintenance of the relationship. The need for confidentiality in the physician–patient relationship gives rise to a legal privilege. This means that, absent a patient authorization or waiver or an overriding law or public policy, medical information is protected from the process known as *discovery*, through which parties to a lawsuit normally can compel disclosure of relevant evidence. In certain states, the physician–patient privilege extends beyond physicians to protect the patient's relationship with other healthcare practitioners (e.g., psychologists, clinical social workers, clinical nurse specialists, nurse midwives, nurse anesthetists, and nurse practitioners). Information that is privileged must satisfy the following conditions:

- It is communicated in the context of the physician–patient relationship.
- It is given with the expectation that it remains confidential.
- It must be necessary for the diagnosis and treatment of the patient.

In understanding the function of the medical record to provide information about the patient's care, treatment, and services and to serve as the method of sharing this information between caregivers, there are monitoring processes to ensure the integrity, accuracy, and completeness of the record and reflect the pertinent clinical documentation. The medical record may be electronic, a hard copy document, or a combination. With legislation demanding that healthcare organizations implement EHRs, the use of electronic records increased.

A written consent or authorization is required to release patient information to anyone outside the organization. A typical release of information form contains the following elements:

- Patient name
- Name of the individual/organization requesting information
- Reason for release of information
- Anticipated use of information released
- Exact material to be released, including reference to PHI
- Period during which the release of information is valid
- Documentation that information is released only to the individual/organization named
- Signature and date of the patient or legal representative (as defined by policy/state law)

National and state statutes regulate the release of information. Medical records and studies may be released without the patient's (or authorized representative's) written authorization for treatment, payment, or healthcare operations. Individuals who may authorize release include the

- representatives from the governing body;
- organization director (chief executive);
- healthcare personnel involved in the care of a patient;
- people responsible for quality, safety, and performance improvement activities; and
- people in the HIM/medical records department.

HIPAA requires healthcare providers (e.g., doctors and health plans) to obtain written authorization from patients to share medical record information. This may be for purposes unrelated to treatment, payment, or routine healthcare operations. The authorization form can originate from the hospital, physician, or health plan, or it can come from the organization requesting the data, such as a researcher, employer, or insurance company. There is no mandated form, but a valid form must include several core elements such as the name, purpose of disclosure, and expiration date.

Utilization management policies and procedures inform practices. A common method to inform and obtain consent is to include a statement on the admission consent form or consent for treatment form. Of concern is provision of the reason for hospitalization, such as treatment of substance use disorders, treatment of mental health disorders, HIV/AIDS, and other PHI as identified by HIPAA or special considerations (e.g., Substance Abuse Confidentiality Regulations, 42 *CFR* Part 2 Revised). These policies are communicated to the third-party payer as part of the contract review process.

**Box 6.4** lists key points pertaining to patient data.

---

**Box 6.4 Key Points: Patient Data**

- PII is a subset of PHI.
- The rules for releasing PHI are determined by national and state statutes and codified in an organization's policies and procedures.
- HIPAA requires healthcare providers (e.g., doctors and health plans) to obtain written authorization from patients to share medical record information for purposes unrelated to treatment, payment, or routine healthcare operations.

---

## Quality Measurement

Performance outcomes measurement or decision support systems can provide a primary focus to determine the quality of healthcare services provided to consumers. By analyzing data and information generated by an effective performance outcomes measurement system, healthcare quality professionals will be able to help identify areas in which to improve quality and resources in their organizations. Other uses for outcomes systems include helping to identify how an organization measures up in relation to its competitors, identifying individual providers and practitioners who meet acceptable levels of quality, allowing providers to respond more rapidly to market changes, paying for exceptional performance, and justifying value-based services.

Chassin and colleagues suggested that quality, safety, and performance improvement programs can focus explicitly on maximizing health benefits to patients, and, to achieve the goal, measures must be included to advance knowledge about whether the goal is being achieved.[46] Four criteria are noted for accountability measures (i.e., process measures; if met, there will be a higher likelihood of improving patient outcomes). These criteria include:

1. Strong evidence shows that the measure associated with the care process leads to improved outcomes.
2. The measure accurately captures the provision of evidence-based care.
3. The measure addresses a process with few intervening steps that must occur before the improved outcome is realized.
4. Implementing the measure has little or no chance of inducing unintended adverse consequences.

Healthcare quality professionals facilitate the analysis and interpretation of outcomes data for an organization. The overall goals for use of outcomes and decision-support data are to improve quality, reduce costs and resource consumption, increase organizational profitability, and develop an information-based strategic plan. Comparisons of length of stay (LOS), costs, complications, and mortality cannot be made legitimately without adjusting severity at the patient level. Severity adjustment and clinical case mix permit effective analysis and eliminate practitioner concerns that their patients are sicker. Evidence to support the focus of measurement is shown as **Table 6.10**.

There are different types of performance measures. Before selecting a measure, one must understand what purpose each measure serves. It is helpful to scan existing quality measures to identify those that are valid and reliable (e.g., CMS, the Agency for Healthcare Research and Quality [AHRQ], the National Quality Forum [NQF], and the National Committee for Quality Assurance [NCQA]). Look for measures vetted through consensus-driven processes involving various stakeholders, including patients and families. The benefit of using an existing and tested measure is there is evidence to support the fidelity in assessing the structure, process, or outcome of care.

- *Structure.* Measures of infrastructure, capacity, systems, and processes (e.g., nurse staffing ratios).

- *Process.* Measures of process performance. They tell whether the parts or steps in the system are performing as planned. This can be in process or at the end of the process (e.g., timely administration of prophylactic surgical antibiotics).
- *Outcomes.* Measures that show results of overall process or system performance (often risk adjusted, e.g., mortality).

Further guidance on evaluating and selecting quality measures is offered by McGlynn[47(p9)] and summarized next.

- *Important.* Is the measure assessing an aspect of efficiency that is important to providers, payers, and policy makers? Is the measure applied at the level of interest to those planning to use the measure? Is there an opportunity for improvement? Is the measure under the control of the provider or health system?
- *Scientifically sound.* Is the measure reliable and reproducible? Does the measure capture the concept of interest? Is there evidence of face, construct, or predictive validity?
- *Feasible.* Are the data necessary to construct this measure available? Is the cost and burden of measurement reasonable?
- *Actionable.* Are the results interpretable? Can the intended audience use the information to make decisions or act?

McGlynn further explains that the ideal healthcare quality measure does not exist and that there are trade-offs when selecting measures for quality assurance, quality control, quality management, or quality improvement.

There are vetted, publicly available quality measures for healthcare quality professionals to employ in improvement efforts. For example, electronic clinical quality measures (eCQMs) are designed to measure many aspects of care, including patient and family engagement, patient safety, care coordination, population/public health, efficient use of healthcare resources, and clinical process/effectiveness for Medicare and Medicaid populations.[48] Implementation of these measures was a requirement for providers to attain Meaningful Use Stage 1 and Stage 2. CMS provides annual updates that document specifications for an evolving set of eCQMs that can be gathered from EHRs.[49] These measures can help providers and organizations report on quality, advancing care information and improvement activities. Further, CMS conditions of participation require a data-driven performance improvement program in hospitals and

**Table 6.10** Evidence-Based Measures

| Measure Type | Evidence | Example of Measure Type and Evidence |
|---|---|---|
| **Structure** Structure of care is a feature of a healthcare organization or clinician related to its capacity to provide high-quality healthcare. | Quantity, quality, and consistency of a body of evidence that the measured healthcare structure leads to desired health outcomes with benefits that outweigh harms (including evidence of the link to effective care processes and the link from the care processes to desired health outcomes). | #0190: Nurse staffing hours. Evidence: increasing nursing hours results in lower mortality or morbidity or leads to provision of effective care processes (e.g., lower medication errors) that lead to better outcomes. |
| **Process** A process of care is a healthcare-related activity performed for, on behalf of, or by a patient | Quantity, quality, and consistency of a body of evidence that the measured healthcare process leads to desired health outcomes in the target population with benefits that outweigh harms to patients. If the measure focus is on inappropriate use, then quantity, quality, and consistency of a body of evidence that the measured healthcare process does *not* lead to desired health outcomes in the target population. | #0551: Angiotensin-converting enzyme (ACE) inhibitor and angiotensin receptor blocker (ARB) use and persistence among members with coronary artery disease at high risk for coronary events. Evidence: use of ACE inhibitor and ARB results in lower mortality or cardiac events. #0058: Inappropriate antibiotic treatment for adults with acute bronchitis. Evidence: antibiotics are not effective for acute bronchitis. |
| **Intermediate clinical outcome** An intermediate outcome is a change in physiologic state that leads to a longer term health outcome. | Quantity, quality, and consistency of a body of evidence that the measured intermediate clinical outcome leads to a desired health outcome. | #0059: Hemoglobin $A_{1c}$ management ($A_{1c} > 9$). Evidence: hemoglobin $A_{1c}$ level leads to health outcomes (e.g., prevention of renal disease, heart disease, amputation, mortality). |
| **Health outcome** An outcome of care is the health status of a patient (or change in health status) resulting from healthcare, desirable or adverse. | Supports the relationship of the health outcome to at least one healthcare structure, process, intervention, or service. In some situations, resource use may be considered a proxy for a health state (e.g., hospitalization may represent deterioration in health status). | #0230: Acute myocardial infarction (AMI). 30-day mortality. Survival is a goal of seeking and providing treatment for AMI. Rationale linking healthcare processes or interventions (aspirin, reperfusion) to mortality or survival. #0171: Acute care hospitalization (risk-adjusted) of home care patients. Improvement or stabilization of condition to remain at home is a goal of seeking and providing home care services. Rationale linking healthcare processes (e.g., medication reconciliation, care coordination) to hospitalization of patients receiving home care services. |
| **Special Considerations by Topic** | | |
| **Experience of care** Patient experience encompasses the range of interactions that patients have with the healthcare system, including their care from health plans, and from doctors, nurses, and staff in hospitals, physician practices, and other healthcare facilities. | Evidence that the measured aspects of care are those valued by patients and for which the patient is the best or only source of information (often acquired through qualitative studies) *or* Evidence that patient experience with care is correlated with desired outcomes such as getting timely appointments and good communication with healthcare providers. | #0166: Hospital Consumer Assessment of Healthcare Providers and Systems (HCAHPS). Evidence that patient or consumer values the aspects of care being measured (e.g., communication with doctors and nurses, responsiveness of hospital staff, pain control, communication about medicines, cleanliness and quiet of the hospital environment, and discharge information). Research shows that when patients are engaged in their healthcare, it can lead to measurable improvements in safety and quality. Forces contributing to the growing imperative to improve patient experience, performance-based compensation systems, board certification, accreditation and licensing, and practice recognition programs. Demand among patients for an enhanced experience and greater participation in their healthcare. |

*(continues)*

**Table 6.10** Evidence-Based Measures                                                                    *(continued)*

| Measure Type | Evidence | Example of Measure Type and Evidence |
|---|---|---|
| **Efficiency**<br>Measures of efficiency combine the concepts of resource use and quality. | Efficiency measured with combination of quality measures and resource-use measures—the right care in the right place at the right time.<br><br>Quality measure component: evidence for the selected quality measures as described in this table.<br><br>Resource-use measure component: does not require clinical evidence as described elsewhere in this table. | Currently, there are no National Quality Forum–endorsed efficiency measures that combine quality and resource use.<br><br>Potential measure: diabetes quality measures or composite used in conjunction with a measure of resource use per episode.<br><br>Activities contributing to high quality and low resource use. Examples are reducing or improving handoffs, teamwork to meet patient needs, and avoiding wasteful or unnecessary medical tests, treatments, and procedures. |

Data from National Quality Forum. Guidance for evaluating the evidence related to the focus of quality measurement and importance to measure and report (pp. 15–16). Published January 2011. www.qualityforum.org/WorkArea/linkit.aspx?LinkIdentifier=id&ItemID=70941; and Agency for Healthcare Research and Quality. What is patient experience? n.d. Accessed February 12, 2022. https://www.ahrq.gov/cahps/about-cahps/patient-experience/index.html

within the next few years will include all healthcare providers.

AHRQ developed a suite of measures called AHRQ Quality Indicators.[50] Software is available for users to apply AHRQ QI to their organizations' administrative data. AHRQ QI modules include prevention, inpatient, patient safety, and pediatric modules. AHRQ also maintains Guidelines and Measures, a place to find legacy guidelines and measures clearinghouses, and the National Guideline Clearinghouse and National Quality Measures Clearinghouse, both resources of evidence-based quality measures and measure sets. Other efforts funded by AHRQ have also brought a focus on more rigorous quality and performance-based data, analytics, improvement science, and implementation research.

Another major source of quality measures can be found on the NQF website. NQF endorsed over 300 measures used in federal public reporting and pay-for-performance programs as well as in private-sector and state programs. NCQA publishes measures that focus specifically on health plans. The Healthcare Effectiveness Data and Information Set (HEDIS) are measures used by more than 90% of America's health plans to assess performance on multiple dimensions of care and service. CMS is working with health plans, purchasers, physicians, provider organizations, and consumers on a Core Quality Measures Collaborative to identify sets of quality measures that payers have committed to using. The guiding principle of the Collaborative was to develop core measure sets that are meaningful to patients, consumers, and physicians,

while reducing variability in measure selection, collection burden, and cost.[51]

In 2014, CMS began the implementation of cross-setting measures as mandated by the Impact Act.[52] The Impact Act requires the submission of standardized data by long-term care hospitals, skilled nursing facilities, home health agencies, and inpatient rehabilitation facilities. Examples of measures include skin integrity and changes in skin integrity; functional status, cognitive function, and changes in function; transfer of health information and care preferences for transitions between levels of care; and all-condition risk-adjusted potentially preventable hospital readmissions rates.

AHRQ is instrumental in advancing the study of measures, especially outcomes and the effectiveness of specific treatments. Criteria developed for the selection of measures based on attributes[53] include the following:

- *Standardization*. Report the same kind of data in the same way.
- *Comparability*. If appropriate, results are risk adjusted for factors (e.g., age, gender, health status).
- *Availability*. Data will be available.
- *Timeliness*. Results will be available when most needed.
- *Relevance*. Results measure concerns of stakeholders and users.
- *Validity*. Measures have been tested so they consistently and accurately reflect the measure.

- *Experience.* Organizations have experience with the measure so it reflects actual performance.
- *Stability.* The measure is not likely to be removed from use.
- *Evaluability.* The measure can be evaluated as better or worse.
- *Distinguishability.* The measure denotes differences between organizations.
- *Credibility.* The measures can be audited.

Other sources of measures are shown in **Table 6.11**. When measures are developed or selected for use, there must be a context in which to determine whether the performance of a specific measure is good. To determine the goodness, there are factors to consider. Does the evidence preestablish the desired or expected performance level? If not, does any regulatory, accreditation, or payer agency identify a desired or expected performance level? The use of comparative data helps set desired targets or goals and provides a method by which to determine how well the organization is performing compared with similar organizations, competitors, best in the industry, and best in class.

To support quality, safety, and performance improvement and other administrative functions, organizations have moved in the direction of building large data warehouses that include information from all systems in the organization. For example, these data warehouses contain clinical, operational, financial, and human resources data. Data warehouses supported by hardware (e.g., servers) and database software combine the information into integrated data tables. The ability to integrate these data allows for robust reporting and analyses.

Data collection can be both expensive and time consuming for any organization. Just enough data are collected. Overmeasurement should be avoided in terms of both number of measures and frequency of measurement and analysis. Healthcare quality professionals can prevent duplicate data collection efforts among diverse groups and departments. It is preferable to evaluate a new data collection process, even if it is new only to the organization. The development of a comprehensive data collection plan for improvement activities can leverage the warehouse and conserve resources. Planning includes the following steps:

**Table 6.11** Sources of Measures

| Source | Examples of Measures |
|---|---|
| Administrative data | <ul><li>Volume, admissions</li><li>Discharges</li><li>Length of stay</li><li>Billing data</li><li>Uniform Hospital Discharge Data Set</li></ul> |
| Medical records | <ul><li>Clinical care</li><li>Medication use</li><li>Surgery and procedural data</li></ul> |
| Patient surveys | Consumer Assessment of Healthcare Providers and Systems |
| Standardized data sets | <ul><li>ORYX</li><li>Outcome and Assessment Information Set</li><li>National Surgical Quality Improvement Program</li><li>HEDIS</li><li>AHRQ (inpatient quality indicators, patient safety indicators, pediatric quality indicators)</li><li>National Hospital Quality Measures</li><li>National Database of Nursing Quality Indicators</li></ul> |
| Other | <ul><li>Culture of safety surveys</li><li>Feedback from patients and families</li><li>Grievance and complaints</li><li>Employee engagement surveys</li><li>Leapfrog Group survey</li><li>National Quality Forum</li></ul> |

- Determine the who, what, when, where, why, and how.
- Structure the design.
- Choose and develop the sampling method.
- Determine and conduct the necessary training.
- Delegate responsibilities and communicate time-lines.
- Facilitate interdepartmental/cross-functional co-ordination.
- Forecast the budget requirements.
- Conduct pilot procedures for the forms and the data collection process.

Usually, at least one business intelligence (BI) tool that allows end users, including quality, safety, and performance improvement staff to create their own reports is connected to the data warehouse.

BI tools have the capability to filter data by diagnosis, location, or provider and produce sophisticated tables, graphs, and analyses. These tools also allow for trending over time and comparisons of different groups. Utilizing the BI tool enables the capability to analyze baseline information before a QI project starts, look at trends over time, and measure the impact of improvement efforts. Further, analytical tools, such as R, SAS, or SPSS can be used on the data available in the warehouse to test for significant changes, control for varying patient characteristics, and build predictive models. See the *Performance and Process Improvement* and *Patient Safety* sections for more information on evaluation and measures.

## Data Specifications

Data collected are aggregated to preserve the confidentiality of information or protect vulnerable patient populations. On the other hand, disaggregated data are divided and broken down into smaller information units. For example, the average LOS of a healthcare system, which is the aggregate data, might be helpful in identifying where the system stands compared to similar hospitals in the region. The average LOS disaggregated by race or gender helps to better understand the disparities that exist among different races or gender groups within the healthcare system's patient population. Such information would help in developing the strategies required to reduce the gaps in disparities among different comparison groups.

Multiple measures sometimes have the same label but vastly different implications depending on the measure construct. For example, reporting on readmission rate without specifying the population and the duration of time between discharge and admission can lead to misleading assumptions. Defining measure specifications is fundamental to both the interpretation of the results and the source data used.

When defining the population, consider clinical and demographic factors (social determinants of health). For example, specify if the clinical cohort is based on DRG, diagnosis (administrative), lab, or X-ray result (clinical), or a combination. Include patient demographics such as age group, gender, insurer, or zip code. The following example uses a formula to calculate the percentage of women in a certain age range who had a screening mammogram. In the formula, the denominator is a subset of the initial cohort and may have exclusions or exceptions to create a more uniform analysis. The numerator is the outcome of the measure's focus (i.e., the subset of the denominator that meets the defining criteria).

*Example:* The Breast Cancer Screening measure CMIT ID: 4005 from the CMS Measure Inventory Tool (CMIT) demonstrates the specifications.[54]

- *Description.* The percentage of women 52–74 years of age who had a mammogram to screen for breast cancer
- *Numerator.* One or more mammograms any time on or between October 1 two years prior to the measurement year and December 31 of the measurement year
- *Denominator.* Women aged 52 to 74 years as of December 31 of the measurement year
- *Denominator exclusion.* Bilateral mastectomy any time during the member's history through December 31 of the measurement year
- *Numerator exclusions.* Evaluation of primary screening, not counting biopsies, breast ultrasounds, or magnetic resonance images because they are not appropriate methods for primary breast cancer screening

Defining the stratification variables is a precursor to structuring the reporting and assures the underlying data model can support the analysis. Reporting a measure in aggregate provides the highest level of measurement and demonstrates compliance. However, stratifying by age range, social risk factors, income, etc., enables a more detailed analysis, informs a deeper level of action, and may detect disparities relative to the measure focus.

### Code Specifications

Most measures require the use of standard code sets to define the patient's condition and status as a means of creating comparable, reliable, consumable measures.

**Table 6.12**  **Commonly Used Code Sets for Measure Development**

| Code Set | Use Case | Measure Examples |
|---|---|---|
| International Classification of Diseases (ICD) | Groups patients into DRGs, Medicare severity DRGs, All Patient Refined Diagnosis Related Groups (APR-DRG), etc. | ■ AHRQ patient safety indicators<br>■ Healthcare-associated conditions |
| SNOMED | Automates the mapping of the problem list in the EHR to a standard nomenclature | ■ Smoking status<br>■ Transitions of care |
| CPT | Standardizes physician documentation of services and procedures | $A_{1c}$ management |
| RxNorm | Normalizes names and unique identifiers of drugs | Appropriate use of anti−methicillin-resistant *Staphylococcus aureus* antibiotics |
| LOINC | Normalizes lab orders and results for clinical exchange | Audiological diagnosis no later than 3 months of age |

**Table 6.12** provides a list of commonly used code sets with a more comprehensive description in the text that follows.

## International Classification of Diseases

On January 16, 2009, the U.S. Department of Health & Human Services (HHS) released the final rule mandating that everyone covered by HIPAA implement International Classification of Diseases ICD-10 for medical coding. The ICD is a diagnostic tool using health data standards (WHO Constitution and Nomenclature Regulations) to classify causes of injury and death. It permits health data analyses, such as the study of mortality and morbidity trends,[55] and is designed to promote international compatibility in health data collecting and reporting. ICD codes form the basis for DRG calculations. Currently, cases are classified into Medicare severity diagnosis related groups for payment under the Inpatient Prospective Payment System (IPPS) based on the following information reported by the hospital: the principal diagnosis, up to 24 additional diagnoses, and up to 25 procedures performed during the stay.[56] ICD-11 was effective January 2022.[57]

## Systemized Nomenclature of Medicine

The Systemized Nomenclature of Medicine-Clinical Terms (SNOMED CT) provides healthcare professionals the ability to use different terms that mean the same thing in their clinical documentation systems. For example, the terms *heart attack*, *myocardial infarction*, and *MI* may mean the same thing to a cardiologist, but to a computer, they are all different.[58] SNOMED CT has been specified in the federal regulations published in September 2012 (see *Federal Register* Vol. 77,

No. 171), for documenting patient problems, encounter diagnosis, procedures, family health history, and smoking status.[59]

SNOMED is used for several purposes, including the problem list and public health reporting. When integrated into the EHR as required for the Office of National Coordinator for Health Information Technology certification, it automates the problem list documentation. For example, when the user types the term *dizzy* to describe a patient's symptom, SNOMED will return a list of suitable options.[60]

SNOMED assists with the electronic exchange of clinical health information and benefits patients, clinicians, and populations to represent clinical information consistently and comprehensively. In quality measurement, smoking status is recorded and whether a summary of care record was provided for each care transition.

## Current Procedural Terminology

Current Procedural Terminology (CPT) codes are a uniform language for coding medical services and procedures to streamline reporting and increase accuracy and efficiency.[61] CPT code descriptors are clinically focused and utilize common standards so that a diverse set of users can have common understanding across the clinical healthcare paradigm. CPT codes are also used for administrative management purposes such as claims processing and developing guidelines for medical care review.[62] Various types of CPT codes are described in **Table 6.13**.

**RxNorm**  RxNorm provides normalized names for clinical drugs and links its names to the drug

**Table 6.13** CPT Categories and Code Examples

| Category | Code Examples |
|---|---|
| **Category I**<br>Codes with descriptors that correspond to a procedure or service. Codes range from 00100 to 99499 and are generally ordered into subcategories based on procedure/service type and anatomy. | ▪ Evaluation and management: 99201–99499<br>▪ Anesthesia: 00100–01999; 99100–99150<br>▪ Surgery: 10000–69990<br>▪ Radiology: 70000–79999<br>▪ Pathology and laboratory: 80000–89398<br>▪ Medicine: 90281–99099; 99151–99199; and 99500–99607 |
| **Category II**<br>Alphanumeric tracking codes are supplemental codes used for performance measurement. Using them is optional and not required for correct coding. However, Category II codes are used in several HEDIS measures (for example in diabetes care and to indicate whether a patient's most recent $A_{1c}$ level is controlled).[63] | Breast cancer screening<br>▪ 3014F: Screening mammography results documented and reviewed<br>Colorectal cancer screening<br>▪ 3017F: Colorectal cancer screening results documented and reviewed<br>Prenatal/postpartum care<br>▪ 0500F: Initial prenatal care visit<br>▪ 0501F: Prenatal flow sheet documented in medical record by first prenatal visit<br>▪ 0503F: Postpartum care visit |
| **Category III**<br>Temporary alphanumeric codes for new and developing technology, procedures, and services. Created for data collection, assessment, and in some instances, payment of new services and procedures that currently don't meet the criteria for a Category I code. | ▪ General Category III codes start from 0003T to 0073T<br>▪ Online medical evaluation codes from 0074T to 0111T<br>▪ Medication therapy management codes from 0115T to 0117T<br>▪ Additional Category III codes, including islet cell transplant codes from 0120T to 0140T |

Data from American Medical Association. CPT® Category II Codes alphabetical clinical topics listing. 2020. Accessed February 12, 2022. https://www.ama-assn.org/system/files/2020-01/cpt-cat2-codes-alpha-listing-clinical-topics.pdf

vocabularies for pharmacy management and drug interaction software, commonly used by healthcare providers and pharmacies. RxNorm normalizes the naming system for generic and branded drugs for supporting semantic interoperation between drug terminologies and pharmacy knowledge base systems. By providing links between these vocabularies, RxNorm can mediate messages between systems not using the same software and vocabulary.[64] RxNorm is produced by the U.S. National Library of Medicine and is one of a suite of designated standards for use in U.S. federal government systems for the electronic exchange of clinical health information.[65] RxNorm is used in a number of quality measures including the Appropriate Use of Anti-Methicillin-Resistant *Staphylococcus Aureus* Antibiotics in the Merit-Based Incentive Payment System (MIPS) measure set.[66,67]

### Logical Observation Identifiers Names and Codes

Logical Observation Identifiers Names and Codes (LOINC) is a clinical terminology for the standardization of laboratory test names in the transactions between healthcare facilities, laboratories, laboratory testing devices, and public health authorities.[68,69] LOINC is one suite of designated standards for use in U.S. federal government systems for the electronic exchange of clinical health information. The exchange of laboratory information is complex, with multiple steps between the order and the results. Standard nomenclature simplifies that complexity when managing multiple test panels, pathology findings, and intermediate microbiology findings as examples. LOINC standardizes quality measure reporting as well. For example, in 2020, the U.S. Department of Health & Human Services used LOINC and SNOMED CT to identify and report SARS-CoV-2 test results in electronic reporting systems to facilitate timely and quality data reporting to state and federal public health agencies.[70]

### Data Protocol

The measure developer must explicitly identify types of data and how to aggregate or link these data so that calculation of the measure is reliable and valid.[71] This information may be of interest to the healthcare quality professional in considering the strength of the measure.

- Define key terms, data elements, codes, and code systems used in the numerator or denominator statement of a calculation, exclusions, and exceptions.
- Describe the level of measurement/analysis to clearly state the procedure for attributing the measure.
- Describe sampling methodology and provide guidance for an appropriate sample size.
- Determine risk adjustment methodology use, specifically for outcome measures.
- Define any time intervals used for inclusion or exclusion as well as the index event used to determine time intervals such as readmission index visit.
- Describe the scoring type (i.e., rates, ratios, composites, categorical value, etc.) and explain how to interpret the results, for example:
  - A higher score indicates better quality; an increase in rate denotes improvement.
  - A lower score indicates better quality; a decrease in median value denotes improvement.
  - A score within a defined interval indicates another classification (i.e., a passing score indicates better quality).
- Develop the measure logic (i.e., the ordered sequence of data retrieval and calculation).

## Measure Documentation

Measure documentation occurs throughout the measure development process. The measure name (or measure title) should be a very brief description of the measure's focus and target population. Measures are documented in the interactive CMIT. An example of breast cancer screening is provided in **Table 6.14**.

## Measure Calculations

Measure calculation is specific to each value-based reporting initiative, the type of measure, and the source of data. For individual measures, the CMIT defines the measure calculation methodology for each measure. During contract negotiations with commercial payers, measure calculation should be an agreed-upon element of the contract. It is important to note two nuances in measure calculation: measures of the same name with different calculation methodologies and single measures using diverse sources of data.

Measures are used in multiple programs. It is important that the quality professional understand when measures of the same name use different calculations. For example, "when a flu shot is administered" can produce different measure results for the

Preventive Care and Screening: Influenza Immunization MIPS measure. Both TJC[72] and CMS[73] require eCQMs, and while TJC strives to maintain alignment with CMS, there are differences in required measures and how they are submitted. **Figure 6.6** describes the alignment of CMS and TJC measures in 2022. Understanding these nuances enables the healthcare quality professional to interpret results and guide stakeholders to better documentation, increased data confidence, and improved outcomes.

Additionally, a measure can produce different results depending on the data source. This is particularly prevalent in the analysis of claims data by the payer versus clinical data by the provider. For example, using claims-only data for measuring compliance with childhood immunizations yields a lower compliance rate than using claims plus clinical data. In one unpublished analysis, only 27% compliance was demonstrated with claims-only data. Once clinical documentation was added, the compliance rate increased to 75%. Hybrid measures introduced by HEDIS combine administrative claims data with data abstracted from member records during a medical record review to create more accurate reporting. NCQA and health plans provide guidelines and both can be a resource for updates.[74]

Risk adjustment is a technique used to consider or to control the fact that different patients with the same diagnosis may have additional conditions or characteristics that can affect how well they respond to treatment. This removes the bias effect that can result when practitioners primarily treat patients who are more likely to experience desirable outcomes, such as those with fewer risk factors or co-occurring illnesses (morbidities). Outcomes measurement systems define the differences between *risk adjustment* and *severity*, whereas other systems use the terms interchangeably. However, there is a difference. Patients in a study population may respond with either "yes" or "no" when asked if they have had certain outcomes; the outcomes variable in this case is binary. The probability of a "yes" answer is the risk of the outcome.

Statistical methodologies are applied to adjust for risk in outcomes. The validity of each risk adjustment model is assessed based on the choice of risk factors, including both potential risk factors and those included in the model, and through measures of how well the predictions match overall experience. This assessment includes indicators such as measures of patient subpopulations, including patients with more than one risk factor, and the concordance statistic, which shows, in percentages, how accurate the model is at predicting the outcome.

**Table 6.14** Breast Cancer Screening Measure Description for MIPS

**CMIT Family ID:** 00093 | **CMIT ID:** 02508-C-MIPS | **Measure Type:** Process
**Date of Information:** Not Available | **Revision:** 7312 | **Program:** Merit-Based Incentive Payment System Program
**Description:** Percentage of women 50–74 years of age who had a mammogram to screen for breast cancer in the 27 months prior to the end of the measurement period.

| Properties | |
|---|---|
| **Date of Information** | Not available |
| **Abbreviated Measure Title** | Not available |
| **Description** | Percentage of women 50–74 years of age who had a mammogram to screen for breast cancer in the 27 months prior to the end of the measurement period. |
| **Numerator** | Women with one or more mammograms during the 27 months prior to the end of the measurement period. |
| **Denominator** | Women 51–74 years of age with a visit during the measurement period. |
| **Denominator Exclusions** | Women who had a bilateral mastectomy or who have a history of a bilateral mastectomy or for whom there is evidence of a right and a left unilateral mastectomy. Hospice services used by patient any time during the measurement period. Patient age 66 or older in Institutional Special Needs Plans (SNP) or residing in long-term care with POS code 32, 33, 34, 54, or 56 for more than 90 consecutive days during the measurement period. Patients 66 years of age and older with at least one claim/encounter for frailty during the measurement period AND a dispensed medication for dementia during the measurement period or the year prior to the measurement period. Patients 66 years of age and older with at least one claim/encounter for frailty during the measurement period AND either one acute inpatient encounter with a diagnosis of advanced illness or two outpatient, observation, ED or nonacute inpatient encounters on different dates of service with an advanced illness diagnosis during the measurement period or the year prior to the measurement period. |
| **Rationale** | Breast cancer is one of the most common types of cancers, accounting for 15% of all new cancer diagnoses in the United States. In 2015, over 3 million women were estimated to be living with breast cancer in the United States and it is estimated that 12% of women will be diagnosed with breast cancer at some point during their lifetime. While there are other factors that affect a woman's risk of developing breast cancer, advancing age is a primary risk factor. Breast cancer is most frequently diagnosed among women ages 55–64; the median age at diagnosis is 62 years. The chance of a woman being diagnosed with breast cancer in a given year increases with age. By age 40, the chances are 1 in 68; by age 50, it becomes 1 in 43; by age 60, it is 1 in 29. |
| **Evidence** | Breast cancer is one of the most common types of cancers, accounting for 15% of all new cancer diagnoses in the United States. In 2015, over 3 million women were estimated to be living with breast cancer in the United States and it is estimated that 12% of women will be diagnosed with breast cancer at some point during their lifetime. While there are other factors that affect a woman's risk of developing breast cancer, advancing age is a primary risk factor. Breast cancer is most frequently diagnosed among women ages 55–64; the median age at diagnosis is 62 years. The chance of a woman being diagnosed with breast cancer in a given year increases with age. By age 40, the chances are 1 in 68; by age 50, it becomes 1 in 43; by age 60, it is 1 in 29. |
| **Denominator Exceptions** | Not applicable |
| **Numerator Exceptions** | Not applicable |
| **Risk Adjusted** | No |
| **Program Status** | Not available |

MIPS = Merit-Based Incentive Payment System Program
CMIT = CMS Measure Inventory Tool
Notes: In addition to Properties, each measure description also includes information about Steward, Characteristics, Groups, Family Measures, Programs, Milestones, Links, Similar Measures, Environmental Scan, and Components.
Centers for Medicare & Medicaid Services. Measures Inventory Tool: measure summary: breast cancer screening measure. Accessed June 20, 2022. https://cmit.cms.gov/cmit/#/MeasureView?variantId=1548&sectionNumber=1

| | CMS | | TJC | | |
|---|---|---|---|---|---|
| | **Status** | **Required for IQR submission?** | **Status** | **Required for ORYX® submission?** | |
| **VTE-1** | Active | Yes (Submit any 3 eCQMs + eOP-1) | Active | Yes (Submit any 4 eCQMs) | **Venous Thromboembolism Prophylaxis** |
| **VTE-2** | Active | Yes (Submit any 3 eCQMs + eOP-1) | Active | Yes (Submit any 4 eCQMs) | **ICU Venous Thromboembolism Prophylaxis** |
| **ED-2** | Active | Yes (Submit any 3 eCQMs + eOP-1) | Active | Yes (Submit any 4 eCQMs) | **Admit Decision Time to ED Departure-Admit** |
| **eOPI-1** | Active | Yes **Required** | Active | Yes (Submit any 4 eCQMs) | **Safe Use of Opioids - Concurrent Prescribing** |
| **PC-01** | Retired | No | Active | Yes (Submit any 4 eCQMs) | **Elective Delivery** |
| **PC-02** | Not available | No | Active | Yes (Submit any 4 eCQMs) | **Cesarean Birth** |
| **PC-05** | Active | Yes (Submit any 3 eCQMs + eOP-1) | Active | Yes (Submit any 4 eCQMs) | **Exclusive Breast Milk Feeding** |
| **PC-06** | Not available | No | Active | Yes (Submit any 4 eCQMs) | **Unexpected Complications in Term Newborns** |
| **PC-07*** | Not available | No | Active | Yes (Submit any 4 eCQMs) | **Severe Obstetric Complications** |
| **STK-2** | Active | Yes (Submit any 3 eCQMs + eOP-1) | Active | Yes (Submit any 4 eCQMs) | **Discharged on Antithrombotic Therapy** |
| **STK-3** | Active | Yes (Submit any 3 eCQMs + eOP-1) | Active | Yes (Submit any 4 eCQMs) | **Anticoagulation Therapy** |
| **STK-5** | Active | Yes (Submit any 3 eCQMs + eOP-1) | Active | Yes (Submit any 4 eCQMs) | **Antithrombotic Therapy / Day 2** |
| **STK-6** | Active | Yes (Submit any 3 eCQMs + eOP-1) | Active | Yes (Submit any 4 eCQMs) | **Discharged on Statin Medication** |

**Figure 6.6** 2022 Measure List for Inpatient eCQM

*New eCQM for 2022

Reproduced from Heilman E. CMS vs TJC: 2022 measure list comparison. Published November 26, 2021. Accessed February 6, 2022. https://blog.medisolv.com/articles/cms-vs-tjc-2022-measure-list-comparison

An important distinction must be made between the statistical analysis of binary and continuous data. Risk adjustment methodologies do not apply to dependent variables that are continuous, like cost or LOS. The answer could be any number on a continuum, not "yes" or "no." Severity adjustment methodologies applied to the cost of LOS data predict severity by using patient-specific variables, called *severity factors*. Frequently, the presence of additional diagnoses helps to define the severity of a group of patients within a

DRG, on an individual patient level, or both. Both risk-adjusted and severity-adjusted data are extremely important outcomes system tools. Using unadjusted or raw data means that all patients in the clinical topic category, regardless of their health status or the existence of varying clinical conditions, are included in the rate calculation. Both raw and risk-adjusted data about the same outcomes topic are available because payers frequently use risk-adjusted data in their initial decision making.

Healthcare quality professionals must be familiar with the ways in which their decision-support databases manage statistical outliers. Are all patients included, or are patients more than two standard deviations (SDs) from the mean removed from data analysis? Most decision-support databases have a consistent approach regarding patients who are outliers. It is critical during data comparisons to make sure that all data sources managed patient outliers in a consistent fashion. For example, a hospital physician group was trying to compare its performance on resource utilization and LOS for community-acquired pneumonia. One patient was hospitalized for more than 100 days because the patient was ventilator dependent and did not have adequate resources to be placed in an extended care facility. This patient's record needed to be removed from the raw data before a fair comparison could be made.

Another factor to consider in the analysis and interpretation of outcomes data is the level of detail. The best system includes clinical and financial information for every payor and practitioner and the patient. This integrated data repository mines data for

- benchmarking quality performance against established standards;
- comparing provider performance within given outcome topics;
- examining details at the patient level;
- viewing patient diagnoses, procedures, and other information;
- determining the impact of managed care on costs and outcomes; and
- analyzing product lines to evaluate their effectiveness and to increase or downsize service offerings.

**Box 6.5** lists key points for design and management of health data analytics techniques.

---

### Box 6.5  Key Points: Design and Management

- Planning for collection and utilization of internally and externally generated data leads to a higher likelihood of success.
- Analyzing data and information generated by an effective performance outcomes measurement system helps identify areas in which to improve quality and resources in their organizations.
- Risk adjustment is a technique used to consider or to control the fact that different patients with the same diagnosis may have additional conditions or characteristics that can affect how well they respond to treatment.

---

# Measurement Concepts

Public repositories of information on evidence-based care quality measures and measure sets are widely used and have proven reliability and validity, such as screening and assessment of substance use and substance use disorders, as well as measurement tools for health and psychosocial studies. Methods that healthcare quality professionals and researchers use include

- interviews (in-person surveys or household surveys),
- focus groups,
- telephone surveys,
- mail-in surveys,
- kiosk surveys, and
- online surveys.

These methods can include instruments such as questionnaires, surveys, rating scales, interview transcripts, and the like. It is critical to use the most credible tools possible (those with proven reliability and validity).

## Reliability

*Reliability* is the extent to which an experiment, test, or measuring procedure yields the same results under similar circumstances by the same or different individuals on repeated trials. It is also referred to as precision, reproducibility, and repeatability. For example, a scale that measures a person's weight as 140 lbs. one minute and then yields a reading of 160 lbs. a minute later would be considered unreliable and not capable of meeting the standards for accuracy or consistency. There are different ways to measure the accuracy of a test or measuring instrument as described below.

- *Reliability coefficient.* The stability of an instrument is derived through procedures referred to as *test–retest reliability.* This is done by administering the test to a sample of people on two occasions and then comparing the scores obtained. The comparison results in a reliability coefficient, which is the numerical index of the test's reliability. The closer the coefficient is to 1.0, the more reliable the tool. In general, reliability coefficients of $\geq 0.70$ are acceptable, although $\geq 0.80$ is desired. The reliability coefficient can be determined by evaluating the internal consistency of a measure. This refers to the degree to which the subparts of an instrument are all measuring the same attribute or dimension. The split-half technique is one of the oldest methods for assessing internal consistency of an instrument and can be done by hand. It correlates scores on half of the measure with scores on the other half. The concept of *reliability by equivalence* compares scores from the various versions of the instrument developed (e.g., parallel forms or alternate forms of a test).

- *Interrater reliability.* This concept refers to the degree to which two raters, operating independently, assign the same ratings in the context of observational research or in coding qualitative materials. The monitoring of the accuracy of a patient acuity system entails interrater reliability. The staff that monitors the system must be able to assign the same classification to the same patient to ensure reliability of their monitoring. Interrater reliability is reported as a degree of concordance, or Cohen's kappa.

## Validity

*Validity* is the degree to which an instrument measures what it is intended to measure. Validity usually is more difficult to establish than reliability. The validity and reliability of an instrument are not wholly independent of each other. An instrument that is not reliable cannot be valid. However, an instrument that is reliable does not have to have validity. For example, a thermometer is a reliable instrument, but it is not valid for measuring height. Valid measures at a high level mean that statistically the instrument is measuring what it is supposed to measure. Several types are described below.

- *Content (face) validity.* This is the degree to which the instrument represents the universe of content. Content validity, although necessary, is not a sufficient indication that the instrument measures what it is intended to measure. For example, a panel of rehabilitation specialists evaluated the Functional Independence Measure tool and identified that it measured the key aspects of the level of disability and change in status. On the other hand, a survey designed to measure patient satisfaction with their primary care provider would be considered inadequate in terms of content validity if it failed to cover the major dimensions of access, waiting time, practitioner–patient interaction, or engagement. Content validity includes judgments by experts or respondents about the degree to which a test measures the relevant construct.
- *Construct validity.* This concept refers to the degree to which an instrument measures the theoretical construct or trait that it was designed to measure.

For example, severity-adjustment scales are tools for measuring staffing needs. Risk-adjustment scales are tools for predicting the probability of outcomes such as morbidity and mortality. If a previously used satisfaction tool had demonstrated validity, a new, abbreviated tool can be compared to the old tool to determine whether the new tool has construct validity. Similarly, two functional status health outcome measures could be compared, such as the SF-36 and SF-12 instruments.

- *Criterion-related validity.* This concept refers to the extent that the score on an instrument can be related to a criterion (the behavior that the instrument is supposed to predict). Criterion-related validity can be either predictive or concurrent, depending on when the criterion variable is measured. If the criterion variable is obtained at the same time as the measurement under study, *concurrent validity* is assessed. If the criterion measure is obtained at some future time (after the predictor instrument was used), *predictive validity* is assessed. A patient acuity system has criterion-related validity because it predicts staffing needs (skill mix and number of staff required).

**Box 6.6** lists key points in measurement concepts.

---

### Box 6.6 Key Points: Measurement Concepts

- Instruments such as questionnaires, surveys, and rating scales are the devices that healthcare quality professionals and researchers use to obtain and record data received from the subjects.
- Reliability is the extent to which an instrument measuring procedure yields the same results under similar circumstances by the same or different individuals on repeated trials. Also referred to as precision, reproducibility, or repeatability.
- The closer the reliability index or reliability coefficient is to 1.0, the more reliable the tool or instrument.
- Validity is the degree to which an instrument measures what it intends to measure and is usually more difficult to establish than reliability.

---

## Data Types

There are two general types of data—categorical and continuous. Methods of sampling, data collection, and analysis are different for each type or level of data. This distinction is critical because quality, safety, and performance improvement work involves both types of data and their associated statistics. The distinction is one of the most significant sources of confusion for people new to performance improvement and data analysis. Data levels are categorical and continuous:

- *Categorical.* A categorical variable is one that has two or more categories, but there is no intrinsic ordering to the categories. For example, a binary variable (such as a yes/no question) is a categorical variable having two categories (yes or no), and there is no intrinsic ordering to the categories. An ordinal variable is like a categorical variable. The difference between the two is that there is a clear ordering of the categories.

- *Continuous.* These are measured data with assigned scales that theoretically have no gaps. The statistical process control (SPC) term for this is *variables data.* The two subtypes of continuous data are interval and ratio. *Continuous data* often converted to count or categorical data. For example, the number of pounds lost by a patient undergoing hemodialysis during treatment in relationship to their desired or dry weight is measurement data. If Mr. Jones was admitted at 170 lbs. and was discharged at his dry weight of 165 lbs., then he measured a 5-lbs. weight loss. If the nurse manager wanted to know the number of patients finishing their treatments at their dry weight for the entire day, then this information would be an example of count data and would be converted into yes/no format.

## Nominal

Nominal data are also called *count*, *discrete*, or *qualitative data.* There are two or more categories, but there is no intrinsic ordering to the categories. In SPC, these are known as *attributes data.* Binary data are categorical data with only two possibilities (e.g., gender). Numerical values can be assigned to each category as a label to facilitate data analysis, but this is purely arbitrary with no quantitative value. If these variables are named, there is no order to the data. Nominal scale is often used in surveys and questionnaires where only the variable label holds significance. Arithmetic operations cannot be performed on them (e.g., addition or subtraction), nor can logical operations like equal to or greater than. Examples of nominal scale data are shown in **Table 6.15**.

## Ordinal

For this type of data, characteristics are categorized and rank ordered. Assignment to categories is not

**Table 6.15** Examples of Nominal Variables

| Nominal Variable | Values |
|---|---|
| Race | ▪ White<br>▪ Black or African American<br>▪ American Indian or Alaska Native<br>▪ Asian<br>▪ Native Hawaiian or other Pacific Islander<br>▪ Some other race |
| Genotype | ▪ Bb<br>▪ BB<br>▪ bB |
| Surgical patient type | ▪ Preoperative<br>▪ Perioperative<br>▪ Postoperative |
| Assigned sex at birth | ▪ Male<br>▪ Female |
| Patient attendance | ▪ Attended video session<br>▪ Did not attend video session |
| Hair color | ▪ Blond<br>▪ Brown<br>▪ Red<br>▪ Other |
| Residence | ▪ Suburbs<br>▪ City<br>▪ Town |
| Marital status | ▪ Married, spouse present<br>▪ Married, spouse absent, not separated<br>▪ Separated<br>▪ Widowed<br>▪ Divorced<br>▪ Never married |
| Occupation | ▪ Management, business, and financial occupation<br>▪ Professional and related occupation<br>▪ Service occupation<br>▪ Sales and related occupation<br>▪ Office and administrative occupations<br>▪ Farming, forestry, and fishing occupation<br>▪ Construction and extraction occupation<br>▪ Installation, maintenance, and repair occupation<br>▪ Production occupations<br>▪ Transportation and material moving occupation |
| Mode of transportation for travel to work | ▪ Car, truck, van as driver<br>▪ Car, truck, van as passenger<br>▪ Public transit<br>▪ Walk<br>▪ Bicycle<br>▪ Other methods |

**Table 6.16** Examples of Ordinal Variables

| Ordinal Variable | Values |
|---|---|
| Nursing staff rank | 1. Nurse level I<br>2. Nurse level II<br>3. Nurse level III |
| Educational attainment | 1. None–8th grade<br>2. 9th–11th grade<br>3. High school graduate<br>4. Some college, no degree<br>5. Associate degree<br>6. Bachelor degree<br>7. Master degree<br>8. Professional degree<br>9. Doctoral degree |
| Patient satisfaction | 1. Very unsatisfied<br>2. Unsatisfied<br>3. Neutral<br>4. Satisfied<br>5. Very satisfied |
| Time of day | 1. Dawn<br>2. Morning<br>3. Noon<br>4. Afternoon<br>5. Evening<br>6. Night |
| Hypertension | 1. Mild<br>2. Moderate<br>3. Severe |

**Table 6.17** Examples of Interval and Ratio Variables

| Interval<br>(natural order, equal intervals) | Ratio<br>(natural order, equal intervals + true zero value) |
|---|---|
| Family income | Height in meters, inches, or feet |
| Time using a 12-hour clock | Body mass index in pounds or kilograms |
| Year | Distance in miles or kilometers |
| Fahrenheit and Celsius temperatures | Kelvin temperature |

arbitrary. If these categories were equally spaced, then the variable would be an interval variable. Examples of ordinal scale data are shown in **Table 6.16**.

## Interval

For interval-level data, the distance between each pair of points is equal and there is no true zero (e.g., the values on a Fahrenheit thermometer). An interval variable is like an ordinal variable, except that the intervals between the values of the numerical variable are equally spaced. Measurements between points have meaning.

## Ratio

For ratio-level data, the distance between each pair of points is equal and there is a true zero (e.g., height and weight). Ratio scale resembles the interval scale, however, in addition to that, it can also accommodate the value of zero on any of its variables. Ratio scale provides the most detailed information to the central tendency using statistical techniques such as mean, median, and mode. Ratio data are calculated by grouping, sorting, adding/subtracting, and multiplying/

dividing, depending on the research. Examples of interval and ratio variables are depicted in **Table 6.17**.

A critical issue is whether the right data are measured or counted. A common criticism of quality, safety, and performance improvement activities is that readily available data, such as patient visits, deaths, infections, falls, cost, and laboratory tests, are analyzed for improvement simply because the data are easy to retrieve.

## Sampling Design

The *population* (N) is the total aggregate or group (e.g., all cases that meet a designated set of criteria for practitioners, all patients who died at a particular hospital, or all registered nurses with a tenure of 10 years or longer). *Sampling* makes research more feasible because it allows researchers to sample a portion of the population to represent the entire population (n). A sample is selected from the accessible population—that is, the population that is available. Sampling has primary purposes, including providing a logical way of making statements about a larger group based on a smaller group and allowing researchers to make inferences or generalize from the sample to the population if the selection process was random and systematic (i.e., unbiased).

## Types of Sampling

There are different methods used to create a sample. Generally, they are grouped into one of two categories described next: probability sampling and nonprobability sampling.

### Probability Sampling

Probability sampling requires every element in the population to have an equal or random chance of being selected for inclusion in the sample. The following are subsets of probability sampling:

1. *Simple random sampling.* Everyone in the sampling frame (all subjects in the population) has an equal chance of being chosen (e.g., pulling a name out of a hat containing all possible names).
2. *Systematic sampling.* After randomly selecting the first case, this method involves drawing every *n*th element from a population, such as picking every third name from a list of names.
3. *Stratified random sampling.* A subpopulation is a *stratum*, and *strata* are two or more homogeneous subpopulations. After the population is divided into strata, each member of a stratum has an equal probability of being selected. Examples of strata include sex, ethnicity, patients with certain diseases, or patients living in certain parts of the country.
4. *Cluster sampling.* This method requires that the population be divided into groups, or clusters. For example, if a researcher is studying medical students, they may not have individual names but may have a list of medical schools in the area. The sample may be randomly derived from this list of medical schools.

## Nonprobability Sampling

Nonprobability sampling provides no way of estimating the probability that each element will be included in the sample. When this approach is used, the results will be representative of the sample only and cannot be generalized to the available population. The following are subsets of nonprobability sampling:

1. *Convenience sampling.* This approach allows the use of any available group of subjects. Because of the lack of randomization in this sampling method, subjects may be atypical in some way. Sending a survey to a list of members of an elder organization may not reflect the opinions of all elders, for example. Convenience sampling may include all patients at an organization who are undergoing a certain procedure over a 12-month period. Selection bias may be present in all convenience sampling because the selected subjects may not accurately reflect the population of interest.
2. *Snowball sampling.* This is a subtype of convenience sampling. This method involves subjects suggesting other subjects for inclusion in the study. The sampling process gains momentum. With this type of sampling, subjects are recruited who are difficult to identify but are known to others because of an informal network.

3. *Purposive or judgment sampling.* This method selects a group or groups based on certain criteria. This method is subjective, and the researcher uses their judgment to decide who is representative of the population. Using a group of nurses, because the researcher believes the group represents a cross-section of women, is an example of this type of sampling. Expert sampling is a type of purposive sampling that involves selecting experts in each area because of their access to the information relevant to the study. Expert sampling is used in the Delphi technique, in which several rounds of questionnaires are distributed on a selected topic and sent to experts to elicit their responses and then sent out again after the initial data analysis. The goal is to achieve rapid group consensus. A conference planning team serves as an example if it uses the Delphi method to identify potential program content that may be of interest to those in the same professions for an upcoming conference.
4. *Quota sampling.* In this type of sampling, the researcher makes a judgment decision about the best type of sample for the investigation. That is, the researcher prespecifies characteristics of the sample to increase its representativeness. The researcher identifies strata of the population and determines the proportions of elements needed from various segments of the population. Stratification may be based on any demographic, such as age or ethnicity.

## Sample Size

Factors may influence the determination of sample size, such as research purpose, design, level of confidence desired, anticipated degree of difference between study groups, and size of the population. Depending on these factors, a small or large sample size may be appropriate. However, except for case studies, the larger the sample, the more valid and accurate the study because a larger sample size is more likely to represent the population. The larger the sample, the smaller the sample error of the mean, which is a measure of fluctuation of a statistic from one sample to another drawn from the same population. Also, as the actual difference between study groups gets smaller, the size of the sample required to detect the difference gets larger. Outcomes that are measured on a continuous scale or using repeated measures require fewer subjects than do categorical outcomes. Using too large a sample to answer a research question is a waste of time and resources.

## Comparison Groups

One of the biggest challenges in making conclusions in the evaluation of QI interventions is the lack of a true comparison group. While looking for changes over time is useful, there is more value in comparing to a group that did not get the intervention (e.g., change in process). Since random assignment to distinct groups is usually not possible, selecting a comparison group is based on convenience. For example, it might be possible to test a new standard of practice (i.e., intervention) to reduce pressure ulcers on several nursing units while maintaining the current practice on other nursing units (i.e., control). The problem is the patients on the units might not be the same. One approach to dealing with this problem is to use propensity score matching.[75] *Propensity score matching* is a multivariate approach to pairing up people with the same characteristics in the intervention and control groups to eliminate potential impact of variation between the groups that are not equal. Propensity score matching is an effective approach to equating groups and a tool that quality, safety, and performance improvement teams consider when analyzing data.

**Box 6.7** lists key points in study design.

---

### Box 6.7  Key Points: Study Design

- Data levels are nominal, ordinal, interval, and ratio.
- Discrete variables are countable in a finite amount of time.
- Sampling makes research more feasible because it allows researchers to sample a portion of the population to represent the entire population.
- Root cause analysis may be initiated when a trend is observed in an unanticipated direction.

---

# Statistical Techniques

The discussion of statistical techniques that follows is in no way a complete account of each topic. Other sources for more information on the various statistical techniques, including Hansen's CAN'T MISS series, are included in *Suggested Readings* and *Online Resources* at the end of this section.

## Statistical Power

Categorical data are the least powerful statistically, and continuous data have the most power. The practical meaning of this when comparing patient outcomes after process change is that fewer data points (and fewer subjects) are needed if data in continuous form are collected. For example, when dealing with blood pressure, a healthcare quality professional might collect the data by categorizing subjects as either hypertensive or nonhypertensive or by recording the measured levels of systolic and diastolic pressure. The latter form is more powerful and allows more flexibility in data analysis.

When designing a quality, safety, and performance improvement project, each step must be planned and accountability assigned. Each organization can adopt an improvement model that facilitates performance improvement and is in alignment with its mission, vision, core values, goals, and strategic plan. See the *Quality Leadership and Integration* and *Performance and Process Improvement* sections.

## Measures of Central Tendency

Measures of *central tendency* are statistical indexes that describe where a set of scores or values of a distribution cluster. *Central* refers to the middle value, and *tendency* refers to the general trend of the numbers. A healthcare quality professional or researcher might ask questions relating to central tendency when answering queries such as, "What is the average LOS for patients with chronic obstructive pulmonary disease?" or "What is the Apgar score of most infants born in the new birthing suites?" The three most common measures of central tendency are the mean, the median, and the mode. The type and distribution of the data determine which measures of central tendency (and spread) are most appropriate.

### Mean

The *mean* (M) of a set of measurements is the sum of all observed scores or values divided by the total number of scores. The mean is also known as the average.

*Example:* If five infants had Apgar scores of 7, 8, 8, 9, and 8, the sum of the values is calculated, and then divided by the total number of infants: $7 + 8 + 8 + 9 + 8 = 40$; $40 \div 5 = 8$; therefore, 8 is the mean.

The mean is the most used of all the measures of central tendency, but it is the most sensitive to extreme scores. In the example just given, if one infant was severely depressed at the time of Apgar scoring and was given a value of 1 instead of 9, the mean then would be 6.4 rather than 8. In this case, the mean is no longer representative of the entire group because it was substantially lowered by just *one* score. The median described shortly, would be a better statistic to use.

It is appropriate to compute the mean for interval or ratio data when variables can be added and the values show a bell-shaped or normal distribution. The mean can be used with ordinal variables with a normal distribution.

## Median

The *median* is the measure of central tendency that corresponds to the middle score. It is the measure of location on a numerical scale above which and below which 50% of the cases fall. To determine the median of data, first arrange the values in rank order. If the total of values is odd, count up (or down) to the middle value. If there are several identical values clustered at the middle, the median is that value. If the total number of values is even, compute the mean of the two middle values.

*Example:* Consider the following set of values: 2 2 2 3 4 5 6 6 8 9. The median for this set of numbers is 4.5, which is the value that divides the set exactly in two. Note that an important characteristic of the median is that the calculation does not consider the quantitative values of the individual scores. An example of this notion can be demonstrated in the sample given. If the last value of 9 was increased to the value 84, the median would remain the same because it does not enter the computation of the median; only the number of values and the values near the midpoint of the distribution enter the computation. The median, consequently, is not sensitive to extreme scores or statistical outliers and is more effective than mean given its intent. It is appropriate to compute the median for ordinal, interval, or ratio data, but not for nominal data.

## Mode

The *mode* is the score or value that occurs most frequently in a distribution of scores. Of the three measures of central tendency, the mode is the easiest to determine; simply determine which value occurs most often in the data set.

*Example 1:* Look at the following distribution of numbers: 30 31 31 32 33 33 33 33 33 34 35 36. It is easy to determine that the mode is 33; the value of 33 appears five times, a higher frequency than for any other number. An easy way to determine the mode is by using a statistical package to run descriptive data frequencies and/or a stem-and-leaf plot. In research studies, the mode is seldom the only measure of central tendency reported. Modes are a quick and easy method to determine an average, but they tend to be unstable. This instability means that the modes tend to fluctuate widely from sample to sample, even when

drawn from the same population. Thus, the mode is reported infrequently, except when used as a descriptor for typical values on nominal data.

*Example 2:* Suppose the administrator of an outpatient clinic intends to measure the typical wait times before the patient meets a clinician for medical help. The administrator collects a sample of 10 wait times in minutes: 7, 14, 20, 3, 6, 10, 8, 4, 7, and 9.

- What statistic should be used to calculate the required value? As the quantitative data collected are measured on the ratio scale (i.e., the person with a wait time of 14 minutes waited two times more than the person with a wait time of 7 minutes), mean or average is the best measure that helps the administrator understand the typical patient wait times. Mean = (7 + 14 + 20 + 3 + 6 + 10 + 8 + 4 + 7 + 9)/10 = 88/10 = 8.8 minutes.
- In the same scenario, calculate median to describe the wait time for a typical patient. Median is the center or midpoint of the distribution. The first step is to order the data values (7, 14, 20, 3, 6, 10, 8, 4, 7, and 9) from smallest to largest (3, 4, 6, 7, 7, 8, 9, 10, 14, 20) or largest to smallest (20, 14, 10, 9, 8, 7, 7, 6, 4, 3). In the next step, since the number of data points is an even number (10), the median for this distribution is the average of the fifth and sixth values (i.e., 7 + 8)/2 or (8 + 7)/2 = 15/2 = 7.5 minutes.
- In the same scenario, calculate mode to describe the wait time for a typical patient. Mode is the value that occurs most frequently in the data. The mode for this distribution is 7 minutes. From a practical perspective, it is important to note that mode is not commonly used as a measure of central tendency because when it comes to continuous variables it is unusual for all the observations to have different values and therefore the entire sample of values may be the mode.

**Box 6.8** lists the key points for discussing measures of central tendency.

---

### Box 6.8 Key Points: Measures of Central Tendency

- The three most common measures of central tendency are mean, median, and mode.
- Mean is also known as the average.
- Median corresponds to the middle score; that is, the point on a numerical scale above which and below which 50% of the cases fall after the data are arranged in rank order.
- Mode is the score or value that occurs most frequently in a distribution of scores.

# Measures of Variability

The purpose of measuring central tendencies of data is to describe the ways subjects or cases group together. In contrast, *variability* looks at the dispersion, or how the measures are spread out. Variability may be further defined as the degree to which values on a set of scores differ. For example, greater variability of age is expected within a hospital than within a nursing home or pediatric intensive care unit. Measures of variability are interpreted as distances on a scale of values, which are unlike averages that are points representing a central value. The three measures of variability presented are the range, interpercentile (including interquartile), and SD.

## Range

The *range* is the difference between the lowest (minimum) and highest (maximum) values in a distribution of scores. Although it indicates the distance on the score scale between the lowest and highest values, the range is best reported as the values themselves and not as the distance between the values. Range offers the advantage of a quick estimate of variability, and it provides information about the two endpoints of a distribution. Disadvantages are its instability because it is based on only two scores and tendency to increase with sample size and its sensitivity to extreme values.

*Example:* Test scores for students range from 98 to 60. The range is 98 minus 60, or 38. When the range is reported in research findings, it normally would be written as a maximum and a minimum, without the subtracted value.

## Interquartile Range

Although there are several interpercentile measures of spread (e.g., interdecile range and interpercentile range), the most common is the *interquartile range*, a stable measure of variability based on excluding extreme scores and using only middle cases. The interquartile range is more stable than the range and is determined by lining up the measures in order of size and then dividing the array into quarters. The range of scores that includes the middle 50% of the scores is the interquartile range; that is, the range between scores composing the lowest quartile, or quarter, and the highest quartile. The interquartile range demonstrates how the middle 50% of the distribution is scattered. The first quartile ends at the 25th percentile. Interquartile range values are often presented in box plots.

*Example:* Growth charts are one of the most used interpercentile measures. Normal growth is represented by measurements between the 25th and 75th percentiles on the National Center for Health Statistics growth charts.

*Example:* Clinical pathways are developed based on the interquartile range of the designated population. Paths are designed around the average patient or those in the middle quartiles.

## Standard Deviation

The variance of a variable is the average of the squared standard deviation from the mean. The *standard deviation* (SD) is the square root of the variance. It is an average of the deviations from the mean and is the most frequently used statistic for measuring the degree of variability in a set of scores. Standard refers to the fact that the deviation indicates a group's average spread of scores or values around their mean; deviation indicates how much each score is scattered from the mean. The larger the spread of a distribution, the greater the dispersion or variability from the mean; consequently, the SD will be a larger value and is said to be heterogeneous. The more the values cluster around the mean, the smaller the amount of variability or deviation and the more homogeneous the group, the smaller the SD. When the distribution deviates from the symmetrical bell curve or normal distribution, then it is known as *skewness*. The relationship that exists between mean, median, and mode is known as the *empirical relationship* and falls into different scenarios such as negatively or positively skewed. Measures of central tendency and spread are useful for summarizing the distribution of data and comparison of two or more data sets. When a normal distribution (or bell-shaped curve) is perfectly symmetrical, the mean, median, and mode all have the same value (as illustrated in **Figure 6.7**). Observed data rarely approach this ideal shape. As a result, the mean, median, and mode usually differ.

The standard bell curve illustrates this measure of variability (**Figure 6.8**). A histogram can be used to display data distribution and to determine if data are normally distributed. When computing the SD, as with the mean, all the scores or values in a distribution are considered. Use of the SD is most appropriate with normally distributed interval or ratio scale data. SDs (and means) may also be calculated for normally distributed values from a broad ordinal scale. SDs can be calculated by hand or with statistical software.

*Example:* The researcher may compare coping-scale scores for two groups of patients, with each group having a different ethnic background. Although each distribution demonstrated a mean score of 30, the SDs were computed at 3 and 8, respectively.

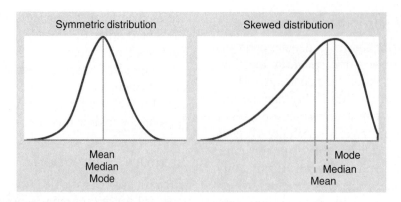

**Figure 6.7** Relation Between Mean, Median, and Mode

Centers for Disease Control and Prevention. *Principles of Epidemiology in Public Health Practice: An Introduction to Applied Epidemiology and Biostatistics*. 3rd ed. Accessed May 4, 2022. https://www.cdc.gov/CSELS/DSEPD/SS1978/Lesson2/Section8.html#TXT210

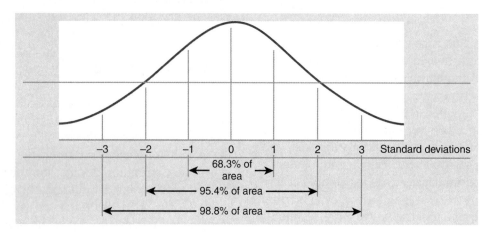

**Figure 6.8** Normal Distribution

The investigator could conclude that although the means were alike, one sample was more homogeneous (or had less variance) in its coping skills.

**Box 6.9** lists the key points of measures of variability.

---

### Box 6.9  Key Points: Measures of Variability

- Three measures of variability are the range, interpercentile, and standard deviation (SD).
- Range is the difference between the highest (maximum) and lowest (minimum) values in a distribution of scores.
- Standard deviation (SD) is an average of deviations from the mean and is the most frequently used statistic for measuring the degree of variability in a set of scores.

---

## Statistical Tests

Significance tests are categorized as either parametric or nonparametric. *Parametric tests* are used with data measured on a continuous scale (i.e., interval or ratio data, which also are known as variables data). *Nonparametric tests* are used with categorical (attributes) data and used with ordinal data, especially if the ordinal categories have a small range of possible values or a nonnormal distribution. **Table 6.18** summarizes statistical options for each type of data and the best types of statistical tests for healthcare studies.

### Parametric Tests

Parametric tests are based on assumptions about the distribution of the underlying population from which the sample was taken. The most common parametric assumption is that data are approximately normally distributed.[76]

**t-Test** The *t*-test assesses whether the means of two groups are statistically different from each other. When determining whether the difference between two group means is significant, a distinction must be made for the two groups. The two groups may be independent; that is, a control group and an experimental

**Table 6.18** Statistical Options for Different Data Types

| | Categorical | Ordinal | Continuous |
|---|---|---|---|
| | **SPC: attribute, nominal, discrete, binary (0/1)** | **Ordinal categorical** | **SPC: variables measured** |
| Examples | Gender, vital status, ethnicity | Age in categories, Functional Independence Measure (FIM) items, patient satisfaction | Age, FIM total, charges, length of stay |
| Usually reported as | Percentage in each category | Percentage in each category (but not always) | Mean, median, minimum, maximum, or percentiles |
| Usual statistical test of differences between groups | Chi-square ($\chi^2$) | $\chi^2$ for most scales; $t$-tests may be appropriate (> 6 levels) if there is a broad scale between groups and data are normally distributed | $t$-tests |
| Control chart* | $p$ if rate > 1/100<br>$u$ if 1/1000 < rate < 1/100<br>$c$ if rate < 1/1000 | Depends on scale, data distribution, and whether data are regrouped | $p$ charts, $c$ charts, $x$ bar and R charts |
| Rules of thumb for sample sizes per plotted point | For $p$ charts; +/− 40 common events; up to 200 for rarer events | (see $p$ chart rules) | Calculate mean based on 2–10 randomly selected values (3–4 optimal) |
| Usual regression technique[†] | Logistic | Logistic (if regrouped as 0/1 outcome) | Ordinary least squares |

\* Most used type; lists not exhaustive.
† Regression is the preferred method for simultaneous control of numerous demographic variables (e.g., gender, age, ethnicity, severity) and is most used in research settings. To control for the influence of a single demographic variable, consider stratifying the analysis by levels of that demographic variable.

group, or they can be dependent, wherein a single group yields pretreatment and posttreatment scores.

*Example:* A healthcare quality professional wants to test the effect of a special educational program on department heads' attitudes toward using graphical or visual displays of data in their performance improvement team meeting. Ten of the 20 department heads are randomly assigned to an experiment group, which will be exposed to videos, discussion groups, and lectures on the use of the basic quality control tools and management and planning tools. The control group comprises the remaining 10 department heads, who will not receive special instruction on using the tools. At the end of the experiment, both groups are administered a scale measuring attitudes toward using these tools. The two-sample independent $t$-test helps the researcher determine if there was a significant statistical difference between the two groups (i.e., whether any difference was due to chance). Alternatively, if all 20 department heads received the training and pretraining and posttraining testing scores, the statistical significance of any changes in average scores would be measured using a paired sample $t$-test.

**Regression Analysis** Regression analysis is based on statistical correlations, or associations among variables. A correlation between two variables is used to evaluate the usefulness of a prediction equation. If this correlation were perfect (i.e., $r = 1$ or $r = -1$), it would be possible to make a perfect prediction about the score on one variable given the score on the other variable. Unfortunately, this is never the case because there never are perfect correlations; consequently, it never is possible to make perfect predictions. The higher the correlation between variables, the more accurate the degree of prediction. If there were no correlation between two variables (i.e., $r = 0$), knowing the score of one would not help to estimate the score on the other. In simple linear regression, one variable ($x$) is used to predict a second variable ($y$). For example, simple regression can be used to predict weight based on height or to predict response to a diabetes management program. Regression analysis is performed with the intent to make predictions about phenomena. The ability to make accurate predictions has substantial implications in the healthcare industry.

**Multiple Regression Analysis** Multiple regression analysis estimates the effects of two or more independent variables ($x$) on a dependent measure ($y$). For example, the objective may be to predict intravenous site infiltration ($y$) based on predictors ($x$), which may include osmolarity of the intravenous solution and addition of an irritating medication, such as potassium, to the intravenous solution.

## Nonparametric Tests

Nonparametric statistical procedures are a class of statistical procedures that do not rely on assumptions about the shape or form of the probability distribution from which the data were drawn.[76]

**Chi-Square Tests and Categorical (Attributes) Data** Much of the data collected by healthcare quality professionals is counted, not measured. Being counted (e.g., 15 male and 30 female patients in the clinic today) means that many arithmetic operations do not apply (it is not possible to calculate the average gender of patients). But it certainly is possible to describe the ratio of the counts (e.g., there were twice as many women as men in the clinic today) or to compare proportions with counted data (50% of male vs. 75% of female patients came for their appointments today). The chi-square test ($\chi^2$) measures the statistical significance of a difference in proportions and is the most reported statistical test in the medical literature. It is the easiest statistical test to calculate manually (see the CAN'T MISS series). It is a statistical test commonly used to compare observed data with data that one would expect to obtain per a specific hypothesis.

*Example:* Using the previously furnished appointment data, 15 of 30 men (50%) with appointments failed to keep them, while only 10 of 40 women (25%) failed to appear. The referent rate of missed appointments in men would be 0.5/0.25 = 2 (i.e., men are twice as likely to not show up as women). While that may or may not fit the hypothesis about men's behavior in this situation, the statistical question is whether this 25% difference in the proportion of no-shows might have happened by chance sampling (in this case, scheduling might be causing the difference). The null hypothesis is that men and women fail to show up for appointments at about the same rate (i.e., rate = 1). Thus, $\chi^2$ tests indicate the likelihood of noting a two-fold difference in no-shows between the groups if, in fact, men and women fail to keep their appointments at the same rate. The actual $\chi^2$ value (test statistic) for these data is 5.84, which corresponds to a statistical

significance ($p$) value of less than 0.02, meaning fewer than 2 out of every 100 days would result in a schedule with which men were twice as likely to not show up. In other words, there is a 2% probability that the difference in no-shows by gender is due to chance, but there is a 98% probability the difference is due to some other factor or factors.

## Tests of Significance

Tests for statistical significance determine the probability that a relationship between two variables is just a chance occurrence. Discussed here are confidence interval and level of significance.

**Confidence Interval** A *confidence interval* (CI) provides a range of possible values around a sample estimate (a mean, proportion, or ratio) calculated from data. CIs are used when comparing groups, but they also have other applications. They reflect the uncertainty that always is present when working with samples of subjects. The sample estimate(s) is a best guess about the true value of interest. Continuing the missed appointment example previously discussed, it is estimated that 50% of men miss their appointments, but the true value may be higher or lower. There is similar uncertainty about the true proportion of women who miss their appointments and about the ratio of the men's and women's proportions. Using the measure of variation from a sample, it is possible to construct a CI that, with a stated level of probability, holds the true value of interest.

*Example:* It was observed (hypothetically) that men are twice as likely to miss their appointments as women. The 95% CI around the referent rate of 2 is (1.27 to 3.13), meaning there is 95% certainty that men are between 1.27 and 3.13 times more likely to miss their appointment. A lower level of confidence would include a narrower range of values. For example, the 90% CI around the referent rate for the appointment data would be (1.44 to 2.77).

**Level of Significance** The level of significance ($p$) gives the probability of observing a difference as large as the one found in a study when, in fact, there is no true difference between the groups (i.e., when the null hypothesis is true). A small $p$-value indicates a small chance that the null hypothesis is true and favors the alternative hypothesis that there is a significance between the two groups. Historically, when the $p$-value is less than 0.05, healthcare quality professional and researchers declared their results statistically significant and rejected the null hypothesis.

*Example:* The $p$-value for the ratio of missed appointment rates above was 0.02, so it was concluded that there was little evidence that men and women had the same rate of missed appointments (the null) and determined that men probably had a higher rate of missed appointments. How much higher? There is 95% confidence that the odds ratio lies between 1.27 and 3.13 times more likely to miss their appointments (see the CI example). Note that if the *p*-value had been > 0.05, the 95% CI would have included 1.0, determining that there was no difference in the proportions of men and women who miss their appointments.

**Box 6.10** lists key points of statistical tests.

---

### Box 6.10  Key Points: Statistical Tests

- Significance tests are parametric or nonparametric.
  - Parametric tests are used with data measured on a continuous scale (i.e., interval or ratio data, which also are known as variables data).
  - Nonparametric tests are used with categorical (attributes) data and with ordinal data, especially if the ordinal categories have a small range of possible values or a nonnormal distribution.
- CI provides a range of possible values around a sample estimate (a mean, proportion, or ratio) that is calculated from data.

---

## Data-Informed Decision Making

The analysis, ultimate interpretation of data, and reporting are meaningful to various audiences. Consider the Data-Information-Knowledge-Wisdom Pyramid (DIKW) that shows data lead to information, information to knowledge, and knowledge to wisdom.[77] The basic premise of this concept is that data in general are abundant and wisdom is rare. Also, data have little or no meaning in isolation. Information is data plus meaning. Knowledge is derived by exploring different patterns within the information, and finally wisdom is understanding the patterns of knowledge and their relationships (**Figure 6.9**).

Good presentation of data creates interest and enhances understanding. Data are reported and analyzed on a regular basis. In this process, it is important to validate the data. Display the data in a summary in an easily understood format. Ask monitored individuals to help with the analysis. There is an analysis of variances and identification of unexpected patterns among caregivers, services, and patients. If there are trends, ask people to identify probable causes and solutions.

## Displaying Data

Healthcare quality professionals can use various charts and diagrams when considering the data collected to make sense of them. These tools typically represent the data in a visual way to assist stakeholders in making decisions about improvement. A challenge for performance improvement or data analytics staff is to display data in a meaningful way for involved departments or interprofessional teams. Graphic display of the data enhances the understanding and use of results. Bader and Bohr describe the use of tables, graphics, infographics, and visuals.[32] Tables are the most familiar format to present information. By highlighting the most pertinent information, readers can quickly and efficiently hone key information. For tables to be most effective, they are understandable and use minimal abbreviations or jargon. They have columns clearly identified, with specific findings highlighted with

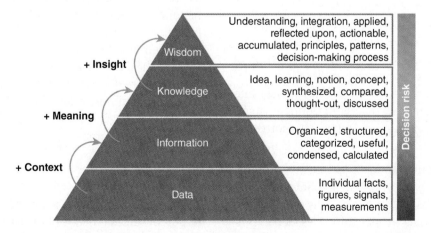

**Figure 6.9** DIKW Pyramid

Reproduced from Tedeschi LO. ASN-ASAS symposium: Future of data analytics in nutrition: mathematical modeling in ruminant nutrition: approaches and paradigms, extant models, and thoughts for upcoming predictive analytics. *J Anim Sci.* 2019;97(5):1921-1944. doi:10.1093/jas/skz092

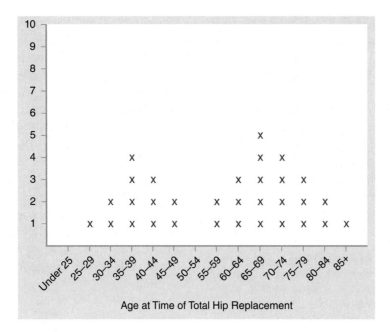

**Figure 6.10** Frequency Distribution

boldface type, underlining, or other distinguishing marks. Graphics and visuals provide a snapshot of an organization's status; where the variations lie; the relative importance of identified problems; and the impact, if any, of changes instituted.[78]

There are publications available on the visual display of data and information. The emphasis is telling stories through graphic representation of data.[79] Common presentations of data include the following:

- *Pareto diagram/chart:* Prioritizes a series of problems or possible causes of problems
- *Histogram:* Illustrates the variability or distribution of data
- *Scatter diagram:* Displays possible cause and effect, illustrates whether one variable might have an impact upon another variable, and can illustrate the strength of that impact
- *Run chart:* Used to monitor processes over time
- *Control chart:* Used to statistically illustrate upper and lower limits of a process and the variation of an organization's process within those limits
- *Stratification:* Breaks down single values into meaningful categories or classifications to focus on improvement opportunities or corrective action[78]

To effectively present data for interpretation and discussion, it is essential to provide a contextual background. Because most people are visually oriented, use a graph to display data. A table of values can accompany the graph. Include an explanation of specifics regarding the data collection (how, when, and where the data are collected, and from whom obtained). The report summarizes the meaning of the values and how computed. State if outliers are removed from the denominator.

## Frequency Distribution

Bell curves, histograms, and 2 × 2 tables are all types of *frequency distributions* (**Figure 6.10**). When people describe a normal distribution, they are referring to a bell curve. Displaying the frequency distribution can help determine if one or more processes are occurring. For example, a frequency distribution can be a bimodal distribution of the ages of patients undergoing a total hip replacement. In other words, the data have two different bell curves present and possibly two different processes. Conceivably, the demographics and risk factors may be different, and each age distribution may need a separate quality, safety, or performance improvement focus.

See the *Performance and Process Improvement* section for more discussion of tools and methods to better understand how to use data, how to translate data to information, and how to use information to drive improvement efforts.

## Histogram

Before further analyzing a data set, review the distribution of values for each of the variables (**Figure 6.11**). The optimal tool for reviewing a distribution depends on the amount of information. A bar chart or bar graph is a way to summarize a set of categorical data and has

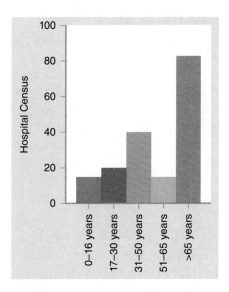

**Figure 6.11** Histogram

different variations such as stacked bar charts, side-by-side bar charts, and clustered bar charts. A *histogram* is a frequency distribution used with numerical data. It is the most-used frequency distribution tool that presents the measurement scale of values along the *x*-axis (each bar is an equal-sized interval) and the frequency scale along the *y*-axis (counts or percentages). Plotting the frequency of each interval reveals the pattern of the data, showing their center and spread (including outliers) and whether there is symmetry or skew. This is important because it may reveal problems in the data and may influence the choice of measure of central tendency and spread.

There is a an important distinction with bar charts and histograms. With a bar chart, the *x*-axis consists of discrete categories (each bar is a separate group). An example of this would be plotting systolic blood pressure > 140 by ethnic group. The height of the bar represents the frequency of elevated blood pressure for each 1 mm Hg change in each ethnic group. A histogram's *x*-axis is divided into categories using equally sized ranges of values along the axis. The variable is measured on a continuous scale, and the bars are not separated by gaps. To continue with the systolic blood pressure example, the groupings of the *x*-axis could be equal sized with ranges defined as 90 to 99, 100 to 119, or 120 to 129 mm Hg. Histograms can be constructed manually or using various statistical software programs.

## Pareto Diagram/Pareto Chart

A *Pareto diagram* (or *Pareto chart*) displays a series of bars with which the priority for problem solving can easily be seen by the varying height of the bars (**Figure 6.12**). The tallest bar is the most frequently occurring issue. The bars are always arranged in descending height. This tool is related to the Pareto principle (named after the 19th-century economist Vilfredo Pareto), which states that 80% of the problems or effects come from 20% of the causes. Therefore, by tackling 20% of the most frequent causes, an 80% improvement can be achieved.

## Pie Chart

Pie charts are useful for understanding all the responses on a measure, usually expressed as percentages (**Figure 6.13**). For example, if a home care

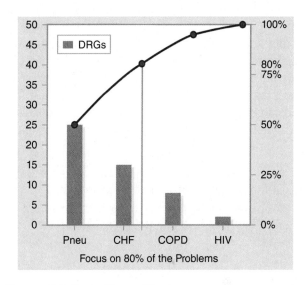

**Figure 6.12** Pareto Diagram/Chart

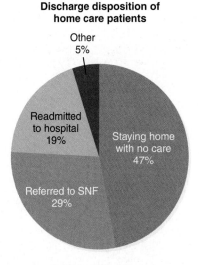

**Figure 6.13** Pie Chart

Data from National Association for Healthcare Quality. *Data Analysis and Reporting: Quick Reference Guide.* Author; 2016; and Centers for Disease Control and Prevention. Evaluation briefs: using graphs and charts to illustrate quantitative data. 2018. Accessed February 16, 2022. https://www.cdc.gov/healthyyouth/evaluation/pdf/brief12.pdf

agency wanted to visualize the discharge disposition of patients when they leave care, the agency would count the number staying home with no care, referred to a skilled nursing facility, readmitted to the hospital, or any other category. The slices of the pie would then represent the percentage in each group. Bigger slices represent a greater proportion of patients.

## Run Chart

When there is an unanticipated pattern or trend, an investigation is initiated to determine the cause (e.g., root cause analysis). For example, if the 30-day readmission rate is climbing 1% every month for a 6-month period, there might be a change in practice. In this case, an interprofessional team may be convened to further analyze and improve the process that is causing the increase. After thorough analysis of the process, the team selects and implements appropriate corrective measures. *Run charts* or *trend charts* are graphic displays of data points over time. Run charts are control charts without the control limits (**Figure 6.14**). Their name

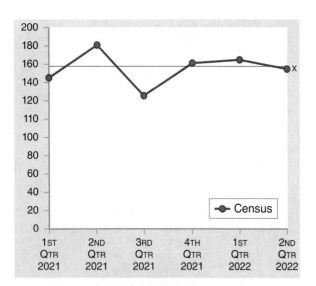

**Figure 6.14** Run Chart

comes from the fact that the user is looking for trends in the data or a substantial number of data points going in one direction or on one side of the average.

Trends indicate a statistically important event that needs further analysis. Resist the tendency to see every variation in the data as significant; wait to interpret the results until at least 10 (or even better, 20) data points are plotted. As indicated in this example, it is best to not analyze data too frequently. For example, looking at quarterly data may more accurately reflect trends over time than reviewing data monthly.

## Scatter Diagram/Scatter Plot

A *scatter diagram* determines the extent to which two variables (quality effects or process causes) relate to one another (**Figure 6.15**). These diagrams often are used in combination with fishbone or Pareto diagrams/charts. The extent to which the variables relate is called *correlation*. Scatter plots can be created manually or with statistical or spreadsheet software.

## Stratification Chart

*Stratification charts* show where a problem does and does not occur or demonstrate underlying patterns (**Figure 6.16**). One such chart is called the Is/Is-Not Matrix. This matrix is used to organize knowledge and information so that patterns can be identified.

## Statistical Process Control

Use of an SPC chart clarifies and interprets a function or process. The performance of functions or processes varies over time. This variation is expected and predictable. It is called *random* or *common-cause variation*. A process is in control if the variation is within the computed upper and lower limits and no trends are evident. There is no need to act if a process is in control. *Special-cause variation* occurs when activity falls outside the control limits or there is an obvious

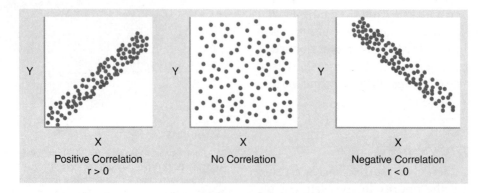

**Figure 6.15** Scatter Diagram/Scatter Plot

nonrandom pattern around the central line. This type of variation is interpreted as a trend and investigated.

SPC is an approach to monitoring quality by looking at whether a process or outcome is within the bounds of the expected. Control charts visualize data

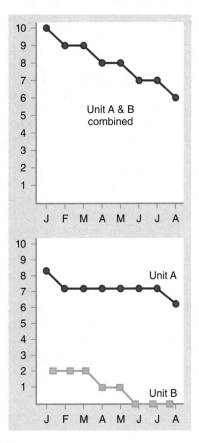

**Figure 6.16** Stratification Chart

to detect and prevent problems. There are two basic types of control charts—a univariate control chart, which is a graphical display (chart) of one quality characteristic and a multivariate control chart, which is a graphical display of a statistic that summarizes or represents more than one quality characteristic. *Control charts* are run charts to which control limits are added above and below the center line (mean). These lines are calculated from the data and show the range of variation in the output of a process. In general, upper control limits and lower control limits are determined by adding and subtracting three SDs to or from the mean. Assuming a normal distribution and no special-cause variation, 99% of data points would be expected to fall between the upper control limit and the lower control limit.

There are types of control charts for both variables and attributes data.

- *Variables data.* 1 Range bar chart, median and range chart, $x$ and $s$ chart, *XmR* chart, moving average chart
- *Attributes data.* P chart, NP chart, U chart, C chart

One common chart presents individual values ($X$) and calculates limits based on the moving range ($mR$); this is the *XmR* chart. The *XmR* chart is used when data are obtained on a periodic basis, such as once a day or once a week, which is common in quality and performance improvement activities. See **Figure 6.17** for an example of a control chart.

By design, control charts are particularly useful in identifying variation in quality measures. The

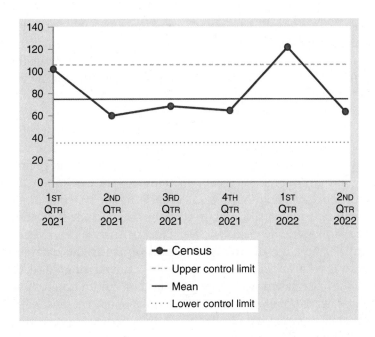

**Figure 6.17** Control Chart

challenge for the healthcare quality professional is determining whether what they are seeing is common or special-cause variation to take the appropriate action.

- *Common-cause variation.* Variation is inherent in any process. Common cause variation is inherent in the design of the process, affects all the outcomes of a process, and results in a stable process that is predictable. On a control chart, this type of variation is exhibited as points between the control limits in no pattern. This is variation that normally would be expected from a process (e.g., due to regular, natural, or ordinary causes). If this type of variation is treated as being unpredictable, it could tamper with the process and, in fact, make things worse. The root cause of the variation must be identified before trying to fix the problem. This is also known as "random" or "unassignable variation."

    *Example:* A hospital system received bad reviews for inadequate patient treatment, and upon investigation, the team identified that most of the problems are related to the poorly maintained equipment. Due to this, the results are somewhat accurate on some days, and highly accurate on other days. This is an example of common-cause variation, as the issue is inherent within the current process.

- *Special-cause variation.* Variation that arises from sources that are not inherent in the process are unpredictable. Special-cause variation is due to irregular or unnatural causes that are not inherent in the design of the process. On a control chart, this type of variation is exhibited as points that fall outside the control limits, or, when inside the control limits, exhibit certain patterns. Special-cause variations are addressed any time they occur with interventions appropriate to eliminate the special cause, if possible. This is also known as "nonrandom" or "assignable variation."

    *Example:* Several patients received cardiac pacemakers at a healthcare system and complained of tiredness after the procedure. Criteria of pacemaker syndrome vary, but symptoms include fatigue, dyspnea on exertion, paroxysmal nocturnal dyspnea, orthopnea, orthostatic hypotension, and syncope. Upon investigation, it is discovered that the surgeon, who was relatively new to the procedure, implanted the pacemakers with the default or factory settings instead of making necessary adjustments. Pacemaker syndrome can be treated with reprogramming of the parameters to

achieve the optimal synchrony of atrial and ventricular contraction.[80(piv)] Once the adjustments were made to fit the patient's needs, they started feeling great. This is an example of special cause variation, as it is an unexpected glitch (on the part of the new surgeon) in the process.

**Box 6.11** lists key points in displaying data.

---

### Box 6.11  Key Points: Displaying Data

- Stratification charts show where a problem does or does not occur or to demonstrate underlying patterns.
- A histogram shows the distribution of the variables and can be used before getting into the additional analysis mode.
- Pie charts are useful for understanding all the responses on a measure, usually expressed as percentages.
- A Pareto chart displays a series of bars that show the most common sources of defects to help prioritize problem solving.
- A scatter plot determines the extent to which two variables relate to one another.
- Statistical process control is an approach to monitoring quality by looking at whether a process or outcome is within the bounds of what is expected. Data are visualized in control charts to detect and prevent problems.
- Variation that is inherent in any process is known as common-cause variation, whereas the variation that arises from sources that are not inherent in the process is known as special-cause variation.

---

## Reporting for Improvement

The management of data, analysis of information, and management through knowledge are necessary to change and improve healthcare organizations. Organizations clarify the difference between data and information. Data are carefully selected, validated, and formatted to make reports useful. This often is easier to mandate than accomplish. However, the goal remains that governing body reports contain only the critical information needed for effective decision making. Achieving this goal would eliminate healthcare data being presented as a pile of computer printouts and various fragmented reports. It is important to keep in mind the data life cycle (**Figure 6.18**) and its functions to frame analysis and reporting for systems, products, and services. Functions may include Envision, Plan, Generate/Acquire, Process/Analyze, Share/Use/Reuse, and Preserve/Discard. Framing the data cycle can be accomplished while considering legal and institutional drivers and data culture to minimize risks and realize value propositions. Lessons learned and insights gleaned from experiences across the cycle can be carried over to future projects.[81]

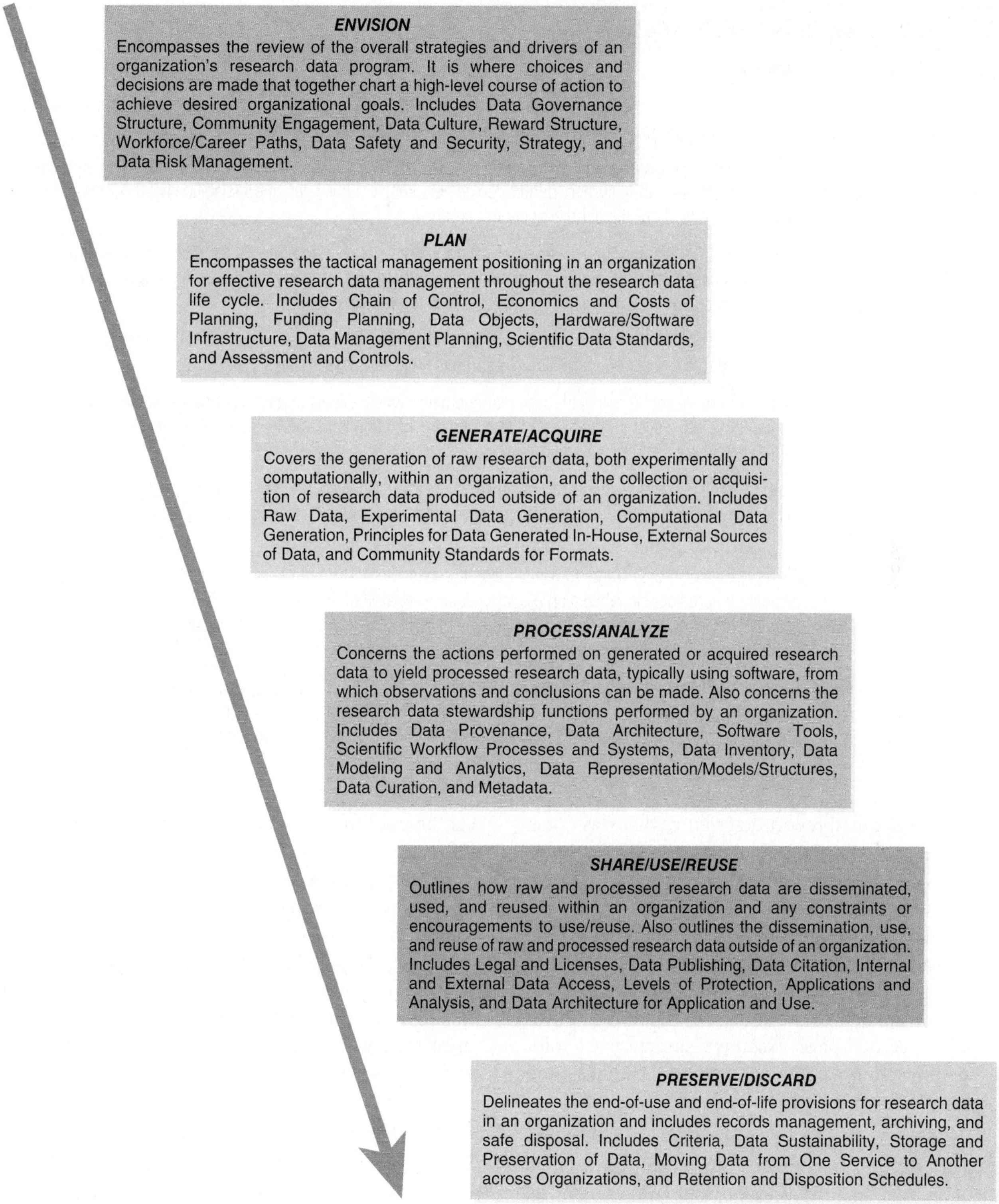

**ENVISION**
Encompasses the review of the overall strategies and drivers of an organization's research data program. It is where choices and decisions are made that together chart a high-level course of action to achieve desired organizational goals. Includes Data Governance Structure, Community Engagement, Data Culture, Reward Structure, Workforce/Career Paths, Data Safety and Security, Strategy, and Data Risk Management.

**PLAN**
Encompasses the tactical management positioning in an organization for effective research data management throughout the research data life cycle. Includes Chain of Control, Economics and Costs of Planning, Funding Planning, Data Objects, Hardware/Software Infrastructure, Data Management Planning, Scientific Data Standards, and Assessment and Controls.

**GENERATE/ACQUIRE**
Covers the generation of raw research data, both experimentally and computationally, within an organization, and the collection or acquisition of research data produced outside of an organization. Includes Raw Data, Experimental Data Generation, Computational Data Generation, Principles for Data Generated In-House, External Sources of Data, and Community Standards for Formats.

**PROCESS/ANALYZE**
Concerns the actions performed on generated or acquired research data to yield processed research data, typically using software, from which observations and conclusions can be made. Also concerns the research data stewardship functions performed by an organization. Includes Data Provenance, Data Architecture, Software Tools, Scientific Workflow Processes and Systems, Data Inventory, Data Modeling and Analytics, Data Representation/Models/Structures, Data Curation, and Metadata.

**SHARE/USE/REUSE**
Outlines how raw and processed research data are disseminated, used, and reused within an organization and any constraints or encouragements to use/reuse. Also outlines the dissemination, use, and reuse of raw and processed research data outside of an organization. Includes Legal and Licenses, Data Publishing, Data Citation, Internal and External Data Access, Levels of Protection, Applications and Analysis, and Data Architecture for Application and Use.

**PRESERVE/DISCARD**
Delineates the end-of-use and end-of-life provisions for research data in an organization and includes records management, archiving, and safe disposal. Includes Criteria, Data Sustainability, Storage and Preservation of Data, Moving Data from One Service to Another across Organizations, and Retention and Disposition Schedules.

**Figure 6.18** Data Life Cycle

Modified from Hanisch RJ, Kaiser DL, Carroll BC. *Research Data Framework (RDaF): Motivation, Development, and a Preliminary Framework Core*. National Institute of Standards and Technology Special Publication 1500-18. Natl. Inst. Stand. Technol. Spec. Publ. 1500-18. February 2021. Accessed June 3, 2022. doi:10.6028/NIST.SP.1500-18

**Table 6.19** provides scenarios of data life cycle steps. Many tools are useful in the analysis of current processes and the design of new processes; this discussion is not meant to be all inclusive. The final product of every quality, safety, or performance improvement project is reporting. For example, reporting can include three types of presentation shared across the organization and used with different audiences.

**Table 6.19** Scenarios for Data Life Cycle Steps

| Life Cycle Step | Scenario |
| --- | --- |
| Generation | A patient shows up for an appointment at a primary care clinic that triggers the beginning of a healthcare encounter. Their information is entered via a self-service kiosk in the waiting area. |
| Collection | The *Ambulatory Surgery Center Survey on Patient Safety Culture* assesses patient safety culture in ambulatory surgery centers (ASCs). A surgery center decides to use this survey designed specifically for ASC staff to ask for their opinions about the culture of patient safety in the facility. |
| Processing | Health plans may want to detect erroneous or fraudulent claims before reimbursing providers. A Medicaid health plan uses administrative and claims data to detect fraud, prescription abuse, upcharges, phantom billings, and other fraud, waste, and abuse events in the revenue cycle. |
| Storage | Providers need to keep medical information accurate, updated, and secure. A hospital decides to migrate data to the cloud to cut costs on maintaining on-premise physical data centers. |
| Management | A comprehensive, real-time health data management system allows providers, patients, and external users to input data into a system. An accountable care organization implements a chain system as a clustering approach to increase transactions throughput. |
| Analysis | A group practice wants to identify unnecessary utilization of the emergency department and uses data mining to look at clinical, financial, and operational patterns for patients with frequent emergency department visits. |
| Visualization | A graphical representation of information and data helps to visualize outliers and patterns. A patient-centered medical home wants to translate test results into risk. Biomarkers (things like blood pressure and cholesterol) predict risk. While high blood pressure is related to risk, the relationship is not linear. Visuals can help a person who has an elevated blood pressure level (e.g., at a doctor's visit) recognize (1) that their risk is elevated *and* (2) that further increases in blood pressure would be harmful.[82] |
| Interpretation | Reviewing current and historical data yields insights on micro and macro levels—patient, organization, and community. This supports informed decision making. A community mental health center may consider past and current risk assessments to determine the level of care for a patient presenting with suicidal ideation. |

- *First.* A detailed report describing what was done. Features all the analyses, tables, and figures; interprets the findings; and offers the specific details about next steps. Share with chairs of departments, quality leaders, and senior administrators.
- *Second.* A high-level presentation to discuss the overall findings and outline suggestions for improvements. Share at team or board meetings.
- *Third.* A one-page executive summary or infographic summarizes the project, findings, and improvement recommendations. Share broadly.

Another avenue of communication to consider is quarterly or semiannual events/forums/town hall meetings that include presentations and posters on recent quality, safety, or performance improvement projects. These events can be offered to a broad audience and widely publicized. Other options for disseminating quality, safety, and performance improvement findings to staff include monthly newsletters, emails, blogs, and other social media distribution outlets.

Myriad data analysis and graphic display tools are available to assist with understanding a process at a point in time and over time. Although no single tool can support an entire process improvement team, tools can be used in combination to facilitate making data-informed decisions. However, the use of tools alone does not guarantee accurate and effective decision making. Quality, safety, and performance improvement teams must be configured to include frontline caregivers, key stakeholders across disciplines, and healthcare quality professionals with expertise in quality, safety, and performance improvement design, implementation, and evaluation (including the tools and statistics described in this section).

## Key Performance Indicators

What gets measured gets done. Key performance indicators (KPIs) are the critical or key indicators to measure performance or progress toward an intended result.[83] They are used to set targets (i.e., desired level of performance) and track progress against the target. Both benchmarking and KPIs allow the management team to identify areas where the company excels as well as areas that need improvement. KPIs are measures of how well an individual or department or organization is performing compared to specific strategic objectives or goals set by the organization. A few examples of KPIs are financial growth and staff retention.

## Benchmarking

Benchmarking compares an organization against other organizations that are well known for best practices within the same domain. A hospital in Florida may compare itself against a top 10 Leapfrog organization to compare performance and chart improvement. In other instances, a hospital within a healthcare system may compare its performance against another hospital within the same system. No matter what data display or reporting tool is used, benchmarking offers the organization to establish performance goals for administrative, financial, and clinical outcomes.

The performance improvement team can determine whether it wants to be average (the industry standard) or raise the bar to a much higher level of performance (the best). When comparison reveals differences, the healthcare organization's management staff can begin to ask questions to determine the factors contributing to variances. Benchmarking includes routinely comparing indicators (structure, process, and outcomes) against best performance and seeking out ways to make improvements with the greatest impact on outcomes. It offers another approach to compare an organization's or individual practitioner's results against a reference point. Ideally, the reference point is a demonstrated best practice.

When looking at potential data for reference points, it is also good to consider evidence-based medicine is the "conscientious, explicit and judicious use of current best evidence in making decisions about the care of individual patients."[84(p71)] However, healthcare quality professionals may more commonly use the term evidence-based practice (EBP). Clinicians base diagnosis, treatment, and decision making on experimental and experiential evidence, patient and professional values, and physiological principles. Benefits to using EBP include the following:

- Promotes quality and patient safety through the provision of effective and efficient healthcare, resulting in less variation in care and fewer unnecessary or nontherapeutic interventions
- Complements the principles of continuous quality, safety, and performance improvement
- Is an essential step for determining the impact of EBPs in outcomes evaluation at the individual and aggregate level

EBPs and QI are based on clinical research and health services research. Clinical research evaluates the impact of interventions on patient outcomes. Outcome measures may include clinical outcomes, functional outcomes, and patient satisfaction or engagement.

Internal or external benchmarks used depend on the measure and what the organization is trying to accomplish. In their discussion about the use of benchmarking and continuous improvement, Ettorchi-Tardy and colleagues noted the advantages of internal benchmarking—it is rapid, it is less expensive, and it offers a learning method.[85(pe110)] For external benchmarking, some advantages might be specificity of the indicators to be used and how these practices might be compared against other healthcare organizations. External sources help develop best practices by implementing the same or similar processes to achieve better results. For example, an organization is focusing on improving vaccination rates among healthcare workers using the "timely and effective care: healthcare worker influenza vaccination" measure. Using a CMS tool called Care Compare, the organization can assess progress in its vaccination rates with data provided by CDC via the National Healthcare Safety Network tool. Another example is using the *Medical Office Survey User Comparative Report* to identify key indicators for benchmarking from the *Survey on Patient Safety Culture*.[86]

One of the most critical decisions an organization makes when launching a benchmarking initiative is selecting the source of comparative data. Organizations have developed benchmarks for various aspects of operations such as efficiency benchmarks (the level of resource required for the completion of a defined number of transactions) and quality benchmarks (the level of consistency applied to similar transactions against recognized standards and the relative level of value of those services). According to Zolelzer, these performance benchmarks define the vision for what is possible in best practice operations and can identify strengths and weaknesses in operations and support operational improvement initiatives.[87] Using administrative performance benchmarking, a health plan can analyze the efficiency of operational areas including claims, medical management, customer service, and administration and look at resource allocations in comparison to peers and competitors.[87]

Healthcare quality professionals often coordinate an organization's benchmarking efforts. Most healthcare regulatory agencies require benchmarking as part of a comprehensive quality, safety, and performance improvement program. Potential data sources for benchmarking include the following:

- Government data available from CMS, CDC, and state government agencies
- Alliances such as large healthcare systems (partnership organizations often provide data extrapolation for their members, frequently providing databases for internal and external benchmarking)

- State peer review organizations and state hospital associations that offer free benchmarking opportunities for hospitals within their state
- For-profit database companies that offer software that helps hospitals or organizations extrapolate and compile their own benchmark data or provide benchmarking data through a centralized database compiled by the company

These data are reported to regulatory and accreditation agencies as part of routine reporting (e.g., ORYX, Outcome and Assessment Information Set, and HEDIS). **Table 6.20** illustrates examples of benchmarking projects.

Balanced scorecards and dashboards are key reporting tools that help organizations track and sustain the improvement of outcomes. However, these tools have subtle differences highlighted in **Table 6.21**.

## Balanced Scorecards

Organizations rely on a bottom-up strategy for performance management where each operating unit (e.g., cardiology, radiology, and dialysis) or key pillar (e.g., finance, quality, and growth) sets its own targets toward meeting the overall organizational strategic goals. Strategy and performance management are key disciplines that help managers and leaders decide and manage important projects to ensure they align with their organizational mission, vision, and values. The measures and indicators for each of these different projects provides the organizational leaders at all

**Table 6.20** Benchmarking Examples

| Type of Benchmarking | Topic | Measure |
|---|---|---|
| Internal | Cesarean section rate | ▪ Physician *A* versus *B* versus *C*; physician group<br>▪ Practice *A* versus *B* versus *C*; physicians versus midwives |
| Internal | Time to administer antibiotic for "XYZ" infection | ▪ Emergency department versus unit *A* versus unit *B*.<br>▪ Emergency department versus urgent care setting |
| Internal | Nursing home resident satisfaction | ▪ Overall satisfaction with nursing care by unit<br>▪ Unit supervisor pays attention to resident safety problems |
| External | Use of ACE inhibitors with acute myocardial infarction | ▪ Health system or proprietary database performance of all hospitals versus region versus similar-size hospital versus own hospital |
| External | Central-line–associated bloodstream infection rates | ▪ Hospital unit versus National Healthcare Safety Network data for similar units; can compare by quartile or median rates for industry standard |
| External | Wrong site/wrong procedure/wrong person surgery | ▪ Inpatient incidence rate versus zero incidence rate |

**Table 6.21** Using Dashboards and Scorecards for Improvement

| Criteria | Dashboard | Scorecard |
|---|---|---|
| Who are the primary users? | Frontline staff | Senior leadership team |
| What is its primary focus or intent? | Operational | Strategic (long-term) |
| What is its format? | In-depth (charts, tables, graphs, gauges) | High-level (one-page overview) |
| How often is it updated? | Real-time or near real-time | Daily, weekly, or monthly |
| Does it enforce accountability? | No | Yes |
| Does it have the drill-down capability? | Yes | No |
| Does it provide actionable information? Data should always be actionable or maybe it is not worth reporting. | Yes | Yes |
| Does it support outcomes improvement? | Yes | Yes |

Data from Lowder D. Healthcare dashboards vs. scorecards: use both to improve outcomes. Published May 22, 2018. Accessed February 15, 2022. https://www.healthcatalyst.com/insights/healthcare-dashboards-vs-scorecards-to-improve-outcomes/

levels with key business and operational insights to track their overall current and expected performance.

The concept of the balanced scorecard is the presentation of a mixture of measures each compared to a target value. The target values can be set by the organization or be based on external benchmarks. In other words, the framework assists leaders in arriving at *agreed-upon criteria,* which focuses on understanding the expectations of the stakeholders and customers; identifying opportunities for growth; and creating value while continuing to improve the existing processes—toward the organizational success.

Balanced scorecards focus on multiple dimensions that underlie care delivery. For example, group key quality metrics into domains: process, outcomes, utilization, and patient experience, and engagement. A balanced scorecard would then have several measures in each of these domains with appropriate targets. One of the biggest benefits is easy communication of the quality measures to executives in the organization (e.g., chief executive officer, chief medical officer, chief nursing officer).

Scorecards provide a brief (usually one-page), high-level overview of a hospital system's long-term strategic outcomes and improvement goals such as reducing readmissions, increasing average patient satisfaction, and reducing turnaround times in operating rooms. Mission and strategy are translated into a set of measures to illustrate a balanced view to the organization's performance as shown in **Figure 6.19**, where the measures are shown for quality patient care. This balanced scorecard also includes indicators for chronic disease management, enhanced care coordination, patient risk, and unplanned emergency room visits, to name a few.

## Dashboards

In the early 1980s, executive information systems, also known as executive support systems, supported senior executives with information necessary for decision making by providing easy access to both internal and external information relevant to meeting strategic goals of the organization. Options available were to purchase a predesigned software package that focuses on a specific industry or creating custom-made software to meet their specific needs. An executive information system could provide summarized information as well as the opportunity to drill down to a more detailed view if necessary.

Executive information systems lost popularity in favor of BI. The ability to comprehensively view into an organization's data and process it to unearth information necessary to eliminate efficiencies and

drive change has become the primary focus for many industries, and more so in healthcare. The advent of large databases to accommodate exponential data growth and the ability of computers and information systems to handle such voluminous data has propelled the growth of the field of BI. It is an overarching term that covers the processes and methods of collecting, storing, and analyzing data from business operations or activities to help organizations optimize their performance by making more data-driven decisions such as identifying issues, tracking performance, comparing data against competitors, identifying ways to increase profit, analyzing customer behavior, identifying market trends, and predicting success. **Table 6.22** illustrates the processes in BI.

Organizations often develop dashboards to represent key management and performance indicators.[88] They are a form of graphical user interface that provides a snapshot of the KPIs that are related to a particular objective or business process. As a decision support or BI reporting tool, the dashboard can provide insights seldom seen with mere gut and intuition using a combination of the right metrics with visualization that will help "provide context and meaning that go beyond the buzzwords and technologies."[89(p1)] Dashboards analyze and forecast organizational systems and processes. These dashboards frequently incorporate external benchmarks, which allow organizations to compare performance to national, state, or regional norms. Benchmarks are available from CMS, state health department websites, medical specialty groups, published literature, and organizations such as The Leapfrog Group. A dashboard example is shown as **Figure 6.20**.

Another example of a dashboard is shown as **Figure 6.21**.[90] In response to an ongoing COVID-19 public health emergency and pandemic, an interactive web-based dashboard was developed and hosted by the Center for Systems Science and Engineering at Johns Hopkins University to provide researchers, public health authorities, and the general public with a user-friendly tool to track the outbreak as it unfolded. There are various dashboards that help visualize the location and number of confirmed COVID-19 cases, deaths, and recoveries for all affected countries.

See the *Performance and Process Improvement, Quality Leadership and Integration, Patient Safety,* and *Quality Review and Accountability* sections for more discussion about data-driven decision making and tools to support performance excellence. Also see **Box 6.12** for key points in reporting for improvement.

ESC CCAC BALANCED SCORECARD

VARIANCE INDICATOR:
Meet or Exceeds | Discuss/Review | Below Target

INDICATOR SOURCE:
M-SAA: Multi-sector Accountability Agreement
QIP: Quality Improvement Plan
ESC: CCAC Performance Indicator

| Domain | Indicator | Baseline Performance | Target Performance | Target Justification and Comment(s) | Performance Corridor | Q1 (2016–17) | Q2 (2016–17) | Q3 (2016–17) | Q4 (2016–17) |
|---|---|---|---|---|---|---|---|---|---|
| | Goals and Objectives for Engaging with community to learn from the patient experience and deliver patient & family centered care [ESC] | 2015/16 100% | ≥90% of goals and objectives on target for completion | Goals and objectives should be achievable within suggested timeframes. | ≥90% / 80–89% / <80% | 90% | 90% | 100% | 100% |
| | Goals and Objectives for Chronic Disease Management [ESC] | 2015/16 88% | ≥90% of goals and objectives on target for completion | Goals and objectives should be achievable within suggested timeframes. | ≥90% / 80–89% / <80% | 90% | 90% | 100% | 100% |
| | Goals and Objectives for Partner of Choice in enhanced Care Coordination [ESC] | 2015/16 92% | ≥90% of goals and objectives on target for completion | Goals and objectives should be achievable within suggested timeframes. | ≥90% / 80–89% / <80% | 90% | 90% | 92% | 100% |
| | Ratio of Admitted Patients to Discharged Patients [ESC] | 2015/16 1.015 | 1.0 | Target set by CCAC as objective to support resource management. | ≤1.00 / 1.01–1.05 / >1.05 | 1.07 | 1.0 | 0.94 | 0.97 |
| | Patient Satisfaction (Overall Experience rating on NRC Picker survey) [QIP] | 2015/16 94.25% | ≥ 95.0% | Stretch target to achieve top performance in province. | ≥95% / 93.2–94.9% / ≤93.1% | 93.5% | 93.5% | Q3/Q4 data not available. | Q3/Q4 data not available. |
| Quality Patient Care | Patient Risk (Falls) [QIP]/[MSAA] | 2015/16 36.9% | ≤30.5% | Target to meet or exceed high performer in Province. | ≤30.5% / 30.7–35.7% / ≥35.7% | 38.3% | 37.7% | 37.2% | 39.6% |
| | % of ALC days (closed cases) [MSAA] | 2013/14 16.4% | ≤15.3% | LHIN MSAA indicator and target (not set). | ≤15.3% / 15.4–16.3% / ≥16.4% | 12.1% | 13.1% | 16.5% | Q4 Data not available |
| | % of palliative/end of life patients who died in their preferred place of death [QIP] | Collecting baseline | Collecting baseline | First year of data collection in QIP. | Provincial average: 61.89% | 70.50% | 63.17% | 70.92% | Q4 Data not available |
| | % of home care patients with unplanned, less urgent ED visit within first 30 days of discharge from hospital [QIP] | 2015/16 Q1 6.88% | ≤3.83% | To be among top quartile among CCAC's. | ≤3.83% / 3.84–6.7% / ≥6.8% | 6.2% | Estimated availability date is Q1. | Estimated availability date is Q1. | Estimated availability date is Q1. |
| | % home care patients who experienced an unplanned readmit to hospital within 30 days of discharge from hospital [QIP] | 2015/16 Q1 14.7% | ≤14.5% | Remain as top performer in province. | ≤14.5% / 14.6–15.6% / ≥15.7% | 15.5% | Estimated availability date is Q1. | Estimated availability date is Q1. | Estimated availability date is Q1. |
| | % complex patients receiving their first Personal Support visit within 5 days [QIP] [MSAA] | 2015/16 90.7% | ≥90.7% | Maintain provincial leadership. | ≥90.7% / 87.4–90.6% / ≤87.3% | 93% | 92.7% | 91.1% | 93.4% |
| | % patients receiving their first nursing visit within 5 days [QIP] [MSAA] | 2015/16 95.0% | ≥95.8% | Achieve top performance in province. | ≥95.8% / 95.5–95.7% / ≤94.5% | 95.4% | 95.8% | 96.1% | 95.4% |

N/A means baseline performance not available.
TBD means indicator to be developed further using historical performance

**Figure 6.19** Balanced Scorecard—an Example

**Table 6.22** **Processes in Business Intelligence**

| Process | What Does This Include? |
| --- | --- |
| Research question | Identifying research question(s) of interest |
| Domains | Identifying domains or data element concepts needed to answer the research question of interest |
| Data sources | Identifying data sources that might contain the data to answer the research question of interest |
| Data preparation | ▪ Compiling data from multiple sources<br>▪ Identifying dimensions and measurements<br>▪ Preparing the data for data analysis |
| Querying | Asking data-specific questions to pull relevant data |
| Descriptive analysis | Performing preliminary data analysis to find out what happened |
| Statistical analysis | Taking the results from descriptive analysis and using statistics to evaluate contributor factors and patterns |
| Reporting | Sharing data with key stakeholders to draw conclusions and support data-informed decisions |
| Performance and benchmarking | ▪ Comparing current performance data to historical data<br>▪ Tracking performance against goals<br>▪ Comparing performance against industry standards and/or competitors |
| Data mining | Utilizing databases, statistics, and machine learning to uncover trends in large data sets |
| Data visualization | Turning data analysis into visual representations such as charts, graphs, and histograms for easier consumption |
| Visual analysis | Utilizing visual storytelling to communicate insights |

Data from Tableau Software. What it is, how it works, its importance, examples, & tools. n.d. Accessed February 10, 2022. https://www.tableau.com/learn/articles/business-intelligence

### Box 6.12 Key Points: Reporting for Improvement

▪ With the DIKW framework, data in general are abundant and wisdom is rare.
▪ Balanced scorecards present mixed measures compared to target values set by the organization or based on external benchmarks.
▪ Use dashboards to monitor key management, clinical, financial, and operational performance indicators.
▪ Benchmarking includes routinely comparing indicators against best performance and seeking out ways to make improvements with the greatest impact.
▪ KPIs are measures of how well an individual, department, or organization is performing compared to strategic objectives or goals set by the organization.
▪ Benchmarking and KPIs allow the management team to identify areas where the company excels as well as areas that need improvement.

## Summary

A historical perspective and new developments in health data analytics puts into context the importance of information management in the work of the healthcare quality professional. The analysis of data and translation to meaningful information are critical given national quality and safety priorities and initiatives. Healthcare reform includes an emphasis on data and information related to individuals, populations, and organizations. Thoughtful strategies foster the use of data in decision making. The public reporting of quality data promotes value-based purchasing where accountability is part of the equation.

Healthcare quality professionals are uniquely positioned to advance the use of data in their organizations and the community through various approaches and strategic thinking, including the following:

• Confidently promoting transparency and trust in gathering and using data with leadership, the workforce, consumers, and external stakeholders
• Leveraging advances in technology (e.g., AI, machine learning, smartphones, smart home systems) to improve engagement of individual and population health improvement and system-level initiatives to improve quality and safety
• Integrating data science and technology strategies to identify individuals and populations at risk

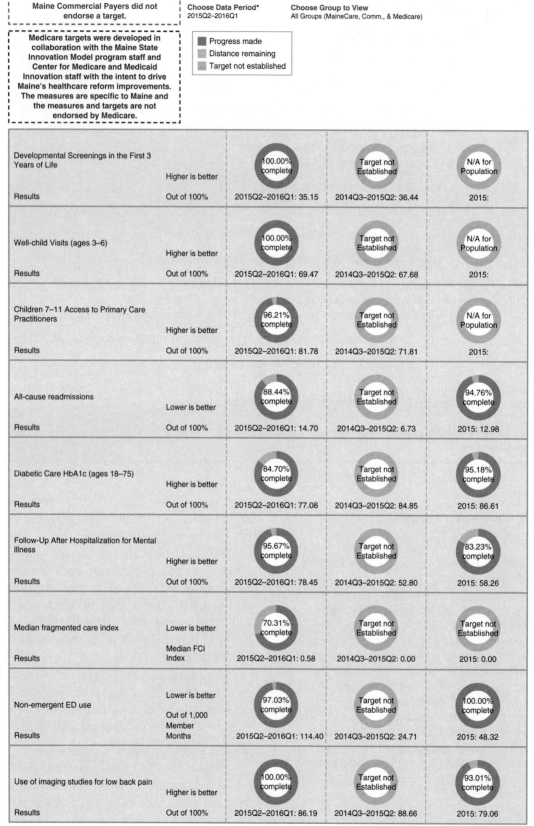

**Figure 6.20** Core Metrics Dashboard

Reproduced from Maine Department of Health and Human Services. Evaluation dashboards. 2016-2017 ME measures (Q4-Q3) V3. Maine State innovation model. n.d. Accessed February 12, 2022. http://www.maine.gov/dhhs/sim/evaluation/dashboard.shtml

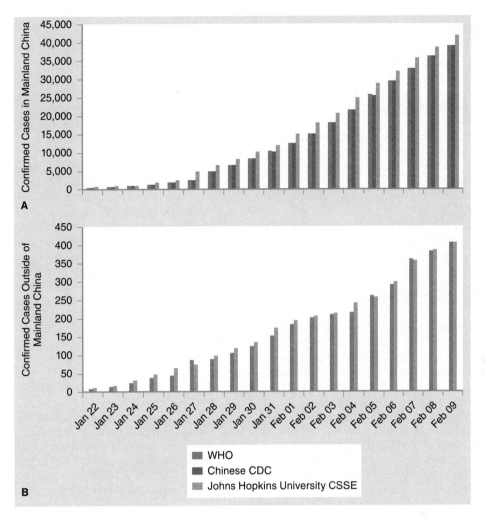

**Figure 6.21** Coronavirus COVID-19 Dashboard

Reprinted from Dong E, Du H, Gardner L. An interactive web-based dashboard to track COVID-19 in real time. *Lancet Infect Dis.* 2020;20(5):533-534. with permission from Elsevier. Accessed February 17, 2022. doi:10.1016/S1473-3099(20)30120-1

(e.g., for chronic conditions or suicide) to inform prevention and treatment interventions

- Ensuring reliable and valid data from diverse sources to design strategies toward equity and equality in healthcare delivery (e.g., patient-generated health data)
- Staying vigilant with bringing forward opportunities to financially reward an organization to connect measures and activities across the quality, cost, and improvement activities performance categories associated with targeted investment and value-based programs (e.g., interoperability and population health measures)

- Realizing moonshot outcomes by bringing together data, people, and technology to effect system and clinical improvements (e.g., reducing the death rate from cancer by at least 50% over the next 25 years)
- Influencing change through advocacy with data to influence pricing, government regulations, and social values encoded in community and individual health behaviors and beliefs

Finally, sound study design and analysis support the healthcare quality professional's efforts to achieve performance excellence and sustain a culture of safety and quality.

# References

1. Juran JM. *Quality and its assurance: an overview. Presented at: 2nd NATO Symposium on Quality and Its Assurance*; 1977; London, England.

2. Juran JM. *Juran on Leadership for Quality: An Executive Handbook*. New York, NY: Free Press; 2003.

3. Deming WE. *The New Economics for Industry, Government, Education*. Cambridge, MA: MIT Press; 2000.

4. Cloud Security. *Alliance Artificial Intelligence in Healthcare*. Published 2021. Accessed March 14, 2022. https://cloudsecurityalliance.org

5. Davenport TH. Competing on analytics. *Harv Bus Rev*. 2006;84(1):98-107, 134.

6. Kayyali B, Knott D, Van Kuiken S. The big-data revolution in US health care: Accelerating value and innovation. Published 2013. Accessed February 22, 2022. http://www.mckinsey.com/industries/healthcare-systems-and-services/our-insights/the-big-data-revolution-in-us-health-care

7. Margolis R, Derr L, Dunn M, et al. The National Institutes of Health's Big Data to Knowledge (BD2K) initiative: capitalizing on biomedical big data. *J Am Med Inform Assoc*. 2014;21(6):957-958. doi:10.1136/amiajnl-2014-002974

8. National Institutes of Standards and Technology. *NIST Big Data Interoperability Framework*: Vol 1, Definitions. NIST special publication 1500-1. Accessed February 15, 2022. https://bigdatawg.nist.gov/_uploadfiles/NIST.SP.1500-1.pdf

9. Firican G. Transforming data with intelligence: the 10 Vs of big data. Published February 8, 2017. Accessed February 12, 2022. https://tdwi.org/articles/2017/02/08/10-vs-of-big-data.aspx

10. The Advisory Board. *Big Data in Health Care: Educational Briefing for Non-IT Executives*. Washington, DC: Author; 2017.

11. President's Information Technology Advisory Committee. Health care delivery and information technology subcommittee: Draft recommendations. Published April 13, 2004. Accessed February 12, 2022. https://www.nitrd.gov/historical/Pitac/meetings/2004/20040413/20040413_draft_hit.pdf

12. Bates DW, Gawande AA. Improving safety with information technology. *N Engl J Med*. 2003;348(25):2526-2534. doi:10.1056/NEJMsa020847

13. Weiner M, Callahan CM, Tierney WM, et al. Using information technology to improve health care of older adults. *Ann Intern Med*. 2003;139:430-436.

14. Office of the National Coordinator for Health Information Technology. Office-based physician electronic health record adoption; Health IT quickstat #50. Published January 2019. Accessed February 12, 2022. https://www.healthit.gov/data/quickstats/office-based-physician-electronic-health-record-adoption

15. El-Yafouri R, Klieb LA. A near complete adoption of electronic health records system in the U.S. lacks interoperability and physician satisfaction. In: *Proceedings of the 14th International Joint Conference on Biomedical Engineering Systems and Technologies* (BIOSTEC 2021). 2021;5:600-604. doi:10.5220/0010320006000604

16. Bates DW, Gawande AA. Improving safety with information technology. *N Engl J Med*. 2003;348(25):2526-2534. doi:10.1056/NEJMsa020847

17. National Committee on Vital and Health Statistics. Letter to the secretary: recommendations for the first set of PMRI standards. Washington, DC: Author. Published February 27, 2002. Accessed February 12, 2022. https://ncvhs.hhs.gov/rrp/february-27-2002-letter-to-the-secretary-recommendations-for-the-first-set-of-pmri-standards/

18. Healthcare Information and Management Systems Society (HIMSS). Evaluating HIT standards: Key principles to support healthcare IT interoperability in the United States. Published 2013. Accessed February 12, 2022. http://www.himss.org/sites/himssorg/files/FileDownloads/2013-09-23-EvaluatingHITStandards-FINAL.pdf

19. Institute of Medicine, Committee on Patient Safety and Health Information Technology. *Health IT and Patient Safety: Building Safer Systems for Better Care*. Washington, DC: National Academies Press; 2012.

20. HealthIT.gov. Promoting interoperability. 2019. Accessed February 12, 2022. www.healthit.gov/providers-professionals/meaningful-use-definition-objectives

21. O'Neill Hayes T. American action forum. Primer: EHR stage 3 meaningful use requirements. Published Oct 28, 2015. Accessed February 12, 2022. https://www.americanactionforum.org/research/primer-ehr-stage-3-meaningful-use-requirements/

22. The Office of National Coordinator for Health Information Technology. About ONC's Cures Act final rule: empowering patients with their health record in a modern health IT economy. Accessed February 12, 2022. https://www.healthit.gov/curesrule/overview/about-oncs-cures-act-final-rule

23. The Office of the National Coordinator for Health Information Technology. The ONC Cures Act Final Rule. Published 2020. Accessed February 15, 2022. https://www.healthit.gov/sites/default/files/cures/2020-03/TheONCCuresActFinalRule.pdf

24. Oracle. What is a data lake? Accessed February 12, 2022. https://www.oracle.com/big-data/what-is-data-lake/

25. Deloitte. Predictive analytics in health care: emerging value and risks. Published 2019. Accessed February 15, 2022. https://www2.deloitte.com/content/dam/insights/us/articles/au22113_predictive-analytics-in-health-care/DI_Predictive-analytics-in-health-care.pdf

26. U.S. Government Accountability Office. Artificial intelligence in health care: benefits and challenges of technologies to augment patient care. Published November 30, 2020. Accessed February 15, 2022. https://www.gao.gov/products/gao-21-7sp

27. Brown S, Ramadoss B. Beyond command centers: how AI-based smart operating systems help achieve outcomes. *Becker's Hospital Review*. Presented at: on-demand webinar. Accessed February 12, 2022. https://go.beckershospitalreview.com/beyond-command-centers-how-ai-based-smart-operating-systems-help-achieve-outcomes

28. Nutley T, Reynolds HW. Improving the use of health data for health system strengthening. *Global Health Action*. 2013;6:1-10. doi:10.3402/gha.v6i0.20001

29. Gudea S. Data, information, knowledge: a healthcare enterprise case. *Perspect Health Inf Manag*. 2005;2:8. doi:10.1.1.104.6709

30. Quality Measurement and Management Project. *Hospital Quality-Related Data: Recommendations for Appropriate Data Requests, Analysis, and Utilization*. Chicago, IL: American Hospital Association; 1991.

31. The Advisory Board. *Big Data in Health Care: Educational Briefing for Non-IT Executives*. Washington, DC: Author; 2017.

32. Bader BS, Bohr D. *Guide to the Interpretation and Use of Quality of Care Data*. Chicago, IL: American Hospital Association, The Hospital Research and Education Trust; 1991.

33. Tweed-Weber, Inc. *Total Quality Management in Home Health Care*. Reading PA: Author; 1992.

34. Higgins TC, Crosson J, Peikes D, et al. *Using Health Information Technology to Support Quality Improvement in Primary Care*. AHRQ Pub. No. 15-0031-EF. Rockville, MD: Agency for Healthcare Research and Quality; 2015.

35. O'Rourke LM, Bader BS. An illustrative quality and performance report for the governing board. *Qual Lett Healthc Lead*. 1993;5(2):15-28.

36. Rontal R. Information and decision support in managed care. *Manag Care Q*. 1993;1(3):3-14.

37. U.S. Department of Health & Human Services, Office of the National Coordinator for Health Information Technology (ONC). Adoption of electronic health record systems among U.S. non-federal acute care hospitals: 2008-2014. Published 2015. Accessed February 12, 2022. https://www.healthit.gov/sites/default/files/data-brief/2014HospitalAdoptionDataBrief.pdf

38. U.S. Department of Health & Human Services, Office of the National Coordinator for Health Information Technology (ONC). Adoption of electronic health record systems among U.S. non-federal acute care hospitals: 2008-2014. Published 2015. Accessed February 12, 2022. https://www.healthit.gov/sites/default/files/data-brief/2014HospitalAdoptionDataBrief.pdf

39. Bright TJ, Wong A, Dhurjati R, et al. Effect of clinical decision-support systems: a systematic review. *Ann Intern Med*. 2012;157(1):29-43.

40. Shahmoradi L, Safdari R, Ahmadi H, Zahmatkeshan M. Clinical decision support systems-based interventions to improve medication outcomes: a systematic literature review on features and effects. *Med J Islam Repub Iran*. 2021;35:27. doi:10.47176/mjiri.35.27

41. Magnuson JA, Dixon BE. Public health informatics: an introduction. In: Magnuson JA, Dixon BE, eds. *Public Health Informatics and Information Systems*. Cham, Switzerland: SpringerNature; 2020:3-16.

42. Popovic JR. Distributed data networks: a paradigm shift in data sharing and healthcare analytics. Published 2015. Accessed February 12, 2022. https://www.pharmasug.org/proceedings/2015/HA/PharmaSUG-2015-HA07.pdf

43. PCORNet. Data. Accessed February 12, 2022. https://pcornet.org/data/

44. Byers JF, Beaudin CL. Critical appraisal tools facilitate the work of the quality professional. *J Healthc Qual*. 2001;23(5):35-38, 40-43. doi:10.1111/j.1945-1474.2001.tb00374.x

45. Data Across Sectors for Health. Adapted from healthcare 101: Healthcare data basics. Published March 2018. Accessed February 12, 2022. https://dashconnect.org/wp-content/uploads/2018/03/Health-Care-Data-101.pdf

46. Chassin MR, Loeb JM, Schmaltz SP, Wachter RM. Accountability measures—using measurement to promote quality improvement. *N Engl J Med*. 2010;363(7):683-688. doi:10.1056/NEJMsb1002320

47. McGlynn EA. *Identifying, Categorizing, and Evaluating Health Care Efficiency Measures*. Final report (prepared by the Southern California Evidence-based Practice Center—RAND Corporation, under contract no. 282-00-0005-21). AHRQ publication 08-0030. Rockville, MD: Agency for Healthcare Research and Quality; April 2008.

48. Centers for Medicare & Medicaid Services. Electronic clinical quality measures. Published 2022. Accessed February 16, 2022. https://www.cms.gov/Regulations-and-Guidance/Legislation/EHRIncentivePrograms/ClinicalQualityMeasures

49. Centers for Medicare & Medicaid Services. eCQM library. Published 2017. Accessed February 12, 2022. https://www.cms.gov/Regulations-and-Guidance/Legislation/EHRIncentivePrograms/eCQM_Library.html

50. Agency for Healthcare Research and Quality. AHRQ quality indicators. Accessed February 12, 2022. https://www.qualityindicators.ahrq.gov/

51. Centers for Medicare & Medicaid Services. Core measures. Published 2016. Accessed February 12, 2022. https://www.cms.gov/Medicare/Quality-Initiatives-Patient-Assessment-Instruments/QualityMeasures/Core-Measures.html

52. Centers for Medicare & Medicaid Services. IMPACT Act of 2014 cross-setting measures drug regimen review. Published 2015. Accessed February 12, 2022. https://www.cms.gov/Medicare/Quality-Initiatives-Patient-Assessment-Instruments/MMS/Downloads/IMPACT-Act-of-2014-Cross-Setting-Quality-Measure-Drug-Regimen-Review_TEP-Member.pdf

53. Agency for Healthcare Research and Quality. Enabling health care decisionmaking through health information technology. Published 2012. Accessed February 12, 2022. https://digital.ahrq.gov/ahrq-funded-projects/enabling-health-care-decisionmaking-through-use-health-information-technology

54. Centers for Medicare & Medicaid Services. Measure Inventory Tool. Last updated June 30, 2021. Accessed February 12, 2022. https://cmit.cms.gov/CMIT_public/ListMeasures

55. World Health Organization. International classification of diseases and related health problems (ICD). Published 2022. Accessed February 17, 2022. https://www.who.int/standards/classifications/classification-of-diseases

56. Centers for Medicare & Medicaid Services (CMS). MS-DRG classifications and software. Page last modified December 22, 2021. Accessed February 12, 2022. https://www.cms.gov/Medicare/Medicare-Fee-for-Service-Payment/AcuteInpatientPPS/MS-DRG-Classifications-and-Software

57. World Health Organization. International classification of diseases (ICD). Updated January 1, 2021. Accessed February 12, 2022. https://www.who.int/standards/classifications/classification-of-diseases

58. National Library of Medicine. Overview of SNOMED CT. Last reviewed October 14, 2016. Accessed February 12, 2022. https://www.nlm.nih.gov/healthit/snomedct/snomed_overview.html

59. The International Health Terminology Standards Development Organization. SNOMED CT—supporting meaningful use. Published February 2014. Accessed February 12, 2022. https://www.snomed.org/SNOMED/media/SNOMED/documents/SnomedCt_MeaningfulUse_20140219-(1).pdf

60. National Library of Medicine. Interactive map-assisted generation of ICD codes (I-MAGIC mapper). Published September 20, 2021. Accessed February 12, 2022. https://imagic.nlm.nih.gov/imagic/code/map?v=5&js=true&pabout=&pinstructions=&init-params=&pat=My+Patient&pat.init=My+Patient&q.f=&q.dob=&p=dce2a9f3z0&p.dce2a9f3z0.e=heart&qadd=

61. American Medical Association. CPT (current procedural terminology). Accessed February 12, 2022. https://www.ama-assn.org/amaone/cpt-current-procedural-terminology

62. American Medical Association. CPT overview and code approval. Accessed February 12, 2022. https://www.ama-assn.org/practice-management/cpt/cpt-overview-and-code-approval

63. American Medical Association. CPT category II codes alphabetical clinical topics listing. Updated January 30, 2020.

Accessed February 12, 2022. https://www.ama-assn.org/system/files/2020-01/cpt-cat2-codes-alpha-listing-clinical-topics.pdf

64. National Library of Medicine. RXNORM overview. Last reviewed July 9, 2021. Accessed February 12, 2022. https://www.nlm.nih.gov/research/umls/rxnorm/overview.html?msclkid=cf408bd5cf4411ecb080730bee6f3583

65. National Library of Medicine. RXNORM source information. Accessed February 12, 2022. https://www.nlm.nih.gov/research/umls/rxnorm/sourcereleasedocs/rxnorm.html?msclkid=cf41246fcf4411ec9b91f8f0719ae401

66. Centers for Medicare & Medicaid Services. Measures Inventory Tool: Measure inventory: RxNorm. Accessed February 12, 2022. https://cmit.cms.gov/CMIT_public/ListMeasures?q=RxNorm

67. Centers for Medicare & Medicaid Services. Measures Inventory Tool: Measure inventory; appropriate use of anti-methicillin-resistant *Staphylococcus aureus* (MRSA) antibiotics. Accessed February 12, 2022. https://cmit.cms.gov/CMIT_public/ViewMeasure?MeasureId=3410

68. National Library of Medicine. Logical Observation Identifiers Names and Codes (LOINC). Last Reviewed February 17, 2015. Accessed February 12, 2022. https://www.nlm.nih.gov/research/umls/loinc_main.html

69. Wolters-Kluwer. LOINC and meaningful use. Last reviewed 12, 2013. Accessed February 12, 2022. https://www.wolterskluwer.com/en/expert-insights/loinc-and-meaningful-use

70. Centers for Disease Control and Prevention. LOINC in vitro diagnostic (LIVD) test code mapping for SARS-CoV-2 tests. Accessed February 12, 2022. https://www.cdc.gov/csels/dls/sars-cov-2-livd-codes.html

71. Centers for Medicare & Medicaid Services. CMS MMS blueprint v17.0 streamlined. Published September 2021. Accessed February 12, 2022. https://www.cms.gov/Medicare/Quality-Initiatives-Patient-Assessment-Instruments/MMS/Downloads/Blueprint.pdf

72. The Joint Commission. Electronic clinical quality measures. Published 2022. Accessed February 12, 2022. https://www.jointcommission.org/measurement/specification-manuals/electronic-clinical-quality-measures/

73. Centers for Medicare & Medicaid Services. Electronic clinical quality measures (eCQMs) specification, testing, standards, tools, and community. Published September 2021. Accessed February 12, 2022. https://www.cms.gov/files/document/blueprint-ecqm-specifications-testing-standards-tools-community.pdf

74. L.A. Care Health Plan. HEDIS MY2020: Hybrid measure quick guide. Published September 2020. Accessed February 12, 2022. https://www.lacare.org/sites/default/files/la3096_hedis_hybrid_measure_guide_202009.pdf

75. Iezzoni L. *Risk Adjustment for Measuring Healthcare Outcomes.* 4th ed. Chicago, IL: Health Administration Press; 2012.

76. Hoskin T. Parametric and nonparametric: demystifying the terms. Published 2012. Accessed February 12, 2022. https://www.mayo.edu/research/documents/parametric-and-nonparametric-demystifying-the-terms/doc-20408960

77. Frické M. Knowledge pyramid: the DIKW hierarchy. Published 2018. Accessed February 12, 2022. https://www.isko.org/cyclo/dikw

78. Brassard M, Ritter D. *The Memory Jogger II.* Methuen, MA: Goal/QPC; 1994.

79. Tufte E. *Beautiful Evidence.* Columbia, MD: Graphics Press; 2006.

80. Ellenbogen KA, Wilkoff BL, Kay GN, Lau CP. *Clinical Cardiac Pacing, Defibrillation and Resynchronization Therapy.* 4th ed. Philadelphia, PA: Elsevier Inc.; 2011. doi:10.1016/C2009-0-44191-6

81. Hanisch RJ, Kaiser DL, Carroll BC. *Research Data Framework (RDaF): Motivation, Development, and a Preliminary Framework Core.* National Institute of Standards and Technology Special Publication 1500-18. Natl. Inst. Stand. Technol. Spec. Publ. 1500-18. February 2021. Accessed June 3, 2022. doi:10.6028/NIST.SP.1500-18

82. Visualizing Health. Our approach: goal-congruent risk visualizations. Accessed February 12, 2022. http://www.vizhealth.org/about/

83. Balanced Scorecard Institute. What is a key performance indicator (KPI)? Accessed January 12, 2022. https://kpi.org/KPI-Basics

84. Sackett DL, Rosenberg WM, Gray JA, Haynes RB, Richardson WS. Evidence-based medicine: what it is and what it isn't. *BMJ.* 1996;312(7023):71-72. doi:10.1136/bmj.312.7023.71

85. Ettorchi-Tardy A, Levif M, Michel P. Benchmarking: a method for continuous quality improvement in health. *Healthcare Policy.* 2012;7(4):e101-e119.

86. Famolaro T, Hare R, Thornton S, et al. *Medical Office Survey: 2020 User Database Report.* April 28, 2021. Rockville, MD: Agency for Healthcare Research and Quality. AHRQ Pub. No. 20-0034; March 2020.

87. Zolelzer N. Managing administrative expenses with operational benchmarking; 2013. Milliman Healthcare Analytics blog. Accessed February 12, 2022. https://info.medinsight.milliman.com/2013/07/managing-administrative-expenses-with-operational-benchmarking/

88. Russell D, Rosenfeld P, Ames S, Rosati RJ. Using technology to enhance the quality of home health care: three case studies of health information technology initiatives at the visiting nurse service of New York. *J Healthc Qual.* 2010;32(5):22-28.

89. Nelson GS. The healthcare performance dashboard: linking strategy to metrics. Published 2010. Accessed February 12, 2022. Paper 167-2010 from SAS Global Forum. http://support.sas.com/resources/papers/proceedings10/167-2010.pdf

90. Dong E, Du H, Gardner L. An interactive web-based dashboard to track COVID-19 in real time. *Lancet Infect Dis.* 2020;20(5):533-534. doi:10.1016/ S1473-3099(20)30147-X

## Suggested Readings

Breen C, Maguire K, Bansal A, et al. Reducing phlebotomy utilization with education and changes to computerized provider order entry. *J Healthc Qual.* 2019;41(3):154-159. doi:10.1097/JHQ.0000000000000150

Brittan MS, Campagna EJ, Keller D, Kempe A. How measurement variability affects reporting of a single readmission metric. *J Healthc Qual.* 2019;41(3):160-164. doi:10.1097/JHQ.0000000000000152

Castaldi M, McNelis J. Introducing a clinical documentation specialist to improve coding and collectability on a surgical service. *J Healthc Qual.* 2019;41(3):e21-e29. doi:10.1097/JHQ.0000000000000146

Dalton AF, Lyon C, Parnes B, Fernald D, Lewis CL. Developing a quality measurement strategy in an academic primary care setting: an environmental scan. *J Healthc Qual.* 2018;40(6):e90-e100. doi:10.1097/JHQ.0000000000000155

Davlyatov G, Borkowski N, Feldman S, et al. Health information technology adoption and clinical performance in federally qualified health centers. *J Healthc Qual.* 2020;42(5):287-293. doi:10.1097/JHQ.0000000000000231

DuGoff EH. Continuity of care in older adults with multiple chronic conditions: how well do administrative measures correspond with patient experiences? *J Healthc Qual.* 2018;40(3):120-128. doi:10.1097/JHQ.0000000000000051

Glauser G, Winter E, Caplan IF, et al. Composite score for outcome prediction in gynecologic surgery patients. *J Healthc Qual.* 2021;43(3):163-173. doi:10.1097/JHQ.0000000000000254

Hansen JP. CAN'T MISS—conquer any number task by making important statistics simple. Part 1. Types of variables, mean, median, variance, and standard deviation. *J Healthc Qual.* 2003;25(4):19-24. doi:10.1111/j.1945-1474.2003.tb01070.x

Hansen JP. CAN'T MISS—conquer any number task by making important statistics simple. Part 2. Probability, populations, samples, and normal distributions. *J Healthc Qual.* 2003;25(4):25-33. doi:10.1111/j.1945-1474.2003.tb01071.x

Hansen JP. CAN'T MISS—conquer any number task by making important statistics simple. Part 3. Standard error, estimation, and confidence intervals. *J Healthc Qual.* 2003;25(4):34-39. doi:10.1111/j.1945-1474.2003.tb01072.x

Hansen JP. CAN'T MISS—conquer any number task by making important statistics simple. Part 4. Confidence intervals with $t$ distributions, standard error, and confidence intervals for proportions. *J Healthc Qual.* 2004;26(4):26-32. doi:10.1111/j.1945-1474.2004.tb00504.x

Hansen JP. CAN'T MISS—conquer any number task by making important statistics simple. Part 5. Comparing two confidence intervals, standard error of the difference between two means and between two proportions. *J Healthc Qual.* 2004;26(4):33-42. doi:10.1111/j.1945-1474.2004.tb00506.x

Hansen JP. CAN'T MISS—conquer any number task by making important statistics simple. Part 6. Tests of statistical significance ($z$ test statistic, rejecting the null hypothesis, $p$ value), $t$ test, $z$ test for proportions, statistical significance

versus meaningful difference. *J Healthc Qual.* 2004;26(4):43-53. doi:10.1111/j.1945-1474.2004.tb00507.x

Hansen JP. CAN'T MISS: conquer any number task by making important statistics simple. Part 7. Statistical process control: $x$–$s$ control charts. *J Healthc Qual.* 2005;27(4):32-43. doi:10.1111/j.1945-1474.2005.tb00566.x

Hansen JP. CAN'T MISS: conquer any number task by making important statistics simple. Part 8. Statistical process control: $n$, $np$, $c$, $u$ control charts. *J Healthc Qual.* 2005;27(4):45-52. doi:10.1111/j.1945-1474.2005.tb00567.x

Hong Y, Kates F, Song SJ, Lee N, Duncan RP, Marlow NM. Benchmarking implications: analysis of Medicare accountable care organizations spending level and quality of care. *J Healthc Qual.* 2018;40(6):344-353. doi:10.1097/JHQ.0000000000000123

Iannello J, Levitt MP, Poetter D, et al. Improving inpatient tobacco treatment measures: outcomes through standardized treatment, care coordination, and electronic health record optimization. *J Healthc Qual.* 2021;43(1):48-58. doi:10.1097/JHQ.0000000000000251

Ozer R, Richards G. Optimizing surgical capacity for a rural hospital through Monte Carlo simulation. *J Healthc Qual.* 2018;40(1):e1-e8. doi:10.1097/01.JHQ.0000462686.55382

Shang J, Russell D, Dowding D, et al. A predictive risk model for infection-related hospitalization among home healthcare patients. *J Healthc Qual.* 2020;42(3):136-147. doi:10.1097/JHQ.0000000000000214

Strockbine VL, Gehrie EA, Zhou QP, Guzzetta CE. Reducing unnecessary phlebotomy testing using a clinical decision support system. *J Healthc Qual.* 2020;42(2):98-105. doi:10.1097/JHQ.0000000000000245

Toumbs R, Dao T, Zhu L, McCullough L, Savitz S, Cossey TC. Stroke templates and trainee education are associated with improved data capture in an academic hospital. *J Healthc Qual.* 2020;42(2):66-71. doi:10.1097/JHQ.0000000000000240

Walsh KE, Secor JL, Matsumura JS, et al. Secure provider-to-provider communication with electronic health record messaging: an educational outreach study. *J Healthc Qual.* 2018;40(5):283-291. doi:10.1097/JHQ.0000000000000115

Whicher D, Ahmed M, Siddiqi S, Adams I, Grossmann C, Carman K, eds. *Health Data Sharing to Support Better Outcomes: Building a Foundation of Stakeholder Trust. NAM special publication.* Washington, DC: National Academy of Medicine; 2020.

# Online Resources

## *Agency for Healthcare Research and Quality*

www.ahrq.gov

- **Guidelines and Measures**
  https://www.ahrq.gov/gam/index.html
- **National Quality Measures Clearinghouse**
  https://www.ahrq.gov/gam/index.html
- **Quality and Patient Safety Resources**
  https://www.ahrq.gov/patient-safety/resources/index.html
- **State Snapshots**
  https://www.ahrq.gov/data/state-snapshots.html
- **Surveys on Patient Safety Culture**
  https://www.ahrq.gov/sops/index.html

## *American Health Information Management Association*

http://www.ahima.org/

## *American Society for Quality*

www.asq.org

*Australian Commission on Safety and Quality in Health Care*

>    www.safetyandquality.gov.au

*Centers for Disease Control and Prevention*

>    https://www.cdc.gov/

- **Behavioral Risk Factor Surveillance System: Annual Survey Data**
  https://www.cdc.gov/brfss/annual_data/annual_data.htm
- **National Center for Health Statistics**
  https://www.cdc.gov/nchs/
- **National Vital Statistics System**
  https://www.cdc.gov/nchs/nvss/

*Centers for Medicare & Medicaid Services—Program Statistics*

>    https://www.cms.gov/research-statistics-data-and-systems/statistics-trends-and-reports/cmsprogramstatistics

*Centre for Effective Practice*

>    https://cep.health/

*Dartmouth Atlas Benchmarking Tool*

>    https://www.ruralcenter.org/resource-library/dartmouth-atlas-benchmarking-tool

*DARTNet Institute—Informing Practice: Improving Care*

>    http://www.dartnet.info/

*eCQI Resource Center*

>    http://ecqi.healthit.gov/

*HealthDeata.gov*

>    https://www.healthdata.gov/

*Health Information Management and Systems Society*

>    http://www.himss.org/

*Health Quality Ontario*

>    https://www.hqontario.ca/

*Health Resources & Services Administration Data Warehouse*

>    https://data.hrsa.gov/

*Institute for Healthcare Improvement*

>    www.ihi.org

*International Society for Quality in Health Care*

>    https://isqua.org/

*The Joint Commission*

>    https://www.jointcommission.org/

*The Leapfrog Group*

>    https://www.leapfroggroup.org/

*National Academies of Sciences, Engineering, and Medicine*

>    https://www.nationalacademies.org/

- **Sharing Health Data**
  https://nam.edu/sharing-health-data-the-why-the-will-the-way-forward/

*National Association for Healthcare Quality*

>    https://nahq.org/

*National Committee for Quality Assurance*

>    https://www.ncqa.org/

*National Health Service-UK*

>    https://www.england.nhs.uk/

*National Institutes of Health*

>    https://www.nih.gov/

*National Quality Forum*

>    https://www.qualityforum.org/Home.aspx

*RAND Corporation*

>    https://www.rand.org/

*Substance Abuse and Mental Health Services Administration*

>    https://www.samhsa.gov/

- **Drug Abuse Warning Network**
  https://www.samhsa.gov/data/data-we-collect/dawn-drug-abuse-warning-network?msclkid=e8b76dd5cf4311ecb656fdb0a8af21ff

- **National Survey on Drug Use and Health**
  https://www.samhsa.gov/data/data-we-collect/nsduh-national-survey-drug-use-and-health?msclkid=04aafca4cf4411eca18c11b9c2d245b9
- **National Mental Health Services Survey**
  https://wwwdasis.samhsa.gov/dasis2/nmhss.htm
- **National Survey of Substance Abuse Treatment Services**
  https://wwwdasis.samhsa.gov/dasis2/nssats.htm
- **Treatment Episode Data Set**
  https://wwwdasis.samhsa.gov/dasis2/teds.htm

## Visualizing Health

http://www.vizhealth.org/

# Population Health and Care Transitions

Patricia Resnik, Jennifer Proctor, Christy L. Beaudin, and Luc R. Pelletier

## SECTION CONTENTS

# Introduction

Population health is rapidly expanding as health systems, healthcare facilities, providers, and payers transition from volume-based to value-based reimbursement models. This section will focus on population health and care transitions, highlighting how the healthcare quality professional is optimally positioned to successfully drive desired care outcomes. The ability to accurately design appropriate data collection tools and analyze vast amounts of population-based data to stratify the population by risk, identify opportunities for improvement, and deploy rapid-cycle process changes is critical to success when operating in a value-based reimbursement arrangement. Care management and care transitions are discussed as they are fundamental to population health management in healthcare.

# Population Health

Healthcare is moving beyond the episode of care to determine health outcomes. Population health is a concept that emerged in Canada when Evans and Stoddart of the Canadian Institute for Advanced Research published a model for analyzing the social determinants of health (SDOH). This model embraced the idea that the social environment determines health. On a macro level, this work influenced health policy, approaches to health promotion, and health services research. On a micro level, it brought into view characteristics of the individual in a group context but did not account for individual behavior changes and health.[1] Population health reached the United States in the late 1990s, with discussions in *Crossing the Quality Chasm: A New Health System for the 21st Century* and then took on more traction with the Affordable Care Act in 2010.

*Population health* can be defined as "the health outcomes of a group of individuals, including the distribution of such outcomes within the group. These populations are often geographic regions, such as nations or communities, but they can also be other groups such as employees, ethnic groups, disabled persons, or prisoners."[2(p381)] Further, population health can be defined as "the health outcomes of a group of individuals, including the distribution of such outcomes within the group."[2(p380)] It considers all the determinants of health, including medical care, social and physical environments and related services, genetics, and individual behavior. An inherent byproduct of population health is the identification, reduction, or elimination of inequity and health disparities.[3] Population health management emerged with healthcare reform. This requires data to guide population care delivery underscoring the importance of possessing knowledge of the healthcare organizations and care delivery, essentials of healthcare quality and safety, regulatory issues, health economics, epidemiology, implementation science, health informatics, and data analytics. For discussion on these areas, see the following sections: *Quality Leadership and Integration; Quality Review and Accountability; Regulatory and Accreditation; Patient Safety; Performance and Process Improvement;* and *Health Data Analytics*.

Determinants of health, such as medical care systems, the social environment, and the physical environment, have biological impact on individuals in part at a population level.[1(p381)] **Figure 7.1** illustrates how an integrated healthcare delivery system contextualized the principles of population health (e.g., policies, programs, determinants, outcomes) into its strategies for improving quality of life and well-being at individual and community levels for physical health, mental health, and substance use services.

Population health shifts thinking from volume-based reimbursement to value-based reimbursement in pursuit of the Triple Aim. In 2007, the Institute for Healthcare Improvement (IHI) introduced the Triple Aim framework, which focused on enhancing the patient experience, improving population health, and reducing healthcare costs accompanied by high-level measures defining the dimension. Since its introduction, the Triple Aim has evolved with changes in healthcare and may now include a fourth aim referred to as "joy in work," "improving the work life of clinicians and staff," "improved clinician/provider experience," or "care team well-being."

Other changes, such as demographics, support the adoption of a population health-based approach. For example, consider that the number of Americans older than age of 65 is projected to reach 80 million by 2040. Add to that the fact that chronic disease prevalence rises as people age. Another consideration is the number of people with multiple chronic conditions. Over the past 2 decades, caring for people with multiple chronic conditions has dramatically driven up healthcare costs. The total economic impact of chronic disease in the United States in 2016 was $4.1 trillion, amounting to 20% of the U.S. gross domestic product.[4]

Population health is another area where data are large volume and high velocity. When the data are available, organizations can assess how they are managing high-risk and high-volume patients, as well as how they are managing the general population. For example, it is often helpful to know what percentage of the population is composed of high utilizers for hospital stays or emergency room visits and to determine the characteristics of these patients so they can be better managed (e.g., more visits to their primary care provider, better diet, behavioral health referrals). In another example, these four features contributed

## Goals

- Address health concerns using trauma-informed, peer-supported integrated behavioral and medical care, treatment and services
- Drive quality and safety through coordinated patient-centered care and engagement (e.g., PCMH, care transitions, clinical pathways, targeted interventions)
- Proactively adapt programs and services to meet changing needs of people based on demographics and socioeconomic factors
- Address the intersectionality of social determinants of health (e.g., housing stability, social isolation, criminal justice involvement, education/literacy, rural/urban)
- Use population data analytics to identify, stratify, and determine risk levels for outreach and interventions
- Redefine ways to deliver care, improve health of individuals, populations, and the community through engagement and partnerships

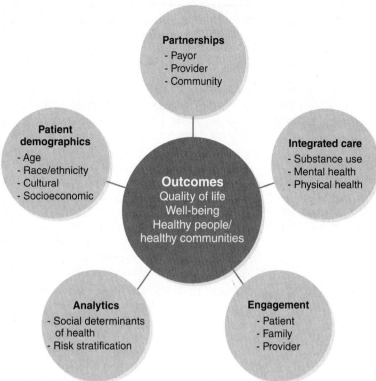

**Figure 7.1** What Is Population Health?

Reproduced from Beaudin CL. *Population Health Model.* Community Bridges, Inc.; 2022.

to better population management of primary care for older adults with chronic illnesses:

1. Comprehensive assessment of the patient's health conditions, treatments, behaviors, risks, supports, resources, values, and preferences
2. Evidence-based care planning and monitoring to meet the patient's health-related needs and preferences
3. Promotion of the patient's and family caregivers' active engagement in care
4. Coordination and communication among all the professionals engaged in a patient's care, especially during transitions from the hospital[5(p1937)]

These population health management activities are amenable to measurement and data analytics. As payment shifts toward value versus volume, it is more common for organizations to be evaluated based on how they are managing entire populations. Payers are putting providers at risk to achieve the best outcomes for these groups of patients. With good data and robust analytics, it is possible to achieve the goal of being a high-performing organization in meeting the needs of specific populations.

How is population health different than public health? It is a reasonable question to ask and important to understand. Population health focuses on the social, cultural, environmental, and physical conditions affecting populations and therefore supports the mission of public health.[6] In 1920, Winslow defined public health as

the science and the art of preventing disease, prolonging life, and promoting physical health and efficiency through organized community efforts for the sanitation of the environment, the control of community infections, the education of the individual in principles of personal hygiene, the organization of medical and nursing services for the early diagnosis and preventive treatment of disease, and the development of the social machinery which will ensure to every individual in the community a standard of living adequate for the maintenance of health, the science and art of preventing disease, prolonging life, and promoting health and efficiency through organized community efforts.[6(p30)]

Public health's mission covers three *Ps*—promotion of health in a population, prevention of disease in a population, and protection of the health of a population.[6(p6)] **Table 7.1** describes the unique features of individual health, population health, and public health.

While equally important, population medicine differs from population health in that the principles relate to the impact of clinical care and individual health outcomes. Eggleston noted that population medicine takes a population perspective from a healthcare system approach. It encompasses the

### Table 7.1 Unique Features of Individual, Public, and Population Health

| | Features |
|---|---|
| *Individual health*<br>Systems for delivering one-on-one individual health services, including those aimed at prevention, cure, palliation, and rehabilitation | ■ Describe an individual's problem, including their symptoms and risks for disease<br>■ Make a diagnosis of their diseases or conditions<br>■ Select individual intervention(s) or treatment(s) tailored to the individual's situation and desires |
| *Public health*<br>Population/community-based prevention perspective utilizing interventions targeting populations or communities as well as defined high-risk or vulnerable groups | ■ Comprises 10 essential services<br>■ Monitor health status to identify and solve community health problems<br>■ Diagnose and investigate health problems and health hazards in the community<br>■ Inform, educate, and empower people about health issues<br>■ Mobilize community partnerships and action to identify and solve health problems<br>■ Develop policies and plans that support individual and community health efforts<br>■ Enforce laws and regulations that protect health and ensure safety<br>■ Link people to needed personal health services and ensure the provision of healthcare when otherwise unavailable<br>■ Ensure the provision of competent public and personal healthcare workforce<br>■ Evaluate effectiveness, accessibility, and quality of personal and population-based health services<br>■ Research for new insights and innovative solutions to health problems<br>■ Group and community-based interventions focusing on communicable disease control, reduction of environmental hazards, food and drug safety, and nutritional and behavioral risk factors |
| *Population health*<br>Systems approach that actively looks for effective points to intervene through the public health system, the healthcare system, or through social interventions or policy solutions | ■ Explicitly and actively engages the public health system, the healthcare system, as well as public policy efforts that address the determinants of health<br>■ Focused on the needs of the population, whether these can be best accomplished through hospitals, home care, hospice, or health department services<br>■ Utilizes interventions designed to improve health outcomes, including reducing death and disability. Interventions include the full spectrum of available options, from prevention to treatment to rehabilitation and palliation.<br>■ Looks at outcomes rather than organizations with outcomes including but not limited to the prevention of disease plus promotion<br>■ Areas of focus<br>  • Describe a population's problem, including the underlying determinants of health and disease<br>  • Make a diagnosis of the problem using a systems approach<br>  • Select intervention(s) utilizing a wide range of available individual, group, and population-based options for intervention |

Data from Riegelman R. *Population Health: A Primer.* Burlington, MA: Jones & Bartlett Learning; 2020:2-3, 10-11, 52.

intersection between the healthcare system and other determinants of population health (e.g., public health and built and social environments). This includes population-specific activities of the healthcare system itself and intersections of the system with other determinants of population health.[7(p7)] Population medicine created a pathway to individualized and precision medicine, which can improve symptom-driven practice using comprehensive patient information with distinguishing factors of illness and health. Population medicine can provide decision support and positively impact patient outcomes.[8] Approaches and techniques to consider in population medicine include artificial intelligence, machine learning, personalized treatment, and data science. See the *Health Data Analytics* section for more information related to data processing and analysis.

**Box 7.1** highlights key points in population health.

### Box 7.1 Key Points: Population Health

- Healthcare quality professionals should understand the fundamentals of population health necessary to create the comprehensive quality infrastructure, which will support population health and value-based reimbursement models.
- Population health considers the health outcomes of a group of individuals, including the distribution of such outcomes within the group keeping in mind the determinants of health (e.g., social and physical environments and related services, genetics, and individual behavior).
- Public health covers promotion of health in a population, prevention of disease in a population, and protection of the health of a population—the three *Ps*.
- Population medicine focuses on specific activities of the medical care system that promote population health beyond the goals of care of the individuals treated encompassing the intersection between the healthcare system and other determinants of population health (e.g., public health and built and social environments).

# Population Health Management

Population health management "is the design, delivery, coordination, and payment of high-quality healthcare services to manage the Triple Aim for a population using the best resources available within the healthcare system."[3(¶11)] The Association of American Medical Colleges (AAMC) describes 10 requirements of a comprehensive population health management program.[9]

1. *Data infrastructure.* This includes the ability to track information in the electronic health record and data registries. Value-based reimbursement is structured around demonstrated improvement in successful outcomes while reducing costs, and it requires effective collection and monitoring of data. Additionally, patient-specific clinical registries are increasingly available directly within the electronic health record, making it easier to identify and collect data on specific patient populations, such as those with chronic health conditions.
2. *Community engagement.* This focuses on understanding the needs of the community and developing relationships with community partners.
3. *Team-based care.* Involves the creation of an interdisciplinary care team, including registered nurses, social workers, and pharmacists.
4. *Panel management.* This refers to caring for the defined population, leveraging evidence-based care for preventive and chronic care, ensuring timely completion of related tasks, identifying and addressing inequities, and engaging with patients to close care gaps.
5. *Patient risk stratification.* This requirement involves the placing of patients into subgroups as determined by the clinic.
6. *Care management.* This requirement involves care for patients with chronic health conditions.
7. *Complex care management.* This refers to identifying high-cost patients and patients with high needs and using a team-based approach to managing the needs of these patients.
8. *Self-management support.* Engaging with patients to provide education and support as the patient actively manages their chronic health condition or preventive health measures.
9. *Addressing social determinants of health.* This identifies social needs that may be affecting the patient's well-being and developing a plan to address those social needs.
10. *Ensuring health equity.* This requirement focuses on identifying and addressing inequities and gaps within the population to reduce health disparities and improve health outcomes.[9(pp1-2)]

Critical to understanding the population is a comprehensive assessment and establishment of a detailed understanding of differences between the types of payers, such as governmental plans and commercial insurers and those who are uninsured. As the National Committee for Quality Assurance (NCQA) describes, "over 60 percent of health and longevity is driven by nonclinical factors"[10(p12)] known as SDOH such as "the conditions in which people are born, grow, live, work, and age—which include socioeconomic status, education, neighborhood and physical environment, employment, social support networks and access to health care."[10(p12)] Addressing social determinants of health is important for health improvement and reduction of long-standing disparities in health and healthcare.[11] **Figure 7.2** provides SDOH examples.

Challenges to addressing SDOH include a lack of concise assessment models, screening tools that are not linked to evidence-based studies, and a lack of provider time and resources to collect information.[12]

Healthy People 2030 addresses the latest health priorities and includes a strong focus on health equity. One of the overarching goals of Healthy People 2030 is to "eliminate health disparities, achieve health equity, and attain health literacy to improve the health and well-being of all."[13(¶2)] Population goals are categorized by health conditions, health behaviors, populations, settings and systems, and SDOH (e.g., economic stability, education access and quality, healthcare access

| Economic stability | Neighborhood and physical environment | Education | Food | Community and social context | Healthcare system |
|---|---|---|---|---|---|
| Employment | Housing | Literacy | Hunger | Social integration | Health coverage |
| Income | Transportation | Language | Access to healthy options | Support systems | Provider availability |
| Expenses | Safety | Early childhood education | | Community engagement | Provider linguistic and cultural competency |
| Debt | Parks | Vocational training | | Discrimination | Quality of care |
| Medical bills | Playgrounds | Higher education | | Stress | |
| Support | Walkability | | | | |
| | Zip code/ geography | | | | |

**Health outcomes**
Mortality, morbidity, life expectancy, healthcare expenditures, health status, functional limitations

**Figure 7.2** Social Determinants of Health

Reproduced from Artiga S, Hinton E. Beyond health care: the role of social determinants in promoting health and health equity. Kaiser Family Foundation. Published May 10, 2018. Accessed March 10, 2022. https://www.kff.org/racial-equity-and-health-policy/issue-brief/beyond-health-care-the-role-of-social-determinants-in-promoting-health-and-health-equity/

and quality, the neighborhood and built environment, and social and community context).[13]

## Data Integration

Data integration from a variety of sources is necessary to perform a thorough evaluation and risk stratification of the population while balancing privacy and security of healthcare data. Sources of data may include the electronic health record, health information exchanges, claims data, patient monitoring devices, screening tools, and other internal and external information technology systems.[10] Stratification should leverage real-time data to the extent possible. The what and how to stratify need clarity. As an example, using test results may depend on demographic characteristics of the population including age, race, and sex where laboratory test results should be interpreted based on similar individuals.[14] Other examples include admission and discharge data that can be integrated to automatically update the population risk stratification.[15] Predictive modeling may help identify certain high-risk situations, such as the risk of readmission within a designated time period; however, predictive modeling does not offer interventions that may help to mitigate the readmission risk. Adding artificial intelligence to predictive modeling could reduce the readmission risk.[15]

Quality, safety, and performance improvement can be enhanced in population health through the application of clinical epidemiology (e.g., case-control studies, cohort studies, propensity score matching) to data collected on many patients for little cost. This comports to a recent emphasis in the healthcare industry related to population health. Comprehensive linked databases have enormous potential to provide information on the influence of tests and treatments on health. The potential value of these data can be realized if the actual receipt of these interventions, health outcomes, and potentially confounding variables can be ascertained accurately for individual patients. Selection bias can be minimized by identifying an appropriate basis for comparison. For example, it is possible to assess changes in patient outcomes after an improvement intervention on a specific nursing unit by comparing those outcomes to a matched group of patients from other units in a hospital or over a prior period for the same unit when adjusting for any confounding variables.

Using data available in electronic records and appropriate statistical methods makes it possible to test for statistical differences related to a quality, safety, or process improvement initiative compared to current practice. This level of analysis makes the results more robust, leading to wider acceptance across an organization and broad adoption of the improvement effort (also known as "spread"). For more information, see the *Health Data Analytics* section.

## Goal Setting

Goal setting should include goals that are specific, measurable, achievable, relevant, and timely (SMART). In addition, consider these key factors when setting goals:

1. Characteristics and needs of the population.
2. Stakeholder obligations, such as alignment of performance measures with accreditation standards, regulatory requirements, and contractual stipulations.
3. The Quadruple Aim, which intends to
   - improve the experience of care,
   - improve the health of populations,
   - reduce the per capita cost of healthcare and incorporate smarter spending, and
   - support positive workforce experiences or joy in work.

Once set, the plan-do-study-act performance improvement cycle may be leveraged to achieve the goals. For more information on the improvement cycle, see the *Performance and Process Improvement* section.

## Targeted Interventions

Targeted interventions include those that are patient centered and evidence based, including a variety of care coordination and care management activities. Targeted interventions are critical for the success of a population health management program and may include wellness and prevention programs with personal coaching and self-management tools (e.g., well-being and resilience), preventive care, and educational activities.[16] Additionally, the care management team can develop patient-specific care plans that consider patient needs, include prioritized goals, and contain a mechanism to track progress toward goals. The care management team also provides the necessary facilitation of care transitions and ensures the patient has self-management support.[15]

Providing practitioner support through partnership is an important driver for success with interventions. Examples of support may include data sharing and analytics, training, embedding care managers, and technical assistance.[17] Informatics and analytics are used to target and reach individuals who are most at risk. Information technology tools such as portals, mobile applications, and telehealth expands the reach of practitioners in engaging patients and their families, and impacts desired outcomes.[18]

## Measurement and Improvement

Value-based care reimbursement models are driving the need for quality measurement and improvement focused on quality, cost, and patient experience. Further, improvement in population health outcomes demands a disciplined and structured approach to measuring health outcomes.[19] For additional information, see the *Quality Review and Accountability* and *Performance and Process Improvement* sections.

The Centers for Medicare & Medicaid Services (CMS) suggests that a population health measure should be defined as a "broadly applicable indicator that reflects the quality of a group's overall health and well-being."[20(p2)] Examples of population health measures include access to care, clinical outcomes, coordination of care and community services, health behaviors, preventive care and screening, and health service utilization.[20] Acknowledging population health depends on a variety of factors, including economic, social, environmental, cultural, and behavioral factors.[20] **Figure 7.3** shows population health's intersections with the Triple Aim.

Further, CMS spells out that population health improvement requires commitment across multiple sectors, including government and tribal agencies, measured entities and payers, community service providers, and private sector partners.

Community health centers are essential partners on any road to population health improvement. The National Association of Community Health Centers encourages quality improvement/performance measurement as one population health management strategy to achieve its Quadruple Aim of improved patient experiences, improved clinical outcomes, and lower costs while improving the work life of healthcare providers.[21(p1)] To help achieve these significant goals, the association calls on quality improvement and performance measurement, which it defines as a "formal methodology that enables health centers to leverage data collection and analysis, process improvement, and performance benchmarking."[21(¶1)]

Viewing measurement and improvement through the additional lens of population health can seem overwhelming. According to IHI,

> a key part of the population health journey is to understand the needs and assets of the patients and individuals in your chosen population. This understanding is core to defining aims; engaging the right partners in the work; and designing effective, equitable, and sustainable care and service delivery systems. While focusing on needs is an important part

**Figure 7.3** Population Health and the Triple Aim

Reproduced from Centers for Medicare & Medicaid Services. Population health measures: supplemental material to the CMS MMS blueprint. Published 2021. Accessed April 4, 2022. https://www.cms.gov/files/document/blueprint-population-health-measures.pdf

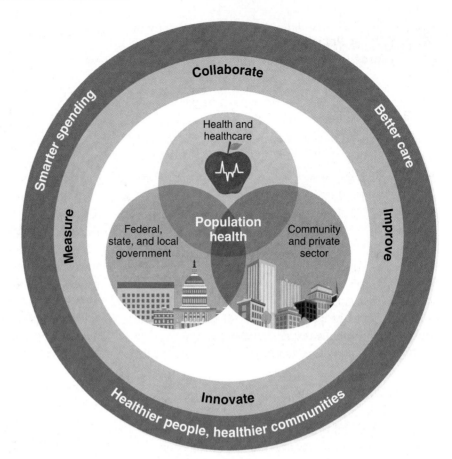

of the process, solely using this approach can focus only on deficiencies within a population. This is why it's also key to consider an assets-based approach, which suggests that all individuals and populations have multiple strengths and capacities, which could be harnessed to make them thrive more fully.[22(p1)]

Using an assets-based approach, IHI proposes a three-part data review process, which follows.

1. Review available data to identify overall patterns that impact the population.
2. Understand the perspectives and experiences of care teams and other professionals providing care or supporting the population to understand a population's greatest needs and assets.
3. Understand the perspectives and experience of the patient to understand what is important to them, the real-world challenges in managing health and living situations, and what might help.[22(p1)]

Healthcare quality professionals should understand how to implement standard performance and process improvement methods, such as the plan-do-study-act cycle to track performance measures in value-based payment arrangements. See the *Performance and Process Improvement* section for more information.

Standardizing workflows across the continuum of care, reducing variation, continuously monitoring performance through data analysis, and providing feedback to providers regularly are key responsibilities of healthcare quality professionals working within population health. The ability to drive change through rapid-cycle improvement and care-gap closure is paramount to achieving successful quality outcomes in value-based risk arrangements. As shared by NCQA, "You can't improve what you don't measure," which is particularly important when payment is tied to performance.[23(p42)]

**Box 7.2** lists key points in population health management.

# Population Health Models and Frameworks

There is a variety of population health models to enable healthcare organizations and public health programs in their efforts to improve the health of populations rather than limiting interventions and improvements to the health of individuals. Friedman and Starfield note that "Although no single public health program can address the wide range of influences on population health, the use of [a variety of models] in public

## Box 7.2 Key Points: Population Health Management

- Healthcare quality professionals should be familiar with and proficient in understanding the different types of population health strategies.
- Professional and government organizations have population health management strategies, frameworks, and models. These can be helpful resources when considering a comprehensive population health management effort.
- Measurement and improvement are the foundation of value-based care and reimbursement models. It is a critical component of driving improvement in health outcomes.

health practice can reorient programs away from more isolated and categorical approaches to more integrated approaches."[15(p367)] Examples of different population health models and frameworks follow.

## American Hospital Association Population Health Framework

The American Hospital Association (AHA), a national organization that represents hospitals, healthcare networks, patients, and communities, presents its framework in support of accountable, equitable care. These groups may include but not be limited to "those who are attributable to or served by a hospital or health care system, those living in a specified geographic area or community, or those experiencing a certain condition or disease."[24(¶8)] The AHA Population Health Framework is shown as **Figure 7.4**.

The importance of driving improvement through integrated models and community partnerships as outlined by AHA was noted in a systematic literature review of hospital–community partnerships. Community or population health improvement is aided by "a better understanding of how health systems engage

**Figure 7.4** Population Health Framework

Reproduced from American Hospital Association. Population Health Framework. Published 2019. © Used with permission of American Hospital Association. Accessed June 12, 2022. https://www.aha.org/system/files/media/file/2019/04/pop-health-framework.pdf

**Health and equity**

Key focus areas

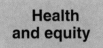

Integrated care models

Community partnerships

Chronic/ complex care

Driving improvement in 2 dimensions

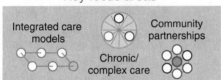

Population health management

Community well-being

Population health foundational capabilities

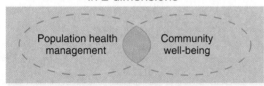

Understanding populations

Engaging in new partnerships

Taking system-level actions

Measuring and sustaining progress

AHA strategies

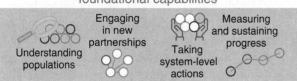

Advocacy | Thought leadership | Knowledge exchange | Agent of change

AHA path forward commitment

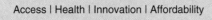

Access | Health | Innovation | Affordability

AHA vision

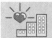   A society of healthy communities where all individuals reach their highest potential for health.

with community partners for population health and should be of interest to hospital administrators focused on population health management [and] organizations interested in collaborating with health systems ...."[25(p2)] Further, healthcare leaders and professionals overseeing population health management activities can

- identify the best partners to support population health efforts,
- leverage and sustain partnerships beyond initial efforts to meet regulatory and accreditation requirements, and
- use partners to support interventions focused on social determinants of health.[25]

The elements of the AHA framework offer population health program developers anchors for transformation initiatives.

## The Care Continuum Alliance Population Health Improvement Model

Another strong voice in population health is the Care Continuum Alliance, which aims to promote health status through the promotion and alignment of population health improvement.[26]

The Care Continuum Alliance identifies the key components of the population health improvement model including strategies and processes, needs assessments (physical, psychological, economic, and environmental needs), health promotion, person-centric health management goals and education (e.g., primary prevention, behavior modification, coordination of care), self-management interventions targeting behavioral changes in the population, evaluation of outcomes (e.g., clinical, humanistic, and economic), and reporting and feedback to the patient, physicians, health plan and ancillary providers.[27(q5)] This population health improvement model highlights three components.

1. Central care delivery and leadership roles of the primary care physician
2. Critical importance of patient activation, involvement, and personal responsibility
3. Patient focus and expansion of care coordination (e.g., wellness, disease, and chronic care management programs)[27(q2)]

The Care Continuum Alliance suggests that the consolidation of these population health dynamics ensures better healthcare quality and patient satisfaction. By extension, the group proposes that, through coordination and integration, healthcare can more effectively address workforce shortages,

access, and affordability. Like population health itself, the focus of this model is the delivery and coordination of appropriate, cost-effective care. The model encourages and rewards improvement and goal achievement.[27]

## Centers for Disease Control and Prevention 6|18 Initiative

In July 2018, the U.S. Centers for Disease Control and Prevention (CDC) introduced its 6|18 Initiative, targeting 6 common and costly health conditions with 18 proven interventions. The 6 conditions and aims are

1. reduce tobacco use;
2. control high blood pressure;
3. improve antibiotic use;
4. control asthma;
5. prevent unintended pregnancy; and
6. prevent type 2 diabetes.

For the project, CDC partners with healthcare purchasers, payers, and providers to improve health and control healthcare costs. CDC provides its partners with "rigorous evidence about high-burden health conditions and associated interventions to inform their decisions to have the greatest health and cost impact. This initiative aligns evidence-based preventive practices with emerging value-based payment and delivery methods," with an intention to improve health and control costs.[28(q1)] The six high-burden health conditions with effective interventions that the CDC is prioritizing are shown in **Figure 7.5**.

CDC also provides fuller descriptions of the conditions, evidence summaries, and resources and tools on the 6|18 website.

## County Health Rankings Model

The County Health Rankings is a program of the University of Wisconsin Population Health Institute. A model of community health was developed by the institute, emphasizing factors and measures that relate to community health. The model can be used by healthcare quality professionals and others to convey the influence of SDOH and to profile the health of a community. Descriptions and statistics show how different health behaviors, clinical care, social and economic factors, and physical environment may determine health status and health outcomes (**Figure 7.6**).

The rankings use more than 30 measures to aid in the understanding of how healthy community residents are today (health outcomes) and the impact of different determinants in the future

**REDUCE TOBACCO USE**

- Increase access to tobacco cessation treatments, including individual, group, and telephone counseling, and Food and Drug Administration-approved cessation medications (in accordance with the 2008 *Public Health Service Clinical Practice Guidelines* and the 2015 *U.S. Preventive Services Task Force* recommendations).
- Remove barriers that impede access to covered cessation treatments, such as cost-sharing and prior authorization.
- Promote increased use of covered treatment benefits by tobacco users.

**CONTROL HIGH BLOOD PRESSURE**

- Implement strategies that improve adherence to anti-hypertensive and lipid-lowering prescription medications via expanded access to:
  - low cost medication copayments, fixed dose medication combinations, and extended medication fills;
  - innovative pharmacy packaging;
  - improved care coordination using standardized protocols, primary care teams, medication therapy management programs, and self-monitoring of blood pressure with clinical support.
- Provide home blood pressure monitors to patients with high blood pressure and reimburse for the clinical support services required for self-measured blood pressure monitoring.

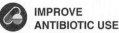
**IMPROVE ANTIBIOTIC USE**

- Require antibiotic stewardship programs in all hospitals and skilled nursing facilities, in alignment with *CDC's Core Elements of Hospital Antibiotic Stewardship Programs and The Core Elements of Antibiotic Stewardship for Nursing Homes.*
- Improve outpatient antibiotic prescribing by incentivizing providers to follow *CDC's Core Elements of Outpatient Antibiotic Stewardship.*

**CONTROL ASTHMA**

- Use the 2007 *National Asthma Education and Prevention Program* as clinical practice guidelines.
- Promote strategies that improve access and adherence to asthma medications and devices.
- Expand access to intensive self-management education by licensed professionals or qualified lay health workers for patients whose asthma is not well-controlled with medical management.
- Expand access to home visits by licensed professionals or qualified lay health workers to provide intensive self-management education and reduce home asthma triggers for patients whose asthma is not well-controlled with medical management and self-management education.

**PREVENT UNINTENDED PREGNANCY**

- Reimburse providers for the full range of contraceptive services (e.g., screening for pregnancy intention; counseling; insertion, removal, replacement, or reinsertion of long-acting reversible contraceptives, and follow-up) for women of childbearing age.
- Reimburse providers for the actual cost of FDA-approved contraceptive methods.
- Unbundle payment for long-acting reversible contraceptives from other postpartum services.
- Remove administrative barriers to receipt of contraceptive services (e.g., pre-approval step therapy restriction, barriers to high acquisition and stocking costs).

**PREVENT TYPE 2 DIABETES**

- Expand access to the National Diabetes Prevention Program, a lifestyle change program to prevent or delay onset of type 2 diabetes.

**Figure 7.5** CDC High-Burden Conditions with Effective Interventions

Reproduced from Centers for Disease Control and Prevention. CDC's 6|18 Initiative: accelerating evidence into action. Published July 2018. Accessed June 19, 2022. https://www.cdc.gov/sixeighteen/docs/6-18-factsheet.pdf

(health factors). The years of data available for each measure vary. **Table 7.2** lists selected measures that are available.

## National Committee for Quality Assurance Population Health Management Conceptual Model

NCQA offers Population Health Program accreditation. NCQA defines *population health management* as "a model of care that addresses individuals' health needs at all points along the continuum of care, including in the community setting, through participation, engagement, and targeted interventions for a defined population."[10(p7)] The goal of population management is to maintain or improve "the physical and psychological well-being of individuals and address health disparities through cost-effective and tailored health solutions."[12(p7)]

Population health management encompasses data integration, understanding the population, population stratification, targeted interventions,

practitioner support, and measurement and quality improvement.[12] The population health management (PHM) conceptual model developed by NCQA outlines the key activities necessary for a comprehensive population health management strategy. As illustrated in **Figure 7.7**, this model may be applied to any entity conducting population health functions.[10]

The patient is at the center of the PHM conceptual model, with a focus on providing care that addresses patient needs, preferences, and values. Considering the components surrounding the patient is vital to the successful implementation of a population health management strategy and creating a comprehensive approach to population health management. Pertaining to the PHM strategy, NCQA highlights four recommendations:

1. Importance of leadership buy-in and strong organizational culture
2. Practitioner leadership
3. Goal setting and alignment
4. Creation and communication of a PHM strategy

**Figure 7.6** County Health Rankings Model

The University of Wisconsin Population Health Institute. County health rankings & roadmaps. Published 2022. Accessed June 18, 2022. www.countyhealthrankings.org

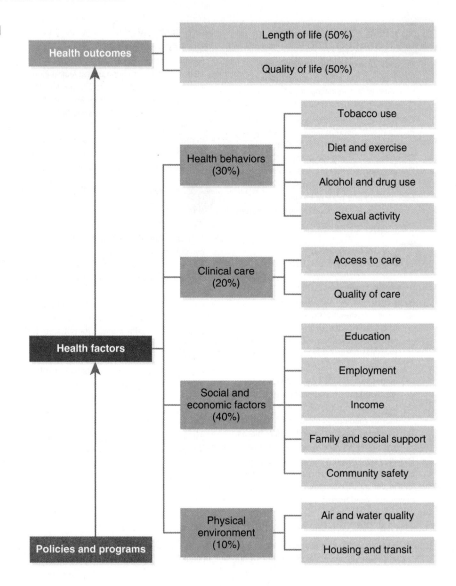

NCQA also developed a road map for population health management that is intended for integrated delivery networks, accountable care organizations, health systems, and other provider entities seeking to understand population health and how it is leveraged for success in value-based care. The road map contains seven milestones configured as a path to value-based care and leverages the activities of the PHM conceptual model (**Figure 7.8**).

## Pathways to Population Health

Aiming to give healthcare leaders pathways to improve the health of the communities served, five organizations—AHA, IHI, the Network for Regional Healthcare Improvement, the Public Health Institute, and Stakeholder Health—came together to create Pathways to Population Health. The experience of the supporting organizations is shown in the pathways framework (**Figure 7.9**). The Pathways to Population Health partnership draws on six foundational

concepts that signal a developing perception of health itself as well as the importance of partnership across healthcare and community sectors.

1. Health and well-being develop over a lifetime.
2. Social determinants drive health and well-being outcomes throughout the life course.
3. Place is a determinant of health, well-being, and equity.
4. The health system needs to address the key demographic shifts out of time.
5. The health system can embrace innovative financial models and deploy existing assets for greater value.
6. Health creation requires partnership because healthcare only holds a part of the puzzle.[29(p1)]

The four portfolios of population health are interconnected and represent a "comprehensive scope of population health-related improvements a health care organization may pursue"[30(p10)] focusing on physical and/or mental health, social and/or spiritual well-being,

Population Health Models and Frameworks

**Table 7.2** Selected Measures from County Health Rankings and Roadmaps

| Ranked Measures | Data Source | |
|---|---|---|
| **Health Outcomes** | | |
| Length of Life | Premature Death | National Center for Health Statistics-Mortality Files |
| Quality of Life | Poor or Fair Health<br>Poor Physical Health Days<br>Poor Mental Health Days | Behavioral Risk Factor Surveillance System |
| | Low Birthweight | National Center for Health Statistics-Natality Files |
| **Health Factors**<br>*Health Behaviors* | | |
| Alcohol and Drug Use | Excessive Drinking | Behavioral Risk Factor Surveillance System |
| | Alcohol-Impaired Driving Deaths | Fatality Analysis Reporting System |
| *Clinical Care* | | |
| Access to Care | Uninsured | Small Area Health Insurance Estimates |
| | Primary Care Physicians | Area Health Resource File/American Medical Association |
| | Dentists | Area Health Resource File/National Provider Identification File |
| | Mental Health Providers | CMS, National Provider Identification |
| Quality of Care | Preventable Hospital Stays<br>Mammography Screening<br>Flu Vaccinations | Mapping Medicare Disparities Tool |
| *Social & Economic Factors* | | |
| Community Safety | Violent Crime | Uniform Crime Reporting-FBI |
| | Injury Deaths | National Center for Health Statistics-Mortality Files |
| **Additional Measures** | **Data Source** | |
| **Health Outcomes** | | |
| Length of Life | COVID-19 Age-Adjusted Mortality<br>Life Expectancy<br>Premature Age-Adjusted Mortality<br>Child Mortality<br>Infant Mortality | National Center for Health Statistics-Mortality Files |
| Quality of Life | Frequent Physical Distress<br>Frequent Mental Distress<br>Diabetes Prevalence | Behavioral Risk Factor Surveillance System |
| | HIV Prevalence | National Center for HIV/AIDS, Viral Hepatitis, STD, and TB Prevention |
| **Health Factors** | | |
| Diet and Exercise | Food Insecurity | Map the Meal Gap |
| | Limited Access to Healthy Foods | USDA Food Environment Atlas |
| Alcohol and Drug Use | Drug Overdose Deaths<br>Motor Vehicle Crash Deaths | National Center for Health Statistics-Mortality Files |

Data from County Health Rankings & Roadmaps. 2022 Measures. Published 2022. Accessed June 19, 2022. https://www.countyhealthrankings.org/2022-measures

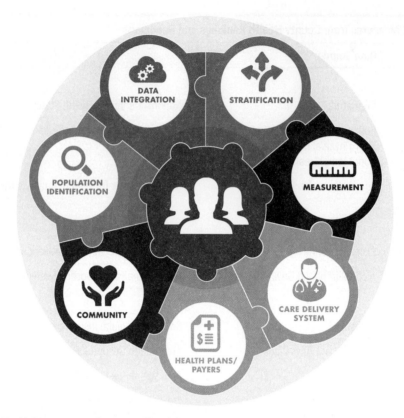

**Figure 7.7** Population Health Management Conceptual Model

Reproduced from National Committee for Quality Assurance. Population health management: resource guide. Published 2018. Accessed June 12, 2022. https://www.ncqa.org/programs/health-plans/population-health-management-resource-guide/

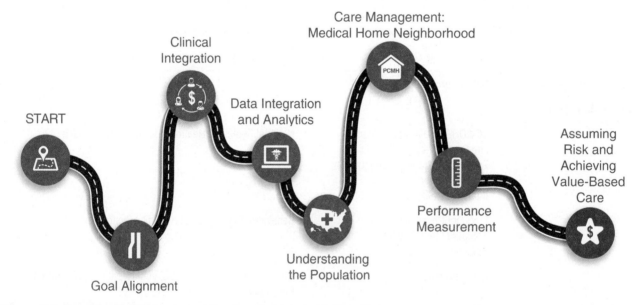

**Figure 7.8** Population Health Management Roadmap for Integrated Delivery Systems

Reproduced from National Committee for Quality Assurance. Population health management: roadmap for integrated delivery health networks. Published 2019. Accessed March 9, 2022. https://www.ncqa.org/wp-content/uploads/2019/11/20191216_PHM_Roadmap.pdf

community health and well-being, and communities of solutions. Together these form meaningful transformation of community well-being creation and population health management with health equity at the core.

## URAC Population Health

URAC established standards for provider and employer-based population health. By adopting its accreditation framework, organizations can demonstrate their

## PATHWAYS TO POPULATION HEALTH

Join health care change agents from across the country as they make practical, meaningful and sustainable advances in population health.

### LEARN
- Understand the key concepts and terms that are foundational for the journey to population health.
- Explore four portfolios of work that health care organizations can do to improve health, well-being and equity.

### ACT
- Celebrate where you are in your population health journey and evaluate your balance across the four portfolios.
- Create and implement a plan to improve your organization's population health initiatives.
- Identify levers that accelerate progress within and across portfolios.

### IMPROVE
- Access a curated set of tools and resources to support your progress.
- Create benchmarks to evaluate and guide your path forward.

### JOIN
- Sign up to stay connected to the larger Pathways to Population Health community.
- Join health care change agents from across the country to share and improve together.

**Pathways to Population Health** is a collaboration among:

**American Hospital Association/ Health Research and Educational Trust**

**Institute for Healthcare Improvement**

**Network for Regional Healthcare Improvement**

**Public Health Institute**

**Stakeholder Health**

Together, these partners leverage their unique assets to help other health care organizations accelerate individual and population health initiatives.

### FOUNDATIONAL CONCEPTS

The six concepts described below help lay the foundation for the **Pathways to Population Health**. They also articulate several reasons why many health care organizations have chosen to embark on this journey. The concepts represent an evolving understanding of what creates health and the ways in which health care organizations can engage.

1. Health and well-being develop over a lifetime.
2. Social determinants drive health and well-being outcomes throughout the life course.
3. Place is a determinant of health, well-being and equity.
4. The health system needs to address the key demographic shifts out of time.
5. The health system can embrace innovative financial models and deploy existing assets for greater value.
6. Health creation requires partnership because health care only holds a part of the puzzle.

What creates health ⟷ How can health care engage?

### TOOLS AND ACTIVITIES

Access a curated set of tools and resources to support and accelerate your progress

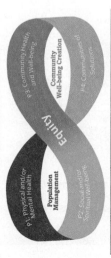

**Framework** — An articulation of foundational concepts and four portfolios of work that health care organizations can undertake to improve health, well-being and equity

**Compass** — A method to catalogue current population health archives and identify opportunities to amplify effort

**Campaign** — An opportunity for health care change agents to share with and learn from one another on this journey

**Oasis** — A curated set of tools and resources to support organizations on their population health journey

### FOUR PORTFOLIOS OF POPULATION HEALTH

Equity — Population Management — Community Well-being Creation

P1: Physical and/or Mental Health
P2: Social and/or Spiritual Well-being
P3: Community Health and Well-being
P4: Communities of Solutions

| | Portfolio 1: Physical and/or Mental Health | Portfolio 2: Social and/or Spiritual Well-Being | Portfolio 3: Community Health and Well-Being | Portfolio 4: Communities of Solutions |
| --- | --- | --- | --- | --- |
| Type of population | Defined | Defined | Place-based and defined | Place-based and defined |
| Focus of work | Proactively address mental and/or physical health for the population for which your organization is directly responsible (e.g., patients, employees) | Proactively address social and spiritual drivers for the population for which your organization is directly responsible (e.g., patients, employees) | Improvement of health, well-being and equity focused on specific topics across a place-based or defined population | Whole community transformation with a focus on long-term structural changes needed for a thriving, equitable community |
| Example activities | Manage diabetes outcomes for a primary care panel; integrate mental health into primary care | Screen for and address social determinants of health in partnership with community social-service agencies; establish peer-to-peer supports | Engage in a multisector partnership to address food insecurity in key neighborhoods | Engage in a multisector partnership to create long-term structure, policy, and systems changes (e.g., preferred purchasing from minority-owned local businesses) |

## PATHWAYS TO POPULATION HEALTH

**For more information please visit:**

http://pathways2pophealth.org/learn.html

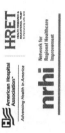

American Hospital Association — Advancing Health in America

HRET — Health Research & Educational Trust

Network for Regional Healthcare Improvement — nrhi

Institute for Healthcare Improvement

PUBLIC HEALTH INSTITUTE

Stakeholder Health

An initiative facilitated by 100 Million Healthier Lives

With generous support provided by Robert Wood Johnson Foundation

---

**Figure 7.9** Pathways to Population Health

approach to achieve the Quadruple Aim as described earlier (e.g., experience of care, health outcomes, satisfaction of healthcare workers, and costs of care). There are two types of population health accreditation—provider based and employer based. They include standards that address areas such as population health (assessment, status, needs, improvement, risk management) and access. Healthcare organizations can evaluate which are best aligned with near-term and long-term needs and with strategic goals and objectives.

## Population Health and Value-Based Care

Success in value-based contracting requires complete buy-in from leadership and practitioners, along with an alignment of goals. Creating and communicating the population health management strategy includes activities such as creating one governing board led by practitioners and employing practitioners under one tax ID to align payment structures. Creating a PHM strategy also includes aligning one strategy across the organization, meeting with practitioners to encourage two-way dialogue and address concerns and including strategy and goals in the network participation agreement. The *Guide to Health Care Partnerships for Population Health Management and Value-Based Care* discusses how "the business model for U.S. healthcare is transforming from a volume-driven model to a consumer-centric, value-driven model."[31(p4)] The focus of the value-based care model is to "improve quality, access, and outcomes, while reducing costs through the effective management of a population's health over the continuum . . ."[31(p6)] This new model of managing the health of a population requires new skills and competencies, "including clinical integration; consumer, clinical, and business intelligence; operational efficiency; customer engagement; and efficient network development."[31(p6)] **Figure 7.10** illustrates this new model.

Hospitals and healthcare systems need to partner with other organizations to capitalize on the capabilities and efficiencies to provide services under care delivery and payment arrangements (i.e., risk-bearing, value-based, targeted investments).[31(p4)] This includes partnerships to address nonmedical factors that impact the health status of a community including SDOH, environmental factors, and economic factors. The types of risk for hospitals and health systems and population health management contracting arrangements fall into two categories as shown in **Table 7.3**.

## Value-Based Reimbursement

Value-based reimbursement requires skill in comprehensive care management, data analytics and predictive modeling, and population risk stratification, along with a full continuum of care and a high-performing network of providers and partners to care for the population. The government also is recognizing the importance of population health, which is addressed

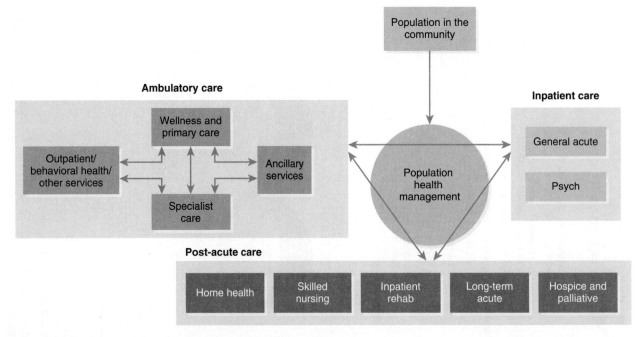

**Figure 7.10** Provider Care Continuum for Population Health Management

Reproduced from Allen PM, Finnerty MJ, Gish RS., et al. *Guide to Health Care Partnerships for Population Health Management and Value-based Care*. Chicago, IL: Health Research & Educational Trust and Kaufman, Hall & Associates, LLC; 2016; 7. Accessed June 9, 2022. www.hpoe.org/healthcarepartnerships

**Table 7.3** Types of Risk Assumed by Hospitals and Health Systems

| Category | Types of Risk |
|---|---|
| Provider risk (assumed by the entities delivering healthcare services) | Clinical or performance risk, which is the ability to deliver patient care that exceeds the targets for safety, quality, compliance, and other measures defined in the risk contract with the payer.<br>▪ Utilization or financial risk, which is incurred by a provider organization through acceptance of a fixed payment in exchange for the provision of care anticipated to have an expected level of utilization and cost.<br>▪ Hospital or insurer-owned plans contracting with providers for the provision of care under capitated arrangements are not technically taking on provider risk but are delegating such risk. |
| Insurance or plan risk | Assumed by hospitals and health systems that have their own insurance plans, with responsibility for attracting and retaining members and the overall costs of plan administration and/or care delivery. |

Data from Kaufman, Hall & Associates, LLC. In: Allen PM, Finnerty MJ, Gish RS, et al., eds. *Guide to Health Care Partnerships for Population Health Management and Value-based Care*. Chicago, IL: Health Research & Educational Trust and Kaufman, Hall & Associates, LLC; 2016. Accessed June 9, 2022. www.hpoe.org/healthcarepartnerships

in the 2010 Affordable Care Act (ACA). The ACA contains four provisions related to population health:

1. Increased access to healthcare through expanded coverage options, Medicaid expansion, and subsidies available through health insurance exchanges
2. Creation of the National Strategy for Quality Improvement
3. Increased focus on preventive health through new payer requirements to cover certain preventive services and the creation of accountable care organizations (ACOs) enabling providers to assume responsibility for the health outcomes of populations
4. Establishment of the National Prevention, Health Promotion, and Public Health Council, in addition to workplace wellness incentives, thus promoting community-based population health[32]

CMS value-based programs include the five original value-based programs that link provider performance of quality measures to provider payment. There are two additional programs that have been added over time, so the programs now include the following:

- End-Stage Renal Disease Quality Incentive Program
- Hospital Value-Based Purchasing Program
- Hospital Readmission Reduction Program
- Value Modifier Program (also called the Physician Value-Based Modifier)
- Hospital Acquired Conditions Reduction Program
- Skilled Nursing Facility Value-Based Purchasing
- Home Health Value Based Purchasing

These programs move pay-for-performance forward based on the quality of patient care versus the quantity of care providers give patients.[33]

The Center for Medicare & Medicaid Innovation has taken steps to incorporate population health and launched 54 payment and service delivery models over the past 10 years. The models enable providers to enter value-based reimbursement arrangements to deliver better care while lowering costs.[34] Population-health models include the traditional Medicare Quality Payment Program, which launched in 2017 as part of the Medicare Access and CHIP Reauthorization Act of 2015 (MACRA). The Medicare Quality Payment Program replaces the Sustainable Growth Rate methodology for payment increases. It enables Medicare to reimburse providers according to high-quality performance while reducing payments to providers not meeting performance expectations.[35] The Quality Payment Program focuses on paying for value and health outcomes.

## Medicare Shared Savings Program and Accountable Care Organizations

Another model conceived by the Center for Medicare & Medicaid Innovation is the Medicare Shared Savings Program (Shared Savings Program), which launched in 2012. The Shared Savings Program focuses on value-based reimbursement and health outcomes, allowing healthcare providers and suppliers to creatively work together under an ACO framework. The Shared Savings Program is an alternative payment model that "promotes accountability of a patient population, coordinates items and services for Medicare fee-for-service beneficiaries, and encourages investment in high-quality efficient services."[36(¶3)] ACOs can share in the cost savings it achieves for Medicare if the ACO is successful in delivering high-quality care, while reducing the overall cost of care. Leadership and culture are important to the success of an ACO.[37]

Accountable care organizations achieve high-quality care and reduced spending when the physicians, hospitals, and other suppliers of healthcare join and provide comprehensive care coordination, ensuring patients receive "the right care at the right time."[38(¶2)] Comprehensive care coordination is vital in a value-based payment arrangement. Understanding the characteristics of the population, identifying those most at risk for costly healthcare utilization, and developing targeted interventions to manage the population across the care continuum are essential components of a population health program focused on providing "better care for individuals, better health for populations, and lowering growth in expenditures."[36(¶1)]

In the early years of the Shared Savings Program, adoption of risk arrangements was slow for ACOs, with most initially opting for risk-free, upside-only risk. According to Daly, the participation in the no-risk accountable care organization track has trended downward since 2017, when 91% of all Shared Savings Program ACOs were in the no-risk track. In 2020, 26% of ACOs were in the no-risk track.[39] As of January 1, 2022, the Shared Savings Program has cared for millions of Medicare beneficiaries while achieving high average overall quality scores and earning millions of dollars in shared savings. CMS offers several types of alternative payment models, "a payment approach that gives added incentives to provide high-quality and cost-efficient care. Alternative payment models can apply to a specific clinical condition, a care episode, or a population."[40(p1)]

In value-based care, there are steps a physician practice can take to prepare for value-based healthcare by promoting the Triple Aim or Quadruple Aim. These steps include:

1. Identify the population and opportunity.
2. Design the care model.
3. Partner for success.
4. Drive appropriate utilization.
5. Quantify impact and continuously improve.[41(p2)]

Identifying the patients who are driving the highest utilization and highest cost of care is critical to successfully identifying and implementing a model of care for high-risk populations. Patients with uncontrolled chronic conditions and multiple health issues may miss follow-up appointments, experience challenges adhering to their treatment plan, and need heightened coordination of care. CMS established a framework for value-based care aligned with empowering patients and clinicians to make decisions about their healthcare using innovative approaches to improve quality, accessibility, and affordability. Areas of focus at the patient and population levels are outlined in **Table 7.4**. These may be instrumental to better manage patient care.

A list of key points for population health and value-based care can be found in **Box 7.3**.

## Care Transitions

Care transitions occur when a patient moves from one healthcare provider or setting to another. Historically, the focus has been from the inpatient hospital setting to another care setting, and improvement efforts have surrounded readmissions due to excessive costs and poor health outcomes. However, given the continuum of care, there are settings across which a person might traverse that require treatment planning and coordination for care (e.g., outpatient surgery to home care, acute hospital care at home). Care transitions can present opportunities and challenges for healthcare providers and systems of care. Some opportunities are seamless handoffs and movement to other levels of care that are better aligned with the needs of the patient and their support system. Some challenges are linkages with downstream providers and lack of systematic care management.

The *ACMA Transitions of Care Standards* serve as a guide for care managers and other healthcare professionals to ensure optimal transitions of care.[42] ACMA refers to the American Case Management Association. Effective care transitions can "prevent medical errors, identify issues for early intervention, avert unnecessary hospitalizations and readmissions, support consumers' preferences and choices and avoid duplication of services"[42(p4)] leading to the improvement in the quality of care and effective utilization of resources. The five transitions of care (TOC) standards were assessed through the ACMA TOC Learning Collaborative with six major health systems participating (**Figure 7.11**). The four primary goals of the collaborative were to

1. test the implementation of the TOC standards in real-world health system environments across a variety of U.S. regions;
2. identify innovative or effective practices as well as challenges and barriers that may impact implementation of the standards;

**Table 7.4** Meaningful Areas of Focus in Value-Based Care

| Area | Focus |
|---|---|
| Promote effective communication and coordination of care | ▪ Medication management<br>▪ Admissions and readmissions to hospitals<br>▪ Transfer of health information and interoperability |
| Promote effective prevention and treatment of chronic disease | ▪ Preventive care<br>▪ Management of chronic conditions<br>▪ Prevention, treatment, and management of mental health<br>▪ Prevention and treatment of opioid and substance use disorders<br>▪ Risk-adjusted mortality |
| Work with communities to promote best practices of healthy living | ▪ Equity of care<br>▪ Community engagement |
| Make care affordable | ▪ Appropriate use of healthcare<br>▪ Patient-focused episode of care<br>▪ Risk-adjusted total cost of care |
| Make care safer by reducing harm caused in the delivery of care | ▪ Healthcare-associated infections<br>▪ Preventable healthcare harm |
| Strengthen person & family engagement as partners in their care | ▪ Personalize care aligned with patient's goals (e.g., voice and choice)<br>▪ End of life care according to preferences<br>▪ Patient's experience of care<br>▪ Patient reported functional outcome |

Reproduced from Moody-Williams, JD. Value-based care. Centers for Medicare & Medicaid Services. Published 2018. Accessed August 4, 2022. https://www.hrsa.gov/sites/default/files/hrsa/advisory-committees/nursing/meetings/2018/nacnep-sept2018-CMS-Value-Based-Care.pdf

---

**Box 7.3 Key Points: Population Health and Value-Based Care**

▪ Value-based care reimbursement models require population-based quality measures.
▪ With good data and robust analytics, it is possible to achieve the goal of being a high-performing organization in meeting the needs of specific populations.
▪ Accountable care organizations under the Centers for Medicare & Medicaid Services enable healthcare providers and suppliers to creatively work together to achieve improved health outcomes at a lower cost of care.
▪ The healthcare quality professional can support value-based reimbursement models through proficiency in risk stratifying the population and leveraging rapid-cycle improvement methodologies to achieve desired outcomes.

3. ask healthcare organizations to assess their compliance with the TOC standards, identify and pursue opportunities for improvement, and then reassess compliance to determine progress made; and

4. share results and lessons learned from the TOC Learning Collaborative to guide broader adoption of ACMA's TOC standards.[42(p5)]

The collaborative provided benchmarking to help identify the standards where improvement efforts can be focused including advance care planning, medication reconciliation, and the electronic health record. The electronic health record contributes to the communication of essential care transition information to stakeholders across the continuum of care.[42(p7)]

| **Standard 1** | **Standard 2** | **Standard 3** | **Standard 4** | **Standard 5** |
|---|---|---|---|---|
| Identify patients at risk for poor transitions | Complete a comprehensive transition assessment | Perform and communicate a medication reconciliation | Establish a dynamic care management plan that addresses all settings throughout the continuum of care | Communicate essential care transition information to key stakeholders across the continuum of care |

**Figure 7.11** Transitions of Care Standards

Reproduced from Bober M, Ferket K. *ACMA Transitions of Care Learning Collaborative.* American Case Management Association. Published 2019. Accessed March 8, 2022. https://transitionsofcare.org/resources/learning-collaborative/

Common issues were identified by the participating organizations, such as

- ensuring longitudinal care management to provide continuity of care across a patient's entire care experience;
- navigating challenges related to postacute care transitions; and
- responding to care management workforce challenges across the continuum.[42(p9)]

## Care Management

Comprehensive care management is essential to population health management. The Agency for Healthcare Research and Quality (AHRQ) describes *care management* as a "promising team-based, patient-centered approach 'designed to assist patients and their support systems in managing medical conditions more effectively.'"[43(p2)] **Table 7.5** describes the

**Table 7.5** Key Care Management Strategies and Recommendations

| | Recommendations for Medical Practice | Recommendations for Health Policy | Recommendations for Health Services Research |
|---|---|---|---|
| Identify populations with modifiable risks* | ■ Use multiple metrics to identify patients with modifiable risks<br>■ Develop risk-based approaches to identify patients most in need of care management (CM) services | ■ Consider return on investment of providing CM services to patients with a broad set of eligibility requirements<br>■ Establish metrics to identify and track CM outcomes to determine success<br>■ Implement value-based payment methodologies through state and federal tax incentives to practices for achieving the Triple Aim | ■ Determine the benefits to different patient segments from CM services<br>■ Investigate the understanding of and parameters affecting modifiable risks<br>■ Develop/refine tools for risk stratification<br>■ Develop predictive models to support risk stratification |
| Align CM services to the needs of the population | ■ Tailor CM services, with input from patients to meet specific needs of populations with different modifiable risks<br>■ Use the electronic medical record to facilitate care coordination and effective communication with patients and outreach to them | ■ Incentivize CM services through CMS transitional CM and chronic care coordination billing codes<br>■ Provide a variety of financial and nonfinancial supports to develop, implement, and sustain CM<br>■ Reward CM programs that achieve the Triple Aim | ■ Evaluate initiatives seeking to foster care alignment across providers<br>■ Create a framework for aligning CM services across the medical neighborhood to reduce potentially harmful duplication of these services<br>■ Determine how best to implement CM services across the spectrum of long-term services and supports |
| Identify and train personnel appropriate to the needed CM services | ■ Determine who should provide CM services given population needs and practice context<br>■ Identify needed skills, appropriate training, and licensure requirements<br>■ Implement interprofessional team-based approaches to care | ■ Incentivize care manager training through loans or tuition subsidies<br>■ Develop CM certification programs that recognize functional expertise | ■ Determine what team-building activities best support delivery of CM services<br>■ Design protocols for workflow that accommodate CM services in different contexts<br>■ Develop models for interprofessional education that bridge trainees at all levels and practicing healthcare professionals |

* Modifiable risk factors are those that an individual has control over and, if minimized, will increase the probability that a person will live a long and productive life.

Data from Agency for Healthcare Research and Quality. Care management: implications for medical practice, health policy, and health services research; ¶12; Published April 2015. Updated August 2018. Accessed June 9, 2022. https://www.ahrq.gov/ncepcr/care/coordination/mgmt.html; The SCAN Foundation. Achieving person-centered care through care coordination. Policy brief No. 8. Published December 2013. Accessed June 9, 2022. http://thescanfoundation. org/achieving-person-centered-care-through-care-coordination; and Institute of Medicine. Health professions education: a bridge to quality. Published 2003. Accessed June 9, 2022. https://www.ncbi.nlm.nih.gov/books/NBK221528/

key care management strategies and recommendations to help organize around appropriate interventions for individuals within a given population that may reduce health risks and decrease the cost of care.

Care management creates the necessary infrastructure to effectively manage the health of a population through the design of appropriate interventions to reduce overall health risks and reduce the cost of care.[43] The functions of care management are implemented by care or case managers, who typically are registered nurses or social workers. For certain chronic disease populations, such as persons with asthma or chronic obstructive pulmonary disease, the case manager may be a respiratory therapist. Interventions span the continuum of care, defined by the Commission for Case Management Certification within its CM Body of Knowledge as matching the "ongoing needs of the individuals being served by the case management process with the appropriate level and type of health, medical, financial, legal, and psychosocial care for services within a setting or across multiple settings."[44(¶3)]

*Case management* "is a term used to refer to management of acute and rehabilitative health care services. Services are delivered under a medical model, primarily by nurses."[45(p273)] Because the continuum of care crosses many healthcare settings, it is imperative for the case manager to engage with the patient across the entire continuum. The roles and functions of case managers are defined in the *Standards of Practice for Case Management*, and when applied to a population of patients, they provide for comprehensive care coordination across the care continuum, defining care coordination as "the deliberate organization of patient care activities between two or more participants (including the patient) involved in a patient's care to facilitate the appropriate delivery of health services."[46(p26)] It is through this care coordination that the case manager is able to engage with patients and their families and caregivers to ensure seamless transition from one level of care to the next, address gaps in care, effectuate necessary follow-up for an established care plan, and ensure the services needed for the patient are implemented. Ten key roles and functions for a case manager are the following:

1. Conducting comprehensive assessments of clients' health and psychosocial needs, including health literacy status and deficits.
2. Developing case management plans for care collaboratively with clients and families or caregivers.
3. Planning with clients, families and caregivers, primary care physicians or providers, other healthcare providers, payers, and communities to maximize healthcare response, quality, and cost-effective outcomes.
4. Facilitating communication and coordination among members of the healthcare team, involving clients in the decision-making process to minimize fragmentation in services and maximize efficiency and cost effectiveness.
5. Educating clients, families or caregivers, and members of healthcare delivery teams about treatment options, community resources, insurance benefits, psychosocial concerns, and case management services, enabling timely and informed decision making.
6. Empowering clients to problem solve by exploring care options, when available, and alternative plans, when necessary.
7. Encouraging the appropriate use of healthcare services and strive to improve quality of care and maintain cost effectiveness on a case-by-case basis.
8. Assisting clients in the safe transitioning of care to next most appropriate levels.
9. Striving to promote client self-advocacy, self-determination, and right to choose including refusal of care.
10. Advocating for clients and payers to facilitate positive outcomes for clients, healthcare teams, and payers; and prioritizing client needs in case of conflict.[45]

## Care Management Infrastructure

A strong care management infrastructure is essential to supporting patients throughout the continuum of care, with defined interventions, care planning, programs, and outcome measures. Often the terms *case manager* and *care manager* are used interchangeably. Titles usually depend on the practice. AHRQ provides the following distinction between case management and care management: "Unlike case management, which tends to be disease-centric and administered by health plans, [care management] is organized around the precept that appropriate interventions for individuals within a given population will reduce health risks and decrease the cost of care."[43(p1)] Refer to the *Glossary* for definitions related to care and case management.

According to the Case Management Society of America (CMSA) *Standards of Practice for Case Management*, "Case managers are recognized experts and vital participants in the care coordination team who empower people to understand and access quality, safe, and efficient health care services."[46(p4)] Case managers practice throughout the continuum of care in a variety of settings including, but not limited to population health, wellness and prevention programs, and disease and chronic care management companies; physician and medical group practices, patient centered medical home (PCMH), accountable care organizations (ACOs), and physician hospital organizations (PHOs); hospitals and integrated care delivery systems, including acute care, sub-acute care, long-term acute care (LTAC) facilities, skilled nursing facilities (SNFs), and rehabilitation facilities; private health insurance programs such as workers' compensation, occupational health, catastrophic and disability management, liability, casualty, automotive, accident and health, long-term care insurance, group health insurance, and managed care organizations; end-of-life, hospice, palliative, and respite care programs.[46(p14)]

Care management that spans the care continuum is a necessary vital function for success in population health and value-based reimbursement arrangements.

## Caring for the Population

The continuum of care includes ambulatory/community-based outpatient settings, acute care hospitalization, rehabilitative or skilled nursing home environments, patient homes with or without home care services, palliative care, and end of life. When a provider enters a value-based risk arrangement or an alternative payment model, it is imperative to create a care management infrastructure that ensures the population is cared for throughout the continuum of care, focusing on health, wellness, and chronic disease prevention. Understanding the characteristics of the population—specifically risk-stratifying the population to best understand patients who need care management intervention to mitigate that risk—is a core element for successful outcomes. Creation of standardized care pathways and protocols to ensure adherence to the most recent evidence-based guidelines reduces variability and provides cost-effective strategies for managing the population. Several examples follow.

### Health and Wellness

Understanding the health of a population is an essential component of population health management. The CDC framework for patient-centered risk assessments aims to do the following:

- Provide guidance to providers offering clinical preventive care, health promotion, and disease management services on ways to use health risk assessments (HRAs) and evidence-based health improvement programs.

- Reduce health disparities by using an HRA and follow-up interventions that are tailored to the person's particular needs (e.g., persons with disabilities).
- Improve health outcomes by identifying modifiable health risks and providing follow-up with patient-targeted behavior change interventions implemented over time.[47(p11)]

While the report focuses on Medicare beneficiaries, the findings can also be applied to non-Medicare populations. Private employers may offer HRAs to understand the types of services to offer employees as part of their benefit plan. The follow-up required after the HRA results are obtained often is coordinated by a care management team, collaborating with the patient's primary care provider, to create an individualized care plan with patient-centered goals. The Patient Protection and Affordable Care Act (P.L.111-148) included wellness programs in the form of grants and technical assistance to help evaluate employer-based wellness programs, and it allowed employers to offer a variety of rewards for participation in wellness programs.[48] Healthy People 2030 "sets data-driven national objectives to improve health and well-being over the next decade,"[49(p1)] including 355 core objectives. There are population-based objectives for a variety of populations. The objectives are also categorized by health conditions, health behaviors, settings, systems, and SDOH.[50] Healthy People 2030 provides evidence-based resources for each objective, as well as the status of each objective, making this a beneficial reference for providers who are managing populations of patients.

Focusing on wellness and disease prevention helps to improve overall health outcomes and appropriately reduce utilization. With certain limitations, CMS reimburses providers for an annual wellness visit that delivers personalized prevention plan services for Medicare beneficiaries who meet other defined criteria.[50] Creating an individualized prevention plan helps the care management team develop activities and interventions to work toward patient-specific health goals.

### Episodic Care

An *episode of care* is a set of services provided to care for an illness or injury during a defined period. There is no one logic for constructing an episode of care, and the structure is often constructed around episode-of-care payments (e.g., case rates, evidence-based case rates, condition-specific capitation, and episode-based bundled payments). Case managers are an integral part of the acute care team, focusing on patient flow and throughput, discharge planning, and the revenue cycle through utilization management activities. Ensuring seamless transitions for individuals and populations, mitigating the risk of readmission, and assisting in the development of the discharge plan begin with case management assessment and risk identification.

Patients in the acute care setting suffer from chronic health conditions such as heart failure, chronic obstructive pulmonary disease, and diabetes. The acute care case manager is responsible for identifying appropriate postacute care services to help the patient manage chronic illnesses. Care managers ensure successful care transitions by coordinating with a variety of postacute providers, including other care management professionals. Given the short length of time patients generally spend in the acute care setting, it is important for the acute care case manager to determine if the patient is a member of a CMS ACO, which enables the patient to have access to additional care management services upon discharge, or if the patient has some other population-based support team to assist with care coordination after discharge.

In 2019, the U.S. Department of Health & Human Services published the *Medicare and Medicaid Programs Revisions to Requirements for Discharge Planning for Hospitals, Critical Access Hospitals, and Health Agencies, and Hospital and Critical Access Hospital Changes to Promote Innovation, Flexibility, and Improvement in Patient Care* final rule.[51] It describes comprehensive revisions to discharge planning requirements. In the acute care setting, the case management professional is responsible for the execution of these requirements, which also consider the patient rights specific to discharge planning.

## Chronic Disease Management

Case managers coordinate care for patients with chronic health conditions such as, but not limited to, asthma, chronic obstructive pulmonary disease, diabetes, and heart failure. Case managers work in a variety of healthcare settings and typically care for patients with chronic health conditions in a population-based model. In a population-based model, case managers primarily focus on helping the patient prevent exacerbations of the chronic illness, seek care in the appropriate setting (primary care vs. emergency department), and educating patients and their families. CMS offers reimbursement for chronic care management for Medicare beneficiaries meeting the eligibility criteria.[52] The chronic care management program requires comprehensive care management, a comprehensive care plan, and care transition management—all within the scope of a case manager's responsibilities. **Table 7.6** illustrates key steps in the case management process.

**Table 7.6** Key Steps in the Case Management Process

| | Step | |
|---|---|---|
| 1. | Client identification and selection | Focuses on identifying clients who would benefit from case management services. This step may include obtaining consent for case management services, if appropriate. |
| 2. | Assessment and problem/opportunity identification | Begins after the completion of the case selection and intake into case management and occurs intermittently as needed throughout the case. |
| 3. | Development of the case management plan | Establishes goals of the intervention and prioritizes the needs of the client, support system, and/or family caregiver, as well. Determines the type of services and resources available to address the established goals or desired outcomes. |
| 4. | Implementation and coordination of care activities | Puts the case management plan into action. |
| 5. | Evaluation of the case management plan and follow-up | Involves the evaluation of the client's status and goals and the associated outcomes. |
| 6. | Termination of the case management process | Brings closure to the care and/or episode of treatment and/or episode of care. The process focuses on discontinuing case management when the client transitions to the highest level of functioning, the best possible outcome is attained, or the needs/desires of the client change. |

Reproduced from Tahan HM, Treiger TM, eds. *CMSA Core Curriculum for Case Management*. Philadelphia, PA: Wolters Kluwer; 2017:296.

In addition to caring for populations of patients with chronic health conditions, case managers provide the necessary care coordination to ensure optimal access to needed services and programs. This initiative demonstrates how leveraging a population health management program can improve overall health outcomes for patients with diabetes.

## Primary Care

The care manager plays a critical role in coordinating services for patients, including navigating the care continuum and practice in a variety of settings, including primary care. They serve targeted and high-risk populations such as persons with cancer, HIV/AIDS, developmental disabilities, high-risk pregnancy, and terminal conditions. Case management may also focus on other demographic characteristics such as age (e.g., geriatrics and pediatrics). The activities of the care manager in primary care are "assessing (and regularly reassessing) patients' care needs; developing, reinforcing, and monitoring care plans; providing education and encouraging self-management; communicating information across clinicians and settings; connecting patients to community resources and social services."[53(p82)] See **Table 7.7** for characteristics of practice facilitators and care managers, which puts primary care in the context of population health.

### AHA Workforce Center—Redesigned Primary Care Model

The care continuum is a central focus of the AHA Workforce Center that used guiding principles to elaborate on workforce roles in primary care and bedside care.[54] **Figure 7.12** summarizes the guiding principles.

These guiding principles encompass four broad categories:

**Table 7.7** Characteristics of Practice Facilitators and Care Managers

| Role | Core Functions | Connection to Practices and Patients | Educational Background |
|---|---|---|---|
| Practice facilitator | Help the practice organize, prioritize, and sequence QI activities | Facilitator is typically employed by an external organization (not the practice) | Social work, nursing, counseling, health management, business, and other areas |
| | Train practice staff to understand and use data to drive QI | Facilitator works with practice staff (not patients) | |
| | Increase practice capacity for QI activities | Facilitator typically works mostly on site at the practice with some interactions by phone, e-mail, or video conference; some facilitators work entirely virtually | |
| | Help build a team orientation among practice staff and a practice culture receptive to change | | |
| | Share best practices and lessons across practices | | |
| Care manager | Assess the patient's care needs | Care manager may be employed by the practice itself, a payer, or state. They are closely integrated into the practice team | Nursing, social work, counseling, and other areas |
| | Develop, reinforce, and monitor individualized care plan | | |
| | Provide patient education and training in self-management skills | Care manager provides services to patients and families | |
| | Coordinate patient's care with other providers and settings, and communicate needed information | Care manager (as we define) works at the practice, and may also interact with patients by telephone, e-mail, in the patient's home, or in other providers' offices | |
| | Connect patient to community resources and social services | | |
| | Participate in practice QI activities | | |

QI = quality improvement.
Reproduced from Taylor EF, Machta RM, Meyers DS, Genevro J, Peikes DN. Enhancing the primary care team to provide redesigned care: the roles of practice facilitators and care managers. *Ann Fam Med.* 2013:81. Accessed June 12, 2022. https://www.ahrq.gov/sites/default/files/wysiwyg/ncepcr/tools/PCMH/enhancing-primary-care-team.pdf

**Guiding Principles Set Forth in "Workforce Roles in a Redesigned Primary Care Model"**

1. In partnership with the patient, the primary healthcare team is guided by what is best, needed, and helpful to the patient and family.

2. The workforce must change how it functions on multiple levels. Care must be provided by interprofessional teams where work is role-based, not task-based, and the team must be empowered to create effective approaches for delivering care.

3. Hospitals can serve as conveners and enablers in primary care delivery. Primary care should be integrated into current and future care systems, and hospitals should form effective partnerships with the community and patients in a way that provides the infrastructure primary care teams need to deliver quality care.

**Guiding Principles Set Forth in "Reconfiguring the Bedside Care Team of the Future"**

1. The patient and family are essential members of the core care team.

2. Bedside care team members are fully engaged at the broadest scope of their practice.

3. The bedside care team is focused, highly effective, and autonomous, coordinating communication with the patient/family.

4. Evidence-based guidelines that improve care are developed and consistently followed by every bedside care team member.

5. Technology replaces some clinical tasks, augmenting decision-making and complementing the clinical judgment of the care team.

6. Patients needing acute care move safely through the healthcare system no matter where they are in the care cycle—whether at the onset of disease, in the middle of community-based care, or at the end of life.

**Figure 7.12** Guiding Principles of the Care Continuum

Reproduced from American Hospital Association. Connecting the dots along the care continuum. 2015:3. © Used with permission of American Hospital Association. Accessed June 12, 2022. https://www.aha.org/system/files/2018-01/15carecontinuum.pdf

1. Patient and family engagement
2. Team-based care
3. New/emerging healthcare models
4. Care coordination and transition management[54(p3)]

The guiding principle for *Care Coordination and Transition Management* states, "Patients needing acute care move safely through the health system no matter where they are in the care cycle—whether at the onset of disease, in the middle of community-based care, or at the end of life."[54(p11)] Five key takeaways related to this guiding principle are

1. training all team members about the value of care coordination;
2. building strong, trusting relationships with patients and families as active participants in addressing their needs so care can be better coordinated;
3. shifting provider mindset from delivering episodic care to practicing a whole person approach;
4. standardizing titles for care coordinators and their competencies will help patients and families better understand who can help when needed; and
5. advocating the value of each care provider for effective care coordination through strong executive leadership.[54(p12)]

## Patient-Centered Medical Home and Medical Neighborhood Concept

Care coordination is one of the five functions and attributes of the patient-centered medical home (PCMH), a model of the organization of primary care that includes comprehensive care, patient-centered care, coordinated care, accessible services, and quality and safety.[55] The medical neighborhood concept is a PCMH, "along with community and social service organizations and State and local public health agencies."[56(p5)] The PCMH serves as the central point of contact and provides the comprehensive care coordination across the care continuum, incorporating aspects of population health into its objectives. Care coordination is a vital component of this model with improved population health management as part of the outcome.[57] **Figure 7.13** represents the key actors and the flow of information in the medical neighborhood.[57]

CMS offers a primary care first (PCF) model through the CMS Innovation Center.[57] This voluntary model is an advanced primary care model, with an alternative payment structure—financial incentives are focused on improved health outcomes. There are two payment model options: general and high-need populations; the latter covers patients with serious illnesses who do not have a primary care physician

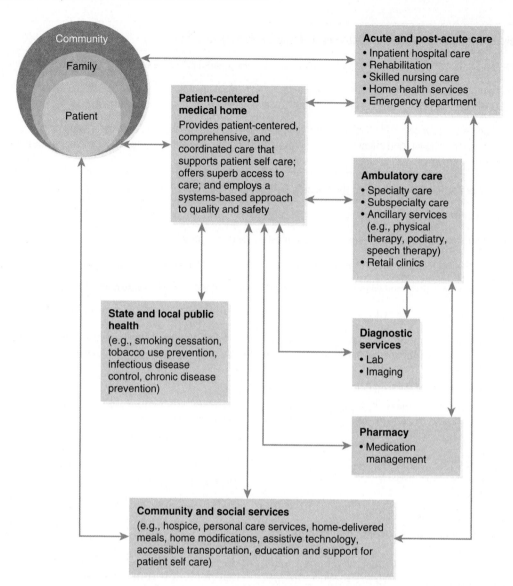

**Figure 7.13** Key Actors and the Flow of Information in the Medical Neighborhood

Reproduced from Taylor EF, Lake T, Nysenbaum J, Peterson G, Meyers D. Coordinating care in the medical neighborhood: critical components and available mechanisms. White paper. Agency for Healthcare Research and Quality; 2011. Accessed June 12, 2022. https://www.ahrq.gov/sites/default/files/wysiwyg/ncepcr/tools/PCMH/coordinating-care-in-the-medical-neighborhood-white-paper.pdf

or who lack effective care coordination.[58] There are currently two cohorts for this primary care model. Cohort 1 started January 2021 and cohort 2 started January 2022. Both include approximately 3000 participating practices and 24 payers. The primary care first model is focused on the following five primary care functions:

1. Access and continuity
2. Care management
3. Comprehensiveness and coordination
4. Patient and caregiver engagement
5. Planned care and population health[57(¶13)]

Primary care first "aims to improve quality, enhance patient experience of care, and reduce expenditures."[59(¶6)] Achievement of the minimum quality threshold for all five quality measures, as listed in **Table 7.8**, is a requirement in the primary care first model.

The role of case managers in primary care supports value-based care and population health management, providing the necessary comprehensive care coordination.

### Behavioral Health Integration

The National Council for Well-Being developed a comprehensive healthcare integration framework, guiding organizations in their integration of physical health (PH) and behavioral health (BH; mental health and substance use conditions). The council placed an

**Table 7.8** Quality Gateway Measures[a] for Practice Risk Groups 1 and 2

| Measure Title (Type) | NQF/Quality ID/ CMS ID | Measure Steward | Performance Years[d] | Benchmark Population | 30th Percentile Benchmark for 2022 |
|---|---|---|---|---|---|
| Diabetes: Hemoglobin A$_{1c}$ (HbA$_{1c}$) poor control (> 9%) (intermediate outcome eCQM) | Quality ID: 001 CMS ID: CMS122 | NCQA | 1–4 | MIPS | 69.42%[e] |
| Controlling high blood pressure (intermediate outcome eCQM) | Quality ID: 236 CMS ID: CMS165 | NCQA | 1–4 | MIPS | 57.08% |
| Colorectal cancer screening (process eCQM) | Quality ID: 113 CMS ID: CMS130 | NCQA | 1–4 | MIPS | 27.52% |
| ACP adapted for PCF (claims-based measure) | NQF ID: 0326[b] | NCQA | Cohort 1: 2–4 Cohort 2: 1–4 | CPC+ and non-CPC+ benchmark population | 3.85% |
| Patient experience of care survey (CAHPS with supplemental items) | NQF ID: 0005[c] | AHRQ | 1–4 | CPC+ and non-CPC+ benchmark population | 79.22% |

ACP = advance care plan; AHRQ = Agency for Healthcare Research and Quality; CAHPS = Consumer Assessment of Healthcare Providers and Systems; CPC+ = Comprehensive Primary Care Plus; eCQM = electronic clinical quality measure; MIPS = measure-based incentive payment system; NCQA = National Committee for Quality Assurance; NQF = National Quality Forum.

[a] The measures in the Quality Gateway are assessed for a given performance year, and the results are applied in the following year. For example, the Quality Gateway applied in Q2 through Q4 of the second performance year is based on performance during the first performance year.

[b] The ACP measure is adapted for use in the PCF model from the Bundled Payments for Care Improvement advanced ACP measure, which is a revised version of the NQF-endorsed ACP measure.

[c] The PCF Patient Experience of Care Survey includes a combination of items from the Clinician and Group CAHPS (NQF ID 0005) as well as from the PCMH CAHPS supplement.

[d] Performance years refers to the measurement periods of the measure. Each measure has a 1-year measurement period. The results of quality measures in the Quality Gateway are applied to the Quality Gateway in the following year.

[e] Diabetes: Hemoglobin A$_{1c}$ (HbA$_{1c}$) poor control (> 9%) is an inverse measure; lower performance scores reflect better quality.

Reproduced from Center for Medicare & Medicaid Innovation. Primary care first: payment and attribution methodologies PY 2022 version II. Published December 2021. Accessed June 14, 2022. https://innovation.cms.gov/media/document/pcf-py22-payment-meth-vol1

intentional emphasis on SDOH and equity in serving disenfranchised and underserved populations.[60] The authors propose the term *integratedness* as

> the degree to which programs or practices are organized to deliver integrated PH and BH prevention and treatment services to individuals or populations, as well as to address SDOH. Integratedness is a measure of development of both structural components (e.g., staffing) and care processes (e.g., screening) that support the extent to which "integrated services" in PH or BH settings are directly experienced by people served and delivered by service providers.[60(p8)]

## Skilled Nursing and Inpatient Rehabilitation Care

Medicare beneficiaries needing extended care services after an inpatient acute care admission may qualify for Medicare coverage in a skilled nursing facility (SNF) or an inpatient rehabilitation facility (IRF).[61] The admission requirements for these types of care settings are different. The acute care case manager or social worker is responsible for facilitating the transition from the acute care setting to the next level of care, including SNF and IRF, and must understand the regulatory and payer requirements for admission to each type of facility. Certain Medicare Shared Savings Programs and the Center for Medicare and Medicaid Innovation models offer waivers to the admission requirements for an SNF. CMS also offered a temporary waiver during the COVID-19 public health emergency, allowing coverage for an SNF admission without a qualifying inpatient hospital admission.[62] The care management team responsible for the population of Medicare beneficiaries participating in the Shared Savings Program tracks or the CMS Innovation Center models should collaborate with the acute care case manager and social worker and the SNF admission team to ensure the SNF waiver requirements are fully understood and met prior to beneficiary admission to the SNF.

To qualify for coverage under Medicare for admission to an SNF, the Medicare beneficiary must meet the CMS 3-day rule, which requires the beneficiary to have a "3-day-consecutive inpatient hospital stay," unless the beneficiary is eligible for one of the SNF 3-day waivers.[62(p3)] The rule does not count the day of discharge or any time prior to the admission, such as the emergency room or as an outpatient. The inpatient hospital admission must be medically necessary, and the beneficiary must need an SNF level of care.[62] CMS requires hospitals to deliver the *Important Message from Medicare (IM)* to Medicare beneficiaries who are admitted to the hospital as an inpatient.[63] This IM notice provides the Medicare beneficiary with important information about their hospital discharge appeal rights.[63] The care management team member facilitating the transition of the Medicare beneficiary from an acute inpatient admission to the next level of care should take the necessary steps to ensure the IM is delivered to the beneficiary in accordance with CMS requirements. **Figure 7.14** shows the relationship between the inpatient admission, SNF, and the patient discharge appeal rights.[64]

Medicare includes benefit coverage for care in an IRF.

The Medicare IRF benefit provides intensive rehabilitation therapy in a resource-intense inpatient hospital environment, including inpatient rehabilitation hospitals and inpatient rehabilitation units. The IRF benefit is for a patient who, due to the complexity of their nursing, medical management, and rehabilitation needs, requires and expects to benefit from an inpatient stay and an interdisciplinary team approach to rehabilitation care.[62(¶5)]

Admission to an IRF for Medicare beneficiaries does not require a 3-day inpatient admission in an acute care setting as a condition of coverage. The care management team responsible for a population of patients participating in the Medicare Shared Savings Program tracks or in one of the Medicare and Medicaid Innovation Models should understand the requirements for coverage for skilled care in an SNF and in the more intensive IRF environment. The care team works collaboratively to understand the most appropriate rehabilitation setting for the patient. Other payers may or may not have the same coverage requirements as Medicare for skilled care in an SNF or intensive inpatient rehabilitation in the IRF. Therefore, the care manager should understand the specific payer requirements when facilitating transitions across the continuum of care.

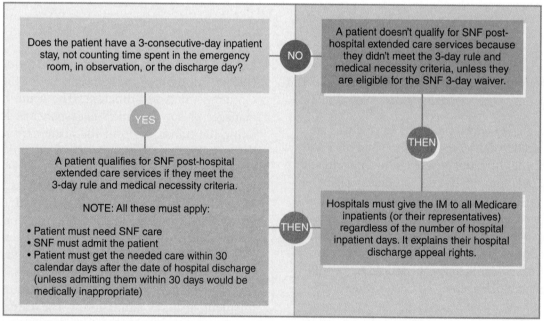

Note: IM = Important Message from Medicare

**Figure 7.14** Relationship Between the Inpatient Admission, SNF, and Patient Discharge Appeal Rights

Reproduced from Centers for Medicare & Medicaid Services. Medicare learning network fact sheet (9730256): skilled nursing facility 3-day rule billing. Published 2022. Accessed June 12, 2022. https://www.cms.gov/Outreach-and-Education/Medicare-Learning-Network-MLN/MLNProducts/Downloads/SNF3DayRule-MLN9730256.pdf#:~:text=To%20qualify%20for%20Skilled%20Nursing%20Facility%20%28SNF%29%20extended,time%20spent%20in%20the%20ER%20or%20outpatient%20observation.?msclkid=9d00662bd0ca11ecbe495039b2cf7880

# Home Healthcare

The patient's home is part of the care continuum, and the hospital-based case manager has a role in assessing the patient's postdischarge needs and working with the patient, family, and care team to arrange for the appropriate community-based services.[65] Patients who may benefit from home healthcare include, but are not limited to, those with chronic health conditions, frail elderly, those with limited cognitive or functional status, patients with debilitating and/or complex illnesses, and patients recovering from stroke or certain types of surgeries.[65]

The AARP Home and Community Preferences Survey found that "77 percent of adults aged 50 and older want to remain in their homes for the long term."[66] This desire to remain in the home provides the case management team with the opportunity to assess patients for needs and set up services for the patient to receive care in their home, including home healthcare. The case manager can facilitate discussions with the care team and family to determine whether the patient or family would accept home healthcare, helping the patient and family to understand the value of home healthcare.

CMS has certain criteria the patient must meet to qualify for home healthcare.[67] Other payers have specific criteria for member home healthcare coverage that may differ from Medicare. The case manager can collaborate with the patient, family, and care team to ensure the payer requirements are understood for home healthcare. That includes confirmation that the prior authorization for the ordered services is obtained.

**Box 7.4** lists key points in care management infrastructure.

---

### Box 7.4 Key Points: Care Management Infrastructure

- Comprehensive care management is necessary for managing populations in value-based reimbursement models.
- Care managers span the continuum of care, collaborating with other healthcare professionals to address patient and family needs.
- Better population management of primary care for older adults with chronic illnesses includes coordination and communication among all the professionals engaged in a patient's care, especially during transitions from the hospital.
- The healthcare quality professional can support population-based care management through a structured care management program and design of standardized workflows, which reduce variability during care transitions and handoffs.

---

# Managing Care Transitions

Transitions of care refers to the movement of patients—between healthcare locations, providers, or levels of care as their conditions and care needs change—and the set of actions designed to ensure coordination and continuity. In any one particular care transition, a variety of factors can make it more difficult for acute, postacute, and ambulatory care providers, as well as payers, to collaborate, coordinate care, and exchange critical information about patients.[68]

Why are transitions of care a population health challenge? More importantly, why are they so important to quality healthcare?

> There is emerging evidence in the healthcare literature that demonstrates the existence of serious quality problems for patients undergoing transitions across multiple sites of care, especially upon discharge from acute care settings to home or other skilled care facilities. Specifically, the current literature describes high rates of readmissions and ED visits as consequences of ineffective care transitions as patients are moving from the acute care environment to discharge to home or community-based care.[69(p1)]

Further, the authors point to evidence of ineffective care transitions in high rates of rehospitalizations and subsequent emergency department visits as patients move from acute care to home or community-based care.[69]

## Case Management

According to the CMSA *Standards of Practice for Case Management,*

> Case Management is a collaborative process of assessment, planning, facilitation, care coordination, evaluation, and advocacy for options and services to meet an individual's and family's comprehensive health needs through communication and available resources to promote patient safety, quality of care, and cost-effective outcomes.[70(p11)]

Transitions of care is included in the many case management roles and responsibilities described within the standards, including the following:

- Collaborating with other healthcare professionals and support service providers across care settings, levels of care, and professional disciplines, with special attention to safe transitions of care.

- Assisting the client in the safe transitioning of care to the next, most appropriate level, setting, and/or provider.[70]

ACMA provides the following definition of case management:

> Case Management in health care delivery systems is a collaborative practice including patients, caregivers, nurses, social workers, physicians, payers, support staff, other practitioners, and the community. The Case Management process facilitates communication and care coordination along a continuum through effective transitional care management. Recognizing the patient's right to self-determination, the significance of the SDOH and the complexities of care, the goals of case management include the achievement of optimal health, access to services, and appropriate utilization of resources.[71(¶3)]

Transitions of care is a central focus of the case manager's role. The case manager is a vital healthcare professional with an expertise in ensuring smooth transitions of care through the coordination of care and services, leveraging a variety of policies, processes, workflows, and assessments, to create the transitional care plan individualized to the patient's needs. Case manager responsibilities may vary by type of organization. As examples, sample responsibilities for PCMH case managers are shown in **Table 7.9**.

## Case Management Models

Case management models that span the continuum of care include acute care hospitals where, according to Zander, there should ideally be a "social worker and RN case manager during all of the prime times when patients enter EDs."[65(p7)] Zander also describes four drivers for building case management across the continuum, including ACOs and value-based purchasing.[65]

### Standardizing Handoffs

Skaret and colleagues describe how "transitions of care have been identified as one of the most dangerous events in a patient's hospitalization,"[72(p274)] citing a review of data from the Centers for Disease Control and Prevention and other medical literature ranking medical errors as the third leading cause of death in the United States.[72] The I-PASS mnemonic (illness severity, patient summary, action list, situation awareness and synthesis by receiver) is a handoff improvement program shown to decrease medical errors and preventable adverse events involving nine tertiary pediatric residency programs.[72] Through the use of technology, Skaret and colleagues created a partially automated, electronic handoff tool that generated a "printable handoff document that includes both automated data and user-generated I-PASS information for each patient on a given inpatient team."[72(p274)] Using the partially automated I-PASS tool demonstrated "a significant reduction in inaccurate data communicated during transitions of care."[72(pp276-277)] This and other tools can be used with special populations such as behavioral health and pediatrics.

---

**Table 7.9** Responsibilities of PCMH Case Managers

- Using clinical decision-support tools, evidence-based care, shared decision making in assessment, treatment planning, and care transitions
- Collaborating with the treatment team (e.g., physicians, advanced practice nurses, physician assistants, nurses, pharmacists, nutritionists, social workers, educators, and care coordinators)
- Understanding and respecting each patient's unique needs, culture, values, and preferences
- Engaging patients/families/support system in decision making about care options
- Coordination of care and services
- Facilitation of patient's timely access to services
- Health education and self-care management
- Monitoring patient conditions and adherence to care regimens
- Following up on tests and procedures
- Consultation with specialty providers
- Facilitating interprofessional care rounds and daily huddles for care planning
- Coordinating transition of care activities
- Engagement and reengagement for appointments
- Responding to patient experiences and patient satisfaction

Data from Tahan HM, Treiger TM, eds. *CMSA Core Curriculum for Case Management*. Philadelphia, PA: Wolters Kluwer; 2017:78.

## Discharge Assessment at Home

Discharge to Assess (D2A), also known as a "flipped" discharge, is an initiative of the Sheffield Teaching Hospitals in the United Kingdom. It focuses on assessing a patient's after-discharge needs in the patient's home, instead of the hospital.[73] This initiative initially started with a focus on the frail elderly population, and it shows reduced length of stay and the safe and timely discharge of patients with complex needs. There has been no increase in readmissions, while at the same time the program has shown decreased costs and increased patient, family, and employee satisfaction.[74]

The D2A results spanned five teaching hospitals with 1920 beds, 16,000 staff, serving a population of 560,000 people.[74] When the discharge assessment occurs in the hospital, it is possible for the discharge to be delayed while that assessment is completed and needed services are coordinated. In the D2A model, patients who are medically cleared are discharged to home, where a team meets them within 2 hours to complete the discharge assessment and ensure needed services are provided.

The two populations of patients served in this model are (1) frail elderly patients, including those with dementia, and (2) other patients exhibiting similar characteristics, such as elderly patients who have had orthopedic surgery and nonelderly patients with dementia.[73] **Figure 7.15** shows the high-level flowchart of the D2A process.

The D2A process has improved and successfully expanded from the frail elderly population to other patient populations. D2A could be useful for care redesign in U.S. healthcare systems such as ACOs and systems seeking to reduce hospital readmissions.[73] Although the setting used in this study was the frail elderly, D2A can also be applied to other subspecialties such as behavioral health and pediatrics. A key measure used to assess the effectiveness of D2A is weekly average wait times for patients between hospital referral and being at home with community-based support services. The following decreases were noted in one study:

- Average wait time decreased from 5.5 days to 3.6 days because of better collaboration between the health and social care teams.
- Average time to transfer a patient from the hospital to active recovery decreased from 5.2 days to 1.2 days.
- Average length of stay declined by more than 4 days following the implementation of the frailty unit in the geriatric medicine department with no increase in readmissions.[73(p10)]

## CMS Acute Hospital Care at Home Program

In 2020, CMS announced an expansion of the Hospital Without Walls program to the Acute Hospital Care at Home program, enabling eligible hospitals to treat patients in their homes through unprecedented regulatory flexibilities. This program, available through a waiver request, requires acute care hospitals to be approved for the Acute Hospital Care at Home waiver.[75] In its announcement of the program, CMS said:

> CMS anticipates patients may value the ability to spend time with family and caregivers at home without the visitation restrictions that exist in traditional hospital settings. It is the patient's choice to receive these services in the home or the traditional hospital setting, and patients who do not wish to receive them in the home will not be required to participate.[75(¶6)]

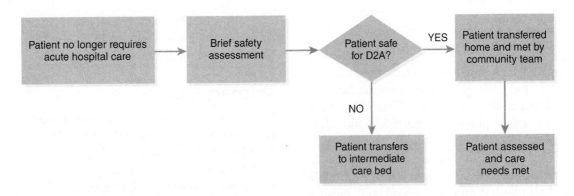

**Figure 7.15** High-Level Flowchart of Discharge to Assess (D2A) Process

CMS accepted requests to waive §482.23(b) and (b)(1) of the Hospital Conditions of Participation, which require nursing services on premises 24 hours a day, 7 days a week, with the immediate availability of a registered nurse for care of any patient.[76] Waiver requests were divided into two categories based on a hospital's prior experience. Hospitals had to submit the waiver request for an entity-specific CMS certification number, not entire systems. For those hospitals that had provided at-home acute hospital services to at least 25 patients previously, an expedited process was conducted that included hospital attestation to specific existing beneficiary protections and reporting requirements. The immediate goal with this group was to allow experienced hospitals to rapidly expand care to Medicare beneficiaries. These hospitals are required to submit monitoring data monthly.[76]

For those hospitals that have treated fewer than 25 patients or have never provided at-home acute hospital services, a more detailed waiver request was required. The request emphasizes internal processes that prove their capability of treating acute hospital at-home patients with the same level of care as traditional inpatients. This group consists of hospitals that are part of a larger, experienced health system, as well as those hospitals without any prior experience that are not part of a larger health system. These hospitals are required to submit monitoring data on a weekly basis.[76] Under this CMS waiver, because the patient is receiving an acute inpatient level of care in their home, the discharge care transition occurs in the patient's home, like the D2A model. In a systematic review by Arsenault-Lapierre and colleagues, persons receiving home care had lower risks for readmission, lower risk for long-term care admissions, and lower scores for depression and anxiety. Home care offers a promising substitute for inpatient hospital stays.[77]

### Readmission Risk Mitigation

According to IHI, "a substantial fraction of all hospitalizations are patients returning to the hospital soon after their previous stay. These rehospitalizations are costly, potentially harmful, and often avoidable."[78(¶1)] To address this challenge, IHI initiated the STate Action on Avoidable Rehospitalizations (STAAR) initiative in May 2009, ending in 2013. STAAR focused on two primary strategies for reducing rehospitalization:

1. Improve transitions of care by cultivating a cross-continuum learning collaborative.

2. Engage state-level leadership to understand and mitigate systemic barriers to change.[79]

As part of the STAAR initiative, IHI created a series of guides to improve transitions of care from the hospital to a variety of care settings. These guides recommended that organizations focus on:

- *Infrastructure and strategy to achieve results.* A review of the necessary leadership support and fundamental improvement methods and resources for testing changes before they are implemented and spread more widely throughout the organization.
- *Measures, resources, and references.* A recommended system of measures to guide improvement, worksheets, and other tools to help hospital teams implement the changes, and a bibliography of selected resources.

Key changes suggested for improving care transitions from hospital to community setting (home health, SNF, clinic office) are summarized in **Table 7.10**.

Mitigating readmission risk is a critical component of care transitions, and it requires the care team to identify and address risk factors that may cause a patient to be readmitted to the hospital. Regarding readmissions, the organization must differentiate between all cause (e.g., a patient discharged after a myocardial infarction and readmitted for a broken leg within 30 days) and risk-adjusted (a patient discharged after a myocardial infarction and readmitted for chest pain or arrhythmias within 30 days) readmissions. **Box 7.5** lists key points in managing care transitions.

# Population Health and Care Transitions in Practice

The following offer examples of leveraging population health and care transition experience competencies to drive improvements in processes and outcomes.

## Primary Care

Burroughs and Smith describe a new model of primary care, which leverages population health to shape the structure of the model. In 1978, the Southeast Georgia Diagnostic and Prevention Center was founded in Vidalia, Georgia. It has grown from a privately owned practice to a regional practice serving payers and employers as far as Nashville, Tennessee. Clients were willing to travel hours for the high-quality, low-cost care offered.[80] The practice consists of general

**Table 7.10** Improving Care Transitions from the Hospital to Community Settings

| Setting | Key Recommendations |
|---|---|
| Hospital to community | Four key recommendations for improving the transition out of the hospital, including typical failures encountered and tools and resources to help teams implement the changes:<br>1. Partner with patient and family to identify posthospital needs.<br>2. Provide teaching and facilitate learning.<br>3. Create and employ posthospital follow-up.<br>4. Provide real-time hand-over. |
| Hospital to home health | Three key recommendations for improving the transition out of the hospital, including typical failures encountered and tools and resources to help teams implement the changes:<br>1. Meet with patient, family, and inpatient caregivers in hospital to review transition plan.<br>2. Assess patient, initiate care plan, and reinforce self-management at postdischarge home visit.<br>3. Engage, coordinate, and communicate with the team. |
| Hospital to skilled nursing facility | Three key recommendations for improving the transition into the SNF from the hospital, including typical failures encountered and tools and resources to help teams implement the changes.<br>1. Ensure SNF staff are ready to and capable of providing care.<br>2. Reconcile the treatment plan and plan for condition changes.<br>3. Engage residents and family caregivers in partnership to create a plan of care. |
| Hospital to clinical office practice | Four recommendations for improving the transition for the patient from the hospital to the clinical office practice setting, including typical failures encountered and tools and resources to help teams implement the changes.<br>1. Provide access to care in a timely way.<br>2. Prepare the patient and clinical team prior to the visit.<br>3. Assess the patient and create a new or revised existing care plan.<br>4. Communicate an ongoing care plan. |

Data from Herndon L, Bones C, Bradke P, Rutherford P. *How-to Guide: Improving Transitions from the Hospital to Skilled Nursing Facilities to Reduce Avoidable Rehospitalizations*. Cambridge, MA: Institute for Healthcare Improvement; June 2013:2. Accessed June 8, 2022. http://www.ihi.org/resources/Pages/Tools/HowtoGuideImprovingTransitionHospitalSNFstoReduceRehospitalizations.aspx; Institute for Healthcare Improvement. Tools: how-to guide: improving transitions from the hospital to community settings to reduce avoidable rehospitalizations; 3. Accessed May 22, 2022. http://www.ihi.org/resources/Pages/Tools/HowtoGuideImprovingTransitionstoReduceAvoidableRehospitalizations.aspx; Sevin C, Evdokimoff M, Sobolewski S, Taylor J, Rutherford P, Coleman EA. *How-to Guide: Improving Transitions from the Hospital to Home Health Care to Reduce Avoidable Rehospitalizations*. Cambridge, MA: Institute for Healthcare Improvement; June 2013:2. Accessed June 8, 2022. http://www.ihi.org/resources/Pages/Tools/HowtoGuideImprovingTransitionsfromHospitaltoHomeHealthCareReduceAvoidableHospitalizations.aspx; and Schall M, Coleman E, Rutherford P, Taylor J. *How-to Guide: Improving Transitions from the Hospital to the Clinical Office Practice to Reduce Avoidable Rehospitalizations*. Cambridge, MA: Institute for Healthcare Improvement; June 2013:3. Accessed June 8, 2022. http://www.ihi.org/resources/Pages/Tools/HowtoGuideImprovingTransitionsHospitaltoOfficePracticeReduceRehospitalizations.aspx

---

**Box 7.5  Key Points: Managing Care Transitions**

- Essential functions of the care management team include managing care transitions and mitigating the risk of return to higher levels of care or readmission.
- The population-based care management team can form collaborative relationships with healthcare professionals across the continuum of care to ensure smooth care transitions for patients.
- Healthcare quality professionals can support care transitions by designing processes to ensure that transition of care quality measures are appropriately monitored and addressed.

internists, physician assistants, registered nurses, licensed practical nurses, a certified coder, support personnel, nutritionists, laboratory technologists, care coordinators, a data analyst, and an information technology specialist. The practice focuses on the right person doing the right job; documentation and coding at the point of care; risk and severity adjustments; and continuous monitoring of quality and cost data to drive performance.

The success of the Southeast Georgia Diagnostic and Prevention Center demonstrates how care providers, health systems, and healthcare entities participating in population health management, risk arrangements, value-based care programs, alternative payment models, and/or ACOs need a comprehensive care management infrastructure to care for the population across the care continuum. This comprehensive infrastructure drives successful health outcomes and reduces the overall cost of care.

## Screening

Quality leaders, physicians, and a senior Lean Six Sigma specialist demonstrate how to integrate population health management strategies into quality through their work in improving diabetic retinopathy screening in their institution's endocrinology clinic. This improvement work was conducted at the Southwestern Health Resources and Southwestern Medical Center in Dallas, Texas. These ambulatory clinics are part of a large ACO with performance goals tied to quality measures.[81] An eye examination and poor control of $HbA_{1c}$ were part of the 2018 Medicare Shared Savings Program composite quality measure for diabetes. Leveraging the define, measure, analyze, improve, and control process improvement methodology, the population health services company for the institution embarked on an initiative to improve retinopathy screening rates for the patient population cared for in the endocrinology clinic. Through a variety of interventions, care gaps can be identified using a population registry, patient outreach via an electronic medical record patient portal, referrals to specialty services, and health maintenance documentation; and by tracking improvement for sustainability.

## Transition Coaching

Balaban and colleagues utilized a social worker transition coach model to improve transitions of care from hospital to home. The program targeted a population of high-risk younger adults who demonstrated a high incidence of comorbid mental health and substance abuse disorders.[82] The work, a collaborative effort of physicians and researchers at Cambridge Health Alliance in Cambridge, Massachusetts, the Department of Population Medicine at Harvard Medical School in Boston, Massachusetts, and the Harvard Pilgrim Health Care Institute in Wellesley, Massachusetts, demonstrated how a social worker–led transitional care program led to reducing the 90-day readmission rate in a nonelderly, high-risk, lower socioeconomic status patient population. The social workers focused on addressing both the medical and personal needs of this low-income population, who might face unstable housing, social isolation, limited education, depression, and substance use.

## Hotspotting

Programs aiming to reduce spending and improve healthcare quality among superutilizers or familiar faces interest healthcare organizations and systems of care. Patients with high use of healthcare services prompted the hotspotting program that was created by the Camden Coalition of Healthcare Providers.[83] The general premise is that in the months after hospital discharge, a team of nurses, social workers, and community health workers visits enrolled patients to coordinate outpatient care and link them with social services.

The coalition looked at 800 hospitalized patients with medically and socially complex conditions and compared the Camden core model with usual care. The model is a care transition program designed to improve patient health and reduce hospital use among vulnerable adults. In looking at the primary outcome measure of hospital readmission within 180 days after discharge, there were not significant findings when comparing the two groups. However, there were takeaways relevant to program development and practices when providing care for persons with complex needs, and program developers suggest that there are challenges for superutilizer programs aimed at medically and socially complex populations. There are mixed results for the effectiveness of care management programs for chronically ill populations. It is suggested that care management approaches connecting patients with existing resources may be insufficient for superutilizers and familiar faces.

## Healthcare Efficiency

Achieving the Triple Aim or the Quadruple Aim is embedded into organizational strategies for quality and safety. In using either aim for improvement, there can be friction between implementing interventions to improve population health when faced with the imperative of increasing productivity.[84] In a 2020 study, an efficiency-focused flow intervention to energize care teams was developed and used in a family practice clinic. The intervention targeted efficiency for quality improvement within the Quadruple Aim framework. The study goals were to increase visit capacity by 50% and complete all administrative and electronic health record activities within an 8-hour workday. Measures were established for each aim.

- *Aim 1: Reducing costs.* Focus on improved efficiency and access to care using clinic outputs, visit capacity, and visits completed.
- *Aim 2: Population health.* Screening for HIV was used as a proxy for population health since the largest gap in care was observed here when considering guidelines.

- *Aim 3: Healthcare team well-being.* A 14-question survey adapted from the Quality Work Competence survey was administered one day pre-intervention, during the intervention, and post-intervention to assess the healthcare team experience (professional fulfilment, skills utilization, stress).
- *Aim 4: Patient experience.* Patients completed a 16-question paper survey at checkout to rate their doctor and whether they would recommend the clinic to others.[84(pp2-3)]

The intervention was associated with improvement in the four aims and productivity. Efficiency significantly correlated with better patient and team experiences. An unintended benefit was positive outcomes associated with HIV screenings. The team also closed or decreased other gaps in care such as immunizations and diabetes mellitus management. While the sample size was small, there appeared to be benefits related to organizing the improvement project around the Quadruple Aim.

See **Box 7.6** for a list of key points in population and care transitions in practice.

---

**Box 7.6  Key Points: Population and Care Transitions in Practice**

- A comprehensive care management infrastructure drives successful health outcomes and reduces the overall cost of care.
- There are challenges with superutilizer programs aimed at medically and socially complex populations that should be considered in program development.
- Through a variety of interventions, care gaps can be identified using a population registry, patient outreach via electronic medical record patient portal, referrals to specialty services, and health maintenance documentation; and by tracking improvement for sustainability.
- While striving to achieve the Triple Aim or Quadruple Aim as part of an organization's improvement strategy, there can be friction between implementing interventions to improve population health when balancing with productivity.

---

## Summary

The healthcare quality professional offers expertise and the unique complement of knowledge and essential competencies when caring for populations of people across the continuum of care while achieving improved health outcomes at lower costs. This can be accomplished by the following:

- Developing and implementing population health policies, programs, and services that align with organizational strategic goals and community needs as well as integrating with the strategic plan, goals, and objectives.
- Supporting organizations in adopting population health approaches and the shift from volume- to value-based care. For example, CMS requires ACOs to demonstrate success in delivering both high-quality care and achievement of cost savings to be eligible for sharing in any savings.[85]
- Driving performance and helping organizations successfully achieve critical performance standards in value-based reimbursement arrangements and alternative payment models to reduce exposure to the negative fiscal impact in downside risk arrangements.
- Exchanging data and information between stakeholder organizations to integrate into improvement initiatives for community and public health initiatives (e.g., SDOH such as housing, employment, food security), continuum of clinical care considerations (e.g., preventive care, acute care, and chronic disease management), and targeted populations with special needs (e.g., veterans, adolescents, and older adults).
- Integrating population health and care management analytic tools/enablers into electronic health records, registries, telemedicine, and analytic tools for providers, organizations, health systems, and community partnerships to better predict and manage illnesses and diseases.
- Developing the expertise to conduct the complex work required to transform quality and safety (e.g., population health management strategies integrated with a quality, holistic approach applied to improvement and collaboration to improve care transitions).[86]

Healthcare quality professionals help leadership develop and maintain a solid infrastructure to support patient engagement and positive clinical outcomes. Through the accurate assessment and understanding of the role of social determinants of health and adoption of population health management principles, organizations can be strengthened in their approaches to the delivery of comprehensive and high-quality care. The results are better care, smarter spending, healthier people, and joy in work where no person is disadvantaged, and individuals and communities achieve health equity.

# References

1. Coburn D, Denny K, Mykhalovskiy E, McDonough P, Robertson A, Love R. Population health in Canada: a brief critique. *Am J Public Health.* 2003;93(3):392-396. doi:10.2105/ajph.93.3.392

2. Kindig D, Stoddart G. What is population health? *Am J Public Health.* 2003;93(3):380-383. doi:10.2105/ajph.93.3.380

3. Lewis N. Populations, population health, and the evolution of population management: making sense of the terminology in US health care today. Published 2014. Accessed May 24, 2017. http://www.ihi.org/communities/blogs/_layouts/15/ihi/community/blog/itemview.aspx?List=81ca4a47-4ccd-4e9e-89d9-14d88ec59e8d&ID=50

4. Centers for Medicare & Medicaid Services. National Health Expenditure data: historical. Published December 15, 2021. Accessed July 21, 2022. https://www.cms.gov/Research-Statistics-Data-and-Systems/Statistics-Trends-and-Reports/NationalHealthExpendData/NationalHealthAccountsHistorical

5. Boult C, Wieland GD. Comprehensive primary care for older patients with multiple chronic conditions. *JAMA.* 2010;304(17):1936-1943.

6. Winslow CEA. The untilled fields of public health. *Science.* 1920;51(1306):23-33.

7. Kindig DA. *Improving population health blog collections 1-4.* University of Wisconsin Population Health Institute. Published 2014. Available at https://www.improvingpopulationhealth.org/

8. Ahmed Z, Mohamed K, Zeeshan S, Dong X. Artificial intelligence with multi-functional machine learning platform development for better healthcare and precision medicine. *Database.* 2020:baaa010. doi:10.1093/database/baaa010

9. Bodenheimer T, Syer S, Fair M, Shipman S. Teaching residents population health management. Association of American Medical Colleges. Published November 2019. Accessed April 5, 2022. https://store.aamc.org/downloadable/download/sample/sample_id/311/

10. National Committee for Quality Assurance. Population health management: Resource guide. Published 2018. Accessed March 9, 2022. https://www.ncqa.org/programs/health-plans/population-health-management-resource-guide/

11. Artiga S, Hinton E. Beyond health care: the role of social determinants in promoting health and health equity. Kaiser Family Foundation. Published May 10, 2018. Accessed March 10, 2022. https://www.kff.org/racial-equity-and-health-policy/issue-brief/beyond-health-care-the-role-of-social-determinants-in-promoting-health-and-health-equity/

12. National Committee for Quality Assurance in Collaboration with Health Management Associates. Population health management: meeting the demand for value-based care. NCQA. Accessed March 31, 2022. https://www.ncqa.org/wp-content/uploads/2021/02/20210202_PHM_White_Paper.pdf

13. U.S. Department of Health & Human Services. Health equity in Healthy People 2030. Accessed April 2, 2022. https://health.gov/healthypeople/priority-areas/health-equity-healthy-people-2030

14. Manrai AK, Patel CJ, Ioannidis JPA. In the era of precision medicine and big data, who is normal? *JAMA.* 2018;319(19):1981-1982. doi:10.1001/jama.2018.2009

15. Friedman DJ, Starfield B. Models of population health: their value for US public health practice, policy, and research. *Am J Public Health.* 2003;93(3):366-369. doi.org/10.2105/AJPH.93.3.366

16. Van Dyke M. In the literature: highlights from commonwealth fund supported studies in professional literature. The Commonwealth Fund. Published August 23, 2016. Accessed April 2, 2022. https://www.commonwealthfund.org/sites/default/files/documents/___media_files_publications_in_the_literature_2016_aug_1896_hibbard_improving_population_hlt_mgmt_hsr_08_23_2016_itl_v2.pdf

17. National Committee for Quality Assurance in Collaboration with Health Management Associates. Population health management: meeting the demand for value-based care. NCQA. Accessed March 31, 2022. https://www.ncqa.org/wp-content/uploads/2021/02/20210202_PHM_White_Paper.pdf

18. Wilson ML. Understanding the technology that supports population health programs. *Amer Nurse Today.* 2017;12(10):28-31.

19. American Hospital Association Center for Health Innovation. AHA population health framework. Accessed April 4, 2022. https://www.aha.org/center/population-health-fundamentals

20. Centers for Medicare & Medicaid Services. Population health measures: supplemental material to the CMS MMS blueprint. Published September 2021. Accessed April 4, 2022. https://www.cms.gov/files/document/blueprint-population-health-measures.pdf

21. National Association of Community Health Centers. Population health management: quality improvement/performance measurement. Published August 2016. Accessed April 5, 2022. https://www.nachc.org/wp-content/uploads/2015/12/NACHC_QI_factsheet_FINAL.pdf

22. Institute for Healthcare Improvement. Guide for undertaking a 3-part data review. Published 2020. Accessed April 4, 2022. http://www.ihi.org/Topics/Population-Health/Documents/IHI_PopulationHealth_GuideforUndertaking3PartDataReview.pdf

23. National Committee for Quality Assurance. Population health management road map for integrated delivery networks. Published November 21, 2019. Accessed March 22, 2022. https://www.ncqa.org/white-papers/population-health-management-roadmap/

24. Hospitals in Pursuit of Excellence. What is population health? American Hospital Association. Published 2014. Accessed March 3, 2022. www.hpoe.org/Reports-HPOE/Population-Health-Definition.pdf

25. Hilts KE, Yeager VA, Gibson PJ, Halverson PK, Blackburn J, Menachemi N. Hospital partnerships for population health: a systematic review of the literature. *J Healthc Manag.* 2021;66(3):170-198. doi:10.1097/jhm-d-20-00172

26. Care Continuum Alliance. Our mission. Accessed May 23, 2022. http://www.carecontinuum.org/about_our_mission.asp

27. Care Continuum Alliance. Advancing the population health improvement model. Accessed April 4, 2022. http://www.carecontinuum.org/Quality/phi_definition.asp#:~:text=The%20Care%20Continuum%20Alliance%20%28CCA%29%20promotes%20a%20proactive%2C,to%20address%20both%20illness%20and%20long%20term%20health

28. Centers for Disease Control and Prevention. CDC's 6|18 Initiative: accelerating evidence into action. Published July 2018. Accessed March 28, 2022. https://www.cdc.gov/sixeighteen/docs/6-18-factsheet.pdf

29. Pathways to population health [poster]. Accessed April 4, 2022. https://www.aha.org/system/files/media/file/2019/04/Poster_PathwaystoPopulationHealth.pdf

30. Saha S, Loehrer S, Cleary-Fishman M, et al.; American Hospital Association. Pathways to population health: an invitation to healthcare change agents. Published 2017. Accessed May 25, 2022. https://www.aha.org/system/files/media/file/2020/09/Pathways-to-Population-Health-Framework.pdf#:~:text=%E2%80%9CPathways%20to%20Population%20Health%3A%20An%20Invitation%20to%20Health,well-being%20of%20the%20patients%20and%20communities%20they%20serve

31. Allen PM, Finnerty MJ, Gish RS, et al. Guide to health care partnerships for population health management and value-based care. American Hospital Association. Published June 2016. Accessed April 1, 2022. http://www.hpoe.org/resources/ahahret-guides/2860

32. National Committee for Quality Assurance in Collaboration with Health Management Associates. Population health management: meeting the demand for value-based care. National Committee for Quality Assurance. Published February 2, 2021. Accessed April 1, 2022. https://www.ncqa.org/white-papers/keys-to-success-in-meeting-the-demand-for-value-in-health-care/

33. Centers for Medicare & Medicaid Services. What are the value-based programs? Published 2022. Accessed June 26, 2022. https://www.cms.gov/Medicare/Quality-Initiatives-Patient-Assessment-Instruments/Value-Based-Programs/Value-Based-Programs

34. Broom T, Gronniger T, Dawe C, Ridlon A, Cavanaugh S. The proven path to re-energizing Medicare innovation. *Health Affairs* [blog], October 14, 2021. doi:10.1377/hblog20211012.117201

35. Centers for Medicare & Medicaid Services. Quality Payment Program overview. Accessed April 2, 2022. https://qpp.cms.gov/about/qpp-overview

36. Centers for Medicare & Medicaid Services. Shared savings program: about the program. Published 2022. Accessed June 19, 2022. https://www.cms.gov/Medicare/Medicare-Fee-for-Service-Payment/sharedsavingsprogram/about

37. Jabbarpour Y, Coffman M, Habib A, et al. Advanced primary care: a key contributor to successful ACOs. Delaware Health Care Commission. Published August 2018. Accessed May 25, 2022. https://dhss.delaware.gov/dhss/dhcc/files/pcpevidencerpt2018.pdf

38. Centers for Medicare & Medicaid Services. Accountable care organizations. Accessed April 2, 2022. https://www.cms.gov/Medicare/Medicare-Fee-for-Service-Payment/ACO

39. Daly R. Number of Medicare ACOs stays flat, but risk-taking increases. Healthcare Financial Management Association. Published 2020. Accessed April 2, 2022. https://www.hfma.org/topics/news/2020/01/number-of-medicare-acos-stays-flat-but-risk-taking-increases.html

40. Centers for Medicare & Medicaid Services. APMs overview. Accessed April 2, 2022. https://qpp.cms.gov/apms/overview

41. Terrell G, Value-based care: promote the Triple Aim. American Medical Association. Published 2019. Accessed May 25, 2022. https://edhub.ama-assn.org/

42. Bober M, Ferket K. ACMA Transitions of Care Learning Collaborative. American Case Management Association. Published 2019. Accessed March 8, 2022. https://transitionsofcare.org/resources/learning-collaborative/

43. Agency for Healthcare Research and Quality. Care management: implications for medical practice, health policy, and health services research. Published 2015. Updated August 2018. Accessed April 2, 2022. https://www.ahrq.gov/ncepcr/care/coordination/mgmt.html

44. Veritas Web Solutions, LLC. Levels of care: CCMC glossary of terms related to levels of care. Accessed June 19, 2022. https://casemanagementstudyguide.com/?s=Levels+of+care%3A+CCMC+glossary+of+terms+related+to+levels+of+care

45. Tahan HM, Treiger TM, eds. *CMSA Core Curriculum for Case Management*. Philadelphia, PA: Wolters Kluwer; 2017.

46. Case Management Society of America. Standards of practice for case management. Published 2016. Accessed June 20, 2022. https://cmsa.org/sop22/

47. Goetzel RZ, Staley P, Ogden L, et al. A framework for patient-centered health risk assessments: providing health promotion and disease prevention services to Medicare beneficiaries. Atlanta, GA: U.S. Department of Health & Human Services, Centers for Disease Control and Prevention; 2011. Accessed August 12, 2022. https://www.cdc.gov/policy/hst/hra/frameworkforhra.pdf

48. Kaiser Family Foundation. Summary of the Affordable Care Act. Updated April 23, 2013. Accessed April 2, 2022. https://files.kff.org/attachment/fact-sheet-summary-of-the-affordable-care-act

49. Office of Disease Prevention and Health Promotion. *Healthy People 2030*. Updated August 2, 2021. Accessed April 2, 2022. https://health.gov/healthypeople

50. Centers for Medicare & Medicaid Services. Medicare wellness visits. Updated February 2021. Accessed April 2, 2022. https://www.cms.gov/Outreach-and-Education/Medicare-Learning-Network-MLN/MLNProducts/preventive-services/medicare-wellness-visits.html

51. Medicare and Medicaid programs; revisions to requirements for discharge planning for hospitals, critical access hospitals, and home health agencies, and hospital and critical access hospital changes to promote innovation, flexibility, and improvement in patient care. *Federal Register*. 2019;84(189):51836-51884. Accessed April 2, 2022. https://www.govinfo.gov/content/pkg/FR-2019-09-30/pdf/2019-20732.pdf

52. Centers for Medicare & Medicaid Services. Chronic care management services. Published 2022. Accessed April 2, 2022. https://www.cms.gov/outreach-and-education/medicare-learning-network-mln/mlnproducts/downloads/chroniccaremanagement.pdf

53. Taylor EF, Machta RM, Meyers DS, Genevro J, Peikes DN. Enhancing the primary care team to provide redesigned care: the roles of practice facilitators and care managers. *Ann Family Med*. 2013;11:80-83. doi:10.1370/afm.1462

54. American Hospital Association. Connecting the dots along the care continuum. Published 2015. Accessed April 2, 2022. https://www.aha.org/system/files/2018-01/15carecontinuum.pdf

55. Agency for Healthcare Research and Quality. Patient centered medical home (PCMH). Published 2021. Updated March 2022. Accessed April 2, 2022. https://www.ahrq.gov/ncepcr/tools/pcmh/index.html

56. Taylor EF, Lake T, Nysenbaum J, Peterson G, Meyers D. Coordinating care in the medical neighborhood: critical components and available mechanisms. Agency for Healthcare Research and Quality. Published 2011. Accessed April 2, 2022. https://www.ahrq.gov/sites/default/files/wysiwyg/ncepcr/tools/PCMH/coordinating-care-in-the-medical-neighborhood-white-paper.pdf

57. Centers for Medicare & Medicaid Services. Primary care first model options. Updated April 5, 2022. Accessed April 9, 2022. https://innovation.cms.gov/innovation-models/primary-care-first-model-options

58. Centers for Medicare & Medicaid Services. Delivering value-based transformation in primary care. Accessed April 2, 2022. https://innovation.cms.gov/files/x/primary-cares-initiative-onepager.pdf

59. Centers for Medicare & Medicaid Services. Primary care first model cohort 2 CY 2021 fact sheet. Published 2021. Accessed April 9, 2022. https://www.cms.gov/newsroom/fact-sheets/primary-care-first-model-cohort-2-cy-2021-fact-sheet

60. National Council for Mental Well-Being. The Comprehensive Healthcare Integration Framework: designing, implementing and sustaining physical health-behavioral health integration. Published 2022. Accessed June 24, 2022. https://www.thenationalcouncil.org/wp-content/uploads/2022/04/04.22.2022_MDI-CHI-Paper_Reduced.pdf

61. Centers for Medicare & Medicaid Services. Medicare benefit policy manual. Published 2021. Accessed June 19, 2022. https://www.cms.gov/Regulations-and-Guidance/Guidance/Manuals/Downloads/bp102c08pdf.pdf

62. Centers for Medicare & Medicaid Services. Medicare provider compliance tips: inpatient rehabilitation hospitals and inpatient rehabilitation units. Medicare Learning Network. Updated September 2021. Accessed April 2, 2022. https://www.cms.gov/Outreach-and-Education/Medicare-Learning-Network-MLN/MLNProducts/medicare-provider-compliance-tips/medicare-provider-compliance-tips.html#IRF

63. Centers for Medicare & Medicaid Services. Important message from Medicare. Modified December 1, 2021. Accessed April 2, 2022. https://www.cms.gov/Medicare/Medicare-General-Information/BNI/HospitalDischargeAppealNotices?msclkid=390bc2e5d0d211ec8802daf5760f695b

64. American Hospital Association. MLN fact sheet skilled nursing facility 3-day rule billing. Published 2020. Updated April 2021. Accessed April 5, 2022. https://www.cms.gov/Outreach-and-Education/Medicare-Learning-Network-MLN/MLNProducts/Downloads/SNF3DayRule-MLN9730256.pdf#:~:text=To%20qualify%20for%20Skilled%20Nursing%20Facility%20%28SNF%29%20extended,time%20spent%20in%20the%20ER%20or%20outpatient%20observation.?msclkid=9d00662bd0ca11ecbe495039b2cf7880

65. Zander K. Population health management: coming of age. *Prof Case Manag.* 2019;24(1):26-38. doi:10.1097/NCM.0000000000000265

66. Davis MR. Despite pandemic percentage of number of older adults who want to age in place stays steady. AARP. Published November 18, 2021. https://www.aarp.org/home-family/your-home/info-2021/home-and-community-preferences-survey.html

67. Centers for Medicare & Medicaid Services. Medicare and home health care. Revised September 2020. Accessed April 1, 2022. https://www.medicare.gov/Pubs/pdf/10969-Medicare-and-Home-Health-Care.pdf

68. Bober M, Ferket, K. ACMA Transitions of Care Learning Collaborative 2019/2020. American Case Management Association. Accessed April 5, 2022. https://issuu.com/collaborativecasemanagement/docs/amca_toc_learningcollaborative

69. Malley A, Kenner C. Transitions in care: a critical review of measurement. *J Periop Crit Intensiv Care Nurs.* 2016;2(4):132. doi:10.4172/2471-9870.1000132

70. Case Management Society of America. Standards of practice for case management. Published 2016. Accessed April 3, 2022. https://www.abqaurp.org/DOCS/2010%20CM%20standards%20of%20practice.pdf

71. American Case Management Association. Definition of case management. Published April 2020. Accessed March 9, 2022. https://www.acmaweb.org/section.aspx?sID=4

72. Skaret MM, Weaver TD, Humes RJ, Carbone TV, Grasso IA, Kumar H. Automation of the I-PASS tool to improve transitions of care. *J Healthc Qual.* 2019;41(5):274-280. doi:10.1097/JHQ.0000000000000174

73. Botwinick L. Discharge to assess: "flipping" discharge assessment from hospital to home. Institute for Healthcare Improvement. Published 2017. Accessed April 21, 2022. http://www.ihi.org/resources/Pages/Publications/Discharge-to-Assess-Flipped-Discharge-Innovation-Case-Study.aspx

74. Institute for Healthcare Improvement. Tools: how-to guide: improving transitions from the hospital to community settings to reduce avoidable rehospitalizations. Published 2013. Accessed June 20, 2022. http://www.ihi.org/resources/Pages/Tools/HowtoGuideImprovingTransitionstoReduceAvoidableRehospitalizations.aspx

75. Centers for Medicare & Medicaid Services. CMS announces comprehensive strategy to enhance hospital capacity amid COVID-19 surge. Published 2020. Accessed April 21, 2022. https://www.cms.gov/newsroom/press-releases/cms-announces-comprehensive-strategy-enhance-hospital-capacity-amid-covid-19-surge

76. Centers for Medicare & Medicaid Services. Acute hospital care at home. Accessed April 21, 2022. https://qualitynet.cms.gov/acute-hospital-care-at-home

77. Arsenault-Lapierre G, Henein M, Gaid D, Le Berre M, Gore G, Vedel I. Hospital-at-home interventions vs in-hospital stay for patients with chronic disease who present to the emergency department: a systematic review and meta-analysis. *JAMA Netw Open.* 2021;4(6):e2111568. doi:10.1001/jamanetworkopen.2021.11568

78. Institute for Healthcare Improvement. Reduce avoidable readmissions. Accessed April 22, 2022. http://www.ihi.org/Topics/Readmissions/Pages/default.aspx

79. Institute for Healthcare Improvement. State action on avoidable rehospitalizations: overview. Accessed April 22, 2022. http://www.ihi.org/Engage/Initiatives/Completed/STAAR/Pages/default.aspx

80. Burroughs J, Smith R. Data-driven population health shapes a new model of primary care. *J Healthc Manage.* 2021;66(1):9-13. doi:10.1097/JHM-D-20-00303

81. Kollipara U, Varghese S, Mutz J, et al. Improving diabetic retinopathy screening among patients with diabetes mellitus using the define, measure, analyze, improve, and control process improvement methodology. *J Healthc Qual.* 2021;43(2):126-135. doi:10.1097/JHQ.0000000000000276

82. Balaban R, Batalden M, Ross-Degnan D, Le Cook B. Using a social worker transition coach to improve hospital-to-home transitions for high-risk nonelderly patients. *J Healthc Qual.* 2020;42(6):315-325. doi:10.1097/JHQ.0000000000000219

83. Finkelstein A, Zhou A, Taubman S, Doyle J. Health care hotspotting—a randomized, controlled trial. *N Engl J Med.* 2020;382:152-162. doi:10.1056/NEJMsa1906848

84. Arnetz BB, Goetz CM, Arnetz JE et al. Enhancing healthcare efficiency to achieve the quadruple aim: an exploratory study. *BMC Res Notes.* 2020;13:362. doi:10.1186/s13104-020-05199-8

85. Centers for Medicare & Medicaid Services. Medicare Shared Savings Program continues to grow and deliver high-quality, person-centered care through accountable care organizations. Published 2022. Accessed May 22, 2022. https://www.cms.gov/newsroom/press-releases/medicare-shared-savings-program-continues-grow-and-deliver-high-quality-person-centered-care-through

86. Miltner R, Pesch L, Mercado S, et al. Why competency standardization matters for improvement: an assessment of the healthcare quality workforce. *J Healthc Qual.* 2021;43(5):263-274. doi:10.1097/jhq.0000000000000316

# Suggested Readings

Ariosto D, Harper EM, Wilson ML, Hull SC, Nahm ES, Sylvia ML. Population health: a nursing action plan. *JAMIA Open.* 2018;1(1):710. doi:10.1093/jamiaopen/ooy003

Balik B, Hilton K, White, K. Conversation and action guide to support staff well-being and joy in work: during and after the COVID-19 pandemic. IHI tool. Cambridge, MA: Institute for Healthcare Improvement; 2020. Available at www.ihi.org

Bristol AA, Schneider CE, Lin, SY, Brody, AA. A systematic review of clinical outcomes associated with intrahospital transitions. *J Healthc Qual.* 2020;42(4):175-187. doi:10.1097/JHQ.0000000000000232

Caron R. *Population Health Principles and Applications for Management.* Chicago, IL: Health Administration Press; 2017.

Dowding DW, Russell D, Onorato N, Merrill JA. Technology solutions to support care continuity in home care: a focus group study. *J Healthc Qual.* 2018;40(4):236-246. doi:10.1097/JHQ.0000000000000104

Evans AC, Bufka LF. The critical need for a population health approach: addressing the nation's behavioral health during the COVID-19 pandemic and beyond. *Prev Chronic Dis.* 2020;17:200261. doi:10.5888/pcd17.200261

Goodrich DE, Kilbourne AM, Nord KM, Bauer MS. Mental health collaborative care and its role in primary care settings. *Curr Psychiatry Rep.* 2013;15(8):383. doi:10.1007/s11920-013-0383-2

Herndon L, Bones C, Bradke P, Rutherford P. *How-to Guide: Improving Transitions from the Hospital to Skilled Nursing Facilities to Reduce Avoidable Rehospitalizations.* Institute for Healthcare Improvement. Published June 2013. http://www.ihi.org/resources/Pages/Tools/HowtoGuideImprovingTransitionHospitalSNFstoReduceRehospitalizations.aspx

Horwitz LI, Chang C, Arcilla HN, Knickman JR. Quantifying health systems' investment in social determinants of health, by sector, 2017–19. *Health Affairs.* 2020;39:2, 192-198. doi:10.1377/HLTHAFF.2019.01246

Institute of Medicine Committee on Assuring the Health of the Public in the 21st Century. Understanding population health and its determinants. *The Future of the Public's Health in the 21st Century.* Washington, DC: National Academies Press; 2002. https://www.ncbi.nlm.nih.gov/books/NBK221225/

Kollipara U, Varghese S, Mutz J, et al. Improving diabetic retinopathy screening among patients with diabetes mellitus using the define, measure, analyze, improve, and control process improvement methodology. *J Healthc Qual.* 2021;43(2):126-135. doi:10.1097/JHQ.0000000000000276

National Academies of Sciences, Engineering, and Medicine. *Population Health Science in the United States: Trends, Evidence, and Implications for Policy: Proceedings of a Joint Symposium.* Washington, DC: The National Academies Press; 2021. doi:10.17226/25631

National Council for Mental Well-Being. The Comprehensive Healthcare Integration Framework: designing, implementing and sustaining physical health-behavioral health integration. Published 2022. Accessed June 24, 2022. https://www.thenationalcouncil.org/wp-content/uploads/2022/04/04.22.2022_MDI-CHI-Paper_Reduced.pdf

Peele P, Keyser D, Lovelace J, Moss D. Advancing value-based population health management through payer–provider partnerships: improving outcomes for children with complex conditions. *J Healthc Qual.* 2018;40(2):e26-e32. doi:10.1097/JHQ.0000000000000101

Perlo J, Balik B, Swensen S, Kabcenell A, Landsman J, Feeley D. *IHI Framework for Improving Joy in Work.* IHI white paper. Cambridge, MA: Institute for Healthcare Improvement; 2017. Accessed June 24, 2022. http://www.ihi.org/resources/Pages/IHIWhitePapers/Framework-Improving-Joy-in-Work.aspx

Reichheld A, Yang J, Sokol-Hessner L, Quinn G. Defining best practices for interhospital transfers. *J Healthc Qual.* 2021;43(4):214-224. doi:10.1097/JHQ.0000000000000293

Riegelman R. *Population Health: A Primer.* Burlington, MA: Jones & Bartlett Learning; 2020.

Rutherford P, Nielsen GA, Taylor J, Bradke P, Coleman E. *How-to Guide: Improving Transitions from the Hospital to Community Settings to Reduce Avoidable Rehospitalizations.* Cambridge, MA: Institute for Healthcare Improvement; 2013. http://www.ihi.org/resources/Pages/Tools/HowtoGuideImprovingTransitionstoReduceAvoidableRehospitalizations.aspx

Schall M, Coleman E, Rutherford P, Taylor J. *How-to Guide: Improving Transitions from the Hospital to the Clinical Office Practice to Reduce Avoidable Rehospitalizations.* Cambridge, MA: Institute for Healthcare Improvement; 2013. http://www.ihi.org/resources/Pages/Tools/HowtoGuideImprovingTransitionsHospitaltoOfficePracticeReduceRehospitalizations.aspx

Sevin C, Evdokimoff M, Sobolewski S, Taylor J, Rutherford P, Coleman EA. *How-to Guide: Improving Transitions from the Hospital to Home Health Care to Reduce Avoidable Rehospitalizations.* Cambridge, MA: Institute for Healthcare Improvement; 2013. http://www.ihi.org/resources/Pages/Tools/HowtoGuideImprovingTransitionsfromHospitaltoHomeHealthCareReduceAvoidableHospitalizations.aspx

Skaret MM, Weaver TD, Humes RJ, Carbone TV, Grasso IA, Kumar H. Automation of the I-PASS tool to improve transitions of care. *J Healthc Qual.* 2019;41(5):274-280. doi:10.1097/JHQ.0000000000000174

Sloand E, VanGraafeiland B, Holm A, MacQueen A, Polk S. Text message quality improvement project for influenza vaccine in a low-resource largely Latino pediatric population. *J Healthc Qual.* 2019;41(6):362-368. doi:10.1097/JHQ.0000000000000190

Smith MA, Yu M, Huling JD, Wang X, DeLonay A, Jaffery J. Impactability modeling for reducing Medicare accountable care organization payments and hospital events in high-need high-cost patients: longitudinal cohort study. *J Med Internet Res.* 2022;24(6):e29420. doi:10.2196/29420

Solar O, Irwin A. *A Conceptual Framework for Action on the Social Determinants of Health.* Social Determinants of Health discussion paper 2 (Policy and Practice). Geneva, Switzerland: WHO; 2010.

Terrell G. *Value-Based Care: Promote the Triple Aim.* American Medical Association; 2019. https://edhub.ama-assn.org/

Warnecke R, Oh A, Breen N, et al. Approaching health disparities from a population perspective: the National Institutes of Health Centers for Population Health and Health Disparities. *Am J Public Health.* 2008;98:1608-1615. doi:10.2105/AJPH.2006.102525

Whittal K, Caldwell A. *Rising risk: Maximizing the odds for care management.* Seattle, WA: Milliman; 2018. Available at https://us.milliman.com/en/

Wyatt R, Laderman M, Botwinick L, Mate K, Whittington J. *Achieving Health Equity: A Guide for Health Care Organizations.* IHI white paper. Cambridge, MA: Institute for Healthcare Improvement; 2016. Available at www.ihi.org

## Online Resources

*Agency for Healthcare Research and Quality*

https://www.ahrq.gov/

- **Patient Centered Medical Home Foundations**
https://www.ahrq.gov/ncepcr/tools/pcmh/implement/foundations.html

*American College of Healthcare Executives*

https://www.ache.org/

*American Hospital Association*

https://www.aha.org/

- **AHA Innovation Center—Population Health**
https://www.aha.org/center/population-health

*American Public Health Association*

https://apha.org/

*Case Management Society of America*

https://cmsa.org/

*Centers for Disease Control and Prevention*

https://www.cdc.gov/

- **6|18 Initiative**
https://www.cdc.gov/sixeighteen/index.html

*Centers for Medicare & Medicaid Services*

https://www.cms.gov/

- **Quality Payment Program**
https://qpp.cms.gov/

*County Health Rankings & Roadmaps*

https://www.countyhealthrankings.org/

*Dartmouth Health Population Health*

https://www.dartmouth-hitchcock.org/about/population-health

*HMP Global Population Health Learning Network*

https://www.hmpgloballearningnetwork.com/site/about-population-health-learning-network

*Institute for Healthcare Improvement*

http://www.ihi.org/

- **Joy in Work**
http://www.ihi.org/Topics/Joy-In-Work/Pages/default.aspx

*KLAS Research Population Health Management*

https://klasresearch.com/compare/population-health-management/256

*National Academy of Medicine*

https://nam.edu/

- **National Plan for Health Workforce Well-Being**
https://nam.edu/initiatives/clinician-resilience-and-well-being/national-plan-for-health-workforce-well-being/#.Yrxkwh82fJE.link

*National Association of Community Health Centers*

https://www.nachc.org/

*National Association for Healthcare Quality*

https://www.nahq.org

- **National Center of Excellence for Integrated Health Solutions**
https://www.samhsa.gov/national-coe-integrated-health-solutions

*National Committee for Quality Assurance*

https://www.ncqa.org

*National Council on Aging*

https://www.ncoa.org/

*National Council on Disability*

https://www.ncd.gov/

*National Council for Mental Wellbeing*

https://www.thenationalcouncil.org/

*Optum Population Health Services*

https://www.optum.com/business/solutions/employer/population-health.html

*Office of the National Coordinator for Health Information Technology*

https://www.healthit.gov/

- **Health IT Playbook—Population Health & Public Health**

  https://www.healthit.gov/playbook/population-public-health/

*Population Health Alliance*

https://populationhealthalliance.org/

*Substance Abuse and Mental Health Services Administration*

https://www.samhsa.gov/

*URAC*

https://www.urac.org/

# Acronyms

## Numbers

| | |
|---|---|
| 5S | *Seiri* (Sort), *Seiton* (Set), *Seiso* (Shine), *Seiketsu* (Standardize), *Shitsuke* (Sustain) |
| 6S | Sort, Set, Shine, Standardize, Sustain, Safety |

## A

| | |
|---|---|
| AAAASF | American Association for Accreditation of Ambulatory Surgery Facilities |
| AAAHC | Accreditation Association for Ambulatory Health Care |
| AAMC | Association of American Medical Colleges |
| ACA | Affordable Care Act |
| ACCME | Accreditation Council for Continuing Medical Education |
| ACE | Angiotensin-converting enzyme |
| ACF | Administration for Children & Families |
| ACGME | Accreditation Council for Graduate Medical Education |
| ACHC | Accreditation Commission for Health Care |
| ACL | Administration for Community Living |
| ACO | Accountable care organization |
| ACR | American College of Radiology |
| ACS | American College of Surgeons |
| ACUG | Accreditation and Certification Users Group |
| AHA | American Hospital Association |
| AHIMA | American Health Information Management Association |
| AHIP | America's Health Insurance Plans |
| AHRQ | Agency for Healthcare Research and Quality |
| AI | Artificial intelligence |
| AIDET | Acknowledge, Introduce, Duration, Explanation, Thank You |
| AIDS | Acquired immune deficiency syndrome |
| ALOS | Average length of stay |
| AMA | American Medical Association |
| AMI | Acute myocardial infarction |
| ANCC | American Nurses Credentialing Center |
| AOTA | American Occupational Therapy Association |
| APA | American Psychiatric Association |
| APA | American Psychological Association |
| APIC | Association for Professionals in Infection Control and Epidemiology |
| APIE | Assess, Plan, Implement, Evaluate |
| APM | Alternative payment model |
| APP | Advanced practice professional |
| APTA | American Physical Therapy Association |
| APR-DRG | All Patient Refined Diagnosis Related Groups |
| ARB | Angiotensin receptor blocker |
| ARRA | American Recovery and Reinvestment Act |
| ASA | American Society of Anesthesiologists |
| ASC | Ambulatory surgery center |
| ASHRM | American Society for Health Care Risk Management |
| ASP | Antibiotic stewardship program |
| ASQ | American Society for Quality |
| ATSDR | Agency for Toxic Substances and Disease Registry |

## B

| | |
|---|---|
| BAA | Business associate agreement |
| BD2K | Big Data to Knowledge |
| BI | Business intelligence |
| BSC | Balanced scorecard |

## C

| | |
|---|---|
| CABG | Coronary artery bypass grafting |
| CAERS | CFSAN Adverse Event Reporting System |
| CAH | Critical access hospital |
| CAHPS | Consumer Assessment of Health Care Providers and Systems |
| CAP | College of American Pathologists |
| CAP | Corrective action plan |
| CARF | CARF International (formerly Commission on Accreditation of Rehabilitation Facilities) |
| CAS | Complex adaptive systems |
| CAUTI | Catheter-associated urinary tract infections |
| CBA | Cost-benefit analysis |
| CCE | Certified Content Expert |
| CCM | Chronic care model |
| CDC | Centers for Disease Control and Prevention |
| CDI | *C. difficile* infection |
| CDM | Common data model |
| CDSS | Clinical decision support systems |
| CEC | Content Expert Certification™ |
| CEO | Chief executive officer |
| CER | Comparative effectiveness research |
| CfC | Conditions for Coverage |
| CFR | Code of Federal Regulations |
| CFSAN | Center for Food Safety and Applied Nutrition |
| CG-CAHPS | CAHPS Clinician & Group Survey |

| | |
|---|---|
| CHAP | Community Health Accreditation Partner |
| CHIP | Children's Health Insurance Program |
| CI | Confidence interval |
| CLABSI | Central line-associated bloodstream infection |
| CLAS | Culturally and Linguistically Appropriate Services |
| CLIA | Clinical Laboratory Improvement Amendments |
| CM | Case management |
| CMIT | CMS Measures Inventory Tool |
| CMO | Chief medical officer |
| CMS | Centers for Medicare & Medicaid Services |
| CMSA | Case Management Society of America |
| CNE | Chief nurse executive |
| CNO | Chief nursing officer |
| COA | Council on Accreditation |
| COLA | Commission of Office Laboratory Accreditation |
| CoP | Conditions of Participation |
| COPD | Chronic obstructive pulmonary disease |
| COPIS | Customer-Output-Process-Input-Supplier |
| CORF | Comprehensive outpatient rehabilitation facility |
| COVID-19 | Coronavirus Disease 2019 |
| COVID-Net | Coronavirus Disease 2019 (COVID-19)–Associated Hospitalization Surveillance Network |
| CPG | Clinical practice guideline |
| CPHQ | Certified Professional in Healthcare Quality |
| CPM | Critical path method |
| CPOE | Computerized prescriber order entry |
| CPR | Cardiopulmonary resuscitation |
| CPRC | Cancer Prevention Research Center |
| CPT | Current Procedural Terminology |
| CQHCA | Committee on Quality of Health Care in America |
| CQI | Continuous quality improvement |
| CQM | Clinical quality measure |
| CRM | Crew Resource Management |
| CSR | Continuous survey readiness |
| CVO | Credentials verification organization |

**D**

| | |
|---|---|
| D2A | Discharge to Assess |
| DHDN | Distributed health data network |
| DHHS | Department of Health & Human Services |
| DIKW | Data-Information-Knowledge-Wisdom Pyramid |
| DM | Disease management |
| DMAIC | Define, Measure, Analyze, Improve, Control |
| DME | Durable medical equipment |
| DMEPOS | Durable Medical Equipment, Prosthetics, Orthotics, and Supplies |
| DNP | Doctor of nursing practice |
| DNSc | Doctor of nursing science |
| DNV | Det Norske Veritas |
| DoD | Department of Defense |
| DOJ | Department of Justice |
| DPH | Department of Public Health |

| | |
|---|---|
| DPMO | Defects per million opportunities |
| DRG | Diagnosis-related group |
| DSM | *Diagnostic and Statistical Manual of Mental Disorders* |

**E**

| | |
|---|---|
| EBP | Evidence-based practice |
| eCQM | Electronic clinical quality measure |
| ED | Emergency department |
| EHR | Electronic health record |
| EMC | Emergency medical condition |
| EMR | Electronic medical record |
| EMTALA | Emergency Medical Treatment and Active Labor Act |
| EP | Eligible professional |
| EQRO | External Quality Review Organization |
| ERISA | Employee Retirement and Income Security Act of 1974 |
| ERM | Enterprise risk management |
| ESC | Evidence of Standards Compliance |
| ESRD | End-stage renal disease |

**F**

| | |
|---|---|
| FAIR | Findable, Accessible, Interoperable, and Reusable |
| FDA | Food & Drug Administration |
| FERPA | Family Educational Rights and Privacy Act |
| FFS | Fee for service |
| FMEA | Failure mode and effects analysis |
| FPPE | Focused professional practice evaluation |
| FQHC | Federally qualified health center |

**H**

| | |
|---|---|
| HAC | Hospital-acquired condition |
| HAI | Healthcare-associated infection |
| HBIPS | Hospital-Based Inpatient Psychiatric Services |
| HCAHPS | Hospital Consumer Assessment of Healthcare Providers and Systems |
| HCDIT | Health Care Delivery and Information Technology |
| HCFAC | Health Care Fraud and Abuse Control Program |
| HCP | Healthcare personnel |
| HCPLAN | Health Care Payment Learning & Action Network |
| HCW | Healthcare worker |
| HEDIS | Healthcare Effectiveness Data and Information Set |
| HEN | Hospital Engagement Network |
| HF | Heart failure |
| HFAP | Healthcare Facilities Accreditation Program |
| HFMEA | Healthcare failure mode and effects analysis |
| HHA | Home health agency |
| HHRP | Hospital readmissions reduction program |
| HHS | U.S. Department of Health & Human Services |
| HIE | Health information exchange |

| | |
|---|---|
| HIIN | Hospital Improvement Innovation Network |
| HIM | Health information management |
| HIMSS | Healthcare Information and Management Systems Society |
| HIP | Health information products |
| HIPAA | Health Insurance Portability and Accountability Act |
| HIPDB | Healthcare Integrity and Protection Data Bank |
| HIT | Health information technology |
| HITECH | Health Information Technology for Economic and Clinical Health Act |
| HIV | Human immunodeficiency virus |
| HMD | Health and Medicine Division of the National Academy of Sciences |
| HMO | Health maintenance organization |
| HPA | Health plan accreditation |
| HQCC | Healthcare Quality Certification Commission |
| HRA | Health risk assessment |
| HRET | Health Research & Education Trust |
| HRM | Healthcare risk management |
| HRO | High reliability organization |
| HRSA | Health Resources & Services Administration |

**I**

| | |
|---|---|
| ICD | International Classification of Diseases |
| ICF/IID | Intermediate Care Facilities for Individuals with Intellectual Disabilities |
| ICU | Intensive care unit |
| IHI | Institute for Healthcare Improvement |
| IHS | Indian Health Service |
| IJ | Immediate jeopardy |
| IMPACT | Improving Medicare Post-Acute Care Transformation Act of 2014 |
| IOM | Institute of Medicine (now Health and Medicine Division of the National Academy of Sciences) |
| IP | Intellectual property |
| IP | Internet protocol |
| IPC | Infection prevention and control |
| IPFCC | Institute for Patient and Family-Centered Care |
| IPPS | Inpatient Prospective Payment System |
| IQI | Inpatient quality indicators |
| IRF | Inpatient rehabilitation facility |
| ISMP | Institute for Safe Medication Practices |
| IT | Information technology |
| ITL | Immediate threat to life |
| IV | Intravenous |

**J**

| | |
|---|---|
| JHQ | *Journal for Healthcare Quality* |
| JIT | Just in time |

**K**

| | |
|---|---|
| KPI | Key performance indicator |
| KRI | Key risk indicator |

**L**

| | |
|---|---|
| LCL | Lower control limit |
| LEP | Low English proficiency |
| LIP | Licensed Independent Practitioner |
| LOC | Level of care |
| LOINC | Logical Observation Identifiers Names and Codes |
| LOS | Length of stay |
| LTAC | Long-term acute care |
| LTC | Long-term care |
| LTCH | Long-term care hospital |

**M**

| | |
|---|---|
| M & M | Morbidity and mortality |
| MACRA | Medicare Access and CHIP Reauthorization Act |
| MAT | Medication-assisted treatment |
| MBHO | Managed behavioral healthcare organization |
| MCO | Managed care organization |
| MD | Medical doctor |
| MDRO | Multidrug-resistant organisms |
| MDS | Minimum data set |
| MGMA | Medical Group Management Association |
| MH | Mental health |
| MIPS | Merit-Based Incentive Payment System |
| MIS | Management information system |
| MMS | Measures Management System |
| MQSA | Mammography Quality Standards Act |
| MRSA | Methicillin-resistant *Staphylococcus aureus* |
| MS | Master of science |
| MSDS | Material safety data sheet |
| MSE | Medical screening examination |
| MU | Meaningful use |

**N**

| | |
|---|---|
| NABP | National Association of Boards of Pharmacy |
| NAHQ | National Association for Healthcare Quality |
| NAIC | National Association of Insurance Commissioners |
| NAM | National Academy of Medicine |
| NASW | National Association of Social Workers |
| NCQA | National Committee for Quality Assurance |
| NCVHS | National Committee on Vital and Health Statistics |
| NEJM | *New England Journal of Medicine* |
| NGC | National Guideline Clearinghouse™ |
| NHIN | Nationwide Health Information Network |
| NHSN | National Healthcare Safety Network |
| NIAHO | National Integrated Accreditation for Healthcare Organizations |
| NIH | National Institutes of Health |
| NIOSH | National Institute for Occupational Safety and Health |
| NPDB | National Practitioner Data Bank |
| NPP | National Priorities Partnership |

| | |
|---|---|
| NPSF | National Patient Safety Foundation |
| NPSG | National Patient Safety Goal |
| NQF | National Quality Forum |
| NQS | National Quality Strategy |
| NSQIP | National Surgical Quality Improvement Program |

**O**

| | |
|---|---|
| OASIS | Outcome and Assessment Information Set |
| OBAE | Obstetric adverse event |
| OCR | Office of Civil Rights |
| OIG | Office of Inspector General |
| OMH | Office of Minority Health |
| ONC | Office of the National Coordinator for Health Information Technology, HHS |
| OPIM | Other potentially infectious materials |
| OPO | Organ procurement organization |
| OPPE | Ongoing professional practice evaluation |
| OPSC | Oregon Patient Safety Commission |
| OR | Odds ratio |
| ORYX | Performance Measurement Reporting (The Joint Commission) |
| OSHA | Occupational Safety and Health Administration |

**P**

| | |
|---|---|
| P4P | Pay for performance |
| PACE | Programs of All-Inclusive Care for the Elderly |
| PCF | Primary Care First |
| PCMH | Patient-centered medical home |
| PCOR | Patient-centered outcomes research |
| PCORI | Patient-Centered Outcomes Research Institute |
| PCP | Primary care physician |
| PCP | Primary care provider |
| PCSP | Patient-centered specialty care |
| PDCA | Plan-Do-Check-Act |
| PDI | Pediatric quality indicators |
| PDSA | Plan-Do-Study-Act |
| PERT | Program Evaluation and Review Technique |
| PFCC | Patient- and family-centered care |
| PFE | Patient and family engagement |
| PfP | Partnership for Patients |
| PH | Physical health |
| PhD | Doctor of philosophy |
| PHI | Protected health information |
| PHM | Population health management |
| PHO | Physician-hospital organization |
| PHQC | Physician and Hospital Quality Certification |
| PHR | Personal health record |
| PI | Performance Improvement |
| PII | Personally identifiable information |
| PICU | Pediatric intensive care unit |
| PIVC | Peripheral IV catheter |
| PN | Pneumonia |
| PoC | Plan of Correction |

| | |
|---|---|
| PPACA | Patient Protection and Affordable Care Act |
| PPE | Personal protective equipment |
| PPPSA | Physician Practice Patient Safety Assessment |
| PPS | Prospective Payment System |
| PQA | Pharmacy Quality Alliance |
| PQI | Prevention quality indicators |
| PQS | Pharmacy Quality Solutions |
| PROM | Patient Reported Outcome Measures |
| PRO-PM | Patient Reported Outcome Performance Measures |
| PSCHO | Patient Safety Climate in Healthcare Organizations |
| PSI | Patient safety indicators |
| PSNet | AHRQ Patient Safety Network |
| PSO | Patient safety organization |
| PSP | Patient safety practice |
| PSQIA | Patient Safety and Quality Improvement Act |
| PSWP | Patient Safety Work Product |

**Q**

| | |
|---|---|
| QA | Quality assurance |
| QC | Quality circle |
| QC | Quality control |
| QCDR | Qualified clinical data registry |
| QFD | Quality function deployment |
| QI | Quality improvement |
| QM | Quality management |
| QPI | Quality and performance improvement |
| QPP | Quality Payment Program |
| QSEN | Quality and Safety Education for Nurses |

**R**

| | |
|---|---|
| RCA | Root cause analysis |
| RCA$^2$ | Root Cause Analysis and Action |
| RFI | Request for improvement |
| RHC | Rural health clinic |
| RM | Risk management |
| RN | Registered nurse |
| ROI | Return on investment |
| RPIW | Rapid Process Improvement Workshop |
| RR | Relative risk |
| RRT | Rapid response team |

**S**

| | |
|---|---|
| SAFER | Survey Analysis for Evaluating Risk |
| SAMHSA | Substance Abuse and Mental Health Services Administration |
| SAQ | Safety Attitudes Questionnaire |
| SBAR | Situation Background Assessment Recommendation |
| SD | Standard deviation |
| SDOH | Social determinants of health |
| SHEA | Society for Healthcare Epidemiology of America |
| SIPOC | Supplier Input Process Output Customer |

| | |
|---|---|
| SMART | Specific, Measurable, Achievable, Relevant, and Time-Bound |
| SNF | Skilled nursing facility |
| SNOMED CT | Systemized Nomenclature of Medicine-Clinical Terms |
| SOM | State Operations Manual |
| SPC | Statistical process control |
| SRE | Serious reportable event |
| SSI | Surgical site infection |
| STAAR | State Action on Avoidable Rehospitalizations |

**T**

| | |
|---|---|
| TeamSTEPPS | Team Strategies and Tools to Enhance Performance and Patient Safety |
| THA | Total hip arthroplasty |
| TJC | The Joint Commission |
| TKA | Total knee arthroplasty |
| TOC | Transitions of care |
| TPM | Total productive maintenance |
| TPO | Treatment, payment or business operations |
| TQM | Total quality management |
| TRIO | Trust, Report, and Improve Organizations |

**U**

| | |
|---|---|
| UCL | Upper control limit |
| UHDDS | Uniform Hospital Discharge Data Set |

| | |
|---|---|
| UM | Utilization management |
| URAC | Utilization Review Accreditation Committee |
| URL | Universal resource locator |
| US | United States |
| USB | Universal Serial Bus |
| USPSTF | U.S. Preventive Services Task Force |

**V**

| | |
|---|---|
| VA | U.S. Department of Veterans Affairs |
| VAERS | Vaccine Adverse Event Reporting System |
| VAP | Ventilator-associated pneumonia |
| VBP | Value-based purchasing |
| VHA | Voluntary Hospital Association |
| VLER | Virtual Lifetime Electronic Record |
| VOC | Voice of the customer |
| VTE | Venous thromboembolism |

**W**

| | |
|---|---|
| WHO | World Health Organization |
| WHP | Wellness and health promotion |
| WIP | Work in progress |

**X**

| | |
|---|---|
| XML | Extensible Markup Language |

# Glossary

The glossary is organized to reflect the nature of healthcare quality—concepts, thinking, applications, methods, and practices. While it is comprehensive, the glossary is not exhaustive. Terms are those found in *HQ Solutions*. Many definitions come from authoritative sources and may also be cited in a section.

**3P** Lean experts typically view this as one of the most powerful and transformative advanced manufacturing tools, and it is typically only used by organizations that have experience implementing other Lean methods. Whereas kaizen and other Lean methods take a production process as a given and seek to make improvements, the production preparation process focuses on eliminating waste through product and process design.

**5S** Quality tool derived from Japanese terms intended to help organizations maintain a safe workplace that supports productivity and reduces waste (*seiri, seiton, seisō, seiketsu,* and *shitsuke*).

**6S** A method used to create and maintain a clean, orderly, and safe work environment. It is based upon the five pillars of the visual workplace in the Toyota Production System, plus another pillar for safety (sort, set, shine, standardize, sustain, and safety). This method is often the first companies implement in their Lean journey since it serves as the foundation of future continuous improvement.

**85/15 Theory** Deming claimed that about 85% of organizational failures are due to system breakdowns involving factors such as management, machinery, or work rules; 85% of the problems detected are process or system-related, whereas only 15% are traceable to workers.

# A

**A3** Lean/Six Sigma tool used to capture an improvement opportunity. A standard format is used to address an improvement process (i.e., seven or nine blocks). This usually includes the background, current condition, goal, analysis, proposal/recommendation/countermeasure, plan, and follow-up.

**Access** Ability to obtain needed healthcare services in a timely manner including the perceptions and experiences of people regarding their ease of reaching health services or health facilities in terms of proximity, location, time, and ease of approach (e.g., timeliness of response or services, time until the next available appointment, and availability of services within a community).

**Accountability** An obligation or willingness to accept responsibility for performance.

**Accountable care organization** A network of healthcare providers who band together to provide the full continuum of healthcare services for patients. The network receives a payment for all care provided to a patient and is held accountable for the quality and cost of care. The goal is to improve quality and reduce costs by allowing them to share in any savings achieved because of these efforts.

**Accreditation** The process in which a local, national, or internationally recognized agency assesses operations and performance of an organization to determine whether a set of recognized and accepted standards are met. The outcome is an official authorization or approval, or recognition for conforming to standards, or to recognize as outstanding.

**Activity network diagram** Sequence of events depicted using an illustration with arrows. It is useful when several simultaneous paths must be coordinated. Also known as an *arrow diagram, program evaluation and review technique (PERT),* or a *critical path method (CPM) chart.*

**Adaptive** The capacity to change and the ability to learn from experience.

**Affinity diagram** Tool that organizes numerous ideas or issues into groupings based on their natural relationships within the groupings. Typically used by teams to analyze or chart a process and to structure and organize issues to provide a new perspective to help solve a problem.

**Agency** Accreditation organization or body or certification organization or body.

**Agility** The capacity to gather and disseminate information about changes in the environment and respond to that information quickly and expediently; the ability to make rapid change and achieve flexibility in operations in response to changes in the external environment or to take advantage of an immediate opportunity.

**Appropriate care** Care that avoids wasteful tests and procedures that provide no benefit to patients, involves a high degree of care coordination to ensure efficient delivery, and encompasses everything patients need to achieve their personal health-related goals.

**Artificial intelligence** A computer applying human intellectual characteristics to problem solve, namely the ability to reason, to generalize, and to learn from previous experiences.

# B

**Balanced scorecard** Approach to performance management where performance measures provide a comprehensive view of organizational performance and not be overly dependent on a few choice indicators. It helps organizations better link long-term strategy with short-term activities.

**Baldrige Award** Competitive award that is given to organizations demonstrating a commitment to quality excellence based on successfully meeting the Baldrige National Health Care Criteria for Performance Excellence.

**Bar chart** Tool to visually demonstrate comparisons among various categories. This visual aid can be organized horizontally or vertically to demonstrate the relationship between one or more categorical variables relative to a single continuous variable. It is a visual tool only and improvement decisions should not be made using this tool.

**Benchmark** Sustained superior performance, which can be used as a reference to raise the mainstream of care by other providers, organizations, and delivery systems. The relative definition of superior will vary situation to situation.

**Benchmarking** Comparison of an organization's or an individual practitioner's results against a reference point. Ideally, the reference point is a demonstrated best practice.

**Best practice** Treatment that is accepted by medical experts as a proper treatment for a certain type of disease and that is widely used by healthcare professionals. Also called *standard medical care*, *standard of care*, and *standard therapy*.

**Biomedical Big Data** The complexity, challenges, and new opportunities presented by the combined analysis of data. In biomedical research, these data sources include the diverse, complex, disorganized, massive, and multimodal data being generated by researchers, hospitals, and mobile devices around the world.

**Black Belt** A practitioner of Six Sigma methods with significant theoretical and practical experience. Mentors individuals newer to this problem-solving framework (e.g., White Belts, Yellow Belts, Green Belts).

**Brainstorming** Instituting a shared method for a team to rapidly and creatively generate many ideas in an efficient way for any topic. The use of this methodology fosters freedom of criticism and judgment while encouraging openness in thinking. Doing this in writing is called brainwriting.

**Budgeting** Formal annual or periodic process through which financial performance goals and actual results are evaluated for the current and previous fiscal years, allowing for the development of formal goals for the next fiscal year.

**Bundle** Small set of evidence-based interventions for a defined patient segment.

**Burnout** A syndrome defined to describe the consequences of severe stress in helping professions. It is characterized by three dimensions—emotional exhaustion, depersonalization, and decreased feelings of personal accomplishment.

**Business intelligence** The processes and methods of collecting, storing, and analyzing data from business operations or activities to help organizations optimize their performance by making more data-driven decisions such as identifying issues, tracking performance, comparing data against competitors, identifying ways to increase profit, analyzing customer behavior, identifying market trends, and predicting success.

# C

**C-Suite** Executives at the highest level of the organization structure. These individuals possess leadership and strategic thinking skills and understand the business fundamentals for healthcare operations. These positions vary by type and size of the healthcare organization but may include the chief executive officer, chief operating officer, chief financial officer, chief medical officer, chief nursing or clinical officer, chief information or technology officer, chief marketing officer, chief human resource officer, and chief quality officer.

**Capital budgeting** The process by which an organization evaluates and selects which long-term investments (or capital expenditures) it will make. Typically, this is an annual activity, but it also may be triggered by events such as requests for new programs or equipment.

**Care bundle** Population and care setting that, when implemented together, result in significantly better outcomes than when implemented individually.

**Care management** Healthcare delivery process that helps achieve better health outcomes by anticipating and linking clients with the services they need in a timely manner. It also helps avoid unnecessary services by preventing medical or other problems from escalating.

**Case management** The process of coordinating medical care provided to patients with specific diagnoses or those with high healthcare needs. These functions are performed by physicians, nurses, or social workers. The process varies depending on the practice setting. Also called *care management*.

**Case management program** An organized approach to the provision of coordinated care services to clients and their support systems. The program is usually described in terms of (1) vision, mission, and objectives; (2) number and type of staff, including roles, responsibilities, and expectations; and (3) a specific model or conceptual framework that delineates the key case management functions, which may include clinical care management, transitional planning, resources utilization and management, bed capacity management, clinical documentation enhancement, quality and variance/delays management, and others, depending on the healthcare organization.

**Case manager** A health and human services professional who is responsible for coordinating the overall care, services, and resources delivered to an individual client or a group of clients and their support systems based on the client's health and human services issues, needs, and interests.

**Cause and effect diagram** Visual aid used to display, explore, and analyze all the potential causes related to a problem or condition and to discover the root causes of variation. Also known as *Ishikawa* or *fishbone diagram*.

**Cellular manufacturing** Production operations in which workstations and equipment are arranged in a sequence that supports a smooth flow of materials and components through the production process with minimal transport or delay. Implementation of this Lean method often represents the first major shift in production activity, and it is the key enabler of increased production velocity and flexibility, as well as the reduction of capital requirements.

**Central tendency** The middle value and the general trend of the numbers. The three most common measures of this are the mean, the median, and the mode.

**Certification** Formal, focused process that an organization, program, individual, or technology undergoes with an assessment by a neutral party or local, national, internationally recognized, or regulatory agency to demonstrate compliance and competency with developed standards. Recognition for meeting special qualifications within a field. It is different from accreditation.

**Certified Professional in Healthcare Quality (CPHQ)** Certification in the healthcare quality field promotes excellence and professionalism. Those with this certification demonstrate their knowledge and expertise in this field by passing a written examination. The designation provides the healthcare employer and the public with the assurance that certified individuals possess the necessary skills, knowledge, and experience in healthcare quality to perform competently.

**Champion** Person who translates the company's vision, mission, goals, and metrics to create an organizational deployment plan; identifies individual projects and resources; and removes roadblocks.

**Change concept** A general approach to developing specific ideas for improvement.

**Checklist** A method that allows complex pathways of care to function with high reliability by giving users the opportunity to pause and take stock of their actions before proceeding to the next step. Also a standard way to ensure completion of critical tasks for a process or activity. It ensures accuracy, accountability, completeness, and efficiency.

**Chi-square ($\chi^2$)** Test of statistical significance that assesses the difference in proportions among two or more variables.

**Chronic disease management** Integrated care approach to addressing illness that includes screenings, checkups, monitoring and coordinating treatment, and patient education.

It can improve quality of life while reducing healthcare costs by preventing or minimizing the effects of a disease.

**Clinical decision support system** Health information technology functionality that builds upon the foundation of an electronic health record to provide persons involved in care processes with general and person-specific information, intelligently filtered and organized, at appropriate times, to enhance health and healthcare.

**Clinical information system** Method designed to support direct patient care processes; automated medical information systems with great potential for analyzing and improving the quality of patient care.

**Clinical pathway** Document-based tools that provide a link between the best available evidence and practice. Also known as a *care pathway*, *critical pathway*, *integrated care pathway*, or *care map*, it is one tool used to manage the quality in healthcare concerning the standardization of care processes.

**Clinical pertinence** An assessment of the documentation in the medical record/electronic health record in terms of the patient's condition, diagnostic results, intervention procedures, vital signs, and other information. This review may determine that documentation was appropriate or not appropriate to the standard of care, key elements of the assessment, treatment plan, interventions, and medication management.

**Clinical practice guideline** A statement that includes recommendations that intend to optimize patient care. They are informed by a systematic review of evidence and an assessment of the benefits and harms of alternative care options.

**Clinical quality measure** A mechanism used for assessing the degree to which a provider competently and safely delivers clinical services that are appropriate for the patient in an optimal timeframe. It is a subset of the broader category of performance measures that conform to practice guidelines, medical review criteria, or standards of quality.

**Clinical risk management** The process of assessing potentially preventable defects in care and acting to mitigate those risks in a comprehensive and multistakeholder way that emphasizes systems thinking. Represents potential monetary losses or gains for providers, based on quality and cost performance that providers can reasonably manage with the proper safeguards in place (e.g., risk adjustment, stop loss, and other mechanisms).

**Cluster sampling** A technique used when natural but relatively heterogeneous groupings are evident in a statistical population. It is often used in marketing research. In this technique, the total population is divided into these groups or clusters and a simple random portion of the groups is selected.

**Common cause variation** Fluctuation caused by unknown factors resulting in a steady but random distribution of output around the average of the data. It is a measure of the process potential, or how well the process can perform when special cause variation is removed.

**Complex** The inclusion of a significant number of elements.

**Complex adaptive systems** Acknowledgment that groups of people create outcomes and effects that are far greater than prediction by summing up the resources and skills available within the group. Three concepts—independent agents, distributed control, and nonlinearity—create conditions for perpetual innovation.

**Complexity science** The study of complex adaptive systems—a field applied to healthcare to understand complex human organizations.

**Compliance** Deliberate and good-faith adherence to regulatory or statutory requirements. Often demonstrated through a program that formalizes processes and procedures to ensure this adherence. Conformity in fulfilling official requirements.

**Composite performance measure** Combination of two or more component quantifications, each of which individually reflects quality of care, into a single quantification with a single score. Also called a *composite measure*.

**Confidence interval** A type of estimate of a population parameter based on sampled data. It offers an estimated range of values likely to include this population parameter and a range wherein the true value is likely to fall based on those samples.

**Construct validity** The degree to which a measurement instrument correctly assesses the theoretical construct or trait that it was designed to measure (e.g., severity adjustment scales are tools for measuring staffing needs).

**Content validity** The degree to which a measurement instrument adequately represents the universe of content; includes judgments by experts or respondents about the degree to which the test measures the relevant construct. Also known as *face validity*.

**Continuous data** Set of data where the values can assume any value within a defined range.

**Continuous quality improvement** A process that continually monitors program performance. When a quality problem is identified, this develops a revised approach to that problem and monitors implementation and success of the revised approach. The process includes involvement at all stages by all organizations, which are affected by the problem and/or involved in implementing the revised approach.

**Continuous survey readiness** Attitude and value demonstrated throughout the organization in goals and practices that yield an uninterrupted state of mental preparedness throughout the organization. Staff are immediately physically ready or available to demonstrate compliance.

**Continuous variable** Measure score in which each individual value for the measure can fall anywhere along a continuous scale and can be aggregated using a variety of methods such as the calculation of a mean or median (e.g., mean number of minutes between presentation to the emergency department to the time of admission).

**Control chart** A type of data display that focuses attention on detecting and monitoring process variation over time; distinguishes special from common causes of variation; provides guidance for ongoing control of a process.

**Convenience sampling** A method of selecting a population that relies on a selection of subjects easily available to the researcher, instead of a randomized portion from the whole population.

**Corrective action plan** A step-by-step plan of action that is developed to achieve targeted outcomes for resolution of identified errors in an effort to (1) identify the most cost-effective actions that can be implemented to correct error causes; (2) develop and implement a plan of action to improve processes or methods so that outcomes are more effective and efficient; (3) achieve measurable improvement in the highest priority areas; and (4) eliminate repeated deficient practices. It is written in response to a survey, inspection, or gap analysis from assessments that define observations as well as recommendations for actions to achieve compliance for a given standard. Also known as a *plan of correction*, *improvement plan*, and *action plan*.

**Correlation** The extent to which variables relate.

**Cost** An amount, usually specified in dollars, related to receiving, providing, or paying for medical care. Things that contribute to it include visits to healthcare providers, healthcare services, equipment and supplies, and insurance premiums. This is a measure of total healthcare spending, which includes total resource use and unit prices, by payer or consumer, for a healthcare service or group of healthcare services, associated with a specified patient population, time, and unit(s) of clinical accountability.

**Cost–benefit analysis** An evaluation performed to determine the viability and broader benefits of proposed capital expenditures. It helps organizations better use financial and human resources and includes a timeframe to demonstrate the costs and benefits of the project over specific periods of time.

**Credentialing** The process of appointing or hiring physicians and other health professionals and granting privileges to licensed independent practitioners utilizing standard, empirically based criteria. These criteria may include peer review information and education and/or board certifications to ensure the practitioner is well qualified and able to deliver the highest quality care.

**Criterion-related validity** An assessment of the relationship between a measure and an outcome. It can be concurrent—referring to the outcome at the point a measure is assessed (i.e., a snapshot in time) or predictive—referring to the positive predictive power of a measure relative to some future event (e.g., the assessment of blood pressure as a predictor of later heart failure).

**Critical path method** A deterministic project management tool used to plan, monitor, and update the project as it progresses. It follows steps, uses network diagrams, schedules individual activities, and determines earliest to latest start and finish times for each activity. It focuses on time/cost tradeoffs.

**Cultural competence** A set of congruent behaviors, attitudes, and policies that come together in a system or agency or among professionals and enables that system, that agency, and those professionals to work effectively in cross-cultural situations.

**Cultural screen** A change management tool identifying and focusing on the aspects of change associated with the culture of the organization that should be assessed to achieve successful change.

**Culture** The set of shared attitudes, values, goals, and practices that characterizes a company or corporation. A system of beliefs and actions that characterize a group. It also refers to norms of behavior and shared values among a group of people. The social "glue" that holds people together. At the heart of this is the notion of shared values (what is important) and behavioral norms (the way things are done). They are described as strong when the core values are intensely held and widely shared.

**Culture of safety** An attitude that encompasses acknowledgment of the high-risk nature of an organization's activities and the determination to achieve consistently safe operations, a blame-free environment where individuals can report errors or near misses without fear of reprimand or punishment, encouragement of collaboration across ranks and disciplines to seek solutions to unsafe conditions, problems, and organizational commitment of resources to address concerns.

**Customer** Actual and potential users of an organization's products, programs, or services. This includes the end users of services as well as others who might be their immediate purchasers or users. These others might include distributors, agents, or organizations that further use services.

# D

**Dashboard** A collection of various individual metrics used to assess the performance of a product, service, or project. Often used to monitor standardized business processes.

**Data** A set of discrete values, either qualitative or quantitative. The abstract representation of things, facts, concepts, and instructions that are stored in a defined format and structure on a passive medium (e.g., paper, computer, microfilm).

**Deeming** Situation that occurs when CMS grants authority to accrediting organizations to determine, on CMS's behalf, whether the organization evaluated by the accrediting organization is following corresponding Medicare regulations.

**Deeming authority** Permission granted by the Centers for Medicare & Medicaid Services to accrediting organizations to determine, on CMS's behalf, whether an organization evaluated by the accrediting organization is following corresponding Medicare regulations.

**Delphi method** A combination of brainstorming, multivoting, and nominal group techniques. This technique is used when group members are not in one location; it is frequently conducted by mail and/or email when a meeting is not feasible.

**Denominator** The lower part of a fraction used to calculate a rate, proportion, or ratio. It can be the same as the initial population or a subset of the initial population to further constrain the population for measurement. Continuous variable measures do not have this, but instead define a measure population.

**Departmentation** How jobs are grouped together such as by function, product, or service, geography, and process or customer.

**Deployment chart** Document used to project schedules for complex tasks and their associated subtasks. It usually is used with a task for which the time for completion is known. The tool also is used to determine who has responsibility for the parts of a plan or project. This tool also is called a *planning grid*. The grid helps the group organize key steps in the project to reach milestones and the desired goal.

**Diagnosis-related group** A classification system that sorts patients by diagnosis, type of treatment, age, and other relevant criteria. Under the prospective payment system, hospitals are paid a set fee for treating patients in a single such category, regardless of the actual cost of care for the individual.

**Diagnostic error** The failure to establish an accurate and timely explanation of the patient's health problem(s) or to communicate that explanation to the patient.

**Diffusion** The process by which an innovation or new idea is communicated through certain channels over time among members of a social system.

**Disruptive innovation** Phenomenon by which an innovation transforms an existing market or sector by introducing simplicity, convenience, accessibility, and affordability where complication and high cost are considered the norm. Initially, this is formed in a specialized market that may appear unattractive or inconsequential to industry insiders, but eventually the new product or idea completely redefines the industry.

# E

**Effective** Producing expected results. Based on scientific knowledge of who will likely benefit and with a philosophy of restraint from providing care unlikely to benefit the patient.

**Efficient** Activities performed effectively with minimum of waste or unnecessary effort or producing a high ratio of results to resources (e.g., equipment, supplies, ideas, and energy). Efficiency of care can be measured by the cost of care associated with a specific level of performance.

**Electronic clinical quality measure** A measure that uses data from electronic health records and/or health information technology systems to measure healthcare quality. The Centers for Medicare & Medicaid Services uses this in a variety of quality reporting and incentive programs.

**Electronic health record** Electronic clinical documentation, results reporting and management, electronic prescribing, clinical decision support, barcoding, and patient engagement tools.

**Engagement** Actions an individual must take to obtain the greatest benefit from the healthcare services available to them.

**Empowerment** Sharing of effective power between formal leaders and lower ranked colleagues. Typically includes a higher level of information sharing, participation in decision making, and delegation of problem-solving authority at the level closest to a situation.

**Enterprise risk management** Comprehensive business decision-making process instituted and supported by the healthcare organization's board, executive management, and medical staff leadership. A comprehensive framework for making decisions that maximize value protection and creation by managing exposure and uncertainty and their connection to total value.

**Episode of care** All care related to a patient's condition over time, including prevention of disease, screening and assessment, appropriate treatment in any setting, and ongoing management.

**Equitable care** All individuals have access to affordable, high quality, culturally and linguistically appropriate care in a timely manner. This includes regular preventive care, in addition to emergency care, as well as mental health support. It does not vary based on a patient's individual characteristics like sex, gender identity, ethnicity, geographic location, or socioeconomic status.

**Evidence-based practice** The conscientious, explicit, and judicious use of current best evidence in making decisions about the care of patients.

**Expert sampling** Type of purposive selection that involves selecting specialists in each area because of their access to the information relevant to the study.

**External Quality Review Organization** An entity that states use to review the care provided by capitated managed care entities. Federal law and regulations require this of the states. These entities may be peer review organizations, another entity that meets peer review organization requirements, or a private accreditation body.

# F

**Failure mode and effects analysis** Preventive approach to identify failures and opportunities for error; can be used for processes as well as equipment. It is a systematic method of identifying and preventing failures before they occur.

**Feasibility** This principle makes sure that the information needed to calculate a measure is readily available so that the effort of measurement is worth it. The measures that best meet this challenge use electronic data that are routinely collected during the delivery of care.

**First-order change** Adjustment of variables (people, processes, technologies) within a system but without altering the structure of the system in which those variables occur.

**Flowchart** Graphical display of a process outlining the sequence and relationship of the pieces of the process.

**Focused professional practice evaluation** Privilege-specific competency assessment of a practitioner that is undertaken for all newly requested privileges and/or whenever a question arises regarding a practitioner's ability to provide safe, high-quality patient care.

**Focused review** An evaluation of processes or outcomes using preestablished criteria or indicators. Also known as *intensive review*.

**Force field analysis** Performance improvement technique to map the nature and relative strength of individual factors leading to, and opposing, the success of an improvement process.

**Frequency distribution** Graphical display indicating whether one or more processes are occurring. Bell curves, histograms, and 2 × 2 tables are all types of this display.

# G

**Goal** Broad, general statement specifying a purpose or desired outcome; may be more abstract than an objective (it can have several objectives). Establishing one of these is an early step in the strategic planning process and sets the direction for the activities to follow.

**Goal congruence** Integration of multiple goals, either within an organization or between multiple groups. It is a result of the alignment of aims to achieve an overarching mission.

**Green Belt** Member of a project team who assists with data collection and helps conduct Six Sigma projects under the direction of a Black Belt.

**Guideline** Systematically developed means of assisting with practitioner and patient decision making about appropriate healthcare for specific clinical circumstances.

# H

**Hawthorne effect** Change in behavior due to awareness of being observed.

**Hazard** Anything that increases the probability of an error, accident, or injury.

**Health data analytics** Approach to quality that converts data into information that is presented through compelling visualizations and journalist style narratives so that any audience, at any level, can clearly understand the stakes and the path.

**Health inequity** Differences in health outcomes between groups within a population that are systematic, avoidable, and unjust.

**Health information technology** Hardware, software, integrated technologies or related licenses, intellectual property, upgrades, or packaged solutions provided as services that are designed for or support the use by healthcare entities or patients for the electronic creation, maintenance, access, or exchange of health details.

**Healthcare Effectiveness Data and Information Set** One of the most widely used performance measure data sets, targeted toward health plans, wellness and health promotion, and disease management programs.

**Healthcare quality** Degree to which health services for individuals and populations increase the likelihood of desired health outcomes and are consistent with current professional knowledge. Quality of care is a measure of performance on specified aims (e.g., safety, timeliness, effectiveness, efficiency, equity, and patient centeredness).

**High reliability** Operating in complex, high-risk environments for extended periods without significant failures, accidents, or avoidable errors. Focus is on standard workflows for more predictable outcomes and level of performance.

**High reliability organization** An organization operating in an industry that is complex with high risk for harm that consistently performs at high levels of safety over long periods of time.

**Histogram** A tool used to illustrate the variability or distribution of data. It presents the measurement scale of values along its *x*-axis (broken into equal-sized intervals) and the frequency scale (as count or percent) along the *y*-axis.

**Hoshin planning** Japanese term for policy deployment; a component of the total quality management/quality improvement system used to ensure that the vision set forth by top management is being translated into planning objectives. Also includes the actions that both management and employees will take to accomplish long-term organizational strategic goals.

**Human factors** Knowledge of people's capabilities and limitations in the design of products, processes, systems, and work environments that affect health and safety. For example, employee attitudes, motivation, health (physical and psychological), education, training, and cognitive functioning can influence the likelihood of a medical error.

# I

**Immediate jeopardy** Mechanism to escalate crisis survey issues immediately within both state and federal agencies and with the healthcare provider. It is determined when a crisis in which the health and safety of individual(s) are at immediate risk is identified.

**Incentive and penalty programs** A series of programs created by healthcare payers that are composed of incentives and reductions for payment (referred to as *adjustments* by the Centers for Medicare & Medicaid Services). At their inception, most programs offer an inducement to participate; currently, however, most of the federal and state programs associated with Medicare and Medicaid are entering the negative adjustment phase of such programs.

**Information** The result of data that are translated into results, as well as statements that are useful for decision making. For it to be meaningful, data must be considered within the context of how they were obtained and how they are to be used.

**Innovation** Making meaningful change to improve an organization's services, processes, and organizational effectiveness and to create new value for stakeholders.

**Instruments** Devices that quality professionals and researchers use to obtain and record data received from the subjects. They can include questionnaires, surveys, rating scales, interview transcripts, and the like. It is critical to use the most credible tools possible (those with proven reliability and validity).

**Insurance/actuarial risk** Unpredictable outcomes or losses that result from outlier patients in a provider's panel who have unusual and expensive conditions.

**Integratedness** The degree to which organized programs and practices deliver physical health and behavioral health prevention, address social determinants of health, and provide therapeutic services to individuals and populations.

**Integration** Harmonization of plans, processes, information, resource decisions, workforce capability and capacity, actions, results, and analyses to support organization-wide goals.

**Interoperability** Ensures that health-related information flows seamlessly; refers to the architecture and standards that make it possible for diverse EHR systems to work compatibly in a true information network.

**Interpercentile measures** Measures of variability; the most common is the *interquartile range*, a stable measure of variability based on excluding extreme scores and using only middle cases. A common example is growth charts. Clinical pathways are developed based on the interquartile range of the designated population.

**Interrater reliability** Degree to which two raters, operating independently, assign the same ratings in the context of observational research or in coding qualitative materials.

**Interrelationship diagram** Drawing that organizes a complex problem by sorting and displaying the cause and effect relationships among its various aspects.

**Interval data** Data that are measured along a scale where there is equal distance between data points (e.g., the values on a Fahrenheit thermometer).

# J

**Journey to zero** Innovative strategies to eradicate hospital-associated infections through a process of laying the foundation (sizing the burden), crafting a multipronged strategy (establishing frontline awareness and minimizing pathogen opportunity), and ensuring sustainable success and promoting long-term gains.

**Just culture** Awareness by everyone throughout the organization about the inevitability of medical errors; but all errors and unintended events are reported, even when the events do not cause patient injury. A culture of safety balances learning and accountability for behavioral choices with organizational and individual values and fosters transparency, trust, and open communication—all which promote the delivery of highly reliable, safe, and quality care. It is further defined as organizational accountability for the systems designed and employee accountability for the choices they make.

**Just in time** Production method that leverages the cellular manufacturing layout to significantly reduce inventory and work in process. It enables a company to produce the products its customers want, when they want them, in the amount they want.

# K

**Kaizen** A long-term approach to work that systematically seeks to achieve incremental changes to improve efficiency and quality. It focuses on removing process waste and maximizing value to the customer (e.g., patient, family).

**Knowledge management** The process of recording, storing, categorizing, and socializing information within an organization.

# L

**Leadership** Ability to influence an individual or group toward achievement of goals; determining the correct direction or path.

**Lean** A fundamental paradigm shift from conventional "batch and queue" mass production to product-aligned "one-piece flow" pull production that rearranges production activities in a way that processing steps of different types are conducted immediately adjacent to each other in a continuous flow.

**Lean enterprise** A system that uses value stream analysis (a tool for exposing waste), root cause analysis (a method for pursuing perfection), and new technologies to facilitate more efficient practices. The major focus is to eliminate waste in the following areas: production, waiting time, inappropriate processing, inventory, transporting, and defects.

**Learning healthcare system** A system designed to generate and apply the best evidence for the collaborative healthcare choices of each patient and provider; to drive the process of discovery as a natural outgrowth of patient care; and to ensure innovation, quality, safety, and value in healthcare.

**Learning organization** A place where people continually expand their capacity to create the results they truly desire, where new and expansive patterns of thinking are nurtured, where collective aspiration is set free, and where people are continually learning to see the whole together.

**Level of significance** The probability of observing a difference ($p$) as large as the one found in a study when, in fact, there is no true difference between the groups (i.e., when the null hypothesis is true).

# M

**Managed care** A plan that integrates the financing and delivery of appropriate healthcare services to covered individuals by means of arrangements with selected providers to furnish a comprehensive set of healthcare services to members, explicit criteria for the selection of healthcare providers, and significant financial incentives for members to use providers and procedures associated with the plan. These plans typically are labeled as health maintenance organizations (staff, group, independent practice association, and mixed models), preferred provider organizations, or point-of-service plans. The services are reimbursed via a variety of methods including capitation, fee for service, and a combination of the two. A healthcare delivery system organized to manage cost, utilization, and quality.

**Management information system** A system that contains both the manual and the automated methods that provide information for decision making. However, the term, as it commonly is used, refers to an automated or computerized system. Other names include *data-processing structure*, *medical information system*, *hospital information system*, and *decision support system*.

**Matrix diagram** Visual aid that permits a team to methodically discover and analyze the relationships between two or more sets of information. A rating system is used, which helps to identify patterns of responsibilities. This visual provides clarity and helps a team reach consensus. Provides structure for decision making.

**Mean** The sum of all scores or values divided by the total number of scores. Also known as the *average*.

**Measure** A mechanism to assign a quantity to an attribute by comparison to a criterion. It may stand alone or belong to a composite, subset, set, and/or collection of measures. In healthcare, it is a way to calculate whether and how often the healthcare system does what it should. Measures are based on scientific evidence about processes, outcomes, perceptions, or systems that relate to high-quality care.

**Measurement** Systematic process of data collection, repeated over time or at a single point in time.

**Median** The number that divides a set of numerically ordered data into a lower and an upper half; also considered the 50th percentile.

**Medical error** An event that caused or could have caused harm to a patient and which could have been prevented given the current state of medical knowledge and processes in place to prevent the event.

**Mission** An organization's purpose or reason for existing. A mission statement answers such questions as "Why are we here?" "Whom do we serve?" and "What do we do?"

**Mistake proofing** Use of process or design features to prevent errors or the negative impact of errors; also known as *poka-yoke*.

**Misuse** Situation that occurs when patients receive appropriate medical services provided poorly, adding to the risk for preventable complications.

**Mode** The value that occurs most frequently within a defined set of numbers.

**Moonshot** A difficult or expensive task, the outcome of which is expected to have great significance.

**Morbidity** In common clinical usage, any disease state, including diagnosis and complications.

**Morbidity rate** Disease rate or proportion of diseased people in a population. The number of people ill during a time period divided by the number of people in the total population.

**Mortality rate** Death rate often made explicit for a characteristic (e.g., gender, sex, or specific cause of death). It contains three essential elements: the number of people in a population exposed to the risk of death, a time factor, and the number of deaths occurring in the exposed population during a certain period.

**Multiple regression analysis** Exercise that estimates the effects of two or more independent variables ($x$) on a dependent measure ($y$).

**Multivoting** An easy method for prioritizing items on a list in a team setting. This method builds consensus using a series of votes to reduce the list to a more manageable size.

# N

**Never event** A medical error that should never occur (e.g., wrong-site surgery); this informal term is often used in place of serious reportable event. Eliminating harm completely is important but difficult to do.

**Nominal data** A set of data distinguished by a name that has no intrinsic relational meaning. For example, ethnicity is nominal whereas temperatures are not.

**Nominal group technique** A collaborative decision-making process for generating many ideas in which people initially work by themselves. Also known as *brainwriting*.

**Nonparametric tests** A type of statistical test that does not require the population's distribution to be characterized by certain parameters. These tests are used when there is no assumption that the population is normally distributed, for example.

**Nonprobability sampling** A method that provides no way of estimating the probability that each element will be included in the sample. When this approach is used, the results will be representative of the sample only and cannot be generalized to the available population. Examples include convenience, snowball, purposive or judgment, expert, and quota.

**Numerator** The upper portion of a fraction used to calculate a rate, proportion, or ratio. Also called *measure focus*; it is the target process, condition, event, or outcome. Criteria are the processes or outcomes expected for each patient, procedure, or other unit of measurement defined in the denominator.

# O

**Objective** A specific statement that details how goals will be achieved and are narrow and concrete. An objective represents the organization's commitment to achieving specific outcomes.

**Ongoing professional practice evaluation** A documented summary of ongoing data collected for assessing a practitioner's clinical competence and professional behavior. The information gathered during this process factors into decisions to maintain, revise, or revoke existing privileges.

**Ordinal data** Statistical ranking such as nursing staff rank (nurse level 1, nurse level 2), educational level (BS, MS, MD), or attitude toward a research scale (strongly agree, agree, neutral, disagree, strongly disagree). No assumption is made that the distances between the points are the same.

**Organizational learning** A pattern of learning carried out in organizations skilled at creating, acquiring, and transferring knowledge and at modifying behavior to reflect new knowledge and insights. Includes both continuous improvement of existing approaches and significant change or innovation, leading to new goals, approaches, products, and markets.

**Outcome** The result of the performance (or nonperformance) of a function or process. The results of care (e.g., increased satisfaction, decreased morbidity, improved quality of life or well-being) or the change in a patient's current and future health status that can be attributed to antecedent healthcare. A measure that assesses the results of healthcare that are experienced by patients: clinical events, recovery and health status, experiences in the health system, and efficiency/cost.

**Outcome measure** A quantified result of healthcare that is experienced by patients: clinical events, recovery and health status, experiences in the health system, and efficiency/cost.

**Overuse** Repeated use of therapy when additional applications have not been proven to be medically necessary or therapeutically beneficial.

# P

**Parametric tests** Statistical tests that assume an underlying data set is normally distributed (i.e., follows the bell curve).

**Pareto chart** A simple bar chart used to prioritize a series of problems or possible causes of problems. It displays a series of bars that are shown in decreasing order of occurrence. The bars clearly display the priority for problem solving. Also known as a *Pareto diagram*.

**Patient** The person who is registered for and/or uses healthcare services such as client, resident, consumer, customer, stakeholder, recipient, or partner.

**Patient and family-centered care** Meaningful interpersonal relationships between the patient and the provider(s) and honoring the whole person and family; respecting individual values, preferences, and choices; and ensuring continuity of care with the goal of ensuring a positive patient experience; also may be referred to as *patient and family-engaged care*.

**Patient safety** Any improvement effort focused on preventing medical errors; prevention and mitigation from harm; the degree to which the healthcare environment is free from hazards or dangers.

**Patient safety organization** An entity that collects and analyzes data, reports, educates, and advocates for the reduction of medical errors; privilege and confidentiality protections are conferred to providers who work with such entities.

**Patient safety practice** Type of process or structure whose application reduces the probability of adverse events resulting from exposure to the healthcare system across the range of diseases and procedures.

**Patient safety solution** Any system design or intervention that has demonstrated the ability to prevent or mitigate patient harm stemming from the processes of healthcare.

**Pay for performance** A healthcare payment system in which providers receive incentives for meeting or exceeding quality—and sometimes cost—benchmarks. Some systems also penalize providers who do not meet established benchmarks. The goal of these programs is to improve the quality of care over time.

**Payment models** Formulas for reimbursing healthcare providers (e.g., hospitals, physicians).

**Peer review** An episode of care assessment that is conducted to improve the quality of patient care or the use of healthcare resources. It is a process protected by statute in most states, although this varies, and by federal statute for federal healthcare facilities. A peer is generally defined as a healthcare professional with comparable education, training, experience, licensure, or similar clinical privileges or scope of practice.

**Peer review organization** An organization funded by the U.S. Department of Health and Human Services to determine the appropriateness and quality of medical care provided to Medicare beneficiaries.

**Percentile** A number that corresponds to one of the equal divisions of the range of a variable in a sample and that characterizes a value of the variable as not exceeded by a specified percentage of all the values in the sample (e.g., a score higher that 95 percent of those attained is said to be in the 95th percentile).

**Performance** The way in which an individual, group, or organization conducts or accomplishes its important functions or processes.

**Performance and process improvement** Setting goals, implementing changes, measuring outcomes and results to achieve better results, and spreading and/or sustaining the better results. This approach applies to any healthcare services.

**Performance assessment** The analysis and interpretation of performance measurement data to transform it into useful information for purposes of continuous performance improvement.

**Performance improvement projects** Projects that examine and seek to achieve better results in major areas of clinical and nonclinical services. These projects are usually based on information such as enrollee characteristics, standardized measures, utilization, diagnosis and outcome information, data from surveys, grievances, appeals, and other processes. A project measures performance at two periods of time to ascertain if improvement has occurred.

**Performance management** Strategy to promote change in organizational culture, systems, and processes by helping to set agreed upon performance goals, allocating and prioritizing resources, informing managers to either confirm or change current policy or program direction to meet those goals, and sharing results of performance in pursuing those goals.

**Performance measures** A gauge used to assess the execution of a process or function of any organization. Quantitative or qualitative measures of the care and services delivered to patients (process) or the result of that care and services (outcomes). They can be used to assess other aspects of an individual or organization such as access and availability of care, utilization of care, health plan stability, patient characteristics, and other structural and operational aspects of healthcare services.

**Performance monitoring** Tracking the impact and effectiveness of a quality improvement action, including collecting and analyzing qualitative or quantitative data.

**Permanent harm** An event or condition that reaches the individual, resulting in any level of harm that permanently alters and/or affects an individual's baseline.

**Person and family-centered care** Respectful care that is responsive to patient preferences, needs, and values and ensures that patient values guide all clinical decisions; meaningful interpersonal relationships between the patient and the provider(s) and honoring the whole person and family; respecting individual values, preferences, and choices; and ensuring continuity of care with the goal of ensuring a positive patient experience. Also referred to as *patient and family-centered care*.

**Pilot testing** Measurement testing that is divided into two main types: alpha testing (also called *formative testing*) and beta testing (also called *field testing*).

**Plan-Do-Check-Act** A four-step process designed to continuously improve quality, originally conceived by Shewhart.

**Plan-Do-Study-Act** A later adaptation by Deming of the plan-do-check-act cycle; also referred to as the *Deming cycle* or the *Deming wheel*.

**Population** Any complete group (e.g., all residents of a community, all cases that meet a designated set of criteria for practitioners, all registered nurses).

**Population health** Outcomes for a group of individuals including outcomes within a group. Maintaining the health and wellness of populations depends on determinants of health, including medical care, public health, genetics, personal behaviors and lifestyle, and a broad range of social, environmental, and economic factors.

**Population health improvement** Efforts to improve health, well-being, and equity for defined or place-based populations.

**Population health management** Design, delivery, coordination, and payment of high-quality healthcare services for a population using the best resources available within the healthcare system; may also be referred to as population medicine.

**Possible, Implement, Challenge, and Kill** Lean tool used to categorize ideas and solutions based on a rough estimate of return on investment. Referred to as PICK chart, it is also called *ease impact matrix* or *impact effort matrix*.

**Preventive care** Healthcare that emphasizes the early detection and treatment of diseases. The focus on prevention is intended to keep people healthier for longer, thus reducing healthcare costs over the long term.

**Prioritization matrix** A tool that organizes tasks, issues, or actions and ranks them based on agreed-upon criteria. The tool combines the tree diagram and the *L*-shaped matrix diagram, displaying the best possible effect.

**Private reporting** Sharing quality measurement results with internal stakeholders only, such as within a single health system.

**Probability sampling** Method of selection in which every item in the population has an equal chance of being selected for inclusion.

**Process** The set of activities that go on within and between practitioners and patients. Goal-directed, interrelated series of actions, events, mechanisms, or steps.

**Process analysis** An industrial quality improvement technique used to improve clinical or administrative outcomes by analyzing its procedures. For example, it occurs whenever a group of individuals diagrams a healthcare course of action.

**Process decision program chart** Map of the identified events and contingencies that can occur between the time a problem is stated and the time it is solved. It attempts to identify potential deviations from the desired process, allowing the team to anticipate and prevent the deviation.

**Process flowchart** See *Flowchart*.

**Process improvement** Methodology utilized to make a course of action better using continuous methods.

**Process map** See *Flowchart*.

**Process measure** A gauge that focuses on a sequence of actions or steps that should be followed to provide high-quality evidence-based care. There should be a scientific basis for believing that the process, when executed well, will increase the probability of achieving a desired outcome.

**Program Evaluation and Review Technique** A probabilistic project management tool used to plan, monitor, and update the project as it progresses. It follows steps, uses network diagrams, schedules individual activities, and determines earliest to latest start and finish times for each activity.

**Project** An endeavor involving a connected sequence of activities and a range of resources designed to achieve specific outcomes considering the constraints of time, costs, and quality used to introduce change.

**Project management** Application of a collection of tools and techniques to direct the use of resources to accomplish a unique, complex, one-time task within time, cost, and quality constraints.

**Project selection matrix** Tool that ranks and compares potential project areas for implementation. Ranking criteria may include organizational and strategic goals, potential fiscal impact to the organization, effect on patient and employee satisfaction, likelihood of success, and completion within a specified timeframe.

**Propensity score matching** A multivariate approach to pairing up people with the same characteristics in the intervention and control groups to eliminate potential impact of variation between the groups due to their not being equal.

**Proportion** A score derived by dividing the number of cases that meet a criterion for quality (the numerator) by the number of eligible cases within a given timeframe (the denominator), where the numerator cases are a subset of the denominator cases (for example, percentage of eligible women with a mammogram performed in the last year).

**Public reporting** Sharing quality measurement results with the general public, such as through a website or printed report.

**Purposive sampling** Method in which a group or groups are selected based on certain criteria. It is subjective, because the researcher uses his or her judgment to decide who is representative of the population. Also known as *judgment sampling*.

# Q

**Quadruple Aim** See *Triple Aim*.

**Quality** Product performance that results in customer satisfaction; freedom from product deficiencies which avoid customer dissatisfaction.

**Quality assurance** The process of looking at how well a healthcare service is provided. The process may include formally reviewing healthcare given to a person or group of persons, locating the problem, correcting the problem, and then checking to see what worked.

**Quality control** A process to ensure that product excellence is maintained or improved. It involves testing units and determining if they are within the specifications for the final product. Charts are used to help standardize processes and limit errors.

**Quality function deployment** Focused methodology for carefully listening to the voice of the customer and then effectively responding to those needs and expectations. Also called *matrix product planning*, *decision matrices*, and *customer-driven engineering*.

**Quality improvement** A means by which high performance is achieved at unprecedented levels by establishing the infrastructure needed; identifying the specific areas for making things better; establishing clear accountability for bringing projects to a successful conclusion; and providing the resources, motivation, and training needed by the teams (e.g., to diagnose the causes, stimulate establishment of a remedy, and establish controls to hold the gains).

**Quality management** A strategic, integrated management system, which involves all managers and employees and uses quantitative methods to continuously improve an organization's processes to meet and exceed customer needs, wants, and expectations.

**Quality measure** Numeric quantification of healthcare quality for a designated accountable healthcare entity, such as a hospital, health plan, nursing home, or clinician. A healthcare performance measure is a way to calculate whether and how often the healthcare system does what it should. Measures are based on scientific evidence about processes, outcomes, perceptions, or systems that relate to care.

**Quality professional** Person who works in a healthcare setting to enhance care delivery, optimize value, and improve outcomes by leading activities in one or more of the following core quality functions: quality leadership and integration, quality review and accountability, regulatory and accreditation, patient safety, performance and process improvement, health data analytics, and population health and care transitions.

**Quantity** Units of medical care production defined by treatments of disease or treated episodes of illness usually used to estimate price, costs, and output of medical care.

**Quota sampling** Method whereby the researcher makes a judgment about the best type of selection for the investigation and specifies characteristics of the selection to increase its representativeness.

# R

**Random sample** A group selected for study, which is drawn at random from the universe of cases by a statistically valid method.

**Range** The difference between the highest and lowest values in a distribution of scores; usually expressed as a maximum and minimum.

**Rapid cycle improvement** The strategy whereby organizations collaborate to identify and prioritize aims for improvement and gain access to methods, tools, and materials that will enable them to conduct sophisticated, evidence-based quality improvement activities that they could not conduct individually.

**Ratio** A score derived by dividing a count of one type of data by a count of another type of data (e.g., the number of patients with central lines who develop infection divided by the number of central line days).

**Ratio data** Values where the distance between each point is equal and there is a true zero (e.g., weight and height).

**Readiness** The state of being prepared mentally or physically for an experience or action, immediately available, or prepared for immediate use.

**Red Rules** Rules that must be followed to the letter; if there is a condition or situation that poses risk, this type of rule stops the line.

**Reengineering** Efforts focused on workforce redesign or on the restructuring of systems and departments into more efficient processes.

**Regression analysis** Statistical procedure to predict outcomes based on the identification of individual variables and how they interact (jointly and severally) with the process being measured.

**Regulations** Requirements issued by various governmental agencies to conduct the intent of legislation enacted by Congress, state legislatures, and local authorities. Compliance with regulations is mandatory by law.

**Reliability** The extent to which an experiment, test, or measuring procedure yields the same results under similar circumstances by the same or different individuals on repeated trials. It is also referred to as *precision*, *reproducibility*, and *repeatability*.

**Reliability coefficient** Numerical index of the test's reliability. The closer the coefficient is to 1.0, the more reliable the tool. In general, reliability coefficients of ≥ 0.70 are considered acceptable, although ≥ 0.80 is desired. The reliability coefficient can be determined by evaluating the internal consistency of a measure.

**Resilience** Process of adapting well in the face of adversity, trauma, tragedy, threats, or even significant sources of stress—such as family and relationship problems, serious health problems, or workplace and financial stressors. It means "bouncing back" from difficult experiences. Represents the ability to use positive mental skills to remain psychologically steady and focused when faced with challenges or adversity and the ability to withstand, recover, and grow in the face of stressors and changing demands.

**Resource use** Combination of goods and services to produce medical care. It can be measured and predicted when a procedure is done many times (e.g., people and things needed to perform cataract surgery are a set of resources). The goods and services are inputs that have a price assigned to them.

**Reversibility** Ability to stop the adoption or use of the innovation and return to a normal or safe position if the innovation is not effective.

**Risk adjustment** Technique used to adjust payments to providers in a manner that adjusts for the fact that different patients with the same diagnosis have conditions or characteristics that affect how well they respond to treatment.

**Risk management** Strategies deployed to protect the organization from unintended negative consequences including financial losses; organized effort to identify, assess, and reduce, where appropriate, risk to patients, visitors, staff, and organizational assets. See also *Enterprise risk management*.

**Robust process improvement** Combination of Lean, Six Sigma, and change management as a new set of tools to achieve high reliability and maintain patient safety

**Root cause analysis** A range of approaches, tools, and techniques used to uncover the true causes of problems.

**Root Cause Analysis and Assessment** To improve the effectiveness and to prevent future harm, necessary actions coupled with the uncovering of the true causes of problems need to be put in place.

**Run chart** A graphic display of data points over time; also called a *trend chart*. Run charts are control charts without the control limits.

# S

**Safe care** Way to reduce harm and avoid patient injury during the process of care or treatment intended to help them.

**Sample** A small number of cases or events that is used to make statements about a population. Researchers use these to make statistical inferences about the population when the population is too large to study in its entirety.

**Sanctions** Administrative remedies and actions (e.g., exclusion, civil monetary penalties) available to the office of the inspector general to deal with questionable, improper, or abusive behaviors of providers under Medicare, Medicaid, or any state health programs.

**SBAR** Acronym for situation, background, assessment, recommendation, which is an evidence-based standardized tool used in healthcare settings to facilitate communication.

**Scatter diagram** A tool used to display possible causes and effects. Can determine the extent to which two variables (quality effects or process causes) relate to one another. Often used in combination with fishbone or Pareto diagrams or charts.

**Scatter plot** A method of graphing two related continuous variables by showing a dot on the perpendicular intersection of values on the *XY* axis where the *x*-axis is a horizontal number line and the *y*-axis is a vertical number line. For example, a patient's temperature may be displayed with a scatter plot by putting the date or time on one axis and the temperature on the other.

**Second-order change** A complex change that requires a significant alteration in thinking and behavior. Also known as an *out-of-the-box change*.

**Sensitivity** The proportion of actual positives that are correctly identified as such (for example, the percentage of people with diabetes who are correctly identified as having diabetes). See also *Specificity*.

**Sentinel event** A patient safety event (not primarily related to the natural course of the patient's illness or underlying condition) that reaches a patient and results in death, severe harm (regardless of duration of harm), or permanent harm (regardless of severity of harm). An event can also be considered sentinel if the event signaled the need for immediate investigation and response.

**Serious reportable adverse events** Also known as *never events*. The Centers for Medicare & Medicaid Services withholds payment to hospitals if any of these events occurs in an acute care facility.

**Severe harm** An event or condition that reaches the individual, resulting in life-threatening bodily injury (including pain or disfigurement) that interferes with or results in loss of functional ability or quality of life that requires continuous physiological monitoring or a surgery, invasive procedure, or treatment to resolve the condition.

**Severity factors** The presence of additional diagnoses that helps to define the severity of a group of patients within a diagnosis-related group, on an individual patient level, or both. A component of risk adjustment.

**Severity of harm** In a failure mode and effects analysis, an estimation of how serious the effects or harm would be if a given failure did occur.

**Simple random sampling** A method in which everyone in the sampling frame (all subjects in the population) has an equal chance of being chosen (e.g., pulling a name out of a hat containing all possible names).

**SIPOC** Means of identifying key drivers of a process using process management (Supplier Input Process Output Customer).

**Six Sigma** An established improvement methodology that uses statistical analysis and other methods to eliminate defects in business processes. It is named after six standard deviations from the mean of a normal curve. At this point on a curve of defects, there are only 3.4 defects per million opportunities.

**Snowball sampling** Subtype of convenience sampling that allows subjects to suggest other subjects for inclusion in the study, so that the sample size increases. This is often used when subjects are difficult to identify but are known to others through an informal network.

**Social determinants of health** Nonmedical factors that influence health outcomes. They are the conditions in which people are born, grow, live, work, and age, as well as a wider set of forces and systems shaping the conditions of daily life.

**Spaghetti diagram** A graphic representation of the flow of traffic or movement. Also called a *layout diagram*.

**Special-cause variation** In statistical process control, a variation in performance that falls outside the control limits or when an obvious nonrandom pattern occurs in a process. This type of variation requires investigation.

**Specification** The technical instructions for how to build and calculate a measure. They describe a measure's building blocks: numerator, denominator, exclusions, target population, how results might be split to show differences across groups (stratification scheme), risk adjustment methodology, how results are calculated (calculation algorithm), sampling methodology, data source, level of analysis, how data are attributed to providers and/or hospitals (attribution model), and care setting.

**Specificity** As a statistical term, this refers to the proportion of negatives that are correctly identified (for example, the percentage of healthy people who are correctly identified as not having the condition). Perfect specificity would mean that the measure recognizes all actual negatives (for example, all healthy people will be recognized as healthy). See also *Sensitivity*.

**Spread** The intentional and methodical expansion of the number and type of people, units, or organizations using the improvements; based on theory and application on diffusion of innovation (knowledge, persuasion, decision, implementation, and confirmation).

**Stakeholder** Any person or group that are or might be affected by an organization's actions and success. Examples include customers, the workforce, partners, collaborators, governing boards, stockholders, donors, suppliers, taxpayers, regulatory bodies, policy makers, funders, and local and professional communities.

**Standard deviation** The dispersion of a data set around the mean. It suggests variability in normally distributed data; lower rates suggest more of the data points cluster around the mean, whereas higher rates suggest broader dispersion of values around the mean. Represented by sigma (e.g., in Six Sigma approaches).

**Standards** Evidence-based guidelines developed and established by consensus or research of an authoritative body. They are used as a guide for optimum achievement and outcomes. Compliance is voluntary, though they may be named in regulations, thereby granting them legal status.

**Statistical process control** Measurement of randomly selected outputs of a process to determine whether the process is affected by special-cause variation. It is applied to monitor and control a process per customer expectations and business science, ensuring that the process operates at its full potential.

**Steward** The person responsible for the fitness and management of data elements within an organization. Also called *measure owner*, this is an individual or organization that owns a measure and is responsible for maintaining the measure. This person is often the same as a measure developer, but not always. They are also the ongoing point of contact for people interested in each measure.

**Strategic goal** A broadly stated or long-term outcome written as an overall statement that relates to a philosophy, a purpose, or a desired outcome.

**Strategic objective** A specific statement written in measurable and observable terms using quantitative and qualitative measurement criteria. Written as an action-oriented statement, it indicates the minimum acceptable level of performance and specific time limit or degree of accuracy.

**Strategic planning** Development and codification of a major direction for an organization's future.

**Strategy** The plans and activities developed by an organization in pursuit of its goals and objectives, particularly about positioning itself to meet external demands relative to its competition.

**Stratification** The division of a population or resource services into distinct, independent groups of similar data, enabling analysis of the specific subgroups. This type of adjustment can show where disparities exist or where there is a need to expose differences in results.

**Stratification chart** A tool designed to show where a problem does and does not occur or to demonstrate underlying patterns.

**Stratified random sampling** Method in which a population is divided into categories (e.g., patients with particular diseases), and each member of every category has an equal probability of being selected.

**Structural measure** Mechanism that assesses features of a healthcare organization or clinician relevant to its capacity for healthcare delivery.

**Structure** The resources available for care delivery and system design.

**System** A group of interacting, interdependent, or interrelated elements that function as independent agents according to a set of rules to form a unified or complex whole influenced by the environment in its functioning.

**Systematic sampling** Method in which, after the first case is randomly selected, every $n$th element from a population is selected (e.g., picking every third name from a list of possible names).

**Systemness** The ability to implement cohesive system-oriented approaches.

**Systems perspective** Managing all the parts of an organization as a unified whole to achieve the mission and strive toward the vision.

# T

**t-Test** Statistical method to analyze the difference between two means to determine whether the difference between them is significant; a distinction must be made regarding the two groups.

**Target population** The numerator (cases) and denominator (population sample meeting specified criteria) of the measure.

**Team** A group of people who are interdependent with respect to information, resources, and skills and who seek to combine their efforts to achieve a common goal.

**Teamwork** A dynamic process involving two or more health professionals with complementary backgrounds and skills, sharing common health goals, and exercising concerted physical and mental effort in assessing, planning, or evaluating patient care.

**Test–retest reliability** An evaluation of a test determined by administering the test to a sample on two occasions and then comparing the scores.

**Timely care** Care in which wait times and harmful delays for those who receive and provide care are eliminated.

**Top box score** The sum of percentages for the top one, two, or three highest points on a purchase intent, satisfaction, or awareness scale. Consumer Assessment of Healthcare Providers and Systems results are publicly reported on the Centers for Medicare & Medicaid Services Care Compare webpage as top-box, bottom-box, and middle-box scores. The top-box is the most positive response.

**Total productive maintenance** Method that seeks to engage all levels and functions in an organization to maximize the overall effectiveness of production equipment. This method further tunes up existing processes and equipment by reducing mistakes and accidents and seeks to involve workers in all departments and levels to ensure effective equipment operation.

**Total quality** An attitude or an orientation that permeates an entire organization and the way that an organization performs its internal and external business. It integrates fundamental management techniques, existing improvement efforts, and the use of technical tools utilizing a disciplined statistical quality control.

**Total quality management** An approach to organizational development and change that ensures that the organization meets or exceeds customer expectations. It is a strategic, integrated management system that involves all managers and employees and uses quantitative methods to continuously improve an organization's processes to meet and exceed customer needs, wants, and expectations. The four principles are: do it right the first time to eliminate costly rework; listen to and learn from customers and employees; make continuous quality improvement an everyday matter; and build teamwork, trust, and mutual respect. Also known as *total quality control*.

**Tracer** A self-assessment methodology designed to follow the care experiences that a patient had while at an organization. It is a way to analyze the organization's system of providing care, treatment, or services using actual patients as the framework for assessing standards compliance. Can be individual, system, or focused.

**Transparency** Communicating and operating in such a way that it is easy for others to see what actions are performed; the full, accurate, and timely disclosure of information. For safe healthcare, such openness and accountability are needed among staff, between caregivers and patients, among institutions, and in public reporting.

**Tree diagram** A method that maps out the full range of paths and tasks involved in a process and must be accomplished to achieve a goal; resembles an organizational chart.

**Trialability** The degree to which an innovation can be tested on a small scale.

**Triple Aim** A framework that includes improving better care, smarter spending, and healthier populations. Workforce engagement may be added as a fourth aim.

**True North** A key concept in Lean process improvement that emerged from Toyota and connotes the compass needle for Lean transformation. True North works like a compass, providing a guide to take an organization from the current condition to where it wants to be.

# U

**Underuse** Situation in which patients do not receive beneficial health services (e.g., heart attack victims not receiving beta-blockers).

**Usability** Principle that checks those users of a measure—employers, patients, providers, hospitals, and health plans—who will be able to understand the measure's results and find them useful for quality improvement and decision making.

**Utilization management** An organized, comprehensive approach to analyze, direct, and conserve organizational resources to provide care that is high quality and cost-effective (e.g., medical necessity appropriateness review; discharge planning and monitoring; overutilization and underutilization surveillance; and identification of overutilization and underutilization).

# V

**Validation** The process by which the integrity and correctness of data are established. These processes can occur immediately after a data item is collected or after a complete set of data is collected.

**Validity** Degree to which an instrument measures what it is intended to measure. It usually is more difficult to establish than reliability.

**Value** A subjective weighing of costs against the health outcomes achieved, including patient satisfaction and quality of life. It is the measure of a specified stakeholder's preference-weighted assessment of a particular combination of quality and cost of care performance (e.g., patients, consumer organizations, payers, providers, governments, or societies).

**Value stream mapping** A map of the process in which only value-added steps for the customer are retained and waste removed. This Lean tool analyzes a process from a systems perspective and creates a visual depiction of the sequential steps in a process from beginning to end.

**Values statement** Written description of what the organization believes in and how it will behave. It defines the deeply held beliefs and principles of the organizational culture. These core values are an internalized framework that is shared and acted on by leadership.

**Variability** Degree to which values on a set of scores differ.

**Variation analysis** Method to identify the contributors to a process that results in consistently inconsistent results.

The contributors to variation include clinical factors, patient characteristics, data collection procedures, or organizational attributes like staffing levels.

**Virtual lifetime electronic record** A digital health record program that tracks the medical history of American soldiers through their entire service, from active duty to veteran status.

**Vision** An organization's statement of its goals for the future, described in measurable terms that clarify the direction for everyone in the organization. Through leadership, it guides an organization's direction, which is built upon its mission.

**Voice of the customer** Tool used at the start of any new product, process, or service design initiative to understand better the customer's wants and needs. It can serve as key input for new product definition, quality function deployment, or the setting of detailed design specifications.

# W

**Wellness** A dynamic and ongoing process involving self-awareness and healthy choices resulting in a successful, balanced lifestyle.

**Work motivation** The psychological forces that determine the direction of a person's behavior in an organization, a person's level of effort, and a person's level of persistence.

# Bibliography

The Advisory Board Company. *The Journey to Zero: Innovative Strategies for Minimizing Hospital-Acquired Infections.* Washington, DC: Author; 2008.

Agency for Healthcare Research and Quality. PSNet: artificial intelligence and diagnostic errors. Published January 31, 2020. Accessed December 14, 2021. https://psnet.ahrq.gov/perspective/artificial-intelligence-and-diagnostic-errors#_ednref1

American Heart Association Center for Workplace Health Research and Evaluation. Resilience in the workplace: an evidence review and implications for practice. Accessed May 15, 2022. https://www.heart.org/-/media/Data-Import/downloadables/5/2/D/RESILIENCE-IN-THE-WORKPLACE-UCM_496856.pdf

American Hospital Association. Checklists to improve patient safety. Accessed May 15, 2022. https://www.aha.org/ahahret-guides/2013-07-10-checklists-improve-patient-safety

American Psychological Association. Resilience. Published 2022. Accessed May 15, 2022. https://www.apa.org/topics/resilience

American Society for Quality. Six Sigma belts, executives and champions. Accessed May 6, 2022. http://asq.org/learn-about-quality/six-sigma/overview/belts-executives-champions.html

Baldrige Performance Excellence Program. *2020-2021 Baldrige excellence framework: (Health care): Proven leadership and management practices for high performance.* Gaithersburg, MD: U.S. Department of Commerce, National Institute of Standards and Technology; 2021:49.

Becher EC, Chassin MR. Improving the quality of healthcare: who will lead? *Health Affairs.* 2001;20:164-179. doi:10.1377/hlthaff.20.5.164

Begun J, Zimmerman B, Dooley K. Health care organizations as complex adaptive systems. In: Mick S & Wyttenbach M, eds. *Advances in Health Care Organization Theory.* San Francisco, CA: Jossey-Bass; 2003:253-258.

Berwick DM, Nolan TW, Whittington J. The Triple Aim: care, health and cost. *Health Affairs.* 2008;27(3):759-769. doi:10.1377/hlthaff.27.3.759

Bodenheimer T, Sinsky C. From triple to quadruple aim: care of the patient requires care of the provider. *Ann Fam Med.* 2014;12(6):573-576.

Business Dictionary. *Goal congruence.* Published October 16, 2021. Accessed May 6, 2022. https://businessdictionary.info/?s=goal+congruence&ct_post_type=post%3Apage%3Adefinition

Center for Advancing Health. *A New Definition of Patient Engagement: What Is Engagement and Why Is It Important?* Washington, DC: Author; 2010.

Centers for Medicare & Medicaid Services. Glossary. Published 2006. Accessed November 11, 2021. https://www.cms.gov/glossary

Centers for Medicare & Medicaid Services. *State operations manual: Appendix Q: Guidelines for determining immediate jeopardy.* Published March 6, 2019. Accessed May 6, 2022. https://www.cms.gov/Regulations-and-Guidance/Guidance/Manuals/downloads/som107ap_q_immedjeopardy.pdf

Chassin MR, Loeb JM. High-reliability health care: getting there from here. *Milbank Q.* 2013;91(3):459-490.

Christensen CM, Bohmer RMJ, Kenagy J. Will disruptive innovations cure health care? *Harvard Bus Rev.* 2000;78(5):102-112, 199.

Commission for Case Manager Certification. About the glossary. Accessed June 8, 2022. https://cmbodyofknowledge.com/content/resources/glossary

Cross TL, Bazron BJ, Dennis KW, Isaacs MR. *Towards a Culturally Competent System of Care.* National Institute of Mental Health, Child and Adolescent Service System Program (CASSP). Washington, DC: Technical Assistance Center, Georgetown University Child Development Center; 1989.

Deming WE. *Out of the Crisis.* Cambridge, MA: MIT Press; 2000.

Donabedian A. *The Definition of Quality and Approaches to Its Assessment.* Ann Arbor, MI: Health Administration Press; 1980:79, 83.

Eckleberry-Hunt J, Van Dyke A, Lick D, Tucciarone J. Changing the conversation from burnout to wellness: physician well-being in residency training programs. *JGME.* 2009;1(2):225-230.

eCQI Resource Center. Glossary. Accessed May 6, 2022. https://ecqi.healthit.gov/glossary

Frampton SB, Guastello S, Hoy L, Naylor M, Sheridan S, Johnston-Fleece M. *Harnessing Evidence and Experience to Change Culture: A Guiding Framework for Patient and Family Engaged Care. Discussion paper.* Washington, DC: National Academy of Medicine; 2015. Accessed November 11, 2021. https://nam.edu/wp-content/uploads/2017/01/Harnessing-Evidence-and-Experience-to-Change-Culture-A-Guiding-Framework-for-Patient-and-Family-Engaged-Care.pdf

Gallup. The real future of work. Published 2018. Accessed November 29, 2021. https://www.gallup.com/workplace/241295/future-work-agility-download.aspx#ite-241304

George JM, Jones GR. *Organizational Behavior.* 3rd ed. Upper Saddle River, NJ: Prentice Hall; 2002.

Graban M, Swartz JE. *Healthcare Kaizen: Engaging Front-Line Staff in Sustainable Continuous Improvement.* Boca Raton, FL: CRC Press; 2012.

Grout JR. *Mistake-Proofing the Design of Health Care Processes.* Rockville, MD: Agency for Healthcare Research and Quality; 2007. AHRQ publication 07-P0020. Accessed May 15, 2022. https://psnet.ahrq.gov/issue/mistake-proofing-design-health-care-processes

Hut N. Amid the COVID-19 pandemic, research finds hospital organizations looking to capitalize on the benefits of systemness. Published April 30, 2021. Accessed November 22, 2021. https://www.hfma.org/topics/news/2021/04/amid-the-covid-19-pandemic--research-finds-hospital-organization.html

Institute of Medicine. *Medicare: A Strategy for Quality Assurance.* Vol. 2. Washington, DC: National Academies Press; 2000:128-129.

Institute of Medicine, Committee on Quality of Health Care in America. *Crossing the Quality Chasm: A New Health System for the 21st Century.* Washington, DC: National Academies Press; 2001.

Institute of Medicine, Roundtable on Evidence-Based Medicine. *The Learning Healthcare System: Workshop Summary.* Washington, DC: National Academies Press; 2007.

Institute of Medicine. *Clinical Practice Guidelines We Can Trust.* Washington, DC: National Academies Press; 2011. Accessed November 11, 2021. https://www.ncbi.nlm.nih.gov/books/NBK209539/

The Joint Commission. SAFER matrix. Accessed May 15, 2022. https://www.jointcommission.org/-/media/tjc/documents/accred-and-cert/safer-matrix/safer-matrix.pdf

The Joint Commission, Joint Commission International, World Health Organization. Patient safety solutions preamble—May 2007. *Jt Comm J Qual Patient Saf.* 2007;33(7):427-429. Accessed May 15, 2022. https://www.jointcommissionjournal.com/article/S1553-7250(07)33126-7/fulltext

The Joint Commission. Sentinel event definition, policy revised. Published 2021. Accessed December 12, 2021. https://www.jointcommission.org/resources/news-and-multimedia/newsletters/newsletters/joint-commission-online/july-21-2021/sentinel-event-definition-policy-revised/

Juran JM. *Juran on Leadership for Quality: An Executive Handbook.* New York, NY: Free Press; 1989.

Kaiser Family Foundation. Health reform glossary. http://www.kff.org/glossary/health-reform-glossary/

Kaplan R, Norton D. Using the balanced scorecard as a strategic management system. *Harvard Bus Rev.* 1996;74:75-85.

Kavaler F, Spiegel A. *Risk Management in Health Care Institutions: A Strategic Approach.* Sudbury, MA: Jones & Bartlett; 1997.

Kindig DA, Stoddart G. What is population health? *Am J Pub Health.* 2003;93:380-383.

Lewis N. Populations, population health, and the evolution of population management: making sense of the terminology in US health care today. Published 2014. Accessed November 11, 2021. http://www.ihi.org/communities/blogs/population-health-population-management-terminology-in-us-health-care

McGlynn EA. *Identifying, Categorizing, and Evaluating Health Care Efficiency Measures.* Final report (prepared by the Southern California Evidence-based Practice Center—RAND Corporation, under contract no. 282-00-0005-21). AHRQ publication 08-0030. Rockville, MD: Agency for Healthcare Research and Quality; 2008.

Medicaid.gov. Managed care. Accessed November 17, 2021. https://www.medicaid.gov/medicaid/managed-care/index.html

Montuori A. Systems approach. In: *Encyclopedia of Creativity.* 2nd ed. Cambridge, MA: Academic Press; 2011:414-421. doi:10.1016/B978-0-12-375038-9.00212-0

National Academies of Sciences, Engineering, and Medicine (NASEM). *Improving Diagnoses in Healthcare.* Washington, DC: NASEM; 2015. Accessed January 10, 2022. https://www.nap.edu/catalog/21794/improving-diagnosis-in-health-care

National Cancer Institute, Dictionary of cancer terms. Best practice. Accessed April 27, 2022. https://www.cancer.gov/publications/dictionaries/cancer-terms/def/best-practice

National Council for Mental Wellbeing. The Comprehensive Healthcare Integration Framework: designing, implementing and sustaining physical health–behavioral health integration. 2022:8. Accessed June 24, 2022. https://www.thenationalcouncil.org/wp-content/uploads/2022/04/04.22.2022_MDI-CHI-Paper_Reduced.pdf

National Institute of Standards and Technology. Baldrige performance excellence core values and concepts. Published 2021. Accessed May 15, 2022. https://www.nist.gov/baldrige/core-values-and-concepts#agility

National Patient Safety Foundation. RCA² improving root cause analyses and actions to prevent harm (version 2). Published 2016. Accessed November 11, 2021. http://www.ihi.org/resources/Pages/Tools/RCA2-Improving-Root-Cause-Analyses-and-Actions-to-Prevent-Harm.aspx

National Quality Forum (NQF). *Phrase Book; A Plain Language Guide to NQF Jargon.* Washington, DC: NQF. Accessed July 29, 2022. https://www.qualityforum.org/Field_Guide/Phrasebook.aspx

Paradiso S, Sweeney N. Just culture: it's more than policy. *Nurs Manage.* 2019;50(6):38-45. doi:10.1097/01.NUMA.0000558482.07815.ae

Pelletier LR, Stichler JE. Patient-centered care and engagement: nurse leaders' imperative for health reform. *J Nurs Admin.* 2014;44(9):473-480. doi:10.1097/NNA.0000000000000102

Pines A, Maslach C. Characteristics of staff burnout in mental health settings. *Hosp Community Psychiatry.* 2006;29:233-237. doi:10.1176/ps.29.4.233

Quality Measurement and Management Project. *Hospital Quality-Related Data: Recommendations for Appropriate Data Requests, Analysis, and Utilization.* Chicago, IL: American Hospital Association; 1991.

Rao MV. Project management—CPM/PERT. Guru Gobind Singh Educational Society's technical campus. Published 2016. Accessed November 11, 2021. https://www.slideshare.net/annaprasad/project-management-cpmpert-61847309

Resar R, Griffin FA, Haraden C, Nolan TW. *Using Care Bundles to Improve Health Care Quality.* IHI Innovation Series white paper. Cambridge, MA: Institute for Healthcare Improvement; 2012. Accessed May 15, 2022. http://www.ihi.org/resources/Pages/IHIWhitePapers/UsingCareBundles.aspx

ReVelle JB. *Quality Essentials: A Reference Guide from A to Z.* Milwaukee, WI: ASQ Quality Press; 2004.

Robbins SP. *Organizational Behavior.* 8th ed. Upper Saddle River, NJ: Prentice Hall; 2001.

Rogers EM. *Diffusion of Innovations.* 4th ed. New York, NY: The Free Press; 1995.

Rokeach M. *The Nature of Human Values.* New York, NY: Free Press; 1973.

Sackett D, Rosenberg WMC, Muir-Gray JA, Haynes RB, Richardson WS. Evidence-based medicine: what it is and what it isn't. *British Med J.* 1996;312(13):71-72. doi:10.1136/bmj.312.7023.71

Saha S, Loehrer S, Cleary-Fisherman M, et al. *Pathways to Population Health: An Invitation to Health Care Change Agents.* Boston, MA: 100 Million Healthier Lives, convened by the Institute for Healthcare Improvement; 2017. Accessed June 18, 2022. www.ihi.org/P2PH

Senge PM. *The Fifth Discipline: The Art and Practice of the Learning Organization.* New York, NY: Doubleday; 1990.

Shatte A, Perlman A, Smith B, Lynch WD. The positive effect of resilience on stress and business outcomes in difficult work environments. *JOEM.* 2017;59(2):135-140.

Shook J. *A3 Templates from Lean Enterprise Institute.* Boston, MA: Lean Enterprise Institute; 2010.

Shortell SM, Morrison E, Robbins S. Strategy-making in health care organizations: a framework and agenda for research. *Med Care Rev.* 1985;2:219-266. doi:10.1177/107755878504200203

Sikka R, Morath JM, Leape L. The quadruple aim: care, health, cost, and meaning in work. *BMJ Qual Saf.* 2015;24(10):608-610. doi:10.1136/bmjqs-2015-004160

Society for Human Resource Management. Mission statement. Published 2022. Accessed May 15, 2022. https://www.shrm.org/resourcesandtools/tools-and-samples/hr-glossary/pages/mission-statement.aspx

Stamatis DH. *Total Quality Management in Healthcare: Implementation Strategies for Optimum Results.* Chicago, IL: Irwin; 1996; p. 58.

Ten Ham-Baloyi W, Minnie K, van der Walt C. Improving healthcare: a guide to roll-out best practices. *Afr Health Sci.* 2020;20(3):1487-1495. doi:10.4314/ahs.v20i3.55

Thompson L. *Making the Team: A Guide for Managers.* Upper Saddle River, NJ: Prentice Hall; 2000.

U.S. Department of Health and Human Services, Office of the National Coordinator. Interoperability basics: defining interoperability. Accessed May 15, 2022. https://www.healthit.gov/public-course/interoperability-basics-training/HITRC_lsn1069/wrap_menupage.htm

U.S. Environmental Protection Agency. Lean thinking and methods. Published 2021. Accessed May 15, 2022. https://www.epa.gov/sustainability/lean-thinking-and-methods-introduction

Watkins MD. What is organizational culture? And why should we care? *Harvard Bus Rev.* Published May 15, 2013. Accessed May 15, 2022. https://hbr.org/2013/05/what-is-organizational-culture

World Health Organization. Social determinants of health. Accessed December 12, 2021. https://www.who.int/healthtopics/social-determinants-of-health#tab=tab_1

Wyatt R, Laderman M, Botwinick L, Mate K, Whittington J. *Achieving Health Equity: A Guide for Health Care Organizations.* IHI white paper. Cambridge, MA: Institute for Healthcare Improvement; 2016. Accessed July 29, 2022. www.ihi.org

Xyrichis A, Ream E. Teamwork: a concept analysis. *J Adv Nursing.* 2008:61:232-241. doi:10.1111/j.1365-2648.2007

# Index

Note: Page numbers followed by *f* or *t* indicate material in figures or tables respectively